HANDBOOK OF

Diagnostic Tests

Third Edition

LIPPINCOTT WILLIAMS & WILKINS
A **Wolters Kluwer** Company
Philadelphia • Baltimore • New York • London
Buenos Aires • Hong Kong • Sydney • Tokyo

STAFF

Publisher
Judith A. Schilling McCann, RN, MSN

Editorial Director
H. Nancy Holmes

Clinical Director
Joan M. Robinson, RN, MSN

Senior Art Director
Arlene Putterman

Clinical Editors
Joanne M. Bartelmo, RN, MSN, CCRN; Wanda H. Jones, RN, BSN, MT

Editors
Jennifer P. Kowalak (senior associate editor), William Welsh (associate editor)

Copy Editors
Kimberly Bilotta (supervisor), Scotti Cohn, Tom DeZego, Heather Ditch, Amy Furman, Shana Harrington, Catherine Kirby, Elizabeth Mooney, Irene Pontarelli, Marcia Ryan, Dorothy P. Terry, Pamela Wingrod

Book Design
Lesley Weissman-Cook

Digital Composition Services
Diane Paluba (manager), Joyce Rossi Biletz (senior desktop assistant), Jan Greenberg, Donna S. Morris

Cover Photograph
Artville Medical Images/Don Carstens

Manufacturing
Patricia K. Dorshaw (senior manager), Beth Janae Orr (book production coordinator)

Editorial Assistants
Danielle J. Barsky, Carol Caputo, Beverly Lane, Linda Ruhf

Librarian
Catherine M. Heslin

Indexer
Barbara Hodgson

The clinical procedures described and recommended in this publication are based on research and consultation with medical and nursing authorities. To the best of our knowledge, these procedures reflect currently accepted clinical practice; nevertheless, they can't be considered absolute and universal recommendations. For individual application, treatment recommendations must be considered in light of the patient's clinical condition and, before administration of new or infrequently used drugs, in light of the latest package-insert information. The authors and the publisher disclaim responsibility for any adverse effects resulting directly or indirectly from the suggested procedures, from any undetected errors, or from the reader's misunderstanding of the text.

HDT3—D N O S A J J M A M
05 04 03 10 9 8 7 6 5 4 3 2 1

Library of Congress Cataloging-in-Publication Data

Handbook of diagnostic tests. — 3rd ed.
p. ; cm.
Includes index.
1. Diagnosis—Handbooks, manuals, etc. 2. Diagnosis, Laboratory—Handbooks, manuals, etc. I. Lippincott Williams & Wilkins.
[DNLM: 1. Laboratory Techniques and Procedures—Handbooks. 2. Laboratory Techniques and Procedures—Nurses' Instruction. 3. Diagnostic Imaging—Handbooks. 4. Diagnostic Imaging—Nurses' Instruction. QY 39 H2368 2003]
RC71.P76 2003
616.07'54—dc21
ISBN 1-58255-203-7 (alk. paper) 2002155964

CONTENTS

CONTRIBUTORS AND CONSULTANTS

Garry Brydges, RN, MSN, ACNP-C, SRNA
Medical Consultant
Houston

Marilyn M. Cooksey, RN, MSN, PhD
Associate Professor of Nursing
William Carey College
Gulfport, Miss.

Jennifer Elizabeth DiMedio, RN, MSN, CRNP
Family Nurse Practitioner
University of Pennsylvania: West Chester (Pa.) Family Practice

Shelba Durston, RN, MSN, CCRN
Adjunct Faculty
San Joaquin Delta College
Stockton, Calif.
Staff Nurse
San Joaquin General Hospital
French Camp, Calif.

René A. Jackson, RN, BSN
Special Procedures Nurse
Charlotte Regional Medical Center
Punta Gorda, Fla.

Kay Luft, RN, MN, CCRN
Assistant Professor
Saint Luke's College
Kansas City, Mo.

Lisa A. Salamon, MSN, CNS, RNC
Clinical Nurse Specialist
Cleveland Clinic Foundation

Bruce Austin Scott, MSN, APRN, BC
Nursing Instructor
San Joaquin Delta College
Stockton, Calif.
Staff Nurse
University of California, Davis, Medical Center
Sacramento

We extend special thanks to the following people who contributed to previous editions:

Charol Abrams, MS, MT(ASCP), CLS(NCA), CLSP(H)

Deborah Becker, RN, MSN, CCRN, CRNP

Susan J. Brown-Wagner, RN, MSN, CRNT, AOCN

Lawrence Carey, BS, PHarmD

Joan T. Converse, MA, CLS(NCA), MT(ASCP)

Ellen Digan, MA, MT(ASCP)

Stanley J. Dudrick, MD

Kathleen Ellstrom, RN, PhD(c), CS

Harriet W. Ferguson, RN,C, MSN, EdD

Ellie Z. Franges, RN, MSN, CCRN, CNRN

Geriann B. Gallagher, ND, APRN

Pamela W. Gitschier, MT, MS

Peggi Guenter, RN, PhD, CNSN

Debra R. Hanna, RN, MSN, CNRN

Michél E. Lloyd, MT(ASCP), SBB
Dawna Martich, RN, MSN
Carol McLimans, MA, MT(ASCP)
Karen E. Michael, RN, MSN
Kambiz Motamedi, MD
Lori Musolf Neri, RN, MSN, CCRN
Gladys Purvis, RN, MSN, CCRN
Linda T. Raichle, PhD, MT(ASCP)
Dorothy L. Rhoads, RN,C, MSN, CRNP
Teresa A. Richardson, BS, MT
Mary Jean Rutherford, MED, MT(ASCP), SC
Sylvia N. Schneider, RN, BSN
Daniele Shollengerger, RN, MSN
Deborah Porter Thornton, MED, MT(ASCP)SC
Karen E. Tumelty, RN, BSN
Patricia Zander, RTR, BS

FOREWORD

Your medical landscape is ever changing. It often seems as if there's a new, ground-breaking advance every day of the week. Because of this, no matter how much you invest in education and how persistent you are in keeping up with the tremendous growth of medical information, there's always more to learn. Your knowledge is never 100% comprehensive. *Handbook of Diagnostic Tests,* Third Edition, was designed with this thought in mind.

In clinical care, there are hundreds of diagnostic tests and procedures to chose from, and tests are constantly being introduced or updated. Without proper reference material, managing the sheer number of available tests would be nearly impossible. Patient preparation would become deficient, results would be read wrong, and interpretations would become unreliable. *Handbook of Diagnostic Tests,* Third Edition, is your solution. It provides the latest information about commonly used tests in a format that's easy to access, and it's dedicated to the laboratory tests and diagnostic procedures that are essential in everyday care.

Handbook of Diagnostic Tests, Third Edition, consists of two major sections. Part One is a compendium of the most important diagnostic findings for more than 500 major disorders arranged alphabetically. View this section from two perspectives. Besides being the perfect quick-reference tool (use it to remind yourself of the key signs and symptoms of the major diseases and to quickly select appropriate diagnostic strategies), it also serves as an ideal cross-reference that links specific disorders to tests.

Part Two provides an in-depth look at more than 550 diagnostic tests in a reader-friendly format that reflects the most current trends in clinical pathology and laboratory medicine. Each entry starts with a general description of the test, including its purpose, then moves onto patient preparation, special equipment needed to perform the procedure, the steps of the procedure, posttest care, precautions, normal findings and reference values, abnormal findings (and their interpretation), and factors that can interfere with proper test administration and accuracy. Many entries include tables, graphs, and illustrations to enhance comprehension. When you find the test you're looking for, you'll have all the information you need within a matter of seconds.

When looking for a specific test, you'll find Part Two's organization to be a great help. The first eight chapters cover the most essential laboratory tests being used today. Chapters 1 through 5 cover tests done on blood samples, including blood chemistry, hematology, coagulation, and endocrine and immunologic assays. Chapters 6 through 8 cover urine, sputum, and bacteriologic testing.

The scope of diagnostic procedures, presented in chapters 9 through 16, includes endoscopic and imaging techniques, the most common tissue biopsy procedures and nuclear medicine scans, and special functional tests and monitoring techniques. The procedures are described in a clear, crisp manner, and most chapters are organized by body system to ensure ease of use. You'll have this section dog-eared according to your specialty in no time.

Valuable information is also provided in the three appendices. You'll find the quick-reference listings of normal laboratory test values and normal and abnormal serum drug levels extremely useful. The illustrated guide to home testing is an extraordinary feature. With its ready-to-copy format, it will become an indispensable part of your instructional materials library.

Handbook of Diagnostic Tests, Third Edition, is an excellent reference tool. Its format is appropriate and convenient, and its size quite portable for an edition of such breadth. I'm sure that all of us in health care — students, new graduates, and experienced professionals — will find it helpful in our everyday professional lives.

Semyon A. Risin, MD, PhD
Assistant Professor
Department of Pathology and Laboratory Medicine
University of Texas–Houston Medical School

PART ONE

Key diagnostic findings in major disorders

Abbreviations used in Part One

These abbreviations are used throughout Part One.

ABG	arterial blood gas	HCT	hematocrit
AFP	alpha-fetoprotein	hGH	human growth hormone
ALT	alanine aminotransferase	HIV	human immunodeficiency virus
ANA	antinuclear antibody	HLA	human leukocyte antigen
ASO	antistreptolysin-O	Ig	immunoglobulin
AST	aspartate aminotransferase	kat	katal
BUN	blood urea nitrogen	kPa	kilopascal
CBC	complete blood count	KS	ketosteroids
CEA	carcinoembryonic antigen	KUB	kidney-ureter-bladder
CK	creatine kinase	LD	lactate dehydrogenase
CO_2	carbon dioxide	LH	uteinizing hormone
CSF	cerebrospinal fluid	MRI	magnetic resonance imaging
CT	computed tomography	$Paco_2$	partial pressure of arterial carbon dioxide
CXR	chest X-ray	Pao_2	partial pressure of arterial oxygen
D&C	dilatation and curettage	Pap	Papanicolaou
DNA	deoxyribonucleic acid	PAWP	pulmonary artery wedge pressure
ECG	electrocardiogram	PET	positron emission tomography
EEG	electroencephalogram	PFT	pulmonary function test
ELISA	enzyme-linked immunosorbent assay	PT	prothrombin time
EMG	electromyography	PTT	partial thromboplastin time
ESR	erythrocyte sedimentation rate	RBC	red blood cell
FEV_1	forced expiratory volume	RF	rheumatoid factor
FSH	follicle-stimulating hormone	T_4	thyroxine
FVC	forced vital capacity	TSH	thyroid-stimulating hormone
GFR	glomerular filtration rate	T_3	triiodothyronine
Hb	hemoglobin	WBC	white blood cell
hCG	human chorionic gonadotropin		

Abdominal aortic aneurysm

- CT scan, MRI, or ultrasonography reveals the size, shape, and location of the aneurysm.
- Anteroposterior and lateral X-rays of the abdomen may detect aortic calcification, which outlines the mass.
- Aortography shows the condition of vessels proximal and distal to the aneurysm and the extent of the aneurysm but may underestimate aneurysm diameter, because it visualizes only the blood flow channel and not the surrounding clot.

Abnormal premenopausal bleeding

- Serum hormone levels reflect adrenal, pituitary, or thyroid dysfunction.
- Urine 17-KS reveal adrenal hyperplasia, hypopituitarism, or polycystic ovarian disease.
- Pelvic ultrasonography rules out uterine masses.
- Hysteroscopy allows visualization of the endometrium.
- Endometrial biopsy rules out malignancy and should be performed in all

patients who experience abnormal premenopausal bleeding.
- Pelvic examination and Pap smear rule out local or malignant causes.

Abruptio placentae
- History includes mild to moderate vaginal bleeding (usually during second half of pregnancy).
- Amniocentesis reveals "port wine" fluid.
- Coagulation tests reveal a rise in fibrin split product levels.
- CBC reveals decreased Hb level and platelet counts.
- Pelvic ultrasonography reveals abnormal echo patterns.

Acceleration-deceleration cervical injuries
- Full cervical spine CT scans or X-rays indicate absence of cervical fracture.
- If the X-rays are negative for obvious cervical fracture, examination emphasizes motor ability and sensation below the cervical spine to detect signs of nerve root compression.

Acquired immunodeficiency syndrome
- ELISA identifies the HIV-1 antibody.
- Western blot test may also reveal the HIV-1 antibody and should be performed after a positive ELISA to confirm the diagnosis (antibody may not be detected in late stages due to inability to mount an antibody response).
- $CD4^+$ T-lymphocyte assay reveals a lymphocyte count < 200 cells/µl in an HIV-infected individual.

Actinomycosis
- Culture of tissue or exudate identifies *Actinomyces israelii.*
- Gram staining of excised tissue or exudates reveals branching gram-positive rods.
- CXR reveals lesions in unusual locations such as the shaft of a rib.

Acute leukemia
- Bone marrow aspiration indicates a proliferation of immature WBCs.
- Bone marrow biopsy reveals cancerous cells.
- CBC indicates pancytopenia with circulating blasts.

Acute poststreptococcal glomerulonephritis
- History includes recent streptococcal infection.
- Serum electrolyte studies show elevated calcium, chloride, phosphate, potassium, and sodium levels.
- BUN and serum creatinine levels are elevated.
- Urinalysis reveals RBCs, WBCs, mixed cell casts, and protein.
- ASO test reveals elevated streptozyme titers, indicating a recent streptococcal infection (in 80% of patients).
- Anti-DNase B titers are elevated, indicating a recent streptococcal infection.
- Serum complement assay levels are low, indicating recent streptococcal infection.
- Throat culture may show group A beta-hemolytic streptococci.
- KUB X-rays show bilateral kidney enlargement.
- Renal biopsy reveals histologic changes indicating glomerulonephritis.

Acute pyelonephritis
- Urinalysis reveals sediment containing leukocytes singly, in clumps, and in casts and, possibly, a few RBCs as well as low specific gravity and osmolality and a slight alkaline urine pH.

- Urine culture reveals more than 100,000 organisms/ml of urine.
- KUB X-rays may reveal calculi, tumors, or cysts in the kidneys and the urinary tract.
- Excretory urography may show asymmetrical kidneys.

Acute renal failure

- History includes renal disease.
- BUN and serum creatinine levels are elevated.
- ABG analysis indicates a blood pH < 7.35 and HCO_3^- level < 22 mEq/L (SI, < 22 mmol/L).

Acute respiratory failure in chronic obstructive pulmonary disease

- ABG measurements show progressive deterioration when compared with normal values for patient; increased HCO_3^- level may indicate metabolic alkalosis or metabolic compensation for chronic respiratory acidosis.
- CXR reveals such pulmonary pathology as emphysema, atelectasis, lesions, pneumothorax, infiltrates, or effusions.
- Hb level and HCT are decreased.
- Serum electrolyte studies reveal hypokalemia.
- WBC count is elevated if bacterial infection is present.
- ECG indicates arrhythmias that suggest cor pulmonale and myocardial hypoxia.

Acute tubular necrosis

- Urinalysis reveals urinary sediment containing RBCs and casts, specific gravity of 1.010 or less, and osmolality < 400 mOsm/kg (SI, < 400 mmol/kg).
- Urine sodium level is between 40 and 60 mEq/L (SI, 40 to 60 mmol/d).
- BUN and serum creatinine levels are elevated.
- Serum electrolyte studies reveal hyperkalemia.
- ABG analysis indicates blood pH < 7.25 and HCO_3^- level < 22 mEq/L (SI, < 22 mmol/L).

Adenoid hyperplasia

- Nasopharyngoscopy or rhinoscopy reveals abnormal tissue mass.
- Lateral pharyngeal X-rays show oblation of the nasopharyngeal air column.

Adrenal hypofunction

- Plasma cortisol levels are decreased.
- Fasting blood glucose and serum sodium levels are decreased (in Addison's disease).
- Serum potassium and BUN levels are increased.
- CBC reveals increased HCT and elevated lymphocyte and eosinophil counts.
- X-rays reveal a small heart.
- Corticotropin level is increased.
- Rapid corticotropin test reveals low cortisol levels.
- Sweat test reveals elevated sodium level (> 46 mmol/L [SI, 46 mEq/L]) and chloride level (> 43 mmol/L [SI, > 43 mEq/L]).
- Urine 17-hydroxycorticosteroid levels and urine 17-KS levels are decreased.

Adrenogenital syndrome

- Physical examination reveals pseudohermaphroditism in females or precocious puberty in patients of either sex.
- Urine 17-KS levels are elevated and can be suppressed by administering oral dexamethasone.
- Levels of urine hormone metabolites (particularly pregnanetriol) and plasma 17-hydroxyprogesterone are elevated.
- Urine 17-hydroxycorticosteroid levels are normal or decreased.
- Symptoms of adrenal hypofunction or adrenal crisis in the first week of life strongly suggest congenital adrenal hyperplasia; elevated serum calcium, chlo-

ride, and sodium levels (in the presence of excessive levels of urine 17-KS and pregnanetriol) and decreased urine aldosterone levels confirm it.

Age-related macular degeneration

- Indirect ophthalmoscopy reveals gross macular changes.
- I.V. fluorescein angiography reveals leaking vessels.
- Amsler's grid reveals visual field loss.

Albinism

- Family history suggests inheritance pattern.
- Inspection shows pale skin (in whites) and white-to-yellow hair.
- Microscopic examination of the skin and of hair follicles reveals the amount of pigment present.
- Pigmentation testing of plucked hair roots by incubating them in tyrosine distinguishes tyrosinase-positive albinism from tyrosinase-negative albinism; tyrosinase-positive hair roots will develop color.

Alcoholism

- History includes chronic and excessive ingestion of alcohol.
- Liver function studies reveal increased levels of serum cholesterol, LD, ALT, AST, and CK in patients with liver damage.
- Serum amylase and lipase levels are elevated (in pancreatitis).

Allergic rhinitis

- Personal or family history includes allergies.
- Sputum and nasal smears reveal a large numbers of eosinophils.
- Skin test for specific allergen is positive, supported by tested response to environmental stimuli.

Alport's syndrome

- Family history includes recurrent hematuria, deafness, and renal failure (especially in men).
- Urinalysis indicates presence of RBCs.
- Renal biopsy reveals histologic changes characteristic of Alport's syndrome.
- Blood tests reveal Ig and complement components.
- Eye examination may reveal cataracts and, less commonly, keratoconus, microspherophakia, myopia, nystagmus, and retinitis pigmentosa.

Alzheimer's disease

- History includes progressive personality, mental status, and neurologic changes.
- PET scan reveals alteration in the metabolic activity of the cerebral cortex.
- Elevated Tau proteins with low levels of soluble amyloid beta-protein precursor in CSF correlate with Alzheimer's disease.
- EEG and CT scan may help diagnose later stages of illness.
- Autopsy reveals neurofibrillary tangles, neuritic plaques, and granulovascular degeneration.

Amebiasis

- Culture of stool, sputum, or aspirates from abscesses, ulcers, or tissue reveal *Entamoeba histolytica* (cysts and trophozoites).
- CT scan may reveal abscess.

Amputation, traumatic

- History and examination reveal trauma to an extremity.
- CBC reveals decreased Hb level and HCT, indicating hemorrhage.

Amyloidosis

- Histologic examination of tissue specimen (rectal mucosa, gingiva, skin,

or nerve biopsy) or abdominal fat pad aspiration using a polarizing or electron microscope and appropriate tissue staining reveals amyloid deposits.
- Liver function studies are generally normal, except for slightly elevated serum alkaline phosphatase levels.
- ECG shows low voltage and conduction or rhythm abnormalities resembling those characteristic of myocardial infarction (with cardiac amyloidosis).
- Echocardiography (M-mode and two-dimensional) may detect myocardial infiltration.

Amyotrophic lateral sclerosis
- Upper and lower motor neuron degeneration occurs without sensory impairment.
- EMG may show abnormalities of electrical activity of involved muscles.
- Muscle biopsy may disclose atrophic fibers interspersed among normal fiber.
- Nerve conduction studies are usually normal.
- CSF analysis reveals increased protein content in one-third of patients.
- CT scan and EEG may help rule out other disorders.

Anal fissure
- Digital examination elicits pain and bleeding.
- Gentle traction on perianal skin allows for visualization of fistula.
- Anoscopy reveals longitudinal tear and confirms the diagnosis.
- Patient may complain of local itching, tenderness, or pain aggravated by bowel movements.

Anaphylaxis
- Patient's history, physical examination, and signs and symptoms establish the diagnosis. They may include a rapid onset of severe respiratory or cardiovascular symptoms after ingestion or injection of a drug, vaccine, diagnostic agent, food, or food additive or after an insect sting.

Ankylosing spondylitis
- Family history includes the disorder.
- X-rays reveal blurring of the bony margins of joints (in early stage), bilateral sacroiliac involvement, patchy sclerosis with superficial bony erosions, squaring of vertebral bodies, and "bamboo spine" (with complete ankylosis).
- Serum HLA-B27 is present in about 95% of patients with primary disease and 80% of patients with secondary disease.
- CBC reveals slightly elevated ESR and alkaline phosphatase and creatine phosphatase levels in active disease.
- Serum IgA levels may be elevated.

Anorectal abscess and fistula
Examination of rectum helps to distinguish type of abscess:
- Perianal abscess produces a red, tender, localized, oval swelling close to the anus, which may drain pus. Sitting or coughing increases pain.
- Ischiorectal abscess involves the entire perianal region on the affected side of the anus. Digital examination reveals a tender induration bulging into the anal canal, which may not produce drainage.
- Patient may report constipation, ribbon-formed stools, and pain with bowel movements.
- Submucous or high intramuscular abscess may produce a dull, aching pain in the rectum, tenderness and, occasionally, induration. Digital examination reveals a smooth swelling of the upper part of the anal canal or lower rectum.
- Pelvirectal abscess produces fever, malaise, and myalgia but no local anal or external rectal signs or pain. Digital examination reveals a tender mass high

in the pelvis, perhaps extending into one of the ischiorectal fossae.

- Sigmoidoscopy, barium enema, and colonoscopy may be performed to rule out other conditions.

Anorectal stricture, stenosis, or contracture

- Visual inspection reveals narrowing of the anal canal.
- Digital examination reveals tenderness and tightness.

Anorexia nervosa

- History includes weight loss of 25% or greater with no organic basis, compulsive dieting and bulimic episodes or gorging and purging, and laxative or diuretic abuse.
- Emaciated appearance is accompanied by maintenance of physical vigor.
- CBC reveals decreased Hb level, platelet count, WBC count, and ESR.
- Bleeding time is prolonged (due to thrombocytopenia).
- Serum creatinine, BUN, uric acid, cholesterol, total protein, albumin, sodium, potassium, chloride, and calcium levels are decreased.
- Fasting blood glucose level is decreased.
- ECG reveals nonspecific ST interval, T-wave changes, prolonged PR interval, and ventricular arrhythmias.
- Additional diagnostic testing may be performed to rule out other disorders that may cause wasting.

Anthrax

- History includes exposure to wool, hides, or other animal products.
- Inspection reveals a large, pruritic, painless skin lesion.
- Tissue culture with Gram stain reveals large gram-positive rods.
- Drainage cultures reveal *Bacillus anthracis*.
- Indirect hemagglutination reveals a fourfold rise in titer.

Aortic insufficiency

- Cardiac catheterization shows reduced arterial diastolic pressure, aortic insufficiency, and valvular abnormalities.
- Echocardiography reveals left ventricular enlargement and changes in left ventricular function; it may show a dilated aortic root, a flail leaflet, thickening of the cusps, or valve prolapse.
- Doppler echocardiography readily detects mild degrees of aortic insufficiency that may be inaudible. It also shows a rapid, high-frequency, diastolic fluttering of the anterior mitral leaflet that results from aortic insufficiency.
- ECG may show left ventricular hypertrophy, ST-segment depression, and T-wave inversion.
- Radionuclide angiography helps to determine the degree of regurgitant blood flow and assess left ventricular function.

Aortic stenosis

- Cardiac catheterization reveals the pressure gradient across the aortic valve (indicating the severity of obstruction), increased left ventricular end-diastolic pressures (indicating left ventricular dysfunction), and the number of cusps.
- CXR shows valvular calcification, left ventricular enlargement, dilation of the ascending aorta, pulmonary venous congestion and, in later stages, left atrial, pulmonary artery, right atrial, and right ventricular enlargement.
- Echocardiography demonstrates a thickened aortic valve and left ventricular wall and possible coexistent mitral valve stenosis.
- Doppler echocardiography allows calculation of the aortic pressure gradient.
- ECG reveals left ventricular hypertrophy and ST-segment and T-wave ab-

normalities. As hypertrophy progresses in severe aortic stenosis, left atrial enlargement is noted. Up to 10% of patients have atrioventricular and intraventricular conduction defects.

Aplastic or hypoplastic anemia

- CBC reveals normochromic and normocytic RBCs with a total count of 1 million or less as well as decreased platelet, neutrophil, and WBC counts.
- Serum iron is elevated. (Hemosiderin is present and tissue iron storage is visible microscopically.)
- Bleeding time is prolonged.
- Bone marrow biopsy yields a "dry tap" or shows severely hypocellular or aplastic marrow, with a varying amount of fat, fibrous tissue, or gelatinous replacement; absence of tagged iron and megakaryocytes; and depression of erythroid elements.

Appendicitis

- History includes right upper quadrant abdominal pain that eventually localizes in lower right quadrant, plus patient complaints of nausea and vomiting, anorexia, and obstipation.
- Temperature is elevated.
- WBC count is elevated, with increased numbers of immature cells.

Arm and leg fractures

- History includes trauma to extremity.
- Physical examination reveals pain and difficulty moving parts distal to the injury.
- Anteroposterior and lateral X-rays of extremity reveal fracture.

Arterial occlusive disease

- Arteriography demonstrates the type (thrombus or embolus), location, and degree of obstruction, and the collateral circulation.
- Doppler ultrasonography and plethysmography show decreased blood flow distal to the occlusion.
- Ophthalmodynamometry helps determine degree of obstruction in the internal carotid artery by comparing ophthalmic artery pressure to brachial artery pressure on the affected side. More than a 20% difference between pressures suggests insufficiency.

Asbestosis

- History includes occupational, family, or neighborhood exposure to asbestos fibers.
- CXR reveals fine, irregular, and linear diffuse infiltrates; extensive fibrosis results in "honeycomb" or "ground glass" appearance. X-rays also show pleural thickening and calcification, with bilateral oblation of costophrenic angles.
- PFTs reveal decreased vital capacity, FVC, and total lung capacity; decreased or normal FEV_1 in 1 second; a normal ratio of FEV_1 to FVC; and reduced diffusing capacity for CO_2.
- ABG analysis may reveal decreased PaO_2 and $PaCO_2$.

Ascariasis

- Stools contain ova or roundworm.
- Vomitus contains roundworm.
- CXR reveals infiltrates, patchy areas of pneumonitis, and widening of hilar shadows.

Aspergillosis

- History includes ocular trauma or surgery.
- CXR reveals crescent-shaped radiolucency surrounding a circular mass.
- Culture of exudate identifies *Aspergillus.*

Asphyxia

- History includes change in mental status and alteration of respiratory pattern.

■ ABG analysis reveals PaO_2 < 60 mm Hg (SI, < 8.02 kPa) and $PaCO_2$ > 50 mm Hg (SI, > 6.64 kPa).
■ CXR may reveal presence of foreign body, pulmonary edema, or atelectasis.
■ Toxicology screening may reveal abnormal Hb level or ingestion of drugs or chemicals.
■ PFTs may indicate respiratory muscle weakness.

Asthma

■ PFTs may reveal:
– forced expiratory flow < 75%
– FEV_1 of 83% or below
– tidal volumes < 5 to 7 ml/ kg of body weight
– residual volume > 35% of total lung capacity.
■ ABG analysis may demonstrate PaO_2 < 75 mm Hg (SI, < 10.03 kPa) and $PaCO_2$ > 45 mm Hg (SI, > 5.3 kPa), indicating severe bronchial obstruction.
■ CBC reveals eosinophil count > 7%.
■ CXR shows hyperinflation.

Asystole

ECG reveals a waveform that's almost a flat line. Characteristic findings include:
■ Atrial rhythm is usually indiscernible; no ventricular rhythm is present.
■ Atrial rate is usually indiscernible; no ventricular rate is present.
■ P wave may be present.
■ PR interval isn't measurable.
■ QRS complex is absent, or occasional escape beats are present.
■ T wave is absent.
■ QT interval isn't measurable.

Ataxia-telangiectasia

■ History and physical examination reveal the presence of ataxia, telangiectasia, and recurrent sinopulmonary infection.
■ Serum analysis shows absent or deficient levels of IgA or IgE.
■ Examination of thymic tissue reveals absence of Hassall's corpuscles.

Atelectasis

■ Chest auscultation reveals decreased or absent breath sounds.
■ CXR reveals characteristic horizontal lines in the lower lung zones (in widespread atelectasis) and dense shadows (with segmental or lobar collapse) with hyperinflation of neighboring lung.

Atopic dermatitis

■ History includes clinical manifestations of allergy symptoms such as asthma, hay fever, or urticaria.
■ CBC reveals elevated eosinophil count.
■ Serum analysis shows elevated IgE levels.
■ Tissue culture may be performed to rule out bacterial, viral, or fungal superinfections.

Atrial fibrillation

ECG findings include:
■ Atrial and ventricular rhythms are grossly irregular.
■ The atrial rate, almost indiscernible, usually exceeds 400 beats/minute. The ventricular rate usually varies from 100 to 150 beats/minute, but can be < 100 beats/minute.
■ P wave is absent. Erratic baseline f (fibrillatory) waves appear instead. These chaotic f waves represent atrial tetanization from rapid atrial depolarizations. When f waves are pronounced, the arrhythmia is called *coarse atrial fibrillation.* When they aren't pronounced, the arrhythmia is called *fine atrial fibrillation.*
■ PR interval is indiscernible.
■ Duration and configuration of QRS complex are usually normal. If ventricular conduction is aberrant, the QRS complex may be wide and abnormally shaped.

- T wave is indiscernible.
- QT interval isn't measurable.
- Atrial fib-flutter, a rhythm that frequently varies between a fibrillatory line and flutter waves, may appear.

Atrial flutter

ECG findings include:

- Atrial rhythm is regular. Ventricular rhythm depends on the atrioventricular (AV) conduction pattern; it's often regular, although cycles may alternate. An irregular pattern may herald atrial fibrillation or indicate a block.
- Atrial rate is 250 to 400 beats/minute. Ventricular rate depends on the degree of AV block; usually, it's 60 to 100 beats/minute, but it may accelerate to 125 to 150 beats/minute.
- P wave is saw-toothed, referred to as flutter or F waves.
- PR interval isn't measurable.
- Usually, duration of QRS complex is within normal limits; however, the complex may be widened if F waves are buried within.
- T wave isn't identifiable.
- QT interval isn't measurable because T wave can't be identified.
- The patient may develop an atrial rhythm that frequently varies between a fibrillatory line and F waves. This is called *atrial fib-flutter;* the ventricular response is irregular.

Atrial septal defect

- Echocardiography measures right ventricular enlargement, may locate the defect, and shows volume overload in the right heart.
- ECG reveals incomplete or complete right bundle-branch block in nearly all cases.
- Cardiac catheterization reveals a left-to-right shunt, determines the extent of shunting and pulmonary vascular disease, detects the size and location of pulmonary venous drainage, and the atrioventricular valves' competence.

Atrial tachycardia

ECG findings include:

- Atrial and ventricular rhythms are regular.
- Atrial rate is characterized by three or more consecutive ectopic atrial beats occurring at a rate between 160 and 250 beats/minute; the rate rarely exceeds 250 beats/minute. The ventricular rate depends on the atrioventricular conduction ratio.
- Usually positive, the P wave may be aberrant, invisible, or hidden in the previous T wave. If visible, it precedes each QRS complex.
- PR interval may be unmeasurable if the P wave can't be distinguished from the preceding T wave.
- Duration and configuration of QRS complex are usually normal.
- T wave usually can't be distinguished.
- QT interval is usually within normal limits, but may be shorter because of the rapid rate.

Atrioventricular (AV) block, third-degree

ECG findings include:

- Atrial and ventricular rhythms are regular.
- Atrial rate, which is usually within normal limits, exceeds the ventricular rate. The slow ventricular rate ranges from 40 to 60 beats/minute, but this rate is determined by the block's location and the origin of the subsidiary impulse.
- P wave has normal size and configuration.
- PR interval isn't measurable because the atria and ventricles beat independently (AV dissociation).
- Configuration of the QRS complex depends on where the ventricular beat

originates. A high AV junctional pacemaker produces a narrow QRS complex; a pacemaker in the bundle of His produces a wide QRS complex; a ventricular pacemaker produces a wide, bizarre QRS complex.
- T wave has normal size and configuration.
- QT interval may or may not be within normal limits.

Basal cell carcinoma
- Inspection reveals skin lesions.
- Tissue biopsy reveals basal cell carcinoma.

B-cell deficiency
- History includes recurrent infections.
- Family history includes infection as cause of death.
- IgM, IgA, and IgG levels are decreased (after age 6 months).
- Tissue biopsy may show B cells but no plasma cells (B cells mature to form plasma cells as part of a normal immune response) in acquired hypogammaglobulinemia.

Bell's palsy
- Inspection reveals facial paresthesia with an inability to raise the eyebrow, close the eyelid, smile, show the teeth, or puff the cheek.
- EEG distinguishes temporary conduction defect from pathologic interruption of nerve fibers (after 10 days).

Benign prostatic hyperplasia
- History includes problems with urination.
- Rectal examination reveals enlarged prostate gland.
- Prostate biopsy reveals histologic changes characteristic of benign prostatic hyperplasia.
- Excretory urography may indicate urinary tract obstruction, hydronephrosis, calculi, or tumors, and filling and emptying defects in the bladder.
- Elevated BUN and creatinine levels suggest impaired renal function.
- Urinalysis and urine culture show hematuria, pyuria, and, when bacterial count exceeds 100,000/ml, infection.
- Cystourethroscopy indicates prostate enlargement (usually performed immediately before surgery to help determine the best operative procedure).

Berylliosis
- History includes occupational, family, or neighborhood exposure to beryllium dust, fumes, or mists.
- In acute berylliosis, CXR reveals acute miliary process or patchy acinous filling, and diffuse infiltrates with prominent peribronchial markings.
- In chronic berylliosis, CXR reveals reticulonodular infiltrates, hilar adenopathy, and large coalescent infiltrates in both lungs.
- PFTs reveal decreased lung capacity.

Bladder cancer
- Cystoscopy with biopsy reveals the presence of malignant cells and may reveal that the bladder is fixed to the pelvic wall or prostate.
- Arylsulfatase A levels are elevated.
- Retrograde cystography evaluates bladder structure and integrity and confirms the diagnosis.
- Excretory urography reveals an early-stage or infiltrating tumor, ureteral obstruction, or a rigid deformity of the bladder wall. This test may also delineate functional problems in the upper urinary tract and help assess the degree of hydronephrosis.
- Urinalysis indicates presence of blood and malignant cytology.
- Ultrasonography may detect metastases in tissue beyond the bladder and can distinguish a bladder cyst from a bladder tumor.

- Pelvic arteriography reveals tumor invasion of the bladder wall.
- CT scan reveals the thickness of the involved bladder wall and detects enlarged retroperitoneal lymph nodes.

Blastomycosis

- Culture of skin lesions, pus, sputum, or pulmonary secretions reveals *Blastomyces dermatitidis.*

Blepharitis

- History includes irritated eyes and rubbing of the eyes.
- Tissue culture of ulcerated lid margin reveals *Staphylococcus aureus* (with ulcerative blepharitis).
- Inspection detects presence of nits (with pediculosis).

Blood transfusion reaction

- Crossmatching reveals conflicting blood types.
- Urinalysis reveals hemoglobinuria.
- Antibody screening reveals anti-A or anti-B antibodies in the blood.
- Serum haptoglobin level falls below pretransfusion level after 24 hours.
- Blood cultures may indicate bacterial contamination.

Blunt and penetrating abdominal injuries

- History includes trauma to abdomen or chest area.
- CXR or abdominal X-ray indicates presence of free air.
- Peritoneal lavage reveals blood, urine, bile, stool, or pus.
- Serum amylase level > 239 U/L (SI, > 4.07 μkat/L) indicates pancreatic injury.
- Hb level and HCT show a serial decrease.
- Excretory urography and retrograde cystography indicate renal and urinary tract damage.
- CT scan indicates abdominal organ rupture.
- Exploratory laparotomy reveals specific injuries when other clinical evidence is incomplete.

Blunt chest injuries

- History includes trauma to chest area.
- With hemothorax, percussion reveals dullness.
- With tension pneumothorax, percussion reveals tympany.
- CXR may indicate rib and sternal injuries, pneumothorax, flail chest, pulmonary contusion, lacerated or ruptured aorta, diaphragmatic rupture, lung compression, or hemothorax.
- CT scan reveals aortic laceration or rupture, or diaphragmatic rupture.
- CK-MB level shows mild elevation.

Bone tumor, primary malignant

- Physical examination detects palpable mass over bony area.
- Biopsy reveals malignant cells.
- Bone X-ray and radioisotope bone scan reveal tumor location and size.
- CT scan reveals tumor location and size.
- MRI reveals tumor.
- Serum alkaline phosphatase level is elevated (in patients with sarcomas).

Botulism

- Offending toxin is detected in the patient's serum, stool, gastric content, or the suspected food.
- EMG shows diminished muscle action potential after a single supramaximal nerve stimulus.

Brain abscess

- History includes congenital heart disease or infection, especially of the middle ear, mastoid, nasal sinuses, heart, or lungs.

- CT scan or MRI reveals site of abscess.
- Arteriography highlights the abscess with a halo.
- Culture of drainage reveals causative organism, such as *Staphylococcus aureus, Streptococcus viridans,* or *Streptococcus hemolyticus.*

Breast cancer

- Breast examination is abnormal.
- Mammography, ultrasonography, or thermography indicates presence of mass.
- Surgical biopsy reveals malignant cells.
- CEA levels are > 20 ng/ml (SI, > 20 µg/L).
- Serum or urine of woman who isn't pregnant contains hCG.

Bronchiectasis

- History includes recurrent bronchial infections, pneumonia, and hemoptysis.
- CXR show pleural thickening, areas of atelectasis, and scattered cystic changes.

Bronchitis, chronic

- CXRs may show hyperinflation and increased bronchovascular markings.
- PFTs demonstrate increased residual volume, decreased vital capacity and forced expiratory flow, and normal static compliance and diffusing capacity.
- ABG analysis reveals decreased PaO_2 and normal or increased $PaCO_2$.
- Sputum culture reveals the presence of microorganisms and neutrophils.
- ECG may detect atrial arrhythmias; peaked P waves in leads II, III, and aV_F; and, occasionally, right ventricular hypertrophy.
- Bronchography reveals location and extent of disease.

Brucellosis

- History includes contact with animals.
- Agglutinin titers within 3 weeks of illness are elevated.
- Multiple blood cultures, bone marrow culture, and biopsy of infected tissue indicate presence of *Brucella* bacteria.

Buerger's disease

- History includes intermittent claudication of the palm of the hand and the instep.
- Doppler ultrasonography reveals diminished circulation in the peripheral vessels.
- Plethysmography reveals decreased circulation in the peripheral vessels.

Burns

- History includes exposure to heat, electricity, or chemicals.
- Examination reveals depth of skin and tissue damage and area affected.
- Urinalysis may reveal myoglobinuria and hemoglobinuria.
- ABG analysis reveals reduced respiratory function.
- Fiber-optic bronchoscopy may reveal epithelial damage to the trachea and bronchi.
- Serum protein studies show increased albumin levels.
- BUN level is increased due to increased protein catabolism.
- Fibrin split products are increased.
- Serum magnesium levels are suppressed.
- Osmotic fragility is high (increased tendency to hemolysis).
- Changes are noted in serum electrolyte levels, including elevated potassium and decreased sodium levels.
- WBC count reveals leukocytosis.

Calcium imbalance

- In hypocalcemia:
  – serum calcium level is < 4.5 mEq/L (SI, < 1.08 mmol/L).

- In hypercalcemia:
  – serum calcium level is > 5.5 mEq/L (SI, > 2.25 mmol/L)
  – urinalysis reveals increased calcium precipitation.

Note: Because approximately one-half of serum calcium is bound to albumin, changes in serum protein must be considered when interpreting serum calcium levels.

Cancer of the vulva

- Pap test reveals abnormal cells.
- Tissue biopsy reveals malignant cells.
- Vulva staining (with toluidine blue dye) indicates diseased tissues.

Candidiasis

- Culture of skin, vaginal scrapings, pus, sputum, blood, or tissue reveals *Candida albicans.*

Cardiac tamponade

- CXR reveals slightly widened mediastinum and cardiomegaly.
- Echocardiography reveals pericardial effusion with signs of right ventricular and atrial compression.
- Pulmonary artery monitoring reveals increased right atrial pressure, right ventricular diastolic pressure, and central venous pressure.

Cardiogenic shock

- Auscultation detects gallop rhythm, faint heart sounds, and a holosystolic murmur (with ruptured ventricular septum or papillary muscles).
- Pulmonary artery pressure monitoring reveals:
  – increased pulmonary artery pressure
  – increased PAWP
  – increased systemic vascular resistance
  – increased peripheral vascular resistance
  – decreased cardiac output.
- Invasive arterial pressure monitoring reveals hypotension.
- CK levels are increased.
- ABG analysis may show metabolic acidosis and hypoxia.
- ECG shows acute myocardial infarction, ischemia, or ventricular aneurysm.

Carpal tunnel syndrome

- Physical examination reveals decreased sensation to light touch or pinpricks in the affected fingers.
- Tinel's sign is positive.
- Wrist-flexion test reveals positive Phalen's sign.
- Compression test provokes pain and paresthesia along the distribution of the median nerve.
- EMG detects a median nerve motor conduction delay of more than 5 milliseconds.

Cataract

- Eye examination reveals the white area behind the pupil (unnoticeable until the cataract is advanced).
- Ophthalmoscopy or slit-lamp examination reveals a dark area in the normally homogeneous red reflex.

Celiac disease

- Tissue biopsy of the small bowel reveals a mosaic pattern of alternating flat and bumpy areas on the bowel surface (due to an almost total absence of villi) and an irregular, blunt, and disorganized network of blood vessels (usually prominent in the jejunum).
- Stool samples (after 72-hour collection) reveal excess fat.
- HLA test reveals presence of HLA-B8 antigen.
- D-xylose absorption test reveals depressed blood and urine D-xylose levels.
- Upper GI series followed by a small-bowel series demonstrates protracted barium passage: Barium shows up in a segmented, coarse, scattered, and clumped pattern; the jejunum shows generalized dilation.

- Glucose tolerance test indicates poor glucose absorption.
- Low serum carotene levels, indicating malabsorption.
- CBC indicates decreased Hb level and HCT as well as decreased WBC and platelet counts.
- Decreased serum albumin, sodium, potassium, cholesterol, and phospholipid levels.
- PT may be shortened.

Cerebral aneurysm

- History includes headache and change in mental status (usually with rupture or leakage).
- Angiography shows location and size of unruptured aneurysm.
- CT scan reveals location of clot, hydrocephalus, areas of infarction, and extent of blood spillage within the cisterns around the brain.

Cerebral contusion

- History includes head trauma.
- CT scan reveals ischemic tissue and hematoma.
- Skull X-ray indicates fracture is absent.

Cerebral palsy

Infant displays:

- difficulty sucking or keeping food in his mouth
- infrequent voluntary movement
- arm or leg tremors with movement
- crossing legs when lifted from behind rather than pulling them up or "bicycling"
- legs difficult to separate to change diapers
- persistent use of one hand, or ability to use hands well but not legs.

Cerebrovascular accident

- Patient reports sudden onset of motor or sensory impairment.
- CT scan detects structural abnormalities, edema, and lesions, such as nonhemorrhagic infarction and aneurysms.
- Cerebral angiography reveals disruption or displacement of the cerebral circulation by occlusion or hemorrhage.
- Ultrasonography of carotid and cerebral arteries may reveal occlusion.
- Digital abstraction angiography evaluates the patency of the cerebral vessels and identifies their position in the head and neck. It also detects and evaluates lesions and vascular abnormalities.
- PET scan provides data on cerebral metabolism and cerebral blood flow changes, especially in ischemic stroke.
- Single-photon emission tomography identifies cerebral blood flow and helps diagnose cerebral infarction.
- EEG may detect reduced electrical activity in an area of cortical infarction.
- Transcranial Doppler studies examine the size of intracranial vessels and the direction of blood flow.
- MRI allows evaluation of the lesion's location and size.

Cervical cancer

- Pap test reveals abnormal cells.
- Cone biopsy of cervical tissue reveals malignant cells.
- Colposcopy determines the source of the abnormal cells seen on the Pap test.

Cesarean birth

These test findings indicate the need for cesarean birth:

- X-ray pelvimetry may reveal cephalopelvic disproportion and malpresentation.
- Ultrasonography may reveal pelvic masses that interfere with vaginal delivery and fetal position.
- Amniocentesis may reveal Rh isoimmunization, fetal distress, or fetal genetic abnormalities.

- Auscultation of fetal heart rate (fetoscope, Doppler unit, or electronic fetal monitor) may reveal acute fetal distress.

Chalazion

- Visual examination and palpation of the eyelid reveal a small bump or nodule.
- Tissue biopsy rules out meibomian gland cancer.

Chancroid

- History includes sexual contact with a partner with chancroid.
- Tissue culture of ulcer exudate, bubo aspirate, or blood reveals *Haemophilus ducreyi.*

Chlamydial infections

- History includes sexual contact with a partner with chlamydial infection.
- Culture of site indicates *Chlamydia trachomatis* (findings may reveal urethritis, cervicitis, salpingitis, endometritis, or proctitis).
- Culture of blood, pus, or CSF reveals *C. trachomatis* (findings may reveal epididymitis, prostatitis, or lymphogranuloma venereum).

Chloride imbalance

- In hypochloremia, serum chloride level is < 98 mEq/L (SI, < 98 mmol/L).
- In hyperchloremia, serum chloride level is > 108 mEq/L (SI, > 108 mmol/L).

Cholelithiasis and related disorders

- Ultrasonography of the gallbladder indicates presence of stones.
- Percutaneous transhepatic cholangiography reveals gallbladder disease.
- Endoscopic retrograde cholangiopancreatography visualizes the biliary tree.
- Hida scan of the gallbladder reveals obstruction of the cystic duct.
- Oral cholecystography shows stones in the gallbladder and biliary duct obstruction.
- Technetium-labeled iminodiacetic acid scan of the gallbladder indicates cystic duct obstruction and acute or chronic cholecystitis if the gallbladder can't be seen.
- Blood studies may reveal elevated serum alkaline phosphatase, LD, AST, and total bilirubin levels and icteric index.
- WBC count is slightly elevated during a cholecystitis attack.

Cholera

- Patient reports voluminous, gray-tinged diarrhea.
- Stool or vomitus culture reveals presence of *Vibrio cholerae.*
- Agglutination and other clear reactions to group- and type-specific antisera provide definitive diagnosis.
- Dark-field microscopic examination of fresh stool shows rapidly moving bacilli.
- Immunofluorescence allows for rapid diagnosis.

Choriocarcinoma

- Radioimmunoassay of hCG levels, performed frequently, provides early and accurate diagnosis; levels that are extremely elevated for early pregnancy indicate gestational trophoblastic disease.
- Histologic examination of possible hydatid vessels confirms the diagnosis.
- Ultrasonography performed after the third month shows grapelike clusters rather than a fetus.
- Amniography reveals the absence of a fetus (performed only when the diagnosis is in question).
- Doppler ultrasonography demonstrates the absence of fetal heart tones.
- Hb level, HCT, and RBC count are abnormal.

- Fibrinogen levels are abnormal.
- PT and PTT are abnormal.
- WBC count and ESR are increased.
- CXR, CT scan, and MRI may identify choriocarcinoma metastasis.
- Lumbar puncture may detect early cerebral metastasis if hCG is in CSF.

Chronic fatigue and immune dysfunction syndrome

- History includes persistent or relapsing debilitating fatigue or tendency to tire easily.
- Average level of activity is < 50% of normal for 6 months or more.
- Fatigue doesn't resolve with bed rest.
- Diagnostic tests rule out other illnesses, such as Epstein-Barr virus, leukemia, and lymphoma.

Chronic glomerulonephritis

- Urinalysis reveals proteinuria, hematuria, cylindruria, and RBC casts.
- BUN level is elevated.
- Serum creatinine level is elevated.
- Kidney X-rays or ultrasonography reveals small kidneys.
- Renal biopsy indicates presence of underlying disease.

Chronic granulomatous disease

- History includes osteomyelitis, pneumonia, liver abscess, or chronic lymphadenopathy in a young child.
- Nitroblue tetrazolium (NBT) test reveals impaired NBT reduction, indicating abnormal neutrophil metabolism.
- Neutrophil function test measures the rate of intracellular killing by neutrophils; in chronic granulomatous disease, killing is delayed or absent.

Chronic lymphocytic leukemia

- CBC reveals numerous abnormal lymphocytes.
- WBC count is mildly but persistently elevated in early stages.
- Granulocytopenia is present.
- Bone marrow aspiration and biopsy reveal lymphocytic invasion.

Chronic mucocutaneous candidiasis

- Inspection reveals large, circular lesions.
- Culture of affected area indicates presence of *Candida*.

Chronic renal failure

- History includes chronic progressive debilitation.
- BUN level is elevated.
- Serum creatinine level is elevated.
- Serum potassium level may be elevated.
- ABG analysis reveals blood pH < 7.35 and HCO_3^- level < 22 mEq/L (SI, < 22 mmol/L).
- Urinalysis may show proteinuria, glycosuria, erythrocytes, leukocytes, and casts.
- Kidney biopsy identifies underlying pathology.

Cirrhosis and fibrosis

- Liver biopsy reveals destruction and fibrosis of hepatic tissue.
- Abdominal X-rays show liver size and cysts or gas within the biliary tract or liver, liver calcification, and massive ascites.
- CT and liver scans determine the liver size, identify liver masses, and reveal hepatic blood flow and obstruction.
- Esophagogastroduodenoscopy reveals bleeding esophageal varices, stomach irritation or ulceration, or duodenal bleeding and irritation.
- ALT, AST, total serum bilirubin, and indirect bilirubin levels are elevated.
- Serum albumin and protein levels are decreased.
- PT is prolonged.
- HCT, Hb, and serum electrolyte levels are decreased.

Coal worker's pneumoconiosis

- History includes exposure to coal dust.
- In simple coal worker's pneumoconiosis (CWP), CXR reveals small opacities (< 1 cm in diameter) prominent in the upper lung fields.
- In complicated CWP, CXR reveals one or more large opacities (1 to 5 cm in diameter), possibly exhibiting cavitation.
- PFTs reveal decreased lung capacity.

Coarctation of the aorta

- Physical examination reveals resting systolic hypertension, absent or diminished femoral pulses, and wide pulse pressure.
- CXR reveals notching of the undersurfaces of the ribs due to collateral circulation.
- Echocardiography reveals left ventricular muscle thickening, coexisting aortic valve abnormalities, and the coarctation site.
- Aortography locates the site and extent of coarctation.
- ECG may reveal left ventricular hypertrophy.

Coccidioidomycosis

- Skin test indicates a positive reaction for coccidioidin.
- Immunodiffusion of sputum and pus from lesions and tissue biopsy reveal presence of *Coccidioides immitis* spores.
- Complement fixation reveals presence of IgG antibodies.
- Serum Ig levels help establish diagnosis.

Colorado tick fever

- History includes recent exposure to ticks.
- Serum studies indicate presence of Colorado tick fever virus.
- Patient may have leukopenia.

Colorectal cancer

- Hemoccult test (guaiac) reveals blood in stools.
- Proctoscopy or sigmoidoscopy reveals presence of mass.
- Colonoscopy reveals lesion.
- Tissue biopsy reveals malignant cells.
- Barium X-ray reveals lesion.
- CEA level is > 5 ng/ml (SI, > 5 μg/L).

Common variable immunodeficiency

- Circulating B-cell count is normal.
- Serum IgM, IgA, and IgG levels are decreased, suggesting diminished synthesis or secretion.
- Antigenic stimulation reveals an inability to produce specific antibodies.
- X-rays may reveal signs of chronic lung disease or sinusitis.

Complement deficiencies

- Total serum complement level is low.
- Specific assays may confirm deficiency of specific complement components.

Concussion

- History includes head trauma, with or without loss of consciousness.
- Patient demonstrates amnesia with regard to traumatic event.
- Patient reports headache.
- Neurologic examination results are normal for patient.
- Skull X-ray and CT scan may be negative.

Congenital hip dysplasia

- Ortolani's or Trendelenburg's sign is positive.
- Inspection reveals extra thigh fold on affected side, higher buttock fold on the affected side, restricted abduction of the affected hip.
- X-ray reveals the location of the femur head and a shallow acetabulum.

Conjunctivitis

- Inspection reveals inflammation of the conjunctiva.
- Stained smear of conjunctival scrapings reveal monocytes (viral conjunctivitis), polymorphonuclear cells (bacterial conjunctivitis), or eosinophils (allergic conjunctivitis).
- Conjunctival culture reveals causative organism.

Corneal abrasion

- History includes eye trauma or prolonged wearing of contact lenses.
- Fluorescein stain of the cornea turns the injured area green during flashlight examination.
- Slit-lamp examination discloses the depth of the abrasion.

Corneal ulcers

- History includes eye trauma or use of contact lenses.
- Flashlight examination reveals irregular corneal surface.
- Fluorescein dye, instilled in the conjunctival sac, stains the outline of the ulcer.

Coronary artery disease

- History includes angina and risk factors for coronary artery disease.
- ECG reveals ischemia and, possibly, arrhythmias during an anginal attack. ECG returns to normal when pain ceases.
- Coronary angiography reveals coronary artery stenosis or obstruction, collateral circulation, and the arteries' condition beyond the narrowing.
- Myocardial perfusion imaging with thallium-201 during treadmill exercise detects ischemic areas.

Cor pulmonale

- Pulmonary artery pressure measurements reveal increased right ventricular and pulmonary artery pressures as well as elevated right ventricular systolic, pulmonary artery systolic, and pulmonary artery diastolic pressures.
- CXR reveals large central pulmonary arteries and rightward enlargement of cardiac silhouette.
- Echocardiography reveals right ventricular enlargement.

Corrosive esophagitis and stricture

- History includes chemical ingestion.
- Oropharyngeal burns (indicated by white membranes and edema of the soft palate and uvula).
- Endoscopy (in the first 24 hours after ingestion) delineates the extent and location of the esophageal injury and assesses depth of the burn; 1 week after ingestion, this test helps assess stricture development.
- Barium swallow, performed 1 week after ingestion and every 3 weeks thereafter, as ordered, identifies segmental spasm or fistula.

Cri du chat syndrome

- History includes cat cry, facial disproportions, microencephaly, small birth size, and poor physical and mental development.
- Karyotype reveals deleted short arms of chromosome 5.

Crohn's disease

- History includes frequent stools and abdominal cramping.
- Barium enema reveals the string sign (segments of stricture separated by normal bowel).
- Sigmoidoscopy and colonoscopy reveal patchy areas of inflammation.
- Biopsy of bowel tissue reveals histologic changes indicative of Crohn's disease.

Cryptococcosis

■ Inspection may reveal signs of meningeal irritation.
■ Sputum, urine, prostatic secretion culture; bone marrow aspirate or biopsy; or pleural biopsy reveals *Cryptococcus neoformans.*
■ Blood culture reveals *C. neoformans* (with severe infection).
■ CXR reveals pulmonary lesion.
■ Cryptococcal antigen and positive cryptococcal culture occurs in 90% of tests.

Cushing's syndrome

■ Serum cortisol levels are consistently elevated.
■ 24-hour urine sample demonstrates elevated free cortisol levels.
■ Dexamethasone suppression test reveals a cortisol level of 5 g/dl (SI, 140 nmol/L) or greater (failure to suppress).
■ Urine 17-hydroxycorticosteroid levels are elevated.
■ Urine 17-KS levels are elevated.
■ Ultrasonography, CT scan, or angiography localize adrenal tumors.
■ CT scan of the head identifies pituitary tumors.

Cutaneous larva migrans

■ Patient displays characteristic migratory lesions.
■ History includes contact with warm, moist soil within the past several months.

Cystic fibrosis

■ Family history includes the disorder.
■ Pulmonary disease or pancreatic insufficiency (absence of trypsin) is present.
■ Sweat test reveals sodium and chloride concentrations of 50 to 60 mEq/L (SI, 50 to 60 mmol/L) or greater.
■ DNA testing may locate the Delta 508 deletion and help to confirm the diagnosis.
■ PFTs evaluate lung function.
■ Sputum culture allows the detection of concurrent infectious disease.
■ ABG analysis helps determine pulmonary status.
■ CXR helps diagnose respiratory obstruction and monitor its progress.

Cystinuria

■ Family history includes renal disease or renal calculi.
■ Chemical analysis of calculi shows cystine crystals, with a variable amount of calcium.
■ Clearance of cystine, lysine, arginine, and ornithine is elevated.
■ Urinalysis with amino acid chromatography indicates aminoaciduria, as evidenced by the presence of cystine, lysine, arginine, and ornithine.
■ Urine pH is usually < 5.
■ Microscopic examination of urine shows hexagonal, flat cystine crystals.
■ Cyanide-nitroprusside test is positive.
■ Excretory urography or KUB X-rays reveal size and location of calculi.

Cytomegalovirus infection

■ Culture of urine, saliva, throat, or blood or biopsy specimens reveal virus.
■ Indirect immunofluorescent test reveals IgM antibody.

Dacryocystitis

■ History includes constant tearing.
■ Culture of discharge from tear sac reveals *Staphylococcus aureus* and, occasionally, beta-hemolytic streptococci in acute dacryocystitis; culture reveals *Streptococcus pneumoniae* or *Candida albicans* in the chronic form.
■ Dacryocystography locates the atresia.

Decompression sickness

- History includes rapid decompression.
- Physical examination reveals incapacitating joint and muscle pain, and neurologic and respiratory disturbance.

Dermatitis

- Family history includes allergy and chronic inflammation.
- Patient demonstrates characteristic distribution of skin lesions.
- Serum IgE levels are elevated.

Dermatophytosis

- Inspection reveals skin lesions.
- Microscopic examination or culture of lesion scrapings reveals infective organism.
- Wood's light examination may reveal types of tinea capitis.

Diabetes insipidus

- History includes head trauma or neurologic surgery.
- Urinalysis reveals almost colorless urine of low osmolality (< 300 mOsmol/kg [SI, < 300 mmol/kg]) and low specific gravity (< 1.005).

Diabetes mellitus

- In nonpregnant adults, findings include:
  – symptoms of uncontrolled diabetes and a random blood glucose level ≥ 200 mg/dl (SI, ≥ 10.6 mmol/L)
  – fasting plasma glucose level ≥ 126 mg/dl (SI, ≥ 7 mmol/L) on at least two occasions
  – in a patient with normal fasting glucose, a blood glucose level > 200 mg/dl (SI, > 10.6 mmol/L) during the second hour of a glucose tolerance test and on at least one other occasion during the glucose tolerance test.
- Ophthalmologic examination may show diabetic retinopathy.
- Urinalysis reveals presence of acetone.

DiGeorge's syndrome

- History includes facial anomalies in infant.
- T-lymphocyte assay shows decreased or absent T cells.
- B-lymphocyte assay shows elevated B cells.
- CT scan or MRI shows thymus is absent.
- Serum calcium levels are < 8 mg/dl (SI, < 2 mmol/L).

Dilated cardiomyopathy

- CXR reveals cardiomegaly, usually affecting all heart chambers, and may also show pulmonary congestion, pleural or pericardial effusion, or pulmonary venous hypertension.
- ECG may reveal ST-segment and T-wave changes.
- Echocardiography reveals left ventricular thrombi, global hypokinesia, and degree of left ventricular dilation.

Diphtheria

- Inspection reveals characteristic thick, patchy grayish green membrane over the mucous membranes of the pharynx, larynx, tonsils, soft palate, and nose.
- Throat culture or culture of other suspect lesions reveals *Corynebacterium diphtheriae.*

Dislocated or fractured jaw

- History includes trauma to jaw or face.
- Maxillary or mandibular mobility is abnormal.
- X-ray of the jaw shows fracture.

Dislocations and subluxations

- Inspection confirms joint deformity.
- X-ray is negative for fracture but may reveal dislocation or subluxation.

- Arthroscopy reveals dislocation or subluxation.

Disseminated intravascular coagulation

- Patient displays abnormal bleeding in the absence of a known hematologic disorder.
- Platelet count is < 100,000/µl (SI, < 100 × 10^9/L).
- Fibrinogen is < 175 mg/dl (SI, < 1.75 g/L).
- PT is > 15 seconds.
- Partial PTT is > 60 seconds.
- Fibrin split products reveal fibrin degradation products > 100 mg/ml.
- D-dimer test (a specific fibrinogen test for disseminated intravascular coagulation) is positive.
- Fibrin degradation products are increased, > 45 µg/ml (SI, > 45 mg/L).

Diverticular disease

- Upper GI series reveals barium-filled pouches in the esophagus and upper bowel.
- Barium enema reveals barium-filled pouches in the lower bowel; barium outlines diverticula filled with stool.

Down syndrome

- History includes hypotonia at birth.
- Karyotype reveals chromosome abnormality.
- Prenatal ultrasonography may suggest Down syndrome if a duodenal obstruction or an atrioventricular canal defect is present.
- Maternal serum AFP levels are reduced.
- Amniocentesis reveals the translocated chromosome.

Dysfunctional uterine bleeding

- History includes excessive vaginal bleeding.
- Organic, systemic, psychogenic, and endocrine causes of bleeding are ruled out.
- D&C and biopsy reveal endometrial hyperplasia.

Dysmenorrhea

- History includes abdominal pain related to menstruation.
- Pelvic examination may reveal the physical cause.
- Laparoscopy may reveal an underlying cause such as endometriosis or uterine leiomyoma.
- D&C may reveal an underlying cause such as cervical stenosis or pelvic inflammatory disease.

Dyspareunia

- History includes discomfort during sexual intercourse.
- Pelvic examination may reveal a physical disorder as underlying cause of discomfort.

Ectopic pregnancy

- Serum pregnancy test shows presence of hCG.
- Real-time ultrasonography (performed if serum pregnancy test is positive) reveals no intrauterine pregnancy.
- Culdocentesis (performed if ultrasonography detects the absence of a gestational sac in the uterus) reveals free blood in the peritoneum.
- Laparoscopy (performed if culdocentesis is positive) reveals pregnancy outside the uterus.

Electric shock

- History includes electrical contact, voltage, and length of contact.
- Physical examination reveals electrical burn.
- ECG reveals ventricular fibrillation or other arrhythmias that progress to fibrillation or myocardial infarction.
- Urine myoglobin test is positive.

Emphysema

■ Examination reveals barrel chest, pursed-lip breathing, and use of accessory muscles of respiration; palpation may reveal decreased tactile fremitus and decreased chest expansion; percussion may reveal hyperresonance; auscultation may reveal decreased breath sounds, crackles and wheezing on inspiration, prolonged expiratory phase with grunting respirations, and distant heart sounds.

■ In advanced disease, CXR may show a flattened diaphragm, reduced vascular markings at the lung periphery, overaeration of the lungs, a vertical heart, enlarged anteroposterior chest diameter, and large retrosternal air space.

■ PFTs indicate increased residual volume and total lung capacity, reduced diffusing capacity, and increased inspiratory flow.

■ ABG analysis usually shows reduced PaO_2 and normal $PaCO_2$ until late in the disease when $PaCO_2$ increases.

■ ECG may reveal tall, symmetrical P waves in leads II, III, and aV_F; a vertical QRS axis; and signs of right ventricular hypertrophy late in the disease.

■ RBC count usually demonstrates an increased Hb level late in the disease, when the patient has persistent severe hypoxia.

Encephalitis

■ Lumbar puncture reveals elevated CSF pressure and clear CSF, with slightly elevated WBC and protein levels.

■ CSF or blood culture reveals virus.

■ Serologic studies (in herpes encephalitis) may show rising titers of complement-fixing antibodies.

■ EEG reveals abnormalities such as generalized slowing of waveforms.

Endocarditis

■ Auscultation reveals a loud, regurgitant murmur.

■ Blood cultures (three or more during a 24- to 48-hour period) reveal infecting organism.

■ WBC count is elevated.

■ ESR is elevated.

■ Serum creatinine level is elevated.

■ Echocardiography or transesophageal echocardiography reveals valvular damage and endocardial vegetation.

Endometriosis

■ Pelvic examination reveals multiple tender nodules on uterosacral ligaments or in the rectovaginal septum, which enlarge and become more tender during menses.

■ Palpation may uncover ovarian enlargement in patients with endometrial cysts on the ovaries or thickened, nodular adnexa (as in pelvic inflammatory disease).

■ Laparoscopy shows small, blue powder burns on the peritoneum or the serosa of any pelvic or abdominal structure.

■ Barium enema rules out malignant or inflammatory bowel disease.

Enterobiasis

■ Collecting a sample from the perianal area with a cellophane tape swab leads to identification of the *Enterobius* ova.

■ History includes pruritus ani as well as recent contact with infected person or infected articles.

Enterocolitis

■ Stool Gram stain reveals numerous gram-positive cocci and polymorphonuclear leukocytes with few gram-negative rods.

■ Stool culture identifies *Staphylococcus aureus* as the causative organism.

■ Blood studies reveal leukocytosis, moderately increased BUN level, and decreased serum albumin level.

Epicondylitis

- History includes traumatic injury or strain associated with athletic activity.
- Examination reveals pain with wrist extension and supination with lateral involvement, or with flexion and pronation with epicondyle involvement.
- X-rays are normal at first, but later bony fragments, osteophyte sclerosis, or calcium deposits appear.
- Arthrography is normal with some minor irregularities on the tendon undersurface.
- Arthrocentesis identifies causative organism if joint infection is suspected.

Epidermolysis bullosa

- Skin biopsy of a freshly induced blister reveals type of epidermolysis bullosa.
- Fetoscopy and biopsy provide prenatal diagnosis of the severe scarring forms (at 20 weeks' gestation).

Epididymitis

- History includes unilateral, dull aching pain radiating to the spermatic cord, lower abdomen, and flank.
- Physical examination shows characteristic waddle, as an attempt to protect the groin and scrotum when walking.
- WBC count in urine is increased.
- Urine culture and sensitivity tests reveal causative organism.
- Elevated serum WBC count indicates infection.

Epiglottiditis

- Throat examination reveals a large, edematous, bright red epiglottis.
- Direct laryngoscopy reveals swollen, beefy-red epiglottis (not done if significant obstruction is suspected or immediate intubation isn't possible).
- Lateral neck X-rays show an enlarged epiglottis and distended hypopharynx.

Epilepsy

- CT scan provides brain density readings indicating abnormalities in internal structures.
- EEG may show paroxysmal abnormalities and helps classify the disorder.
- MRI helps identify the cause of the seizure by providing clear images of the brain in regions where bone normally hampers visualization.

Epistaxis

- History includes trauma to the nose, chemical irritation, sinus infection, or coagulopathy.
- Inspection with a bright light and nasal speculum locates the site of bleeding.

Erectile dysfunction

- Detailed sexual history reveals persistent or recurrent partial or complete failure to attain or maintain erection until completion of sexual activity or a persistent or recurrent lack of a subjective sense of sexual excitement and pleasure during sexual activity.
- Urologic screening rules out urogenital problems.
- Neurologic evaluation rules out neurologic dysfunction.
- Drug history rules out medication use as a causative factor.

Erysipeloid

- History includes occupational exposure to *Erysipelothrix insidiosa* and skin injury.
- Examination reveals purple erythema of the skin, persisting over several days.
- Full-thickness skin biopsy taken from the edge of the lesion results in isolation of *E. insidiosa*.

Erythroblastosis fetalis

- Maternal history reveals risk factors for incompatibility of fetal and maternal blood, such as erythroblastotic stillbirths, abortions, previously affected children, previous anti-Rh titers, and blood transfusions.

- Maternal blood typing indicates mother is Rh-negative (titers determine changes in the degree of maternal immunization).
- Amniocentesis reveals an increase in bilirubin levels (indicating possible hemolysis) and elevations in anti-Rh titers.
- Radiologic studies may show edema and, in hydrops fetalis, the halo sign (edematous, elevated, subcutaneous fat layers) and the Buddha position (fetus's legs are crossed).
- Direct Coombs' test of umbilical cord blood confirms maternal-newborn Rh incompatibility.
- An umbilical cord Hb count < 10 g/dl (SI, < 100 g/L) signals severe disease.
- Stained RBC examination reveals many nucleated peripheral RBCs.

Esophageal cancer

- X-rays of the esophagus, with barium swallow and motility studies, reveal structural and filling defects and reduced peristalsis.
- CXR or esophagography reveals pneumonitis.
- Esophagoscopy, punch-and-brush biopsies, and exfoliative cytologic tests confirm esophageal tumors.
- Bronchoscopy may reveal tumor growth in the tracheobronchial tree.
- Endoscopic ultrasonography (combined with endoscopy and ultrasonography) identifies depth of tumor penetration.
- Mediastinoscopy reveals lesion and extent of disease.
- Esophageal biopsy reveals malignant cells.

Esophageal diverticula

- Barium swallow reveals characteristic out-pouching in esophagus.
- Esophagoscopy rules out other lesions as cause.

Exophthalmos

- Physical examination reveals forward displacement of the eyeballs.
- Exophthalmometer readings reveal the degree of anterior projection and asymmetry between the eyes to be > 12 mm.
- X-rays show orbital fracture or bony erosion by an orbital tumor.
- CT scan identifies lesions in optic nerve, orbit, or ocular muscle within the orbit.

Extraocular motor nerve palsies

- Neuroophthalmologic examination reveals third nerve palsy (ptosis, exotropia, pupil dilation, and unresponsiveness to light, inability to move and accommodate), fourth nerve palsy (diplopia and inability to rotate eye downward and upward), or sixth nerve palsy (one eye turning, with the other eye unable to abduct beyond midline).
- Skull X-rays rule out intracranial tumor.
- CT scan and MRI rule out tumor.
- Cerebral angiography rules out vascular abnormalities.
- Blood studies rule out diabetes.
- Culture and sensitivity tests reveal infective organism (for sixth nerve palsy resulting from infection).

Extrapulmonary tuberculosis

- Acid-fast smear reveals *Mycobacterium tuberculosis.*
- Tuberculin skin test is positive.
- CXR reveals primary pulmonary nodular infiltrates and cavitations (often, however, CXR is negative in extrapulmonary tuberculosis).
- Fluid specimen culture (urine, synovial fluid) reveals *M. tuberculosis.*

Fallopian tube cancer

- History includes unexplained postmenopausal bleeding.
- Pap test reveals abnormal cells.
- Ultrasonography defines tumor mass.
- Barium enema rules out intestinal obstruction.
- Laparotomy and biopsy reveal malignant cells.

Fanconi's syndrome

- 24-hour urine testing reveals excessive excretion of glucose, phosphate, amino acids, HCO_3^-, and potassium.
- Phosphorus and nitrogen levels are elevated (with increased renal dysfunction).
- Serum alkaline phosphatase levels are elevated (with rickets).
- Serum potassium level is decreased.
- Serum HCO_3^- level is < 22 mEq/L (SI, < 22 mmol/L).

Fatty liver

- Examination reveals large, tender liver.
- Liver function studies reveal low albumin, elevated globulin, elevated total bilirubin, low aminotransferase and, commonly, elevated cholesterol levels.
- PT is prolonged.
- Liver biopsy reveals excessive fat.

Femoral and popliteal aneurysms

- Palpation reveals a pulsating mass above or below the inguinal ligament (in femoral aneurysm) or in the popliteal space (in popliteal aneurysm).
- Arteriography or ultrasonography reveals location and size of aneurysm.

Folic acid deficiency anemia

- Serum folate level is decreased.
- Reticulocyte count is decreased.
- Schilling test is positive.
- Serum blood studies show macrocytosis, increased mean corpuscular volume, and abnormal platelets.

Folliculitis, furunculosis, and carbunculosis

- Examination reveals pustule, painful nodule, or abscess on areas with hair growth.
- Wound culture identifies *Staphylococcus aureus*.
- CBC may reveal leukocytosis.
- In carbunculosis, history includes preexistent furunculosis.

Galactorrhea

- History includes milk secretion more than 21 days after weaning.
- Breast palpation results in expression of secretions.
- Microscopic examination reveals fat droplets in fluid.
- Prolactin levels are > 200 ng/ml (SI, > 200 μg/L).
- CT scan rules out pituitary tumor.
- Mammography rules out tumor.

Galactosemia

- Deficiency of the enzyme galactose-1-phosphate uridyl transferase in RBCs indicates classic galactosemia; decreased galactokinase level in RBCs indicates galactokinase deficiency.
- Serum and urine galactose levels are increased.
- Ophthalmoscopy reveals punctate lesions in the fetal lens nucleus.
- Liver biopsy reveals acinar formation.
- Liver enzyme levels (AST and ALT) are elevated.
- Urinalysis reveals presence of albumin.
- Amniocentesis provides prenatal diagnosis (recommended for heterozygous and homozygous parents).

Gallbladder and bile duct carcinoma

- Liver function test may show elevated urobilirubin levels and may show elevated levels of bile and bilirubin.
- Serum bilirubin levels are elevated (5 to 390 mg/dl [SI, > 90 μmol/L]).
- Patient may be jaundiced.
- PT is prolonged.
- Serum alkaline phosphatase levels are consistently elevated.
- Liver-spleen scan identifies abnormality.
- Cholecystography shows stones or calcifications.
- MRI may show areas of tumor growth.
- Cholangiography outlines common bile duct obstruction.
- Ultrasonography of the gallbladder shows a mass.
- Endoscopic retrograde cholangiopancreatography identifies tumor site.
- Biopsy reveals malignant cells.

Gas gangrene

- History includes recent surgery or a deep puncture wound with rapid onset of pain and crepitation around the wound.
- Anaerobic cultures of wound drainage reveal *Clostridium perfringens.*
- Gram stain of wound drainage reveals large, gram-positive, rod-shaped bacteria.
- X-rays reveal gas in tissues.
- Blood studies reveal leukocytosis and, later, hemolysis.

Gastric carcinoma

- Barium X-rays with fluoroscopy reveal tumor or filling defect in the outline of the stomach, loss of flexibility and distensibility, and abnormal gastric mucosa with or without ulceration.
- Gastroscopy with fiber-optic endoscope visualizes mucosal lesions and allows gastroscopic biopsy (biopsy reveals malignant cells).
- Photography with fiber-optic endoscope provides a permanent record of gastric lesions that may help determine disease progression and effect of treatment.
- CT scans, CXR, liver and bone scans, and liver biopsy may rule out specific organ metastasis.

Gastritis

- History includes gastric discomfort or bleeding.
- Gastroscopy demonstrates inflammation of mucosa and confirms diagnosis.
- Stools or vomitus may contain occult blood.
- Hb level and HCT are decreased if bleeding has occurred.

Gastroenteritis

- History includes acute onset of diarrhea accompanied by abdominal pain and discomfort.
- Stool or blood culture reveals causative bacteria, parasites, or amoebae.
- Barium enema reveals inflammation.

Gastroesophageal reflux

- Barium swallow with fluoroscopy may be normal except in patients with advanced disease; in children, barium esophagography under fluoroscope reveals reflux.
- Esophageal acidity test reveals pH of 1.5 to 2.0.
- Acid perfusion test elicits pain or burning.
- Gastroesophageal reflux scanning detects radioactivity in the esophagus.
- Endoscopy and biopsy identify pathologic mucosal changes.

Gaucher's disease

- Bone marrow aspiration reveals Gaucher's cells.

- Direct assay of glucocerebrosidase activity, which can be performed on venous blood, shows absent or deficient activity.
- Liver biopsy reveals increased glucosylceramide accumulation.
- Serum acid phosphatase levels are increased.
- Platelet count and serum iron level are decreased.

Genital herpes

- History includes oral, vaginal, or anal sexual contact with an infected person or other direct contact with lesions.
- Examination reveals vesicles on the genitalia, mouth, or anus.
- Tissue culture and histologic biopsy of vesicular fluid reveals herpes simplex virus type 2.

Genital warts

- Dark-field examination of scrapings from wart cells shows marked vascularization of epidermal cells, which helps to differentiate genital warts from condylomata lata.
- Applying 5% acetic acid (white vinegar) to the warts turns them white, indicating papillomas.

Giardiasis

- History includes such risk factors as recent travel to an endemic area, participation in sexual activity involving oral-anal contact, ingestion of suspect water, or institutionalization.
- Stool specimen shows cysts.
- Duodenal aspirate or biopsy shows trophozoites.
- Small-bowel biopsy shows parasitic infection.

Glaucoma

- History includes gradual loss of peripheral vision.
- Tonometry (using an applanation, Schiøtz, or pneumatic tonometer) reveals increased intraocular pressure.
- Gonioscopy determines the angle of the anterior chamber of the eye, differentiating between chronic open-angle glaucoma and acute angle-closure glaucoma.
- Ophthalmoscopy reveals cupping and atrophy of the optic disk.
- Slit-lamp examination visualizes anterior structures of the eye, demonstrating effects of glaucoma.
- Perimetry or visual field tests evaluate the extent of visual field loss of open-angle deterioration.
- Fundus photography reveals changes in the optic disk.

Glycogen storage diseases

- Type Ia:
  - Liver biopsy reveals normal glycogen synthetase and phosphorylase enzyme activities but reduced or absent glucose-6-phosphatase activity.
  - Liver biopsy reveals normal glycogen structure, but elevated amounts.
  - Serum glucose levels are low.
  - Plasma studies reveal high levels of free fatty acids, triglycerides, cholesterol, and uric acid.
  - Injection of glucagon or epinephrine increases pyruvic and lactic acid levels but doesn't increase blood glucose levels.
  - Glucose tolerance test curve reveals depletional hypoglycemia and reduced insulin output.
- Type II (Pompe's):
  - Muscle biopsy reveals increased concentration of glycogen with normal structure and decreased alpha-1, 4-glucosidase level.
  - ECG (in infants) shows large QRS complexes in all leads, inverted T waves, and a shortened PR interval.

– EMG (in adults) demonstrates muscle fiber irritability and myotonic discharges.
– Amniocentesis reveals a deficiency in alpha-1,4-glucosidase level.
– Placenta or umbilical cord examination shows an alpha-1,4-glucosidase deficiency.
– Liver biopsy shows deficient debranching activity and increased glycogen concentration.

- Type III (Cori's):

– Laboratory tests (in children only) may reveal elevated AST or ALT levels and an increase in erythrocyte glycogen.

- Type IV (Andersen's):

– Liver biopsy demonstrates deficient branching enzyme activity and that the glycogen molecule has longer outer branches.

- Type V (McArdle's):

– Serum studies indicate no increase in venous levels of lactate in sample drawn from extremity after ischemic exercise.
– Muscle biopsy reveals a lack of phosphorylase activity and an increased glycogen content.

- Type VI (Hers'):

– Liver biopsy shows decreased phosphorylase beta activity and increased glycogen concentration.

- Type VII:

– Serum studies indicate no increase in venous levels of lactate in sample drawn from extremity after ischemic exercise.
– Blood studies reveal low erythrocyte phosphofructokinase activity and reduced half-life of RBCs.
– Muscle biopsy shows deficient phosphofructokinase with a marked rise in glycogen concentration with normal structure.

- Type VIII:

– Liver biopsy shows deficient phosphorylase beta activity and increased liver glycogen levels.
– Blood studies show deficient phosphorylase beta kinase in leukocytes.

Goiter, simple

- History includes residence in an area known for nutritionally related risk factors (such as iodine-depleted soil or malnutrition) or ingestion of goitrogenic medications or foods.
- Serum TSH or T_3 concentration is high or normal.
- T_4 concentrations are low to normal.
- Uptake of ^{131}I is normal or increased.
- Protein-bound iodine is low to normal.
- Urinary excretion of iodine is low.

Gonorrhea

- History includes sexual contact with a partner with gonorrhea.
- Culture from site of infection (urethra, cervix, rectum, pharynx) reveals *Neisseria gonorrhoeae.*
- Culture of joint fluid and skin lesions reveals gram-negative diplococci (gonococcal arthritis).
- Culture of conjunctival scrapings confirms gonococcal conjunctivitis.
- Complement fixation and immunofluorescent assays of serum reveal antibody titers four times the normal rate.

Goodpasture's syndrome

- Immunofluorescence of alveolar basement membrane shows linear deposition of Ig as well as complement 3 and fibrinogen.
- Immunofluorescence of glomerular basement membrane (GBM) shows linear deposition of Ig combined with detection of circulating anti-GBM antibody.
- Lung biopsy shows interstitial and intra-alveolar hemorrhage with hemosiderin-laden macrophages.
- CXR reveals pulmonary infiltrates in a diffuse, nodular pattern.

- Renal biopsy reveals focal necrotic lesions and cellular crescents.
- Serum creatinine and BUN levels typically increase two to three times normal.
- Urinalysis may reveal RBCs and cellular casts, granular casts, and proteinuria.

Gout

- Microscopic analysis of synovial fluid obtained by needle aspiration reveals needlelike intracellular crystals of sodium urate; presence of monosodium urate monohydrate crystals confirms diagnosis.
- Serum uric acid levels are normal, but may be increased; the higher the level, the more likely a gout attack.
- Urine uric acid levels are increased (in approximately 20% of patients).
- X-rays reveal damage to the articular cartilage and subchondral bone (in chronic gout).

Granulocytopenia

- Patient demonstrates marked neutropenia.
- WBC count is markedly decreased.
- CBC reveals few observable granulocytes.
- Bone marrow aspiration reveals a scarcity of granulocytic precursor cells beyond the most immature forms.

Guillain-Barré syndrome

- History includes minor febrile illness 1 to 4 weeks before current symptoms.
- Examination reveals progressive muscle weakness.
- CSF analysis reveals normal WBC count, rising protein levels (peaks in 4 to 6 weeks), and increasing pressure.
- EMG reveals repeated firing of the same motor unit instead of widespread sectional stimulation.
- Electrophysiologic studies may reveal marked slowing of nerve conduction velocities.

Haemophilus influenzae infection

- Blood culture reveals *H. influenzae* infection.
- CBC reveals polymorphonuclear leukocytosis and, in young children with severe infection, leukopenia.

Hearing loss

- Audiometry identifies and quantifies hearing loss.
- The Weber, the Rinne, and Schwabach tests differentiate between conductive and sensorineural hearing loss.
- Auditory brain stem response and behavioral tests may help to identify neonatal or infant hearing loss.
- CT scan evaluates vestibular and auditory pathways.
- Pure tone audiometry identifies the presence and degree of hearing loss.
- MRI detects acoustic tumors and lesions.

Heart failure

- Auscultation reveals dyspnea or crackles.
- CXR reveals increased pulmonary vascular markings, interstitial edema, or pleural effusion and cardiomegaly.
- Pulmonary artery monitoring reveals elevated pulmonary artery and capillary wedge pressures and elevated left ventricular end-diastolic pressure in left-sided heart failure, and elevated right atrial pressure or central venous pressure in right-sided heart failure.

Hemochromatosis

- Serum or plasma iron concentration is elevated.
- Transferrin levels are increased to 70% to 100% saturation.
- 24-hour urine collection shows excretion of iron after administration of deferoxamine, an iron-chelating agent.

■ Liver biopsy may also confirm diagnosis.

Hemophilia

■ History suggests disorder runs in family.
■ History includes prolonged bleeding after surgery or trauma or of episodes of spontaneous bleeding into muscles or joints.
■ Hemophilia A:
– Factor VIII assay is 0% to 55% of normal.
– PTT is prolonged.
– Platelet count and function, bleeding time, and PT are normal.
■ Hemophilia B:
– Factor IX assay is deficient.
– PTT is prolonged.
■ Hemophilia C:
– Assay testing reveals deficient factor XI but normal factors VIII and IX levels (rules out hemophilias A and B).
– PTT is prolonged.
■ CT scan rules out intracranial bleeding.
■ Arthroscopy rules out joint bleeding.
■ Endoscopy rules out GI bleeding.

Hemorrhoids

■ History includes intermittent rectal bleeding after defecation.
■ Examination reveals hemorrhoids protruding from rectum.
■ Proctoscopy reveals internal hemorrhoids.
■ Anoscopy and flexible sigmoidoscopy identify internal hemorrhoids and rule out polyps or fistulae.

Hemothorax

■ History includes recent trauma to chest area.
■ Chest percussion reveals dullness.
■ Chest auscultation reveals decreased to absent breath sounds on the affected side.
■ Thoracentesis reveals blood or serosanguineous fluid.
■ CXR reveals pleural fluid with or without mediastinal shift.
■ ABG studies show respiratory failure.
■ Hb levels may be decreased depending on the degree of blood loss.

Hepatic encephalopathy

■ History includes liver disease, with symptoms beginning with slight personality changes progressing to mental confusion and coma.
■ Serum ammonia levels are > 33 μmol/L (SI, > 33 μmol/L).
■ EEG shows slowing waves as the disease progresses.

Hepatitis, viral

■ Hepatitis profile identifies serum antigens and antibodies (serum markers) specific to the causative virus, establishing the type of hepatitis (types A, B, C, D, and E).
■ PT is prolonged (more than 3 seconds longer than normal indicates liver damage).
■ AST and ALT levels are elevated.
■ Serum alkaline phosphatase levels are elevated.
■ Serum and urine bilirubin levels are elevated (with jaundice).
■ Serum albumin is decreased and serum globulin is increased.
■ Liver biopsy and liver scan show patchy necrosis.

Hereditary hemorrhagic telangiectasia

■ History includes an established family pattern of bleeding disorders.
■ Examination reveals localized aggregations of dilated capillaries on the skin of the face, ears, scalp, hands, arms, and feet, and under the nails; characteristic telangiectases are raised or flat, nonpulsatile, violet in color, blanche under pressure, and bleed easily.

- Bone marrow aspiration shows depleted iron stores, which confirms secondary iron deficiency anemia.
- Platelet count may be abnormal.

Herniated disk

- History includes unilateral low back pain radiating to the buttocks, legs, and feet, often associated with a previous traumatic injury or back strain.
- X-rays show degenerative changes and rule out other abnormalities.
- MRI also rules out spinal compression.
- Lasègue's test causes resistance and pain, as well as loss of ankle or knee-jerk reflex.
- Myelography pinpoints the level of herniation and reveals spinal canal compression by herniated disk material.
- CT scan identifies soft tissue and bone abnormalities.
- EMG confirms nerve involvement.
- Neuromuscular tests identify motor and sensory loss and leg muscle weakness.

Herpangina

- Examination reveals vesicular lesions on the mucous membranes of the soft palate, tonsillar pillars, and throat.
- Cultures of mouth washings or stool reveal the coxsackieviruses.
- Antibody titers are elevated.

Herpes simplex

- Examination reveals edema with small vesicles on an erythematous base that rupture, leaving a painful ulcer followed by yellow crusting.
- Isolation of virus from local lesions and biopsy reveal *Herpesvirus hominis*.

Herpes zoster

- Examination reveals small red, nodular skin lesions that spread unilaterally around the thorax or vertically over the arms or legs and vesicles filled with clear fluid or pus.
- Examination of vesicular fluid and infected tissue reveals eosinophilic intranuclear inclusions and varicella virus.
- Lumbar puncture shows increased CSF pressure; CSF analysis shows increased protein levels and, possibly, pleocytosis (with central nervous system involvement).

Hiatal hernia

- CXR reveals air shadow behind the heart (with large hernia).
- Barium swallow with fluoroscopy reveals outpouching at lower end of the esophagus and identifies diaphragmatic abnormalities.
- Serum Hb level and HCT may be decreased (with paraesophageal hernia).
- Endoscopy and biopsy rule out varices and other small gastroesophageal lesions.
- Esophageal motility studies reveal esophageal motor or lower esophageal pressure abnormalities.
- pH studies reveal reflux of gastric contents.
- Acid perfusion test reveals heartburn resulting from esophageal reflux.

Hirschsprung's disease

- Rectal biopsy reveals absence of ganglion cells.
- Barium enema studies reveal a narrowed segment of distal colon with a sawtooth appearance and a funnel-shaped segment above it; barium is retained longer than the usual 12 to 24 hours.
- Rectal manometry detects failure of the internal anal sphincter to relax and contract.
- Upright films of the abdomen show marked colonic distention.

Histoplasmosis

- History includes an immunocompromised condition or exposure to contaminated soil in an endemic area.
- Tissue biopsy and sputum culture reveal *Histoplasma capsulatum* (in acute primary and chronic pulmonary histoplasmosis).
- Histoplasmosis skin test is positive.
- Complement fixation test results and agglutination titers are increased.

Hodgkin's disease

- Lymph node biopsy reveals Reed-Sternberg's abnormal histiocyte proliferation and nodular fibrosis and necrosis.
- CT scan shows lymph node abnormality.
- Lymphangiography shows lymph node abnormality.
- Bone marrow, liver, mediastinal, and spleen biopsies; abdominal CT scan; and lung and bone scans identify organ involvement.
- Blood studies show normochromic anemia (in 50% of patients) and elevated, normal, or reduced WBC count and differential showing any combination of neutrophilia, lymphocytopenia, monocytosis, and eosinophilia.
- Serum alkaline phosphatase levels are increased.

Hookworm disease

- Stool specimen reveals hookworm ova.
- Blood studies show decreased Hb level (in severe cases) and markedly increased WBC count with eosinophil count elevation.

Huntington's disease

- History includes family inheritance pattern along with progressive chorea and dementia, with usual onset between ages 35 and 40.
- PET scan identifies disease.
- DNA analysis identifies marker for gene linked to the disease.
- Evoked potential studies reveal bilateral abnormal P100 latencies.
- Pneumoencephalography reveals the characteristic butterfly dilation of the brain's lateral ventricles.
- CT scan reveals brain atrophy.

Hydatidiform mole

- History includes vaginal bleeding, ranging from brownish red spotting to bright red hemorrhage.
- Examination reveals an abnormally enlarged uterus; pelvic examination reveals grapelike vesicles.
- Histologic identification of hydatid vesicles after passage helps confirm diagnosis.
- Ultrasonography shows grapelike structures rather than a fetus; use of a Doppler ultrasonic flowmeter demonstrates the absence of fetal heart tones.
- Amniography reveals the absence of a fetus.
- WBC count and ESR are increased.
- Hb level, HCT, RBC count, PT, PTT, fibrinogen levels, and hepatic and renal function studies are abnormal.
- Serum hCG levels are elevated 100 days or more after the last menstrual period.
- Serum human placental lactogen levels are subnormal.

Hydrocephalus

- Examination reveals an abnormally large head size for age.
- Skull X-rays reveal thinning of the skull with separation of sutures and widening of the fontanels.
- Ventriculography reveals enlargement of the brain's ventricles.
- Angiography, CT scan, or MRI of the brain reveals areas of altered density and rules out intracranial lesions.

Hydronephrosis

- KUB X-rays reveal bilateral kidney enlargement.
- Renal ultrasonography reveals large, echo-free, central mass that compromises the renal cortex.
- Excretory urography reveals abnormal kidneys.
- Urine studies reveal the inability to concentrate urine, a decreased GFR and, possibly, pyuria (if infection is present).

Hyperaldosteronism

- Serum potassium levels are persistently low (in the absence of edema, diuretic use, GI loss, or abnormal sodium intake).
- Low plasma renin level after volume depletion by diuretic administration and upright posture and a high plasma aldosterone level after volume expansion by salt loading confirms primary hyperaldosteronism in a hypertensive patient without edema.
- Serum HCO_3^- level is elevated with ensuing alkalosis resulting from the loss of hydrogen and potassium in the distal tubules.
- Serum and urine aldosterone levels are increased.
- Plasma volume levels are increased.
- Adrenal angiography or CT scan reveals adrenal tumor.
- Suppression testing reveals decreased plasma aldosterone and urine metabolites (secondary hyperaldosteronism) or normal plasma aldosterone and urine metabolites (primary hyperaldosteronism).
- ECG reveals ST-segment depression and the presence of U waves, indicating hypokalemia.
- CXR shows left ventricular hypertrophy from chronic hypertension.
- CT scan, ultrasonography, or MRI identifies tumor location.

Hyperbilirubinemia

- Patient is jaundiced.
- Serum bilirubin levels are > 10 mg/dl (SI, > 180 μmol/L).

Hyperemesis gravidarum

- History includes uncontrolled nausea and vomiting that persists beyond the first trimester of pregnancy.
- Examination reveals substantial weight loss.
- Serum sodium, chloride, potassium, and protein levels are decreased.
- BUN level is elevated.
- Urinalysis reveals ketonuria and proteinuria.

Hyperlipoproteinemia

- Type I (Fredrickson's hyperlipoproteinemia, fat-induced hyperlipemia, idiopathic familial):
  - Chylomicrons (very-low-density lipoproteins [VLDL], low-density lipoproteins [LDL], high-density lipoproteins [HDL]) are present in plasma 14 hours or more after last meal.
  - Serum chylomicron and triglyceride levels show high elevation; serum cholesterol levels are slightly elevated.
  - Serum lipoprotein lipase levels are decreased.
  - Leukocytosis is present.
- Type II (familial hyperbetalipoproteinemia, essential familial hypercholesterolemia):
  - Plasma concentrations of LDL are increased.
  - Serum LDL and cholesterol levels are elevated.
  - Increased LDL levels are detected by amniocentesis.
- Type III (familial broad-beta disease, xanthoma tuberosum):
  - Serum beta-lipoprotein levels are abnormal.
  - Cholesterol and triglyceride levels are elevated.
  - Glucose levels are slightly elevated.

- Type IV (endogenous hypertriglyceridemia, hyperbetalipoproteinemia):
  - Plasma VLDL levels are elevated.
  - Plasma triglyceride levels are moderately increased.
  - Serum cholesterol levels are normal or slightly elevated.
  - Glucose tolerance is mildly abnormal.
  - History includes early coronary artery disease.
- Type V (mixed hypertriglyceridemia, mixed hyperlipidemia):
  - Chylomicrons are present in plasma.
  - Plasma VLDL levels are elevated.
  - Serum cholesterol and triglyceride levels are elevated.

Hyperparathyroidism

- Serum parathyroid hormone levels are increased.
- Serum calcium levels are increased.
- Urine cyclic adenosine monophosphate test reveals failure to respond to parathyroid hormone.
- X-rays show diffuse demineralization of bones, bone cysts, outer cortical bone absorption, and subperiosteal erosion of the radial aspect of the middle fingers.
- X-ray spectrophotometry demonstrates increased bone turnover.
- Radioimmunoassay shows increased concentration of parathyroid hormone with accompanying hypercalcemia.
- Serum phosphorus levels are increased.
- Serum and urine chloride, uric acid, creatinine, and alkaline phosphatase levels are increased; basal acid secretion is present.
- Serum immunoreactive gastrin levels are increased.

Hyperpituitarism

- Growth hormone (GH) immunoassay shows increased plasma GH levels.
- Glucose suppression test shows failure to suppress GH level to below accepted norm of 5 ng/ml (SI, 5 µg/L).
- Skull X-rays, CT scan, arteriography, and pneumoencephalography reveal the presence and extent of a pituitary lesion.
- Bone X-rays reveal a thickening of the cranium (especially of frontal, occipital, and parietal bones) and of the long bones, as well as osteoarthritis in the spine.

Hypersplenism

- I.V. infusion of chromium-labeled RBCs or platelets reveals high spleen-liver ratio of radioactivity, indicating splenic destruction or sequestration.
- CBC shows decreased Hb levels, WBC count, and platelet count, and elevated reticulocyte count.
- Examination reveals splenomegaly.

Hypertension

- Serial blood pressure measurements on a sphygmomanometer are more than 140/90 mm Hg.
- Urinalysis reveals presence of protein, RBCs, WBCs, or glucose.
- Excretory urography may reveal renal atrophy.
- BUN and serum creatinine levels are normal or elevated, suggesting renal disease.

Hyperthyroidism

- Radioimmunoassay shows increased serum T_4 and T_3 levels.
- Thyroid scan reveals increased uptake of ^{131}I.
- Thyroid-releasing hormone (TRH) stimulation test reveals failure of the TSH level to rise within 30 minutes after administration of TRH.
- Autoantibody tests reveal presence of thyroid-stimulating Ig.

Hypervitaminoses A and D

- History includes accidental or misguided use of supplemental vitamin preparations.
- Serum vitamin A level is > 90 µg/dl (SI, > 2.8 µmol/L) in hypervitaminosis A.
- Serum vitamin D level is > 100 ng/ml (SI, > 250 nmol/L) in hypervitaminosis D.
- Serum carotene level is > 250 µg/dl (SI, > 4.74 µmol/L) in hypercarotenemia.
- X-rays show calcification of tendons, ligaments, and subperiosteal tissues in hypervitaminosis D.

Hypoglycemia

- Blood glucose studies reveal abnormally low levels (< 45 mg/dl [SI, < 2.6 mmol/L]).
- C-peptide assay identifies fasting hypoglycemia.

Hypogonadism

- Serum and urine gonadotropin levels are increased in primary, or hypergonadotropic, hypogonadism and decreased in secondary, or hypogonadotropic, hypogonadism.
- Chromosomal analysis identifies the cause.
- Testicular biopsy and semen analysis reveal impaired spermatogenesis and low testosterone levels.
- X-rays and bone scans show delayed closure of epiphyses and immature bone age.

Hypoparathyroidism

- Radioimmunoassay shows decreased serum parathyroid hormone levels.
- Urine and serum calcium levels are decreased.
- Serum phosphorus levels are increased.
- Urine creatinine levels are decreased.
- X-rays show increased bone density and malformation.
- Cyclic adenosine monophosphate test demonstrates a 10- to 20-fold increase.
- ECG shows increased QT and ST intervals due to hypercalcemia.

Hypopituitarism

- Radioimmunoassay shows decreased plasma levels of some or all pituitary hormones.
- Serum T_4 levels are decreased (with thyroid dysfunction).
- Arginine test reveals failure of hGH levels to rise after arginine infusion (with pituitary dysfunction).
- Insulin tolerance test reveals failure of stimulation or a blunted response of hGH levels (with hypothalamic-pituitary-adrenal axis dysfunction).
- Urine 17-KS levels are decreased (with hypoadrenalism).
- Levels of serum pituitary hormones (FSH, LH, and TSH) are decreased.
- CT scan, pneumoencephalography, or cerebral angiography confirms the presence of tumors inside or outside the sella turcica.

Hypothermic injuries

- History includes severe and prolonged exposure to cold.
- Core body temperature is < 95° F (35° C).
- Physical examination shows burning, tingling, numbness, swelling, pain, and mottled blue-gray skin in exposed areas.

Hypothyroidism in adults

- Radioimmunoassay shows low serum levels of thyroid hormones.
- Serum TSH level may be increased (due to thyroid insufficiency) or decreased (due to hypothalamic or pituitary insufficiency).
- Radioactive iodine uptake test reveals below normal percentages of iodine uptake.

- Radionuclide thyroid imaging reveals "cold spots."
- Thyroid ultrasonography identifies cysts or tumors.
- Serum antithyroid antibodies are elevated (in autoimmune thyroiditis).

Hypothyroidism in children

- Elevated serum TSH levels are associated with low T_3 and T_4 levels.
- Thyroid scan (^{131}I uptake test) shows decreased uptake levels and confirms the absence of thyroid tissue in athyroid children.
- Gonadotropin levels are increased and compatible with sexual precocity in older children.
- Hip, knee, and thigh X-rays reveal absence of the femoral or tibial epiphyseal line and delayed skeletal development that's markedly inappropriate for the child's chronological age.

Hypovolemic shock

- History includes recent loss of blood volume.
- Blood pressure auscultation reveals mean arterial pressure under 60 mm Hg in adults and a narrowing pulse pressure.
- Blood studies show low Hb level and HCT, low RBC count, and low platelet levels.
- Serum potassium, sodium, LD, creatinine, and BUN levels are elevated.
- Urine specific gravity is > 1.020.
- Urine osmolality is elevated.
- Urine creatinine levels are decreased.
- ABG measurements show decreased pH, decreased PaO_2, and increased $PaCO_2$ levels.

Idiopathic hypertrophic subaortic stenosis

- Echocardiography shows increased thickness of the intraventricular septum and abnormal motion of the anterior mitral leaflet during systole, occluding left ventricular outflow in obstructive disease.
- Cardiac catheterization reveals elevated left ventricular end-diastolic pressure and, possibly, mitral insufficiency.
- ECG usually demonstrates left ventricular hypertrophy, T-wave inversion, left anterior hemiblock, Q waves in precordial and inferior leads, ventricular arrhythmias and, possibly, atrial fibrillation.
- Phonocardiography confirms an early systolic murmur.

Idiopathic thrombocytopenic purpura

- Platelet count is markedly decreased.
- Bleeding time is prolonged.
- Bone marrow studies show an abundance of megakaryocytes (platelet precursors) and a shortened circulating platelet survival time.

IgA deficiency

- Serum IgA levels are < 15% of total Ig or < 60 mg/dl (SI, < 0.60 g/L).
- IgA is usually absent from secretions.

Impetigo

- Inspection reveals characteristic lesions.
- Microscopic visualization, Gram stain, or culture of exudate identifies *Staphylococcus aureus* as causative organism.
- WBC count may be elevated.

Inactive colon

- History includes dry, hard, infrequent stools.
- Digital rectal examination reveals stools in the lower portion of the rectum and a palpable colon.
- Proctoscopy reveals unusually small colon lumen, prominent veins, and an abnormal amount of mucus.
- Upper GI series and barium enema rule out tumor.
- Fecal occult blood test is negative.

Inclusion conjunctivitis

- History includes sexual contact with a partner infected with *Chlamydia trachomatis.*
- Examination reveals swollen, reddened lower eyelids, excessive tearing, and a moderately purulent discharge.
- Conjunctival scraping reveals cytoplasmic inclusion bodies in conjunctival epithelial cells and many polymorphonuclear leukocytes; culture for bacteria is negative.

Infantile autism

- History includes symptom development before age 30 months.
- Denver Developmental Screening Test shows delayed development, especially of social and language skills.
- IQ testing indicates retardation.
- Evaluation reveals impairment in social interaction skills, verbal and nonverbal communication, and imaginative activity and a markedly restricted range of activities and interests.

Infectious mononucleosis

- WBC count is elevated during 2nd and 3rd week of illness, with lymphocytes and monocytes making up 50% to 70% of WBCs (10% of lymphocytes are abnormal).
- Heterophil agglutination tests indicate the presence of heterophil antibodies; testing at 3- to 4-week intervals reveals a rise to four times normal levels.
- Indirect immunofluorescence shows antibodies to Epstein-Barr virus and cellular antigens.
- Liver function studies are abnormal.

Infectious myringitis

- Otoscopic examination shows small, reddened, inflamed blebs in the ear canal, on the tympanic membrane, and in the middle ear (with bacterial invasion).
- Culture of exudate identifies infective organism.

Infertility, female

- History includes inability to achieve pregnancy after having regular intercourse, without contraception, for at least 1 year.
- Progesterone blood levels reveal a luteal phase deficiency.
- FSH levels are decreased.
- Hysterosalpingography reveals tubal obstruction or uterine abnormalities.
- Endoscopy shows tubal obstruction or uterine abnormalities.
- Laparoscopy visualizes abdominal and pelvic areas and may reveal peritubular adhesions or ureterotubal obstruction.
- Postcoital (Sims Huhner) test shows inadequate motile sperm cells in cervical fluid after intercourse.
- Immunologic or antibody testing detects spermicidal antibodies in the sera of the female.

Infertility, male

- History includes abnormal sexual development, delayed puberty, or infertility in previous relationships.
- Medical history also includes prolonged fever, mumps, impaired nutritional status, previous surgery, or trauma to genitalia.
- Semen analysis reveals subnormal sperm counts, decreased sperm motility, abnormal morphology, or absence of viable spermatozoa.
- Urine 17-KS levels are decreased.
- Serum testosterone levels are decreased.

Influenza

- Nose and throat culture identifies the causative virus.
- Cold agglutinin titers are elevated.
- Serum antibody titers are increased.

■ WBC count is decreased and lymphocytes are increased (uncomplicated cases).

Inguinal hernia

■ History includes sharp or "catching" pain when lifting or straining, with excessive coughing, or following a recent pregnancy.
■ Examination reveals a swelling or lump in the inguinal area.
■ Palpation of the inguinal area, while the patient is performing Valsalva's maneuver, reveals pressure against the fingertip (indirect hernia) or pressure against the side of the finger (direct hernia).
■ Abdominal X-ray rules out obstruction.
■ WBC count may be elevated.

Insect bites and stings

■ Tick:
– History reveals exposure in woods and fields and complaints of itching.
– After several days, tick paralysis (acute flaccid paralysis, starting as paresthesia and pain in legs and resulting in respiratory failure from bulbar paralysis) occurs.
■ Bee, wasp, or yellow jacket:
– History reveals painful sting.
– Examination reveals protruding stinger (bees), edema, urticaria, or pruritus.
– Systemic reaction (anaphylaxis), indicating hypersensitivity, usually appears within 20 minutes and may include weakness, chest tightness, dizziness, nausea, vomiting, abdominal cramps, and throat constriction.
■ Brown recluse (violin) spider:
– History reveals exposure to dark areas (outdoor privy, barn, woodshed) in south-central United States with reaction within 2 to 8 hours of the bite.
– Examination reveals localized vasoconstriction with ischemic necrosis at bite site and small, reddened puncture wound forming a bleb and becoming ischemic, proceeding to a dark, hard center in 3 to 4 days and an ulcer within 2 to 3 weeks.
– Pain is minimal initially, but increases over time.
– Commonly, fever, chills, malaise, weakness, nausea, vomiting, edema, seizures, joint pains, petechiae, cyanosis, and phlebitis develop.
– Rarely, thrombocytopenia and hemolytic anemia develop and lead to death within 24 to 48 hours (usually in a child or patient with previous history of cardiac disease).
■ Scorpion:
– In nonlethal types, history reveals symptoms lasting from 24 to 78 hours and including local swelling and tenderness, sharp burning sensation, skin discoloration, paresthesia, lymphangitis with regional gland swelling, and anaphylaxis (rare).
– In lethal types, history reveals symptoms including immediate sharp pain, hyperesthesia, drowsiness, itching (nose, throat, mouth), impaired speech, and generalized muscle spasms (including jaw muscle spasms, laryngospasm, incontinence, seizures, nausea, and vomiting).
■ Black widow spider:
– History reveals exposure to dark areas (outdoor privy, barn, woodshed) in southern United States between April and November and report of pinprick sensation followed by dull, numbing pain.
– Examination reveals edema and tiny red bite marks, rigidity of stomach muscles, and severe abdominal pain (10 to 40 minutes after bite).
– Muscle spasms develop in extremities.
– Ascending paralysis occurs, causing difficulty in swallowing and labored, grunting respirations.

– Other symptoms include extreme restlessness, vertigo, sweating, chills, pallor, seizures (especially in children), hyperactive reflexes, hypertension, tachycardia, thready pulse, circulatory collapse, nausea, vomiting, headache, ptosis, eyelid edema, urticaria, pruritus, and fever.

Intestinal obstruction

- History includes progressive, colicky abdominal pain and distention.
- Abdominal X-ray reveals the presence and location of intestinal gas or fluid.
- In X-ray, small-bowel obstruction appears as a typical "stepladder" pattern of alternating gas and fluid levels.
- In X-ray, large-bowel obstruction reveals a distended, air-filled colon or a closed loop of sigmoid with extreme distention.
- Serum sodium, chloride, and potassium levels may decrease because of vomiting.
- WBC count may be normal or slightly elevated if necrosis, peritonitis, or strangulation occurs.
- Serum amylase level may increase.
- Sigmoidoscopy, colonoscopy, or barium enema may help identify the cause of obstruction.

Intussusception

- Barium enema reveals characteristic coiled spring sign and delineates the extent of intussusception.
- Upright abdominal X-rays may show a soft-tissue mass and signs of complete or partial obstruction, with dilated loops of bowel.
- Elevated WBC count may indicate obstruction, strangulation, or bowel infarction.

Iodine deficiency

- Serum T_4 levels are low, with high ^{131}I uptake.
- 24-hour urine collection reveals low iodine levels.
- Serum TSH levels are high.
- Radioiodine uptake test traces ^{131}I in the thyroid 24 hours after administration.

Iron deficiency anemia

- Bone marrow studies reveal depleted or absent iron stores and normoblastic hyperplasia.
- Hb level is decreased.
- HCT is decreased.
- Serum iron levels are low, with high iron binding capacity.
- Serum ferritin levels are low.
- RBC count is low, with microcytic and hypochromic cells.
- GI studies rule out or confirm the bleeding.

Irritable bowel syndrome

- History includes diarrhea alternating with constipation and bowel upset related to diet or psychological stress.
- Sigmoidoscopy may reveal spastic contraction.
- Barium enema may reveal colonic spasm and tubular appearance of descending colon.
- Colonoscopy, rectal examination, or rectal biopsy may rule out other disorders.
- Fecal tests for occult blood, parasites, and pathogenic bacteria are negative.

Junctional tachycardia

ECG findings include:

- Atrial and ventricular rhythms are usually regular. The atrial rhythm may be difficult to determine if the P wave is absent or hidden in the QRS complex or preceding T wave.
- Atrial and ventricular rates exceed 100 beats/minute (usually between 100 and 200 beats/minute). The atrial rate may be difficult to determine if the P wave is absent or hidden in the QRS complex, or precedes the T wave.

■ P wave is usually inverted. It may occur before or after the QRS complex, be hidden in the QRS complex, or be absent.
■ If the P wave precedes the QRS complex, the PR interval is shortened (< 0.12 second). Otherwise, the PR interval can't be measured.
■ Duration of QRS complex is within normal limits. The configuration is usually normal.
■ T-wave configuration is usually normal, but may be abnormal if the P wave is hidden in the T wave. Fast rate may make the T wave indiscernible.
■ QT interval is usually within normal limits.

Juvenile angiofibroma
■ Nasopharyngeal mirror or nasal speculum reveals a blue mass in the nose or nasopharynx.
■ Nasal X-rays reveal a bowing of the posterior wall of the maxillary sinus.
■ Angiography reveals the size and location of the tumor and also shows the source of vascularization.

Keratitis
■ History includes recent infection of the upper respiratory tract accompanied by cold sores.
■ Slit-lamp examination reveals one or more small branchlike (dendritic) lesions (caused by herpes simplex virus).
■ Touching the cornea with cotton reveals reduced corneal sensation.

Kidney cancer
■ Renal ultrasonography and CT scan identify renal tumor.
■ Excretory urography, nephrotomography, and KUB X-ray identify renal tumor.
■ Liver function studies show increased alkaline phosphatase, bilirubin, and transaminase levels.
■ PT is prolonged.
■ Blood studies show anemia, polycythemia, hypercalcemia, and increased ESR.
■ Urinalysis reveals hematuria.
■ Antegrade urography and cytologic studies reveal malignancy.
■ Renal biopsy reveals malignant cells.
■ Radionuclide renal imaging reveals malignant tumor.

Klinefelter syndrome
■ Karyotype obtained by culturing lymphocytes from the patient's peripheral blood shows chromosome abnormality.
■ Testosterone level is depressed after puberty.
■ Urine 17-KS levels are decreased.
■ FSH levels are increased.

Kyphosis
■ History includes severe pain.
■ Examination reveals curvature of the thoracic spine and bone destruction.
■ X-rays reveal vertebral wedging, Schmorl's nodes, irregular plates and, possibly, mild scoliosis of 10 to 20 degrees.

Labyrinthitis
■ History includes nausea and vomiting, hearing loss, and severe vertigo from any movement of the head.
■ Examination reveals spontaneous nystagmus with jerking movements of the eyes toward the unaffected ear.
■ Culture of drainage identifies infective organism.
■ Audiometry reveals sensorineural hearing loss.
■ CT scan rules out brain lesion.

Laryngeal cancer
■ History includes hoarseness that lasts longer than 2 weeks.
■ Laryngoscopy reveals lesion.

- Laryngeal tomography, CT scan, or laryngography defines the borders of a lesion.
- Laryngeal biopsy reveals malignant cells.
- CXR identifies metastasis.

Laryngitis
- History includes hoarseness, ranging from mild to complete loss of voice.
- Indirect laryngoscopy reveals red, inflamed and, occasionally, hemorrhagic vocal cords, with rounded rather than sharp edges, and exudate; bilateral swelling may be present, which restricts movement but doesn't cause paralysis.

Lassa fever
- History includes recent travel to an endemic area.
- Throat washings, pleural fluid, or blood cultures reveal Lassa virus.
- Antibody titer reveals Lassa Ig.

Legg-Calvé-Perthes disease
- Examination reveals restricted abduction and rotation of the hip.
- Hip X-rays (taken every 3 to 4 months) reveal flattening of the femoral head or deformity, new bone formation, and eventually regeneration of the joint.
- Bone scan reveals involvement of anterolateral portion of the femoral head.
- Aspiration and culture of synovial fluid rule out joint sepsis.

Legionnaires' disease
- Cultures of respiratory tract secretions and tissue culture identify *Legionella pneumophila.*
- Direct immunofluorescence testing reveals *L. pneumophila.*
- Indirect fluorescent serum antibody testing shows convalescent serum with a fourfold or greater rise in antibody titer for *L. pneumophila.*
- CXR reveals patchy, localized infiltration, which progresses to multilobar consolidation, pleural effusions and, in fulminant disease, opacification of the entire lung.
- Blood studies show leukocytosis, increased ESR, and increases in alkaline phosphatase, ALT, and AST levels.
- ABG measurements show decreased PaO_2 and, initially, decreased $PaCO_2$.
- Bronchial washings, blood and pleural fluid cultures, and transtracheal aspirate studies rule out pulmonary infections.

Leishmaniasis
- Scrapings from edges of lesion identify species of *Leishmania.*
- *Leishmania* skin test is positive.

Leprosy
- Examination reveals skin lesions and muscular and neurologic deficits.
- Biopsy of skin lesions, peripheral nerves, or smear of skin or ulcerated mucous membranes allows identification of *Mycobacterium leprae.*

Lichen planus
- Examination reveals generalized eruptions of flat, glistening purple papules marked with white lines or spots appearing linearly or coalescing into plaques.
- Skin biopsy reveals lichen planus.

Listeriosis
- Cultures of blood, CSF, cervical or vaginal lesion drainage, or lochia from a mother with an infected fetus reveal *Listeria monocytogenes.*
- CBC reveals monocytosis.

Liver abscess
- Liver scan reveals filling defects at the area of the abscess longer than ¾″ (1.9 cm).

- Hepatic ultrasonography reveals defects caused by abscess.
- CT scan reveals a low-density, homogenous area with well-defined borders.
- CXR reveals the diaphragm on the affected side to be raised and fixed.
- Blood tests show elevated levels of AST, ALT, alkaline phosphatase, and bilirubin.
- Serum albumin is decreased.
- WBC count is elevated.
- Blood cultures and percutaneous liver aspiration identify causative organism.
- Stool cultures and serologic and hemagglutination tests isolate *Entamoeba histolytica* (in amoebic abscesses).

Liver cancer

- Needle biopsy or open biopsy reveals malignant cells.
- AFP levels are elevated in 70% of patients with hepatocellular carcinoma.
- Liver scan shows filling defects.
- Liver function tests are abnormal.
- CXR rule out metastasis to lungs.
- Arteriography may define large tumors.
- Serum electrolyte measurements show increased levels of sodium.
- Serum glucose and cholesterol levels are decreased.

Lower urinary tract infection

- Microscopic urinalysis reveals RBC and WBC counts > 10 per high-power field.
- Clean-catch urinalysis reveals bacterial count of more than 100,000/ml.
- Voiding cystoureterography or excretory urography shows congenital anomalies predisposing the patient to urinary tract infections.

Lung abscess

- Auscultation of the chest may reveal crackles and decreased breath sounds.
- CXR shows a localized infiltrate with one or more clear spaces, usually containing air or fluid.
- Percutaneous aspiration of an abscess or bronchoscopy may be used to obtain cultures to identify the causative organism.
- Blood and sputum cultures and Gram stain identify causative organism.
- WBC count is elevated.

Lung cancer

- CXR reveals lesion or mass.
- Sputum cytology reveals malignant cells.
- Bronchoscopy reveals site of mass.
- Biopsy reveals malignant cells.
- Tissue biopsy reveals evidence of metastasis.

Lupus erythematosus

- Examination reveals classic butterfly rash occurring over the nose and cheeks.
- ANA, anti-DNA, and lupus erythematosus cell tests are positive.
- Urine studies may show RBCs, WBCs, urine casts, sediment, and protein loss.
- CXR reveals pleurisy or lupus pneumonitis.
- Blood studies may show decreased serum complement 3 and complement 4 levels, indicating active disease; ESR is usually elevated; leukopenia, mild thrombocytopenia, and anemia also may be evident.
- ECG may show a conduction defect (with cardiac involvement or pericarditis).
- Renal biopsy identifies progression and extent of renal involvement.

Lyme disease

- History includes recent travel to endemic areas or exposure to ticks.
- Examination reveals the classic skin lesion called *erythema chronicum mi-*

grans, beginning as a red macule or papule at the tick bite site growing in size to as large as 2″ (5 cm), described as hot and pruritic, with bright red outer rims and white centers.

- Mild anemia and elevated ESR, leukocyte count, serum IgM level, and AST level support the diagnosis.
- Antibody titers, ELISA, or blood culture may reveal *Borrelia burgdorferi;* lumbar puncture with CSF analysis allows for identification of antibodies to *B. burgdorferi* (if Lyme disease involves the central nervous system).

Lymphocytopenia

- Lymphocyte count is markedly decreased.
- Bone marrow aspiration and lymph node biopsies identify the cause.

Magnesium imbalance

- Hypomagnesemia:
  - Serum magnesium levels are < 1.5 mEq/L (SI, < 15 mg/L).
  - Serum potassium and calcium levels are decreased.
  - ECG shows tachyarrhythmias, slightly prolonged PR interval, prolonged QT interval, slightly prolonged QRS complex, ST-segment depression, prominent U waves, and broad flattened T waves.
- Hypermagnesemia:
  - Serum magnesium levels are > 2.5 mEq/L (SI, > 25 mg/L).
  - Serum potassium and calcium levels are elevated.
  - ECG shows prolonged PR interval, prolonged QRS complex, and elevated T wave.

Malaria

- History includes travel to an endemic area, recent blood transfusion, or I.V. drug use.
- Blood smears reveal parasites in RBCs.
- Indirect immunofluorescent serum antibody tests reveal malaria (2 weeks after onset).
- CBC shows decreased Hb level and a normal or decreased WBC count.
- Urinalysis reveals protein and WBCs in urine sediment.
- Serum blood studies show a reduced platelet count, prolonged PT, prolonged PTT, and decreased plasma fibrinogen levels (in falciparum malaria).

Malignant brain tumor

- Skull X-ray, brain scan, CT scan, or MRI reveals lesion.
- Biopsy of lesion reveals malignant cells.
- Lumbar puncture shows increased protein levels and decreased glucose levels in CSF; increased CSF pressure, indicating increased intracranial pressure; and, occasionally, tumor cells in CSF.

Malignant lymphoma

- Examination reveals enlarged lymph nodes.
- Biopsy of lymph nodes, tonsils, bone marrow, liver, bowel, or skin reveals malignant cells.
- CXR; lymphangiography; liver, bone, and spleen scans; CT scan of the abdomen; and excretory urography show disease progression.
- Serum uric acid level is normal or elevated.
- Serum calcium level may be elevated, indicating bone lesions.

Malignant melanoma

- Examination reveals skin lesion or nevus with recent changes in appearance.
- Excisional biopsy and full-depth punch biopsy reveal malignant cells.
- Urine test reveals melanin.

Mallory-Weiss syndrome

- History includes recent bout of forceful vomiting followed by vomiting

blood or passing blood rectally (after a few hours to several days).
- Endoscopy identifies esophageal tear.
- Angiography reveals bleeding site.
- Serum HCT is decreased. (Measurements help to quantify blood loss.)

Marfan syndrome
- History includes disease in close relatives.
- Examination reveals skeletal deformities and ectopia lentis.
- X-rays reveal skeletal abnormalities.
- Echocardiography detects aortic root dilation.

Mastitis and breast engorgement
- History includes breast discomfort or other symptoms of inflammation in a lactating woman.
- Examination reveals redness, swelling, warmth, hardness, tenderness, cracks or fissures of the nipple, and enlarged lymph nodes.
- Cultures of expressed milk identify infective organism (generalized mastitis).
- Cultures of breast skin identify infective organism (localized mastitis).

Mastoiditis
- X-rays of the mastoid area reveal hazy mastoid air cells, and the bony walls between the cells appear decalcified.
- Otoscopy reveals a dull, thickened, and edematous tympanic membrane, if the membrane isn't concealed by obstruction.
- Culture and sensitivity tests identify causative organism.
- Audiometry shows a conductive hearing loss.

Medullary cystic disease
- Family history includes medullary cystic disease.
- Arteriography and excretory urography reveal small kidneys.
- Kidney biopsy shows structural abnormalities.
- Blood studies show profound anemia.
- Serum alkaline phosphatase level is elevated (in young patients).

Medullary sponge kidney
- Excretory urography reveals a characteristic flowerlike appearance of the pyramidal cavities when they fill with contrast material.
- Urinalysis is normal, but may show increased WBC count and casts (with infection) or an increased RBC count (with hematuria).

Ménière's disease
- History includes vertigo, tinnitus, and hearing loss or distortion.
- Audiometric studies indicate a sensorineural hearing loss and loss of discrimination and recruitment.
- MRI rules out brain lesions or tumors.
- Auditory brain stem response test rules out cochlear or retrocochlear lesion as the cause of hearing loss.

Meningitis
- Lumbar puncture reveals cloudy CSF, elevated CSF pressure, high protein level, and depressed glucose concentration.
- CSF culture and sensitivity tests reveal gram-positive or gram-negative organisms.
- CXR shows pneumonitis or lung abscess, tubercular lesions, or granulomas (secondary to fungal infection).
- Sinus and skull X-rays may help identify cranial osteomyelitis, paranasal sinusitis, or skull fracture.
- WBC count shows leukocytosis.
- CT scan rules out cerebral hematoma, hemorrhage, or tumor.

- Brudzinski's and Kernig's signs are positive.

Meningococcal infection

- Blood, CSF, or lesion culture reveals *Neisseria meningitidis*.
- Platelet and clotting levels are decreased (with skin or adrenal hemorrhages).

Menopause

- History includes menstrual cycle irregularities.
- Pap test results show changes indicating the influence of estrogen deficiency on vaginal mucosa.
- Radioimmunoassay blood studies show decreased estrogen levels and plasma estradiol level of 0 to 30 pg/ml (SI, 9 to 92 pmol/L).
- Pelvic examination, endometrial biopsy, and D&C rule out suspected organic disease.
- Serum FSH level is 30 to 100 mIU/ml (SI, 30 to 100 IU/L).
- Plasma LH level is 20 to 100 mIU/ml (SI, 20 to 100 IU/ml).

Metabolic acidosis

- ABG analysis reveals:
  - pH < 7.35 (in severe acidosis, pH may fall to 7.10)
  - $PaCO_2$ normal or < 34 mm Hg (SI, < 5.3 kPa)
  - HCO_3^- level may be < 22 mEq/L (SI, < 22 mmol/L).
- Anion gap is > 14 mEq/L (SI, > 14 mmol/L).
- Serum potassium levels are usually elevated.
- Blood glucose and serum ketone body levels are elevated (in diabetes mellitus).
- Plasma lactic acid levels are elevated (in lactic acidosis).

Metabolic alkalosis

- ABG analysis reveals:
  - pH > 7.45
  - $PaCO_2$ may be > 45 mm Hg (SI, > 5.3 kPa) (indicating respiratory compensation)
  - HCO_3^- level > 29 mEq/L (SI, > 29 mmol/L).
- Serum electrolyte levels usually show decreased potassium, calcium, and chloride levels.
- ECG shows a low T wave merging with a P wave and atrial or sinus tachycardia.

Mitral insufficiency

- Cardiac catheterization may indicate signs of mitral insufficiency, including increased left ventricular end-diastolic volume and pressure, increased PAWP and atrial pressure, and decreased cardiac output.
- CXR may demonstrate left atrial and ventricular enlargement, pulmonary venous congestion, and calcification of the mitral leaflets.
- Echocardiography may reveal abnormal motion of the valve leaflets, left atrial enlargement, and a hyperdynamic left ventricle.
- ECG may show left atrial and ventricular hypertrophy, sinus tachycardia, or atrial fibrillation.

Mitral stenosis

- Cardiac catheterization shows a diastolic pressure gradient across the mitral valve and elevated left atrial and pulmonary artery pressures as well as an elevated PAWP. Catheterization may also reveal elevated right ventricular pressure, decreased cardiac output, and abnormal contraction of the left ventricle. Note that this test may not be indicated in patients who have isolated mitral stenosis with mild symptoms.
- CXR shows left atrial and left ventricular enlargement (in severe mitral stenosis), straightening of the left border of the cardiac silhouette, enlarged

pulmonary arteries, dilation of the pulmonary veins of the upper lobes of the lungs, and mitral valve calcification.
- Echocardiography may disclose thickened mitral valve leaflets and left atrial enlargement.
- ECG can reveal atrial fibrillation, right ventricular hypertrophy, left atrial enlargement (in sinus rhythm), and right axis deviation.

Motion sickness
- History includes nausea, vomiting, dizziness, headache, fatigue, diaphoresis, or difficulty breathing related to a sensation of motion.
- If problem is persistent and affects the person's lifestyle, audiometry and vestibular tests may rule out vertigo.

Multiple endocrine neoplasia
- Family history reveals inheritance pattern, confirmed by genetic testing.
- Evaluation of signs and symptoms suggests multiple endocrine neoplasia.
- Diagnostic tests reveal hyperplasia, adenoma, or carcinoma in two or more endocrine glands, confirmed by biopsy.

Multiple myeloma
- CBC shows moderate to severe anemia; differential may show 40% to 50% lymphocytes but seldom more than 3% plasma cells.
- Rouleaux formation is seen on differential smear results.
- Analysis of urine proteins reveals Bence Jones protein, proteinuria, and hypercalciuria.
- Serum calcium levels are elevated.
- Serum electrophoresis shows an elevated globulin spike, which is electrophoretically and immunologically abnormal.
- Excretion tests show phenolsulfonphthalein level > 25% in 15 minutes, > 80% in 2 hours.
- Bone marrow aspiration detects myelomatous cells.
- KUB X-rays reveal bilateral renal enlargement.
- X-rays reveal multiple, sharply circumscribed osteolytic lesions, especially on the skull, pelvis, and spine.

Multiple sclerosis
- History includes multiple neurologic attacks with characteristic remissions and exacerbations.
- EEG results are abnormal.
- CSF analysis reveals elevated gamma globulin fraction of IgG (with normal serum gamma globulin levels).
- MRI reveals multifocal white matter lesions resulting from demyelination.
- Evoked potential studies show slowed conduction of nerve impulses (in 80% of patients).
- CT scan may show lesions within the brain's white matter.

Mumps
- History includes inadequate immunization and exposure to person infected with mumps.
- Examination reveals swelling and tenderness of the parotid glands and one or more of the other salivary glands.
- Antibody titer increases fourfold 3 weeks after acute phase of illness.
- Serum amylase level may be elevated.

Muscular dystrophy
- History includes progressive muscle weakness and evidence of genetic transmission.
- Muscle biopsy reveals fat and connective tissue deposits, degeneration and necrosis of muscle fibers and, in Duchenne's and Becker's dystrophies, a deficiency of the muscle protein dystrophin.
- EMG shows short, weak bursts of electrical activity in affected muscles.

- Genetic testing identifies the gene defect (in some patients).
- Urine creatinine, serum CK, LD, ALT, and AST levels are elevated.

Myasthenia gravis

- History includes progressive muscle weakness and muscle fatigability that improves with rest.
- Tensilon test is positive, showing improved muscle function after an I.V. injection of edrophonium or neostigmine.
- Serum acetylcholine receptor antibodies test is positive in symptomatic adults.
- EMG reveals motor unit potentials that are initially normal but progressively diminish in amplitude with continuing contractions.
- CXR or CT scan may show a thymoma.

Mycosis fungoides

- History includes multiple, varied, and progressively severe skin lesions.
- Biopsy of lesions reveals lymphoma cells.
- Fingerstick smear reveals Sézary cells (abnormal circulating lymphocytes), found in the erythrodermic variants of mycosis fungoides (Sézary syndrome).

Myelitis and acute transverse myelitis

- WBC count is normal or slightly elevated.
- CSF analysis may show normal or increased lymphocyte and protein levels and allows for isolation of the causative agent.
- Throat washings may reveal the causative virus (in poliomyelitis).
- CT scan or MRI may rule out spinal tumor.
- Examination may reveal focal neck and back pain with development of paresthesia and sensory loss.

Myocardial infarction

- History includes substernal chest pain, with radiation.
- Serial 12-lead ECG may be normal or inconclusive during the first hours after a myocardial infarction (MI); may reveal serial ST-segment depression (in subendocardial MI) and ST-segment elevation and Q waves (in transmural MI).
- Cardiac enzyme tests reveal elevated CK levels, with CK-MB isoenzyme >5% of total CK over a 72-hour period.
- Cardiac protein tests reveal elevated troponin T and I levels. Elevations of troponin I are specific for myocardial injury.
- Echocardiography shows ventricular wall dyskinesia (with a transmural MI).
- Radioisotope scans using I.V. technetium 99m pertechnetate show "hot spots," indicating damaged muscle.
- Myocardial perfusion imaging with thallium-210 reveals a "cold spot" in most patients during the first few hours after a transmural MI.

Myocarditis

- History includes recent febrile upper respiratory tract infection, viral pharyngitis, or tonsillitis.
- Cardiac examination reveals supraventricular and ventricular arrhythmias, S_3 and S_4 gallops, a faint S_1, possibly a murmur of mitral insufficiency, and a pericardial friction rub (in patients with pericarditis).
- Endomyocardial biopsy reveals histologic changes consistent with myocarditis.
- Cardiac enzyme levels, including CK, CK-MB, serum AST, and LD, are elevated.
- WBC count and ESR are elevated.
- Antibody titers such as ASO are elevated.

■ ECG shows diffuse ST-segment and T-wave abnormalities, conduction defects, and other ventricular and supraventricular arrhythmias.
■ Cultures of stool, throat, pharyngeal washings, or other body fluids identify the causative bacteria or virus.

Nasal papillomas

■ Examination reveals inverted papillomas as large, bulky, highly vascular, and edematous; color varies from dark red to gray; consistency, from firm to friable.
■ Examination may also reveal exophytic papillomas that are raised, firm, and rubbery; color varies from pink to gray; papillomas are securely attached by a broad or pedunculated base to the mucous membrane.
■ Biopsy reveals histologic findings characteristic of papillomas.

Nasal polyps

■ X-rays of sinuses and nasal passages reveal soft tissue shadows over the affected areas.
■ Examination with a nasal speculum reveals nasal obstruction and a dry, red surface with clear or gray growths; large growths may resemble tumors.

Near-drowning

■ History includes recent water submersion.
■ Auscultation of the lungs reveals rhonchi and crackles.
■ ABG analysis reveals:
–pH < 7.35
–PaO_2 < 75 mm Hg (SI, < 10.03 kPa)
–HCO_3^- level < 22 mEq/L (SI, < 22 mmol/L).
■ ECG may show supraventricular tachycardia, premature ventricular contractions, and nonspecific ST-segment and T-wave abnormalities.

Necrotizing enterocolitis

■ Anteroposterior and lateral abdominal X-rays reveal nonspecific intestinal dilation and, in later stages, gas or air in the intestinal wall.
■ Platelet count is decreased.
■ Serum sodium levels are < 135 mEq/L (SI, < 135 mmol/L).
■ Serum bilirubin levels (indirect, direct, and total) may be elevated.
■ Blood and stool cultures are positive for *Escherichia coli, Clostridia, Salmonella, Pseudomonas,* or *Klebsiella.*
■ Hb level is decreased.
■ PT and PTT are prolonged.
■ Fibrin degradation products are increased.
■ Guaiac test detects occult blood in stool.

Nephrotic syndrome

■ Urinalysis shows marked proteinuria and reveals increased number of hyaline, granular, and waxy, fatty casts and oval fat bodies.
■ Renal biopsy provides histologic identification of the lesion.
■ T_3 resin uptake percentage is high with a low or normal free T_4 level.
■ Serum protein electrophoresis reveals decreased albumin and gamma globulin levels and markedly increased $alpha_2$ and beta globulin levels.
■ Serum triglyceride, phospholipid, and cholesterol levels are elevated.

Neurofibromatosis

■ Examination reveals café-au-lait spots and multiple pedunculated nodules (neurofibromas) of varying sizes on the nerve trunks of the extremities and on the nerves of the head, neck, and body.
■ X-rays and CT scan reveal widening internal auditory meatus and intervertebral foramen.
■ Myelography reveals spinal cord tumors.

- Lumbar puncture with CSF analysis reveals elevated protein concentration.

Neurogenic arthropathy

- History includes painless joint deformity.
- X-rays reveal soft-tissue swelling or effusion (early stage), articular fracture, subluxation, erosion of articular cartilage, periosteal new bone formation, and excessive growth of marginal new bodies or resorption.
- Vertebral examination reveals narrowing of vertebral disk spaces, deterioration of vertebrae, and osteophyte formation.
- Synovial biopsy reveals bony fragments and bits of calcified cartilage.

Neurogenic bladder

- History includes neurologic disease or spinal cord injury.
- CSF analysis shows increased protein level indicating cord tumor; increased gamma globulin level may indicate multiple sclerosis.
- X-rays of the skull and vertebral column show fracture, dislocation, congenital anomalies, or metastasis.
- Myelography shows spinal cord compression.
- EMG confirms presence of peripheral neuropathy.
- Cystometry reveals abnormal micturition and vesical function.
- External sphincter EMG reveals detrusor-external sphincter dyssynergia.
- Voiding cystourethrography reveals neurogenic bladder.
- Whitaker test reveals bladder abnormality.

Nezelof syndrome

- History includes failure to thrive, poor eating habits, weight loss, and recurrent infections in children.
- Family history may reveal genetic transmission.
- T-lymphocyte assay reveals defective T cells that are moderately to markedly decreased in number.

Nocardiosis

- History reveals progressive pneumonia despite antibiotic therapy.
- Culture of sputum or discharge identifies *Nocardia.*
- Biopsy of lung or other tissue identifies *Nocardia.*
- CXR shows fluffy or interstitial infiltrates, nodules, or abscesses.

Nonspecific genitourinary infections

- History includes sexual contact with a partner with a nonspecific genitourinary infection.
- Cultures of prostatic, cervical, or urethral secretions reveal excessive polymorphonuclear leukocytes but few, if any, specific organisms.

Nonviral hepatitis

- History includes exposure to hepatotoxic chemicals or drugs.
- Serum ALT levels are > 56 U/L (SI, > 0.96 μkat/L).
- Serum AST levels are > 40 U/L (SI, > 0.68 μkat/L).
- Serum total and direct bilirubin levels are elevated (with cholestasis).
- Serum alkaline phosphatase levels are elevated.
- Differential WBC count reveals elevated eosinophils.

Nystagmus

- Inspection reveals involuntary eye movement.
- Positional testing causes nystagmus to occur.
- Electronystagmography reveals nystagmus.
- Vestibular acuity tests may rule out a vestibular lesion as the cause.

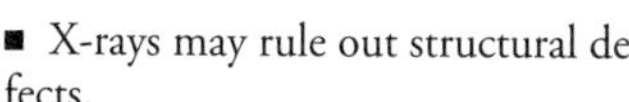

■ X-rays may rule out structural defects.

Obesity

■ Observation and comparison of height and weight to a standardized table reveals weight exceeding ideal body weight by 20% or more. In morbid obesity, body weight $> 200\%$ of standard range.

■ Measurement of the thickness of subcutaneous fat folds with calipers reveals excess body fat.

Optic atrophy

■ Slit-lamp examination reveals a pupil that reacts sluggishly to direct light stimulation.

■ Ophthalmoscopy shows pallor of the nerve head from loss of microvascular circulation in the disk and deposit of fibrous or glial tissue.

■ Visual field testing reveals a scotoma and, possibly, major visual field impairment.

Orbital cellulitis

■ Examination reveals eyelid edema and purulent discharge.

■ Culture of eye discharge identifies *Streptococcus, Staphylococcus,* or *Pneumococcus* as the causative organism.

Ornithosis

■ History includes recent exposure to birds.

■ *Chlamydia psittaci* is recovered from mice, eggs, or tissue culture inoculated with the patient's blood or sputum.

■ Comparison of acute and convalescent sera shows a fourfold rise in antibody titers during convalescent phase.

■ CXR reveals patchy lobar infiltrate.

Osgood-Schlatter disease

■ Examination reveals pain during internal rotation of the tibia while extending the knee from 90 degrees flexion, which subsides immediately with external rotation of the tibia.

■ X-rays may reveal epiphyseal separation and soft tissue swelling (up to 6 months after onset) and eventual bone fragmentation.

Osteoarthritis

■ History includes deep, aching joint pain, particularly after exercise or weight bearing, usually relieved by rest; and morning stiffness that lasts < 30 minutes.

■ Examination may reveal nodes in the distal and proximal joints that become red, swollen, and tender.

■ X-rays reveal narrowing of the joint space or margin, cystlike bony deposits in joint space and margins, sclerosis of the subchondral space, joint deformity due to degeneration or articular damage, bony growths at weight-bearing areas, and fusion of joints.

Osteogenesis imperfecta

■ Examination reveals blue sclera and deafness.

■ X-rays reveal multiple old fractures and skeletal deformities.

■ Skull X-ray shows wide sutures with small, irregularly shaped islands of bone (wormian bones).

Osteomyelitis

■ History includes sudden pain in the affected bone accompanied by tenderness, heat, swelling, and restricted movement.

■ Blood cultures identify *Staphylococcus aureus, Streptococcus pyogenes, Pneumococcus, Pseudomonas aeruginosa, Escherichia coli,* or *Proteus vulgaris* as the causative organism.

■ Bone scan shows infection site in early stages of illness.

■ X-ray reveals abnormal areas of calcification (may not be evident until 2 to 3 weeks).

- ESR is elevated (> 20 mm/hour; SI, > 20 mm/hour).
- WBC count reveals leukocytosis.

Osteoporosis

- X-rays may reveal typical degeneration in the lower thoracic and lumbar vertebrae; vertebral bodies may appear flattened and more dense than normal.
- Photon absorptiometry reveals deterioration of bone mass.
- Bone biopsy reveals thin, porous, but otherwise normal-looking bone.
- Bone densitometry reveals decreased bone density.

Otitis externa

- Examination reveals pain on palpation of the tragus or auricle.
- Otoscopy reveals a swollen external ear canal (sometimes to the point of complete closure), periauricular lymphadenopathy (tender nodes in front of the tragus, behind the ear, or in the upper neck) and, occasionally, regional cellulitis.
- In fungal otitis externa, examination reveals thick, red epithelium after removal of growth.
- Microscopic examination or culture and sensitivity tests identify *Aspergillus niger* or *Candida albicans* as the causative organism for fungal otitis externa; *Pseudomonas, Proteus vulgaris, Streptococcus,* or *Staphylococcus aureus* as the causative organism for bacterial otitis externa.
- In chronic otitis externa, examination of the ear canal reveals a thick red epithelium.

Otitis media

- In acute suppurative otitis media:
  – Otoscopy reveals obscured or distorted bony landmarks of the tympanic membrane.
  – Pneumatoscopy may show decreased tympanic membrane mobility.
  – Examination shows that pulling on the auricle doesn't exacerbate the pain.
- In acute secretory otitis media:
  – Otoscopy demonstrates tympanic membrane retraction, causing the bony landmarks to appear more prominent, with clear or amber fluid detected behind the tympanic membrane, possibly with a meniscus and bubbles.
  – If hemorrhage into the middle ear has occurred, the tympanic membrane appears blue-black.
- In chronic otitis media:
  – History discloses recurrent or unresolved otitis media; otoscopy shows thickening, and sometimes scarring, and decreased mobility of the tympanic membrane.
  – Pneumatoscopy reveals decreased or absent tympanic membrane movement.
- History of recent air travel or scuba diving suggests barotitis media.

Otosclerosis

- Rinne test reveals bone conduction lasting longer than air conduction (normally, the reverse is true); as otosclerosis progresses, bone conduction deteriorates.
- Audiometric testing reveals hearing loss ranging from 60 dB in early stages to total loss as the disease advances.
- Weber's test reveals sound lateralizing to the more affected ear.

Ovarian cancer

- Examination reveals abdominal mass.
- CT scan shows the abdominal tumor.
- Pelvic ultrasonography reveals mass.
- Exploratory laparotomy with biopsy reveals malignant cells.
- Transvaginal ultrasonography shows ovarian enlargement and growth.
- Transvaginal Doppler color flow imaging reveals ovarian growth.

- CEA levels are > 20 ng/ml (SI, > 20 µg/L).
- Serum hCG levels are elevated in a nonpregnant woman.
- Barium enema reveals obstruction and size of tumor.

Ovarian cysts

- Pelvic ultrasonography reveals ovarian mass.
- Laparoscopy reveals a bubble on the surface of the ovary, which may be clear, serous, or mucus-filled.
- hCG titers are highly elevated (with theca-lutein cysts).
- Progesterone levels are elevated.

Paget's disease

- X-rays reveal increased bone expansion and density (before overt symptoms appear).
- Bone scan reveals radioisotope concentrates in areas of active lesions (early pagetic lesions).
- Bone biopsy reveals characteristic mosaic pattern.
- Serum alkaline phosphatase level is highly elevated.
- Urine hydroxyproline levels are increased.

Pancreatic cancer

- Ultrasonography, CT scan, or MRI reveals mass size and locations.
- Laparotomy and biopsy reveal malignant cells.
- Barium swallow shows neoplasm or changes in the duodenum or stomach indicating carcinoma of the head of the pancreas.
- Endoscopic retrograde cholangiopancreatography shows mass and abnormalities of the pancreatic ducts.
- Cholangiography shows obstructed bile ducts caused by carcinoma of the pancreas.
- Secretin test reveals an abnormal volume of secretions, HCO_3^-, or enzymes.
- Serum alkaline phosphatase and serum bilirubin levels are markedly elevated with biliary obstruction.
- Plasma insulin immunoassay reveals measurable serum insulin (with islet cell tumors).
- Stool guaiac testing shows presence of occult blood, suggesting ulceration in GI tract or ampulla of Vater.

Parainfluenza

- History includes symptoms of respiratory illness.
- Serum antibody titers differentiate parainfluenza from other respiratory illnesses.
- Blood culture reveals virus (rarely done).

Parkinson's disease

- History and examination reveal muscle rigidity, akinesia, and pill-roll tremors increasing during stress or anxiety.
- Urinalysis reveals decreased dopamine levels.
- Evoked potential studies reveal bilateral abnormal P100 latencies.

Pediculosis

- In pediculosis capitis, examination reveals oval, grayish nits that can't be shaken loose.
- In pediculosis corporis, examination reveals characteristic skin lesions and nits found on clothing.
- In pediculosis pubis, examination reveals nits attached to pubic hairs, which feel coarse and grainy to the touch.

Pelvic inflammatory disease

- History includes recent sexual intercourse, intrauterine device insertion, childbirth, or abortion.
- Cultures and Gram stain of secretions from the endocervix or cul-de-sac identify *Neisseria gonorrhoeae* or

Chlamydia trachomatis as the infective organism.
- Ultrasonography reveals an adnexal or uterine mass.
- Laparoscopy reveals infection or abscess.

Penetrating chest wounds
- Examination reveals chest wound and a sucking sound during breathing.
- Hb level and HCT are markedly decreased, indicating severe blood loss.
- CXR reveals pneumothorax and possible lung laceration.

Penile cancer
- Tissue biopsy reveals malignant cells.
- Examination reveals small circumscribed lesion, pimple, or sore on the penis, which may be accompanied by pain, hemorrhage, dysuria, purulent discharge, and urinary meatal obstruction (in late stages).

Peptic ulcers
- History includes heartburn, midepigastric pain, or gastric bleeding.
- Endoscopy reveals ulcer.
- Upper GI X-rays show abnormalities in the mucosa.
- Gastric secretory studies show hyperchlorhydria.
- Biopsy rules out malignancy.
- Stool guaiac testing reveals presence of occult blood.

Perforated eardrum
- History includes trauma to the ear accompanied by severe earache and bleeding from the ear.
- Direct visual inspection of the tympanic membrane with an otoscope confirms perforation; flaccid, thin areas indicate previous perforation.
- Audiometric testing reveals hearing loss.

Pericarditis
- Chest auscultation reveals pericardial friction rub.
- Pericardial fluid culture identifies infecting organism (in bacterial or fungal pericarditis).
- ECG reveals ST-segment elevation in the standard limb leads and most precordial leads without the significant changes in QRS morphology that occur with myocardial infarction.
- ECG may also reveal atrial ectopic rhythms and diminished QRS voltage (with pericardial effusion).
- Echocardiography reveals an echofree space between the ventricular wall and the pericardium (with pericardial effusion).

Peritonitis
- Examination reveals severe abdominal pain with direct or rebound tenderness.
- Abdominal X-rays reveal edematous and gaseous distention of the small and large bowel, or air in the abdominal cavity (with perforation of a visceral organ).
- Paracentesis reveals bacteria in fluid, exudate, pus, blood, or urine.
- CXR may show elevation of the diaphragm.
- Elevated WBC count indicates leukocytosis.

Pernicious anemia
- Hb level is markedly decreased.
- RBC count is decreased.
- Mean corpuscular volume is increased.
- Serum vitamin B_{12} assay reveals levels < 190 pg/ml (SI, < 162 pmol/L).
- Schilling test reveals < 3% excretion of radioactive B_{12} in urine in 24 hours.
- Bone marrow aspiration reveals erythroid hyperplasia with increased numbers of megaloblasts but few normally developing RBCs.

- Gastric analysis reveals absence of free hydrochloric acid after histamine or pentagastrin injection.

Pharyngitis

- Examination reveals generalized redness and inflammation of the posterior wall of the pharynx and red, edematous mucous membranes studded with white or yellow follicles.
- Exudate is usually confined to the lymphoid areas of the throat, sparing the tonsillar pillars.
- Throat culture identifies the infective organism, most commonly *Streptococcus.*

Phenylketonuria

- Family history indicates presence of autosomal recessive gene.
- Guthrie screening test reveals elevated serum phenylalanine levels.
- Drops of 10% ferric chloride solution added to a wet diaper turns a deep, bluish-green color, indicating phenylpyruvic acid in the urine.
- Low serum tyrosine level in neonates age 1 week or less.
- Urine testing reveals presence of phenylpyruvic acid.

Pheochromocytoma

- History includes acute episodes of hypertension, headache, sweating, and tachycardia, particularly in a patient with hyperglycemia, glycosuria, and hypermetabolism.
- 24-hour urine test reveals increased excretion of total free catecholamine and its metabolites, vanillylmandelic acid, and metanephrine.
- Total plasma catecholamines may show levels 10 to 50 times higher than normal.
- Angiography reveals an adrenal medullary tumor.
- Excretory urography with nephrotomography, adrenal venography, or CT scan helps localize a tumor.

Phosphate imbalance

- Hypophosphatemia: Serum phosphate level is $<$ 2.7 mg/dl (SI, $<$ 0.87 mmol/L) in adults and $<$ 4.5 mg/dl (SI, $<$ 1.45 mmol/L) in children.
- Hyperphosphatemia: Serum phosphate level is $>$ 4.5 mg/dl (SI, $>$ 1.45 mmol/L) in adults and $>$ 6.7 mg/dl (SI, $>$ 1.78 mmol/L) in children.

Photosensitivity reactions

- History includes recent exposure to light or certain chemicals.
- Examination reveals erythema, edema, desquamation, and hyperpigmentation (characteristic skin eruptions).
- Photopatch test for ultraviolet A and B may identify the causative light wavelength.

Pilonidal disease

- Examination reveals a series of openings along the midline of the intergluteal fold with thin, brown, foul-smelling drainage or a protruding tuft of hair; pressure on the sinus tract produces purulent drainage.
- Culture of discharge from the infected sinus reveals staphylococci or skin bacteria (usually not bowel bacteria).

Pituitary tumors

- Skull X-rays with tomography reveal enlargement of the sella turcica or erosion of its floor and enlargement of the paranasal sinuses and mandible, thickened cranial bones, and separated teeth (if growth hormone predominates).
- Carotid angiography reveals displacement of the anterior cerebral and internal carotid arteries (with enlarging tumor mass).
- Intracranial CT scan may confirm the existence of the adenoma and accurately depict its size.
- Orbital radiography shows superior orbital fissure enlargement.

- MRI of the brain differentiates healthy, benign, and malignant tissues and blood vessels.
- Tangent screen examination reveals bitemporal hemianopia.
- Urine free cortisol levels are > 108 μg/24 hours (SI, > 276 mmol/ 24 hours).
- HGH levels are > 5 ng/ml (SI, > 5 μg/L) in men, > 10 ng/ml (SI, > 10 μg/L) in women.
- Urine 17-hydroxycorticosteroid levels are > 10 mg/24 hours (SI, > 27.6 μmol/ 24 hours as cortisol) in men, > 6 mg/ 24 hours (SI, > 16.5 μmol/24 hours as cortisol) in women, and > 5 mg/ 24 hours (SI, > 13.8 μmol/24 hours as cortisol) in children.

Pityriasis rosea

- Examination reveals slightly raised oval lesion, approximately 2 to 6 cm in diameter, changing to yellow-tan or erythematous patches with scaly edges approximately 0.5 to 1 cm in diameter on the trunk and extremities.

Placenta previa

- History includes painless bleeding during third trimester of pregnancy.
- Pelvic ultrasonography reveals abnormal echo patterns.
- Pelvic examination (performed only immediately before delivery) reveals only cervix and minimal descent of fetal presenting part.

Plague

- History includes exposure to rodents (bubonic plague).
- Culture of skin lesion reveals *Yersinia pestis.*
- WBC count is elevated; WBC differential reveals increased polymorphonuclear leukocytes.
- CXR reveals fulminating pneumonia (with pneumonic plague).

Platelet function disorders

- History includes excessive bleeding or bruising.
- Bleeding time is prolonged.
- PT and PTT are normal.
- Platelet count is normal.
- Platelet function tests measure platelet release reaction and aggregation to identify defective mechanism.

Pleural effusion and empyema

- CXR reveals radiopaque fluid in dependent regions.
- Lung auscultation reveals decreased breath sounds.
- Percussion detects dullness over the effused area, which doesn't change with respiration.
- Pleural fluid analysis reveals:
  – transudative effusions with decreased specific gravity
  – empyema with acute inflammatory WBCs and microorganisms
  – empyema or rheumatoid arthritis with extremely decreased pleural fluid glucose levels.

Pleurisy

- Auscultation of the chest reveals characteristic pleural friction rub — a coarse, creaky sound heard during late inspiration and early expiration, directly over the area of pleural inflammation.
- Palpation may reveal coarse vibration.

Pneumocystis carinii pneumonia

- History includes an immunocompromising condition (such as HIV infection, leukemia, and lymphoma) or procedure (such as organ transplantation).
- Histologic studies of sputum specimen confirm presence of *P. carinii.*

- CXR shows slowly progressing, fluffy infiltrates and occasional nodular lesions or a spontaneous pneumothorax.
- Gallium scan of the chest shows increased uptake over the lungs even if the CXR appears relatively normal.

Pneumonia

- Percussion reveals dullness; auscultation discloses crackles, wheezing, or rhonchi over the affected lung area as well as decreased breath sounds and decreased vocal fremitus.
- CXR discloses infiltrates, confirming the diagnosis.
- Gram stain and culture of sputum show acute inflammatory cells.
- WBC count indicates leukocytosis in bacterial pneumonia and a normal or low count in viral or mycoplasmal pneumonia.
- Blood cultures reflect bacteremia and help determine the causative organism.

Pneumothorax

- History includes sudden, sharp pain and shortness of breath.
- CXR reveals air in the pleural space and, possibly, mediastinal shift.
- Examination reveals overexpansion and rigidity of the affected chest side; in tension pneumothorax, examination may reveal neck vein distention.
- Palpation of chest reveals crackling beneath the skin and decreased vocal fremitus.
- Chest auscultation reveals decreased or absent breath sounds on the affected side.
- ABG measurements reveal pH <7.35, $PaO_2 < 80$ mm Hg (SI, 10.6 kPa), and $PaCO_2 > 45$ mm Hg (SI, 5.3 kPa).

Poisoning

- History includes ingestion, inhalation, injection of, or skin contact with a poisonous substance.
- Toxicologic studies (including drug screens) reveal poison in the mouth, vomitus, urine, stool, or blood or on the victim's hands or clothing.
- CXR (with inhalation poisoning) reveals pulmonary infiltrates or edema, or aspiration pneumonia (with petroleum distillate inhalation).

Poliomyelitis

- Throat culture or stool examination reveals poliovirus.
- Convalescent serum antibody titers rise fourfold from acute titers.
- CSF pressure and protein levels may be slightly increased.
- WBC count may be elevated initially, mostly due to polymorphonuclear leukocytes, which constitute 50% to 90% of the total count; thereafter, the number of cells is diminished with mononuclear leukocytes accounting for most of them.

Polycystic kidney disease

- Family history includes polycystic kidney disease.
- Physical examination reveals large bilateral, irregular masses in the flanks.
- Excretory or retrograde urography reveals enlarged kidneys, with elongation of pelvis, flattening of the calyces, and indentations caused by cysts.
- Excretory urography of the neonate shows poor excretion of contrast agent.
- Ultrasonography, CT scan, and radioisotope scans of the kidney show kidney enlargement and presence of cysts. CT scan also demonstrates multiple areas of cystic damage.

Polycythemia, secondary

- RBC mass is increased.
- Hb level, HCT, mean corpuscular volume, and mean corpuscular Hb level are increased.
- Urine erythropoietin and blood histamine levels are elevated.

- Arterial oxygen saturation may be decreased.
- Bone marrow biopsies reveal hyperplasia confined to the erythroid series.

Polycythemia, spurious

- Hb level, HCT, and RBC count are elevated.
- RBC mass is normal.
- WBC count is normal.

Polycythemia vera

- Laboratory studies confirm polycythemia vera by showing increased RBC mass and normal arterial oxygen saturation in association with splenomegaly or two of the following:
  – elevated platelet count
  – elevated WBC count
  – elevated leukocyte alkaline phosphatase level
  – elevated serum B_{12} elevation or unbound B_{12}-binding capacity.
- Bone marrow biopsy reveals panmyelosis.
- Serum and urine uric acid levels are increased.

Polymyositis and dermatomyositis

- Muscle biopsy reveals necrosis, degeneration, regeneration, and interstitial chronic lymphocytic infiltration.
- Muscle enzyme levels (CK, aldolase, AST) are elevated and not attributable to hemolysis of RBCs or hepatic or other diseases.
- Urine creatine level is markedly increased.
- EMG reveals polyphasic short-duration potentials, fibrillation, and bizarre high-frequency repetitive changes.
- ANA test is positive.

Porphyrias

- Screening tests reveal porphyrins or their precursors (such as aminolevulinic acid and porphobilinogen) in urine, stool, blood, or skin biopsy.
- Urinary lead level is > 400 mg/ 24-hour collection.

Potassium imbalance

- Hypokalemia:
  – Serum potassium levels are < 3.5 mEq/L (SI, < 3.5 mmol/L).
  – ECG shows flattened T waves, elevated U waves, and depressed ST segment.
- Hyperkalemia:
  – Serum potassium levels are > 5 mEq/L (SI, > 5 mmol/L).
  – ECG shows tall, tented T waves; widened QRS complex; prolonged PR interval; flattened or absent P waves; and depressed ST segment.

Precocious puberty in females

- X-rays of hands, wrists, knees, and hips reveal advanced bone age and possible premature epiphyseal closure.
- Androstenedione level is > 3 ng/ml.
- Radioimmunoassays for estrogen levels and FSH levels are abnormally high for age.
- Vaginal smear for estrogen secretion reveals abnormally high levels.
- Urinary test for gonadotropic activity and excretion of 17-KS show abnormally high levels.

Precocious puberty in males

- Detailed patient history reveals recent growth pattern, behavior changes, family history of precocious puberty, or hormonal ingestion.
- In true precocious puberty:
  – Serum levels of LH, FSH, and corticotropin are elevated.
  – Plasma tests for testosterone demonstrate elevated levels (equal to those of an adult male).
  – Evaluation of ejaculate indicates true precocity by revealing presence of live spermatozoa.

– Skull and hand X-rays reveal advanced bone age.
- In pseudoprecocious puberty:
– Chromosome analysis may demonstrate an abnormal pattern of autosomes and sex chromosomes.
– Steroid excretion levels, such as testosterone and 24-hour 17-KS levels, are elevated.

Pregnancy

- Serum hCG level is elevated.
- Urine hCG level is elevated.
- Pelvic examination reveals changes to uterus consistent with pregnancy.
- Ultrasonography reveals presence of fetus in the uterus.

Pregnancy-induced hypertension

- Mild preeclampsia:
– Systolic blood pressure is 140 mm Hg or shows a rise of 30 mm Hg or more above the patient's normal systolic pressure (measured on two occasions, 6 hours apart).
– Diastolic blood pressure is 90 mm Hg or shows a rise of 15 mm Hg or more above the patient's normal diastolic pressure (measured on two occasions, 6 hours apart).
– Proteinuria (urine protein level is > 500 mg/24 hours).
- Severe preeclampsia:
– Blood pressure measurements are 160/110 mm Hg or higher (measured on two occasions, 6 hours apart) on bed rest.
– Proteinuria is increased (urine protein level ≥ 5 g/24 hours).
– Patient has oliguria (urine output ≤ 400 ml/24 hours).
– Deep tendon reflexes are hyperactive.
- Eclampsia:
– History and examination reveal signs of severe preeclampsia and seizure activity.
– Ophthalmoscopic examination may reveal vascular spasm, papilledema, retinal edema or detachment, and arteriovenous nicking or hemorrhage.

Premature labor

- Physical examination reveals rhythmic uterine contractions, cervical dilation and effacement, possible rupture of membranes, expulsion of cervical mucus plug, and bloody discharge occurring before expected date of delivery.
- Vaginal examination reveals progressive cervical effacement and dilation.
- Pelvic ultrasonography identifies fetus' position in the mother's pelvis.

Premature rupture of the membranes

- History includes passage of amniotic fluid before the expected date of delivery.
- Examination reveals amniotic fluid in the vagina.
- Nitrazine paper test of fluid from posterior fornix turns deep blue.
- Fluid from posterior fornix smeared on slide and allowed to dry takes on a fernlike pattern.

Premenstrual syndrome

- History includes menstruation-related symptoms, including mild to severe personality changes, nervousness, irritability, fatigue, lethargy, depression, breast tenderness or bloating, joint pain, headache, diarrhea, and exacerbations of skin, respiratory, or neurologic problems recorded for 2 to 3 months.
- Serum estrogen and progesterone levels are normal (ruling out hormonal imbalance).

Pressure ulcers

- History includes immobility, malnutrition, or skin irritation.
- Inspection reveals skin breakdown.

- Wound culture and sensitivity identify the infecting organisms.

Proctitis

- In acute proctitis, sigmoidoscopy reveals edematous, bright-red or pink rectal mucosa that's thick, shiny, friable, and possibly ulcerated.
- In chronic proctitis, sigmoidoscopy reveals thickened mucosa, loss of vascular pattern, and stricture of the rectal lumen.
- Biopsy reveals absence of malignant cells.

Progressive systemic sclerosis

- History includes Raynaud's phenomenon.
- ANA test is positive, revealing low titer and speckled pattern.
- Hand X-rays reveal terminal phalangeal tuft resorption, subcutaneous calcification, and joint space narrowing and erosion.
- CXR shows bilateral basilar pulmonary fibrosis.
- RF is positive in approximately one third of patients.
- ESR is elevated.
- Urinalysis reveals proteinuria, microscopic hematuria, and casts (with renal involvement).

Prostatic cancer

- Digital rectal examination reveals small, hard nodule in prostate area.
- Serum prostate-specific antigen levels are elevated.
- Serum prostatic acid phosphatase is > 3.7 ng/ml (SI, > 3.7 μg/L).
- Serum alkaline phosphatase level is elevated.
- Biopsy reveals malignant cells.

Prostatitis

- Examination reveals tender, indurated, swollen, and warm prostate.
- Urine samples, taken at start of voiding, midstream, after a physician massages the prostate, and final specimen, reveal a significant increase in colony count of the prostatic specimens.

Protein-calorie malnutrition

- History includes poor diet lacking in protein.
- Examination reveals a small, gaunt, and emaciated appearance with no adipose tissue; dry and "baggy" skin; general weakness; sparse hair and dull brown or reddish yellow eyes; and slow pulse rate and respirations.
- Anthropometry reveals height and weight < 80% of standard for the patient's age and sex, and below standard arm circumference and triceps skinfolds.
- Serum albumin and pre-albumin levels are markedly decreased.

Pruritus ani

- History includes perianal itching, irritation, or superficial burning.
- Rectal examination identifies no fissures or fistulas.
- Biopsy rules out carcinoma.

Pseudomembranous enterocolitis

- History includes sudden onset of copious, watery or bloody diarrhea; abdominal pain; and fever.
- Rectal biopsy reveals characteristic histologic changes, such as plaquelike lesions on the colonic mucosal surface consisting of fibrinopurulent exudate and necrotic epithelial debris.
- Stool cultures identify *Clostridium difficile*.

Pseudomonas infections

- Culture of blood, spinal fluid, urine, exudate, or sputum identifies the *Pseudomonas* organism.

■ Gram stain reveals gram-negative bacillus.

Psoriasis

■ Examination reveals dry, cracked, encrusted lesions (erythematous plaques) accompanied by itching on the scalp, chest, elbows, knees, back, or buttocks.
■ Skin biopsy reveals psoriasis.
■ Serum uric acid level is elevated, without indications of gout.

Psoriatic arthritis

■ Examination reveals psoriatic lesions.
■ X-rays reveal erosion of terminal phalangeal tufts, "whittling" of the distal end of the terminal phalanges, "pencil-in-cup"' deformity of the distal interphalangeal joints, sacroiliitis, and atypical spondylitis with syndesmophyte formation, resulting in hyperostosis and vertebral ossification.
■ Rheumatoid screening test is nonreactive.
■ ESR is elevated.
■ Serum uric acid levels are increased.

Ptosis

■ Examination reveals drooping of the upper eyelid.
■ Measurement of palpebral fissure widths, range of lid movement, and relation of lid margin to upper border of the cornea reveal the severity of illness.

Puerperal infection

■ History includes fever within 48 hours after delivery or abortion.
■ Culture of lochia, blood, incisional exudate (from cesarean incision or episiotomy), uterine tissue, or material collected from the vaginal cuff reveals *Streptococcus,* coagulase-negative staphylococci, *Clostridium perfringens, Bacteroides fragilis,* or *Escherichia coli* as the causative organism.
■ Elevated WBC count shows leukocytosis and an increased sedimentation rate.
■ Pelvic examination reveals induration without purulent discharge (parametritis).
■ Culdoscopy shows adnexal induration and thickening.

Pulmonary edema

■ Examination reveals respiratory distress.
■ Chest auscultation reveals crackles in the lung fields.
■ ABG analysis usually shows decreased PaO_2 (hypoxia) and variable $PaCO_2$. Profound respiratory alkalosis and acidosis may occur; metabolic acidosis occurs when cardiac output is low.
■ CXR shows diffuse haziness of the lung fields and, often, cardiomegaly and pleural effusions.
■ Pulmonary artery catheterization reveals elevated pulmonary wedge pressures.

Pulmonary embolism and infarction

■ Lung scan reveals perfusion defects in areas beyond occluded vessels.
■ Pulmonary angiography reveals emboli.
■ CXR shows areas of atelectasis, elevated diaphragm and pleural effusion, prominent pulmonary artery and, occasionally, a wedge-shaped infiltrate suggesting pulmonary infarction.
■ ECG may show right axis deviation; right bundle-branch block; tall, peaked P waves; ST-segment depression; T-wave inversion; and supraventricular tachycardia.
■ Auscultation reveals right ventricular gallop, increased intensity of the pulmonic component of S_2, crackles, and pleural rub at the site of the embolism.
■ ABG analysis may show decreased PaO_2 and $PaCO_2$ levels.

Pulmonary hypertension

- Pulmonary artery catheterization reveals elevated pulmonary systolic pressure and PAWP.
- Pulmonary angiography reveals filling defects in pulmonary vasculature.
- PFTs may show decreased flow rates and increased residual volume (with underlying obstructive disease); total lung capacity may be decreased (with underlying restrictive disease).
- ABG analysis reveals decreased PaO_2.
- ECG shows right axis deviation and tall or peaked P waves in inferior leads (with right ventricular hypertrophy).

Pulmonic insufficiency

- Cardiac catheterization shows pulmonic insufficiency, increased right ventricular pressure, and associated cardiac defects.
- CXR shows enlargement of the right ventricle and pulmonary artery.
- Echocardiography shows right ventricular or right atrial enlargement.
- ECG may be normal in mild cases or show right ventricular or right atrial hypertrophy.

Pulmonic stenosis

- Cardiac catheterization reveals increased right ventricular pressure, decreased pulmonary artery pressure, and an abnormal valve orifice.
- CXR usually reveals a normal heart size and normal lung vascularity, although the pulmonary arteries may be evident. With severe obstruction and right-sided heart failure, CXR may reveal right atrial and ventricular enlargement.
- Echocardiography reveals the abnormality in the pulmonic valve.
- ECG results may be normal in mild cases, or they may indicate right axis deviation and right ventricular hypertrophy. High amplitude P waves in leads II, III, aV_F, and V_1 indicate right atrial enlargement.

Rabies

- History reveals recent animal bite.
- Throat and saliva culture identifies virus.
- Serum fluorescent rabies antibody test is positive.
- WBC count is elevated, with increased polymorphonuclear and large mononuclear cells.
- Urine glucose, acetone, and protein levels are elevated.

Radiation exposure

- History includes exposure to radiation and nausea and vomiting.
- CBC reveals decreased Hb level and HCT, and decreased WBC, platelet, and lymphocyte counts.
- Bone marrow studies reveal blood dyscrasias.
- X-rays may show bone necrosis.
- Geiger counter measurement reveals the amount of radiation in an open wound.

Rape-trauma syndrome

- History includes rape or attempted rape, accompanied by feelings of anxiety, grief, anger, fear, or revenge.
- Examination shows signs of physical trauma.
- X-rays reveal fractures.
- Vaginal specimen is positive for semen.
- Fingernail and pubic hair scrapings and semen analysis may help to identify alleged rapist.

Raynaud's disease

- History and examination reveal changes in skin color induced by cold or stress, bilateral involvement, minimal cutaneous gangrene or absence of gangrene, and clinical symptoms of 2 years' duration or more.

- Cold stimulation test demonstrates Raynaud's syndrome.
- Arteriography reveals no underlying secondary disease.

Rectal polyps
- Proctosigmoidoscopy or colonoscopy reveals type, size, and location of polyps.
- Biopsy reveals histologic changes consistent with polyps.
- Barium enema reveals polyps high in the colon.
- Stool guaiac testing reveals presence of occult blood.

Rectal prolapse
- In complete prolapse, visual examination reveals the full thickness of the bowel wall and, possibly, the sphincter muscle protruding and mucosa falling into bulky, concentric folds.
- In partial prolapse, visual examination reveals only partially protruding mucosa and a smaller mass of radial mucosal folds.

Reiter's syndrome
- History includes venereal or enteric infection.
- HLA testing reveals presence of HLA-B27.
- Analysis of urethral discharge and synovial fluid reveals numerous WBCs, mostly polymorphonuclear leukocytes.
- Synovial fluid analysis reveals increased complement and protein; fluid is grossly purulent.
- WBC count and ESR are elevated.

Relapsing fever
- History includes recurrent fever for 5 to 15 days.
- Blood smear shows spirochetes.
- WBC count is elevated, with increase in lymphocytes (although WBC count may be within normal limits).
- ESR is increased.

Renal calculi
- KUB X-rays reveal renal calculi.
- Excretory urography reveals size and location of calculi.
- Kidney ultrasonography reveals obstructive changes.
- Urine culture may reveal urinary tract infection.
- Urinalysis may be normal or may show increased specific gravity, acid or alkaline pH (depending on the type of stone), hematuria, crystals, casts, and pyuria (with or without WBCs).
- 24-hour urine collection shows presence of calcium oxalate, phosphorus, or uric acid.

Renal infarction
- Urinalysis reveals proteinuria and microscopic hematuria.
- Urine enzyme levels, especially LD and alkaline phosphatase, are elevated.
- Serum ALT, AST, and LD levels are elevated.
- Excretory urography shows diminished or absent excretion of contrast dye (with vascular occlusion or urethral obstruction).
- Isotopic renal scan demonstrates absent or reduced blood flow to the kidneys.
- Renal arteriography reveals infarction.

Renal tubular acidosis
- Urine studies reveal pH > 6, low titratable acids and ammonia content, increased HCO_3^- and potassium levels, and low specific gravity (< 1.005).
- Blood pH is < 7.35.
- Serum HCO_3^- level is < 22 mEq/L (SI, < 22 mmol/L).
- Serum potassium and phosphorus levels are decreased.

Renal vein thrombosis
- Excretory urography reveals enlarged kidneys and diminished excretory func-

tion (in acute thrombosis); urography contrast medium seems to "smudge" necrotic renal tissue.
- In chronic thrombosis, excretory urography may show ureteral indentations that result from collateral venous channels.
- Renal venography reveals filling defects.
- Renal biopsy reveals characteristic histologic changes.
- Urinalysis reveals gross or microscopic hematuria, proteinuria (> 2 g/day in chronic disease), casts, and oliguria.
- Blood studies show leukocytosis, hypoalbuminemia, hyperlipemia, and thrombocytopenia.

Renovascular hypertension
- Isotopic renal blood flow scan and rapid-sequence excretory urography demonstrate abnormal renal blood flow and discrepancies in kidney size and shape.
- Renal arteriography reveals the arterial stenosis or obstruction.
- Samples from both the right and left renal veins allow for comparison of plasma renin levels with those in the inferior vena cava; renin level is increased in the affected kidney.

Respiratory acidosis
- ABG measurements reveal:
  - pH < 7.35
  - $PaCO_2$ > 45 mm Hg (SI, > 5.3 kPa)
  - HCO_3^- level of 22 to 26 mEq/L (SI, 22 to 26 mmol/L) in the acute stage and > 26 mEq/L (SI, > 26 mmol/L) in the chronic stage.

Respiratory alkalosis
- ABG measurements reveal:
  - pH > 7.45
  - $PaCO_2$ < 35 mm Hg (SI, < 4.7 kPa) in acute stage
  - HCO_3^- level normal in acute stage and < 22 mEq/L (SI, < 22 mmol/L) in chronic stage.

Respiratory distress syndrome, adult
- Initial ABG measurements reveal:
  - pH > 7.45
  - PaO_2 < 60 mm Hg (SI, < 8.02 kPa)
  - $PaCO_2$ < 35 mm Hg (SI, 4.7 kPa).
- ABG measurements following progression of illness reveal:
  - pH < 7.35
  - decreased PaO_2 (despite oxygen therapy)
  - $PaCO_2$ level > 45 mm Hg (SI, > 5.3 kPa)
  - HCO_3^- level < 22 mEq/L (SI, < 22 mmol/L).
- Serial CXRs initially show bilateral infiltrates; later X-rays reveal ground glass appearance and eventually "white-outs" of both lungs.

Respiratory distress syndrome, child
- CXR reveals fine reticulonodular pattern (may be normal for first 6 to 12 hours after birth).
- ABG measurements reveal pH < 7.35 and PaO_2 < 75 mm Hg (SI, < 10.03 kPa).
- Chest auscultation reveals normal or diminished air entry and crackles (rare in early stages).
- Amniocentesis reveals lecithin-sphingomyelin ratio of < 2 (used to assess risk of respiratory distress syndrome).

Respiratory syncytial virus infection
- Cultures of nasal and pharyngeal secretions identify respiratory syncytial virus infection (not always reliable).
- Serum antibody titers elevated (maternal antibodies may impair results before age 6 months).
- CXR may reveal pneumonia.

- Indirect immunofluorescence and ELISA tests are positive.

Restrictive cardiomyopathy

- CXR reveals massive cardiomegaly, affecting all four chambers of the heart, pericardial effusion, and pulmonary congestion (advanced stage).
- Echocardiography detects increased left ventricular muscle mass and differences in end-diastolic pressures between the ventricles.
- Carotid palpation reveals blunt carotid upstroke with small volume.
- Cardiac catheterization demonstrates increased left ventricular end-diastolic pressure.
- ECG may show low-voltage complexes, hypertrophy, atrioventricular conduction defects, or arrhythmias.

Retinal detachment

- Ophthalmoscopy reveals the usually transparent retina to be gray and opaque.
- In severe detachment, ophthalmoscopy reveals folds in the retina and a ballooning out of the area.
- Indirect ophthalmoscopy reveals retinal tears.
- Ocular ultrasonography shows a dense sheetlike echo on a B-scan.

Retinitis pigmentosa

- Family history indicates a possible predisposition to retinitis pigmentosa.
- Electroretinography shows a retinal response time slower than normal or absent.
- Visual field testing (using a tangent screen) detects ring scotomata.
- Fluorescein angiography shows white dots (areas of dyspigmentation) in the epithelium.
- Ophthalmoscopy may initially show normal fundi but later reveals characteristic black pigmentary disturbance.

Reye's syndrome

- History includes recent viral disorder with varying degrees of encephalopathy and cerebral edema.
- ALT level is > 56 U/L (SI, > 0.96 μkat/L).
- AST level is > 40 U/L (SI, > 0.68 –2 to +13 kat/L.
- Liver biopsy reveals fatty droplets uniformly distributed throughout cells.
- PT and PTT are prolonged.
- CSF analysis reveals WBCs < 10/ml; in coma, CSF pressure is increased.
- Serum ammonia levels are elevated.
- Serum fatty acid and lactate levels are elevated.
- Serum glucose levels are normal or low.

Rheumatic fever and rheumatic heart disease

- History includes streptococcal infection.
- Examination reveals joint pain and swelling and one or more of these symptoms: carditis, polyarthritis, chorea, erythema marginatum, or subcutaneous nodules.
- C-reactive protein is positive.
- ASO titer is elevated (within 2 months of onset).
- Echocardiography and cardiac catheterization reveal valvular damage.
- Cardiac enzymes may be elevated (in severe carditis).

Rheumatoid arthritis, adult

- Serum RF titer is above 1:80.
- X-rays reveal bone demineralization and soft-tissue swelling (in early stages), loss of cartilage and narrowing of joint spaces, and cartilage and bone destruction, erosion, subluxations, and deformities.
- Synovial fluid analysis reveals increased volume and turbidity but decreased viscosity and complement 3

and complement 4 levels, and elevated WBC count.

- ESR is increased.
- CBC shows moderate decrease in RBC count, Hb level, and HCT and slight leukocytosis.

Rheumatoid arthritis, juvenile

- History includes persistent joint stiffness and pain in the morning or after periods of inactivity.
- ANA test may be positive in patients who have pauciarticular juvenile rheumatoid arthritis (JRA) with chronic iridocyclitis.
- RF is present in 15% of patients with JRA, as compared with 85% of patients with rheumatoid arthritis.
- Early changes seen on X-ray include soft-tissue swelling, effusion, and periostitis in affected joints.
- In later X-ray studies, osteoporosis and accelerated bone growth may appear, followed by subchondral erosions, joint space narrowing, bone destruction, and fusion.
- CBC usually shows decreased Hb levels, increased neutrophil count, increased platelet levels, and elevated ESR.
- Blood studies reveal elevated C-reactive protein, serum haptoglobin, Ig, and complement 3 levels.
- HLA testing reveals presence of HLA-B27, forecasting later development of ankylosing spondylitis.

Rocky Mountain spotted fever

- History includes tick bite or travel to a tick-infested area.
- Complement fixation test shows a fourfold rise in convalescent antibodies compared to acute titers.
- Blood culture identifies *Rickettsia rickettsii.*
- Decreased platelet count indicates thrombocytopenia during second week of illness.
- WBC count is elevated during second week of illness.

Rosacea

- Examination reveals vascular and acneiform lesions without the comedones characteristically associated with acne vulgaris; in severe cases, rhinophyma is seen.

Roseola infantum

- History includes high fever (103° to 105° F [39.4° to 40.4° C]) followed by rash 48 hours after fever subsides.
- Examination reveals maculopapular, nonpruritic rash that blanches on pressure.

Rubella

- History includes exposure to infected person.
- Examination reveals maculopapular rash, beginning on the face and spreading to the trunk and extremities.
- Examination also reveals lymphadenopathy.
- Cell cultures of throat, blood, urine, and CSF reveal rubella virus.
- Convalescent serum antibody titers rise fourfold from acute titers.

Rubeola

- History includes exposure to person infected with the measles virus (patient may be unaware of contact).
- Examination reveals the pathognomonic Koplik's spots.
- Cultures of blood, nasopharyngeal secretions, and urine identify measles virus (during the febrile period).
- Serum antibody titers appear within 3 days after onset of the rash and reach peak titers 2 to 4 weeks later.

Salmonellosis

■ Culture of blood, stool, urine, bone marrow, pus, or vomitus identifies gram-negative bacilli of the genus *Salmonella*.
■ Widal's test reveals a fourfold rise in titer.

Sarcoidosis

■ Kveim skin test confirms discrete epithelioid cell granuloma.
■ CXR reveals bilateral hilar and right paratracheal adenopathy with or without diffuse interstitial infiltrates; occasionally, large nodular lesions appear in lung parenchyma.
■ Lymph node, skin, or lung biopsy reveals noncaseating granulomas with negative cultures for mycobacteria and fungi.
■ PFTs show decreased total lung capacity and compliance and decreased diffusing capacity.
■ Tuberculin skin test, fungal serologies, and sputum cultures for mycobacteria and fungi and biopsy cultures are negative.

Scabies

■ Visual examination of the contents of the scabietic burrow may reveal itch mite.
■ Mineral oil placed over the burrow, followed by superficial scraping and examination of expressed material, reveals ova or mite feces.
■ Pediculicide administration to affected area clears skin.

Scarlet fever

■ History includes recent streptococcal pharyngitis.
■ Examination reveals strawberry tongue and fine erythematous rash that blanches on pressure.
■ Pharyngeal culture identifies group A beta-hemolytic streptococci.
■ CBC reveals granulocytosis and, possibly, a reduced RBC count.

Schistosomiasis

■ History includes travel to endemic areas.
■ Urine, stool, or lesion biopsy reveals ova.
■ WBC count reveals eosinophilia.

Scoliosis

■ Examination reveals unequal shoulder height, elbow levels, and heights of iliac crests and asymmetry of the paraspinal muscles.
■ Scoliosometer (an apparatus for measuring curvature of the spinal column) reveals angle of trunk rotation to be abnormal.
■ Anterior, posterior, and lateral spinal X-rays reveal degree of curvature and flexibility of the spine.

Septal perforation and deviation

■ History and examination reveal whistle on inspiration, rhinitis, epistaxis, nasal crusting, and watery discharge.
■ Inspection of the nasal mucosa with bright light and a nasal speculum reveals perforation or deviation.

Septic arthritis

■ Synovial fluid Gram stain and culture or biopsy of synovial membrane reveals gram-positive cocci *(Staphylococcus aureus, Streptococcus pyogenes, Streptococcus pneumoniae,* or *Streptococcus viridans)*, gram-negative cocci *(Neisseria gonorrhoeae* or *Haemophilus influenzae)*, or gram-negative bacilli (*Escherichia coli, Salmonella,* or *Pseudomonas)* as the causative organism.
■ Joint fluid analysis reveals gross pus or watery, cloudy fluid of decreased viscosity, with markedly elevat-

ed WBCs/ml, containing primarily neutrophils.

- Culture of skin exudate, sputum, urethral discharge, stool, urine, blood, or nasopharyngeal secretions is positive for causative organism.
- Skeletal X-rays show distention of joint capsules, followed by narrowing of joint space (indicating cartilage damage), and erosions of bone (joint destruction).
- WBC count may be elevated with many polymorphonuclear cells; ESR is increased.

Septic shock

- History includes infection accompanied by fever, confusion, nausea, vomiting, and hyperventilation.
- Blood cultures identify gram-negative bacteria (*Escherichia coli, Klebsiella, Enterobacter, Pseudomonas, Proteus,* or *Bacteroides*) or gram-positive bacteria (*Streptococcus pneumoniae, S. pyogenes,* or *Actinomyces*) as the causative organism.
- WBC count is elevated.
- Pulmonary artery catheterization reveals decreased central venous pressure, pulmonary artery pressures, wedge pressure, cardiac output (may be initially elevated), and systemic vascular resistance.
- ABG measurements reveal decreased $PaCO_2$, low or normal HCO_3^- level, and pH > 7.45 (in early stages); as shock progresses, decreasing $PaCO_2$, PaO_2, HCO_3^- level, and pH indicate the development of metabolic acidosis with hypoxemia.
- Serum BUN and creatinine levels increase; creatinine clearance decreases.
- Urine osmolality is < 400 mOsm/kg serum water (SI, < 400 mmol/kg serum water); ratio of urine osmolality to plasma osmolality is < 1.5.
- ECG reveals ST-segment depression, inverted T waves, and arrhythmias.

Severe combined immunodeficiency disease

- History includes overwhelming infections during the first year of life.
- T-cell count and function are severely diminished.
- Lymph node biopsy reveals absence of lymphocytes.

Shigellosis

- Microscopic examination of a fresh stool may reveal mucus, RBCs, and polymorphonuclear leukocytes.
- Stool culture identifies *Shigella.*
- Hemagglutinating antibodies may be present, indicating severe infection.

Sickle cell anemia

- Family history includes homozygous inheritance.
- Stained blood smear reveals sickle cells.
- Hb electrophoresis reveals HbS.
- CBC may reveal decreased RBC count and elevated WBC and platelet counts.
- ESR is decreased.
- Serum iron levels are increased.

Sideroblastic anemias

- Bone marrow aspirate reveals ringed sideroblasts.
- Microscopic examination reveals RBCs that are hypochromic or normochromic and slightly macrocytic; red cell precursors may be megaloblastic, with anisocytosis and poikilocytosis.
- Hb levels are decreased.
- Serum iron and transferrin levels are increased.

Silicosis

- History includes occupational exposure to silica dust.
- Examination reveals decreased chest expansion, diminished intensity of breath sounds, areas of hyporesonance and hyperresonance, fine to medium

crackles, and tachypnea (with chronic silicosis).
- CXR reveals the following:
– small, discrete, nodular lesions distributed throughout both lung fields but typically concentrated in the upper lung zones
– enlarged hilar lung nodes that exhibit "eggshell" calcification (in simple silicosis)
– one or more conglomerate masses of dense tissue (in complicated silicosis).
- PFTs reveal:
– reduced FVC (in complicated silicosis)
– reduced FEV_1 (in obstructed disease)
– reduced maximal voluntary ventilation (in restrictive and obstructive disease)
– reduced diffusing capacity for carbon monoxide when fibrosis destroys alveolar walls and oblates pulmonary capillaries, or when fibrosis thickens the alveolar capillary membrane.
- ABG measurements reveal:
– significantly decreased PaO_2 (in the late stages of chronic or complicated disease)
– decreased or normal $PaCO_2$ in early stages; may increase as restrictive pattern develops.

Sinus bradycardia

- ECG reveals:
– regular atrial and ventricular rhythm
– atrial and ventricular rates < 60 beats/minute
– P wave of normal size and configuration with a P wave preceding each QRS complex
– PR interval within normal limits and constant
– QRS complex of normal duration and configuration
– T wave of normal size and configuration
– QT interval within normal limits, but possibly prolonged.

Sinus tachycardia

- ECG reveals:
– regular atrial and ventricular rhythms
– atrial and ventricular rates > 100 beats/minute (usually between 100 and 160 beats/minute)
– P wave of normal size and configuration with a P wave preceding each QRS complex
– PR interval within normal limits and constant
– QRS complex of normal duration and configuration
– T wave of normal size and configuration
– QT interval within normal limits, but commonly shortened.

Sinusitis

- Nasal examination reveals inflammation and pus.
- Sinus X-rays reveal cloudiness in the affected sinus, air-fluid levels, or thickened mucosal lining.
- Transillumination allows inspection of the sinus cavities by passing a light through them; in sinusitis, purulent drainage prevents passage of light.

Sjögren's syndrome

- History and examination reveal two of the following three conditions: xerophthalmia, xerostomia (with salivary gland biopsy showing lymphocytic infiltration), and associated autoimmune or lymphoproliferative disorder.
- ESR is elevated.
- Hypergammaglobulinemia is present.
- RF test is positive (75% to 90% of patients).
- ANA test is positive (50% to 80% of patients).
- Schirmer's tearing test is positive for tearing deficiency.
- Lower lip biopsy shows salivary gland infiltration by lymphocytes.

Skull fractures

- History includes recent head trauma.
- Skull X-ray shows fracture (minor vault fractures may not be visible)
- Neurologic examination evaluates cerebral function.
- Cerebral angiography reveals vascular disruption from internal pressure and injury.
- CT scan, echoencephalography, air encephalography, MRI, and radioactive scanning reveal cranial nerve injury or intracranial hemorrhage from ruptured blood vessels. These tests also help to localize subdural or intracerebral hematomas.

Snakebites, poisonous

- Examination reveals fang marks.
- Bleeding time and PTT are prolonged.
- Hb level and HCT are decreased.
- Platelet count is sharply decreased.
- Urinalysis may reveal hematuria.
- CXR may show pulmonary edema or emboli.
- ECG may reveal tachycardia and ectopic beats.

Sodium imbalance

- Hyponatremia:
  - Serum sodium level is < 135 mEq/L (SI, < 135 mmol/L).
  - Urine sodium level is > 100 mEq/24 hours (SI, > 100 mmol/d).
  - Serum osmolality is low.
- Hypernatremia:
  - Serum sodium level is > 145 mEq/L (SI, > 145 mmol/L).
  - Urine sodium level is < 40 mEq/24 hours (SI, < 40 mmol/d).
  - Serum osmolality is high.

Spinal cord defects

- Examination reveals a protruding sac on the spine.
- Transillumination of sac reveals meningocele.
- Spinal X-ray shows bone defect (in spina bifida occulta).
- CT scan reveals hydrocephalus (in 90% of patients).

Spinal injuries without cord damage

- History includes trauma, metastatic disease, infection, or endocrine disorder.
- Physical examination reveals the location and level of injury.
- Spinal X-rays reveal fracture.
- Myelography reveals spinal mass.
- Lumbar puncture reveals increased CSF pressure, indicating spinal trauma or lesion.

Spinal neoplasms

- Lumbar puncture reveals clear yellow CSF with increased protein levels.
- X-rays show distortions of intervertebral foramina, changes in vertebrae or collapsed areas in the vertebral body, and localized enlargement of the spinal canal indicating an adjacent block.
- Myelography identifies the level of the lesion.
- CT scan and MRI show cord compression and tumor location.
- Radioisotope bone scan reveals evidence of metastatic invasion of the vertebrae by showing increased osteoblastic activity.
- Biopsy reveals malignant cells.

Sporotrichosis

- Examination reveals small, painless, movable subcutaneous nodules with discoloration and ulceration.
- Cultures of either sputum, pus, or bone drainage identify *Strongyloides schenckii.*

Sprains and strains

- History includes recent injury or chronic overuse of extremity.

■ Examination reveals pain (local with a sprain, sharp and transient with a strain), swelling, and ecchymoses (rapid onset with a sprain; may take several days with a strain).
■ X-ray of the extremity doesn't indicate fracture.

Squamous cell carcinoma
■ Examination reveals ulcerated nodule with indurated base.
■ Biopsy reveals squamous cell carcinoma.

Staphylococcal scalded skin syndrome
■ Examination reveals three-stage progression of erythema, exfoliation, and desquamation.
■ Skin lesions are positive for Group 2 *Staphylococcus aureus*.

Stomatitis and other oral infections
■ Examination reveals inflammation of the oral mucosa or surrounding area.
■ Smear of ulcer exudate reveals fusiform bacillus or spirochete as the causative organism (in Vincent's angina).

Strabismus
■ Visual acuity test reveals the degree of visual defect.
■ Hirschberg's method detects malalignment.
■ Retinoscopy identifies refractive error.
■ Maddox rods test identifies specific muscle involvement.
■ Convergence test shows distance at which convergence is sustained.
■ Duction test reveals limitation of eye movement.
■ Cover-uncover test demonstrates eye deviation and the rate of recovery to original alignment.
■ Alternate-cover test shows intermittent or latent deviation.

Strongyloidiasis
■ History includes travel to endemic area.
■ Stool specimen contains *Strongyloides stercoralis* larvae.
■ Sputum specimen contains eosinophils and larvae.
■ Hb level is decreased.
■ WBC count with differential shows eosinophils at 450 to 700/µl (SI, 4.5 to 7×10^9/L).

Stye
■ Visual examination reveals abscess of the lid glands.
■ Abscess culture reveals a staphylococcal organism.

Sudden infant death syndrome
■ Autopsy reveals:
– small or normal adrenal glands
– petechiae over the visceral surface of the pleura, within the thymus, and in the epicardium
– well-preserved lymphoid structures
– pathologic changes suggesting chronic hypoxemia
– edematous, congestive lungs fully expanded in the pleural cavities
– liquid blood in the heart (not clotted)
– curd from the stomach inside the trachea.

Syndrome of inappropriate antidiuretic hormone
■ History includes recent weight gain despite anorexia, nausea, and vomiting.
■ Serum osmolality is < 280 mOsm/kg of water.
■ Serum sodium level is < 123 mEq/L (SI, < 123 mmol/L).
■ Urine sodium level is > 20 mEq/L without diuretics (SI, > 20 mmol/L).

Syphilis

- History includes sexual contact with partner with syphilis.
- Culture of lesion identifies *Treponema pallidum*.
- The fluorescent treponemal antibody-absorption test identifies antigens of *T. pallidum* in tissue, ocular fluid, CSF, tracheobronchial secretions, and exudates from lesions.
- Venereal Disease Research Laboratory (VDRL) slide test and rapid plasma reagin test are positive, detecting nonspecific antibodies.
- In neurosyphilis:
  – CSF analysis reveals elevated total protein level.
  – VDRL slide test is reactive.
  – Cell count > 5 mononuclear cells/ml.

Taeniasis

- History includes travel to endemic areas; exposure to eating undercooked, infected beef, pork, or fish; or in dwarf tapeworm, exposure to an infected person.
- Laboratory observation reveals tapeworm ova or body segments in stool.
- Beef tapeworm reveals:
  – crawling sensation in perianal area
  – intestinal obstruction and appendicitis.
- Pork tapeworm reveals:
  – seizures, headaches, personality changes (often overlooked in adults).
- In fish tapeworm:
  – anemia (Hb as low as 6 to 8 g/dl; SI, 60 to 80 g/L).
- Dwarf tapeworm reveals:
  – no symptoms (mild infestation)
  – anorexia, diarrhea, restlessness, dizziness, and apathy (severe infestation).

Tay-Sachs disease

- Family history includes Eastern European Jewish ancestry or history of the disease. Diagnostic screening may detect carriers of autosomal recessive gene.
- Serum analysis shows deficiency of hexosaminidase A.
- Ophthalmic examination reveals optic nerve atrophy and a distinctive cherry-red spot on the retina.

Tendinitis and bursitis

- History includes unusual strain or injury 2 to 3 days before onset of pain or heat-aggravated joint pain.
- Examination reveals localized pain and inflammation at joint.
- X-rays (in late stages) reveal bony fragments, osteophyte sclerosis, or calcium deposits.
- Arthrography is usually normal, with occasional small irregularities on the undersurface of the tendon.

Testicular cancer

- Physical examination reveals testicular mass.
- Transillumination confirms tumor.
- Biopsy reveals malignant cells.
- Excretory urography reveals ureteral deviation (indicates node involvement).
- Testosterone levels are > 1,200 ng/dl (SI, > 41.6 nmol/L) or < 300 ng/dl (SI, < 10.4 nmol/L).
- Urine testing indicates presence of hCG.
- Serum AFP and beta-hCG levels are increased.

Testicular torsion

- Physical examination reveals tense, tender swelling in the scrotum or inguinal canal and hyperemia of the overlying skin.
- Doppler ultrasonography reveals testicular torsion.

Tetanus

- History includes trauma and absence of tetanus immunization.
- Meningitis, rabies, phenothiazine or strychnine toxicity, or other conditions that mimic tetanus are ruled out.

■ Cultures are positive for an anaerobic spore forming rod clostridium tetani.

Tetralogy of Fallot

■ Echocardiography reveals septal overriding of the aorta, the ventricular septal defect (VSD), and pulmonic stenosis, and detects hypertrophy of walls of the right ventricle.
■ Cardiac catheterization shows pulmonic stenosis, the VSD, and the overriding aorta and rules out other cyanotic heart defects.
■ Auscultation reveals a loud systolic heart murmur, which may diminish or obscure the pulmonic component of S_2.
■ Palpation may reveal a cardiac thrill at the left sternal border and an obvious right ventricular impulse.
■ ECG shows right ventricular hypertrophy, right axis deviation and, possibly, right atrial hypertrophy.
■ CXR reveals decreased pulmonary vascular marking (depending on the severity of pulmonary obstruction) and a boot-shaped cardiac silhouette.

Thalassemia

■ Thalassemia major reveals:
– lowered RBC count and Hb level
– elevated reticulocyte level
– elevated bilirubin and urinary and fecal urobilinogen levels
– low serum folate level
– X-rays of the skull and long bones showing a thinning and widening of the marrow space
– Hb electrophoresis revealing a significant rise in HbF and a slight increase in HbA_2
– peripheral blood smear revealing extremely thin and fragile RBCs, pale nucleated RBCs, and marked anisocytosis.
■ Thalassemia intermedia reveals:
– hypochromic and microcytic RBCs.
■ Thalassemia minor reveals:
– hypochromic and microcytic RBCs
– Hb electrophoresis revealing a significant increase in HbA_2 and a moderate rise in HbF.

Thoracic aortic aneurysm

■ CXR reveals widening of the aorta.
■ CT scan or MRI reveals location and size of aneurysm.
■ Aortography reveals the lumen of the aneurysm, its size and location and, in dissecting aneurysm, the false lumen.

Throat abscesses

■ History includes staphylococcal or streptococcal infection.
■ Examination reveals swelling of the soft palate on the abscessed side of the throat, with displacement of the uvula to the opposite side; red, edematous mucous membranes; and tonsil displacement toward the midline.
■ Retropharyngeal abscess is indicated by:
– history of nasopharyngitis or pharyngitis
– soft, red bulging of the posterior pharyngeal wall
– X-rays that reveal the larynx pushed forward and a widened space between the posterior pharyngeal wall and vertebrae
– pharyngeal culture that identifies infective organism.
■ Throat culture reveals streptococcal or staphylococcal infection.

Thrombocytopenia

■ Platelet count is markedly decreased.
■ Bleeding time is prolonged.
■ PT and PTT are normal.
■ Bone marrow studies reveal an increased number of megakaryocytes (platelet precursors) and shortened platelet survival.

Thrombophlebitis

■ Homans' sign is positive.

- Doppler ultrasonography reveals reduced blood flow to a specific area and obstruction to venous flow.
- Plethysmography reveals decreased circulation distal to affected area.
- Phlebography reveals filling defects and diverted blood flow.

Thyroid cancer

- History includes exposure to radiation therapy or a family history of thyroid cancer.
- Examination reveals an enlarged, palpable node in the thyroid gland, neck, lymph nodes of the neck, or vocal cords.
- Thyroid scan reveals a "cold," nonfunctioning nodule.
- Thyroid biopsy reveals a well-encapsulated, solitary nodule of uniform but abnormal structure.
- Serum calcitonin assay reveals an elevated fasting calcitonin and an abnormal response to calcium stimulation (with medullary cancer).

Thyroiditis

- Autoimmune thyroiditis reveals:
  – positive precipitin test
  – high titers of thyroglobulin
  – microsomal antibodies present in serum.
- Subacute granulomatous thyroiditis reveals:
  – elevated ESR
  – increased thyroid hormone levels
  – decreased thyroidal radioiodine uptake.

Tic disorders

- History identifies stressors that may be related to symptoms.
- Examination reveals recurrent, involuntary movements involving the facial muscles, coughing, sniffling, or jerking head movements.
- Psychogenic tics are ruled out.

Tinea versicolor

- Wood's light examination reveals lesions.
- Microscopic examination of skin scrapings shows hyphae and clusters of yeast.

Tonsillitis

- Examination reveals generalized inflammation of the pharyngeal wall and swollen tonsils that project from between the pillars of the fauces and exude white or yellow follicles, with inflamed uvula.
- Purulent drainage appears when pressure is applied to the tonsillar pillars.
- Throat culture identifies infective organism, commonly beta-hemolytic streptococci.

Torticollis

- History includes painless neck deformity.
- Examination reveals enlargement of the sternocleidomastoid muscle.
- Cervical spine X-rays are negative for bone or joint disease but may reveal an associated disorder such as tuberculosis, scar tissue formation, or arthritis (in acquired torticollis).

Toxic epidermal necrolysis

- Examination reveals scalded skin with no history of burn.
- Nikolsky's sign (skin sloughs off with slight friction) appears in erythematous areas.
- Culture and Gram stain identify infective organism.
- WBC count reveals leukocytosis.

Toxic shock syndrome

- Culture of vaginal discharge or lesions identifies *Staphylococcus aureus.*
- CK level is elevated.
- BUN level is elevated.
- Serum creatinine level is elevated.

- AST level is > 56 U/L (SI, > 0.95 –2 to + 3 kat/L) and ALT level is > 40 U/L (SI, > 0.68 µkat/L).
- Platelet count is markedly decreased.

Toxocariasis

- History includes pica, eosinophilia, or recent exposure to a dog.
- Massive leukocytosis develops.
- Hypereosinophilia develops.
- Antibodies to *Toxocara canis* are present in serum.
- Liver biopsy contains *T. canis* larvae.

Toxoplasmosis

- History includes exposure to a cat or ingestion of uncooked meat.
- Blood, body fluid, or tissue tests positive for *Toxoplasma gondii* antibodies.
- *T. gondii* is identified in mice after their inoculation with specimens of patient's body fluids, blood, and tissue.

Tracheoesophageal fistula and esophageal atresia

- Examination reveals respiratory distress and drooling in a newborn.
- Catheter (#10 or #12 French) meets obstruction when passed through the nose at 4″ to 5″ (10 to 12.5 cm) distal from the nostrils.
- CXR demonstrates the position of the catheter and can show a dilated, air-filled upper esophageal pouch, pneumonia in the right upper lobe, or bilateral pneumonitis.
- Abdominal X-ray reveals gas in the bowel in a distal fistula (but none in a proximal fistula or atresia without fistula).
- Cinefluorography defines the upper pouch by allowing visualization on a fluoroscopic screen and differentiates between overflow aspiration from a blind end (atresia) and aspiration due to passage of liquids through a tracheoesophageal fistula.

Trachoma

- Examination reveals follicular conjunctivitis with corneal infiltration and upper lid or conjunctival scarring, with symptoms persisting for 3 weeks.
- Microscopic examination of a Giemsa-stained conjunctival scraping reveals cytoplasmic inclusion bodies, some polymorphonuclear reaction, plasma cells, Leber's cells (large macrophages containing phagocytosed debris), and follicle cells.

Transposition of the great arteries

- Echocardiography reveals the reversed position of the aorta and the pulmonary artery and records echoes from both semilunar valves simultaneously, due to the aortic valve displacement.
- Cardiac catheterization reveals decreased oxygen saturation in left ventricular blood and aortic blood; increased right atrial, right ventricular, and pulmonary artery oxygen saturation; and right ventricular systolic pressure equal to systemic pressure.
- Dye injection during catheterization reveals the transposed vessels and the presence of any other cardiac defects.
- CXR shows right atrial and ventricular enlargement causing the heart to appear oblong (within days to weeks) and increased vascular markings, except when pulmonic stenosis exists.
- ECG reveals right axis deviation and right ventricular hypertrophy (may be normal in a neonate).
- ABG measurements reveal hypoxia and secondary metabolic acidosis.

Trichinosis

- History includes ingestion of raw or improperly cooked pork or pork products.
- Stools contain mature worms and larvae during the invasion stage.

- Skeletal muscle biopsy reveals encysted larvae 10 days after ingestion.
- Antibody titers are elevated during acute and convalescent stage.
- During acute stages, serum liver enzymes (AST, LD, and CK) are elevated.
- Eosinophil count is elevated.

Trichomoniasis

- History includes sexual contact with person with trichomoniasis.
- Examination reveals vaginal erythema; edema; frank excoriation; a frothy, malodorous, greenish yellow vaginal discharge; and, rarely, a thin, gray pseudomembrane over the vagina.
- Cervical examination shows punctate cervical hemorrhages, giving the cervix a strawberry appearance.
- Microscopic examination of vaginal or seminal discharge identifies *Trichomonas vaginalis.*
- Culture of clear urine specimens may also reveal *T. vaginalis.*

Trichuriasis

- History includes ingestion of food contaminated with nematoid ova.
- Stool specimen contains whipworm ova.

Tricuspid insufficiency

- Cardiac catheterization shows markedly decreased cardiac output; mean right atrial and right ventricular end-diastolic pressures may be elevated.
- CXR reveals right atrial and ventricular enlargement.
- Echocardiography shows right ventricular dilation and paradoxical septal motion. It may show prolapsing or flailing of the tricuspid valve leaflets. Doppler echocardiography provides estimates of pulmonary artery and right ventricular systolic pressure.
- ECG reveals right atrial hypertrophy and right or left ventricular hypertrophy. ECG also may reveal atrial fibrillation or incomplete right bundle-branch block.

Tricuspid stenosis

- Cardiac catheterization shows increased right atrial pressure and decreased cardiac output; it may also show an increased pressure gradient across the tricuspid valve.
- CXR reveals right atrial and superior vena cava enlargement.
- Echocardiography reveals a thick tricuspid valve with reduced mobility and right atrial enlargement.
- ECG shows right atrial hypertrophy and right ventricular hypertrophy. Atrial fibrillation may be present. Tall, peaked P waves are seen in lead II and prominent, upright P waves are seen in lead V_1, indicating right atrial enlargement.

Trigeminal neuralgia

- History includes pain in the superior mandibular or maxillary area, without sensory or motor impairment.
- Examination reveals splinting on the affected side of the face while talking.
- Skull X-rays, tomography, and CT scans rule out sinus or tooth infections and tumors.

Tuberculosis

- Stains and cultures of sputum, CSF, urine, and abscess drainage reveal heat-sensitive, nonmotile, aerobic, acid-fast bacilli.
- CXR shows nodular lesions, patchy infiltrates, cavity formation, scar tissue, and calcium deposits.
- Auscultation reveals crepitant crackles, bronchial breath sounds, wheezes, and whispered pectoriloquy.
- Chest percussion reveals a dullness over the affected area.
- Tuberculin skin test reveals that the patient has been infected with tuberculosis.

Tularemia

- History includes exposure to animals or ticks.
- Lymph nodes, sputum, or gastric washings identify *Francisella tularensis.*
- Agglutination test reveals a rise in antibody titers.
- Skin test (with a diluted specimen of *F. tularensis*) has a positive reaction (90% of patients).

Typhus, epidemic

- Weil-Felix reaction reveals a fourfold rise in agglutination titer 8 to 12 days after infection.
- Complement fixation for group-specific typhus antigens is positive 8 to 12 days after infection.

Ulcerative colitis

- History includes recurrent bloody diarrhea and GI disturbances.
- Sigmoidoscopy shows increased mucosal friability, decreased mucosal detail, and thick inflammatory exudate.
- Biopsy reveals histologic changes characteristic of ulcerative colitis.
- Colonoscopy identifies the extent of the disease.
- Barium enema identifies the extent of the disease and detects complications.
- ESR increases, correlating with severity of attack.
- Serum potassium and magnesium levels are decreased.
- CBC shows decreased Hb level and leukocytosis.
- Serum albumin level is decreased.
- PT is prolonged.

Undescended testes

- Examination of scrotum reveals unpalpable testes, either unilateral or bilateral.
- Buccal smear identifies genetic sex by showing a male sex chromatin pattern.
- Serum gonadotropin levels confirm the presence of testes.

Urticaria and angioedema

- History includes exposure to medications, food, and environmental influences.
- Skin testing reveals specific allergens.
- Serum complement 4 and complement 1 esterase inhibitor levels are decreased (confirming hereditary angioedema).
- CBC, urinalysis, ESR, and CXR rule out inflammatory infections.

Uterine cancer

- Endometrial, cervical, and endocervical biopsies reveal malignant cells.
- Schiller's test shows cancerous tissues resisting stain.
- Cervical biopsies and endocervical curettage identify degree of cervical involvement.
- Barium enema reveals bladder or rectal involvement.

Uterine leiomyomas

- History includes abnormal endometrial bleeding.
- Pelvic palpation reveals round or irregular mass.
- Ultrasonography shows a dense mass.
- Hysterosalpingography reveals asymmetric uterus.
- Laparoscopy reveals lumps on the uterus.
- CBC reveals decreased RBC count, Hb level, and HCT.

Uveitis

- Slit-lamp examination reveals a "flare and cell" pattern, which looks like light passing through smoke, and an increased number of cells over the inflamed area.
- Examination with a special lens, slit-lamp, and ophthalmoscope identifies

active inflammatory fundus lesions involving the retina and choroid.
■ Serologic tests indicate toxoplasmosis (in posterior uveitis).

Vaginal cancer
■ Pap test reveals abnormal cells.
■ Vaginal examination, aided by Lugol's solution, reveals lesion.
■ Lesion biopsy reveals malignant cells.
■ Gallium scan shows abnormal gallium activity.

Vaginismus
■ History and examination rule out physical disorders causing muscle constriction.
■ Pelvic examination reveals involuntary constriction of the musculature surrounding the outer portion of the vagina.
■ Detailed sexual history reveals involuntary spastic contraction of the lower vaginal muscles, possibly coexisting with dyspareunia, preventing intercourse.

Varicella
■ History includes exposure to person infected with chickenpox, although the patient may be unaware of contact.
■ Examination reveals crops of small, erythematous macules on the trunk or scalp progressing to papules and then clear vesicles on a erythematous base; vesicles become cloudy and break, and then form a scab.
■ Vesicular fluid tests positive for herpesvirus varicella-zoster.

Variola
■ History includes exposure to infected person.
■ Aspirate from vesicles and pustules reveals variola virus.
■ Complement fixation detects antibodies to variola virus.
■ Microscopic examination of smears from lesions shows variola virus.

Vascular retinopathies
■ Central retinal artery occlusion:
– Ophthalmoscopy (direct or indirect) shows emptying of retinal arterioles.
– Slit-lamp examination reveals, within 2 hours of occlusion, clumps or segmentation in the artery. Later examination shows a milky white retina around the optic disk (resulting from swelling and necrosis of ganglion cells caused by reduced blood supply). Other findings include a cherry-red spot in the macula (which subsides after several weeks).
– Ophthalmodynamometry measures approximate relative pressures in the central retinal arteries and indirectly assesses internal carotid artery blockage.
– Ultrasonography reveals blood vessel conditions in the neck.
– Digital subtraction angiography identifies carotid occlusion.
– MRI helps identify the reason for obstruction by revealing carotid or other obstruction.
– Contrast-enhanced CT scan discloses the diseased carotid artery.
■ Central retinal vein occlusion:
– Ophthalmoscopy (direct or indirect) reveals retinal hemorrhage, retinal vein engorgement, white patches among hemorrhages, and edema around the optic disk.
– Ultrasonography confirms or rules out occluded blood vessels.
■ Diabetic retinopathy:
– Slit-lamp examination shows thickening of retinal capillary walls.
– Indirect ophthalmoscopy demonstrates retinal changes, such as microaneurysms (earliest change), retinal hemorrhages and edema, venous dilation and beading, exudates, vitreous hemorrhage, proliferation of fibrin into vitreous from retinal holes, growth of new

blood vessels, and microinfarctions of nerve fiber layer.
– Fluorescein angiography shows leakage of fluorescein from dilated vessels and differentiates between microaneurysms and true hemorrhages.
■ Hypertensive retinopathy:
– History reveals hypertension and decreased vision.
– Ophthalmoscopy (direct or indirect) performed in early disease discloses hard and shiny deposits, tiny hemorrhages, narrowed arterioles, nicking of the veins where arteries cross them (referred to as arteriovenous nicking), and elevated arterial blood pressure. The same test in later disease shows cotton wool patches, exudates, retinal edema, papilledema caused by ischemia and capillary insufficiency, hemorrhages, and microaneurysms.

Vasculitis

■ Polyarteritis nodosa:
– History includes hypertension, abdominal pain, myalgia, headache, joint pain, and weakness.
– ESR is elevated.
– Leukocytosis, anemia, and thrombocytosis are present.
– C_3 complement is depressed.
– RF titer is > 1:80.
– Circulating immune complexes are present.
– Tissue biopsy shows necrotizing vasculitis.
■ Allergic angiitis and granulomatosis:
– History includes asthma.
– Eosinophilia is present.
– Tissue biopsy may show granulomatous inflammation with eosinophilic infiltration.
■ Polyangiitis overlap syndrome:
– History includes allergy.
– Eosinophilia is present.
– Tissue biopsy that may show granulomatous inflammation with eosinophilic infiltration.
■ Wegener's granulomatosis:
– Leukocytosis is present.
– Tissue biopsy reveals necrotizing vasculitis with granulomatous inflammation.
– ESR and IgA and IgG levels are elevated.
– RF titer is low.
– Circulating immune complexes are present.
■ Temporal arteritis:
– Hb level is decreased.
– ESR is elevated.
– Tissue biopsy shows panarteritis with infiltration of mononuclear cells, giant cells within vessel wall, fragmentation of internal elastic lamina, and proliferation of intima.
■ Takayasu's arteritis:
– Hb level is decreased.
– Leukocytosis is present.
– Lupus erythematosus cell preparation is positive and ESR is elevated.
– Arteriography shows calcification and obstruction of affected vessels.
– Tissue biopsy shows inflammation of adventitia and intima of vessels and thickening of vessel walls.
■ Hypersensitivity vasculitis:
– History includes exposure to an antigen, such as a microorganism or a drug.
– Tissue biopsy may show leukocytoclastic angiitis (usually in postcapillary venules), with infiltration of polymorphonuclear leukocytes, fibrinoid necrosis, and extravasation of erythrocytes.
■ Mucocutaneous lymph node syndrome:
– History and examination reveal fever, nonsuppurative cervical adenitis, edema, congested conjunctivae, desquamation of fingertips, and erythema of oral cavity, lips, and palms.
– Tissue biopsy may show intimal proliferation and infiltration of vessel walls with mononuclear cells.

Velopharyngeal insufficiency

■ Examination reveals unintelligible speech.
■ Fiber-optic nasopharyngoscopy permits monitoring of velopharyngeal patency during speech and may identify the insufficiency.
■ Ultrasonography shows air-tissue overlap reflecting the degree of velopharyngeal sphincter incompetence; an opening of > 20 mm^2 results in unintelligible speech.

Ventricular aneurysm

■ History includes persistent arrhythmias, onset of heart failure, or systemic embolization in a patient with left ventricular failure and a history of myocardial infarction.
■ CXR reveals an abnormal bulge distorting the heart's contour (with large aneurysm).
■ Left ventriculography reveals left ventricular enlargement, with an area of akinesia or dyskinesia and diminished cardiac function.
■ Echocardiography reveals abnormal motion in the left ventricular wall.

Ventricular fibrillation

■ ECG findings include:
– Atrial rhythm isn't measurable.
– Ventricular rhythm has no pattern or regularity.
– Atrial and ventricular rates aren't measurable.
– P wave and PR interval aren't measurable.
– Duration of the QRS complex isn't measurable; configuration is wide and irregular.
– T wave isn't measurable.

Ventricular septal defect

■ Echocardiography or MRI reveals a large defect and its location in the septum, estimates the size of a left-to-right shunt, suggests pulmonary hypertension, and identifies associated lesions and complications.
■ Cardiac catheterization determines the size and exact location of the defect, calculates the degree of shunting, determines the extent of pulmonary hypertension, and detects associated defects.
■ CXR is normal with small defects; in large defects, it shows cardiomegaly, left atrial and ventricular enlargement, and prominent pulmonary vascular markings.
■ ECG is normal with small defects; in large defects, it shows left and right ventricular hypertrophy.

Ventricular tachycardia

■ ECG findings include:
– Atrial rhythm isn't measurable. Ventricular rhythm is usually regular, but may be slightly irregular.
– Atrial rate can't be measured. Ventricular rate is usually rapid (140 to 220 beats/minute).
– P wave is usually absent. It may be obscured by and is dissociated from the QRS complex. Retrograde and upright P waves may be present.
– PR interval isn't measurable.
– QRS complex has a duration > 0.12 second, has a bizarre appearance, and usually has increased amplitude.
– T wave occurs in the opposite direction of the QRS complex.
– QT interval isn't measurable.

Vesicoureteral reflux

■ History includes symptoms of urinary tract infection.
■ Examination reveals hematuria or strong-smelling urine (in infants).
■ Palpation may reveal a hard, thickened bladder (if posterior urethral valves are causing an obstruction in male infants).
■ Cystoscopy reveals reflux.

■ Urinalysis reveals bacterial count > 100,000/ml; specific gravity < 1.010, and increased pH.
■ Excretory urography may show dilated lower ureter, ureter visible for its entire length, hydronephrosis, calyceal distortion, and renal scarring.
■ Voiding cystourethrography identifies and determines the degree of reflux, shows when reflux occurs, and may also pinpoint the cause.
■ Bladder catheterization identifies the amount of residual urine.

Vitamin A deficiency
■ History includes inadequate dietary intake of foods high in vitamin A.
■ Ocular examination reveals xerophthalmia, Bitot's spots, perforation, and scarring.
■ Serum levels of vitamin A are < 20 µg/dl (SI, < 0.70 µmol/L).
■ Carotene levels are < 40 µg/dl (SI, < 0.76 µmol/L).

Vitamin B deficiencies
■ History includes inadequate dietary intake of foods high in vitamin B.
■ Serum vitamin B_2 is < 2 µg/dl.
■ 24-hour urine test reveals:
– thiamine deficiency
– riboflavin deficiency
– niacin deficiency
– pyridoxine deficiency.

Vitamin C deficiency
■ History includes inadequate intake of ascorbic acid.
■ Serum ascorbic acid levels are < 0.2 mg/dl (SI, < 11.5 µmol/L).

Vitamin D deficiency
■ History includes inadequate dietary intake of preformed vitamin D.
■ Serum vitamin D_3 levels are low or undetectable.
■ Serum calcium levels are < 7.5 mg/dl (SI, < 1.88 mmol/L).
■ Alkaline phosphatase levels are < 4 Bodansky units/dl.
■ X-rays reveal characteristic bone deformities and abnormalities such as Looser's zones.

Vitamin E deficiency
■ History includes diet high in polyunsaturated fatty acids fortified with iron but not vitamin E.
■ Serum vitamin E levels are < 5 µg/ml (SI, < 12 µmol/L).
■ Serum CK levels are increased.
■ Platelet levels are increased.

Vitamin K deficiency
■ PT is 25% longer than the normal range of 10 to 20 seconds (in the absence of anticoagulant therapy or hepatic disease).
■ Capillary fragility test is positive.

Vitiligo
■ Examination reveals stark white skin patches.
■ Wood's light examination in a darkened room detects vitiliginous patches; depigmented skin reflects the light, while pigmented skin absorbs it.

Vocal cord nodules and polyps
■ History includes persistent hoarseness.
■ Indirect laryngoscopy initially shows small red nodes; later, white solid nodes appear on one or both cords.
■ Indirect laryngoscopy shows unilateral or, occasionally, bilateral, sessile or pedunculated polyps of varying size anywhere on the vocal cords.

Vocal cord paralysis
■ History and examination reveal hoarseness or airway obstruction.

■ Indirect laryngoscopy reveals one or both cords fixed in an adducted or partially abducted position.

Volvulus

■ History includes sudden onset of severe abdominal pain.
■ Examination reveals palpable abdominal mass.
■ Abdominal X-rays reveal obstruction and abnormal air-fluid levels in the sigmoid and cecum (in midgut volvulus, abdominal X-rays may be normal).
■ Barium enema findings include:
– In cecal volvulus, barium fills the colon distal to the section of cecum.
– In sigmoid volvulus in children, barium may twist to a point; in adults, barium may take on an "ace of spades" configuration.
■ In midgut volvulus, upper GI series reveals obstruction and possibly a twisted contour in a narrow area near the duodenojejunal junction where barium won't pass.
■ WBC count is elevated, indicating strangulation or bowel infarction.

Von Willebrand's disease

■ History reveals family inheritance pattern.
■ Bleeding time is prolonged.
■ PTT is prolonged.
■ Factor VIII-related antigens are decreased and factor VIII activity level is low.
■ Clot retraction and platelet aggregation are normal.

Vulvovaginitis

■ Examination reveals vaginal discharge and inflammation of the vulva.
■ Culture of vaginal exudate identifies presence of *Trichomonas vaginalis, Candida albicans, Gardnerella vaginitis, Neisseria gonorrhoeae,* or *Phthirus pubis.*

Warts

■ Visual examination reveals evidence of irregular growth on skin.
■ Sigmoidoscopy may rule out internal involvement in recurrent anal warts.

Whooping cough

■ Examination reveals forceful coughing that ends in a characteristic whoop.
■ Nasopharyngeal swabs and sputum cultures identify *Bordetella pertussis* (in the early stages of illness).
■ WBC count is markedly elevated, with 60% to 90% lymphocytes.

Wilms' tumor

■ Examination reveals palpable abdominal mass in early childhood.
■ Gallium scan reveals abnormal activity.
■ Percutaneous renal biopsy reveals malignant cells.
■ Excretory urography doesn't indicate neoplasm or extrarenal mass.

Wilson's disease

■ Slit-lamp ophthalmic examination reveals Kayser-Fleischer rings (in advanced disease).
■ Liver biopsy reveals excessive copper deposits and tissue changes indicative of chronic active hepatitis, fatty liver, or cirrhosis.
■ Serum ceruloplasmin is < 22.9 mg/dl (SI, < 0.22 g/L).
■ Urine copper is > 100 μg/24 hours (SI, > 1.6 μmol/24 hours); may be as high as 1,000 μg (SI, > 16 μmol).

Wiskott-Aldrich syndrome

■ History includes thrombocytopenia, bleeding disorders at birth, and recurrent infections.
■ Platelet count is markedly decreased.
■ IgE levels are normal or elevated, IgG and IgA levels are normal, and IgM levels are decreased.

■ Isohemagglutinin levels are low or absent.
■ Sputum and throat cultures commonly identify *Streptococcus pneumoniae,* meningococci, or *Haemophilus influenzae* as the causative organisms.

Wounds, open trauma

■ History includes injury.
■ Examination reveals open wound.
■ X-rays show bone damage, extent of injury to the area and surrounding tissue, and retention of injuring object.
■ EMG reveals isolated, irregular motor unit potentials with increased amplitude and duration indicating peripheral nerve injury.
■ Nerve conduction studies reveal abnormal nerve conduction time indicating peripheral nerve injury.
■ CBC reveals decreased Hb and HCT levels and increased WBC count.

X-linked infantile hypogammaglobulinemia

■ Serum IgM, IgA, and IgG are decreased or absent (in patient at least age 9 months).
■ Antigenic stimulation testing confirms an inability to produce specific antibodies, although cellular immunity remains intact.

Yellow fever

■ Blood culture reveals presence of arbovirus.
■ Urine albumin levels are increased (in 90% of patients).
■ Antibody titer is elevated.

Zinc deficiency

■ History includes excessive intake of foods containing iron, calcium, vitamin D, and the fiber and phytates in cereals.
■ Serum zinc levels are < 121 µg/dl (SI, < 18.4 µmol/L).

PART TWO

Diagnostic tests

1

Hematology and coagulation tests

Red Blood Cells

Red Blood Cell Count

The red blood cell (RBC) count, also called an erythrocyte count, is part of a complete blood count. It's used to detect the number of RBCs in a microliter (µl), or cubic millimeter (mm^3), of whole blood.

Purpose

- To provide data for calculating mean corpuscular volume and mean corpuscular hemoglobin, which reveal RBC size and hemoglobin content
- To support other hematologic tests for diagnosing anemia or polycythemia

Patient preparation

- Explain to the patient that this test is used to evaluate the number of RBCs and to detect possible blood disorders.
- Tell the patient that a blood sample will be taken. Explain who will perform the venipuncture and when.
- Explain to the patient that he may feel slight discomfort from the needle puncture and the tourniquet.
- If the patient is a child, explain to him (if he's old enough) and his parents that a small amount of blood will be taken from the finger or earlobe.
- Inform the patient that he need not restrict food and fluids.

Procedure and posttest care

- For adults and older children, draw venous blood into a 3- or 4.5-ml (EDTA) sodium metabisultite solution tube.
- For younger children, collect capillary blood in a microcollection device.
- Ensure that subdermal bleeding has stopped before removing pressure.
- If a hematoma develops at the venipuncture site, apply warm soaks.

Precautions

- Completely fill the collection tube.
- Invert the tube gently several times to mix the sample and the anticoagulant.
- Handle the sample gently to prevent hemolysis.

Reference values

Normal RBC values vary, depending on the type of sample and on the patient's age and sex, as follows:

- adult males: 4.5 to 5.5 million RBCs/µl (SI, 4.5 to 5.5 $\times$ 10^{12}/L) of venous blood
- adult females: 4 to 5 million RBCs/µl (SI, 4 to 5 $\times$ 10^{12}/L) of venous blood
- children ages from 4.6 to 4.8 million/µl (SI, 4.6 to 4.8 $\times$ 10^{12}/L) of venous blood
- full-term neonates: 4.4 to 5.8 million/µl (SI, 4.4 to 5.8 $\times$ 10^{12}/L) of capillary blood at birth, decreasing to 3 to 3.8 million /µl (SI, 3 to 3.8 $\times$ 10^{12}/L) at age 2 months, and increasing slowly thereafter.

Normal values may exceed these levels in patients living at high altitudes or those who are very active.

Abnormal findings

An elevated RBC count may indicate absolute or relative polycythemia. A depressed count may indicate anemia, fluid overload, or hemorrhage beyond 24 hours. Further tests, such as stained cell examination, hematocrit, hemoglobin, red cell indices, and white cell studies, are needed to confirm the diagnosis.

Interfering factors

- Failure to use the proper anticoagulant or to adequately mix the sample and the anticoagulant
- Hemoconcentration due to prolonged tourniquet constriction
- Hemodilution due to drawing the sample from the same arm used for I.V. infusion of fluids
- High white blood cell count (false-high test results in semiautomated and automated counters)
- Diseases that cause RBCs to agglutinate or form rouleaux (false decrease)
- Hemolysis due to rough handling of the sample or drawing the blood through a small-gauge needle for venipuncture

HEMATOCRIT

A hematocrit (HCT) test may be done separately or as part of a complete blood count. It measures percentage by volume of packed red blood cells (RBCs) in a whole blood sample; for example, an HCT of 40% indicates that a 100-ml sample of blood contains 40 ml of packed RBCs. Packing is achieved by centrifuging anticoagulated whole blood in a capillary tube so that red cells are tightly packed without hemolysis.

Purpose

- To aid diagnosis of polycythemia, anemia, or abnormal states of hydration
- To aid calculation of erythrocyte indices

Patient preparation

- Explain to the patient that HCT is tested to detect anemia and other abnormal blood conditions.
- Tell the patient that the test requires a blood sample. Explain who will perform the venipuncture and when.
- Tell the patient he may experience transient discomfort from the needle puncture and pressure of the tourniquet.
- If the patient is a child, explain to him (if he's old enough) and his parents that a small amount of blood will be taken from the finger or earlobe.
- Inform the patient that he need not restrict food and fluids.

Procedure and posttest care

- Perform a fingerstick using a heparinized capillary tube with a red band on the anticoagulant end.
- Fill the capillary tube from the red-banded end to about two-thirds capacity; seal this end with clay.
- Alternatively, perform a venipuncture and fill a 3- or 4.5-ml EDTA tube.
- Ensure subdermal bleeding has stopped before removing pressure.
- If a hematoma develops at the venipuncture site, apply warm soaks. If the hematoma is large, monitor pulses distal to the venipuncture site.

Precautions

- Send the sample to the laboratory immediately.
- If you perform the test, place the tube in the centrifuge with the red end pointing outward.
- Fill the collection tube completely.
- Invert the tube gently several times to mix the sample.

Reference values

HCT is usually measured electronically. The results are 3% lower than manual measurements, which trap plasma in the column of packed RBCs.

Reference values vary, depending on the type of sample, the laboratory performing the test, and the patient's age and sex, as follows:

- neonates: 55% to 68% (SI, 0.55 to 0.68)
- neonates age 1 week: 47% to 65% (SI, 0.47 to 0.65)
- infants age 1 month: 37% to 49% (SI, 0.37 to 0.49)
- infants age 3 months: 30% to 36% (SI, 0.3 to 0.36)
- age 1 year: 29% to 41% (SI, 0.29 to 0.41)
- age 10 years: 36% to 40% (SI, 0.36 to 0.4)
- adult males: 42% to 52% (SI, 0.42 to 0.52)
- adult females: 36% to 48% (SI, 0.36 to 0.48)

Abnormal findings

Low HCT suggests anemia, hemodilution, or massive blood loss. High HCT indicates polycythemia or hemoconcentration due to blood loss and dehydration.

Interfering factors

- Failure to fill the tube properly, to use the proper anticoagulant, or to adequately mix the sample and the anticoagulant
- Hemolysis due to rough handling of the sample or drawing the blood through a small-gauge needle for venipuncture
- Hemoconcentration due to tourniquet constriction for longer than 1 minute (increase, typically 2.5% to 5%)
- Hemodilution due to drawing the blood from arm above an I.V. infusion

RED CELL INDICES

Using the results of the red blood cell (RBC) count, hematocrit (HCT), and total hemoglobin (Hb) tests, red cell indices (erythrocyte indices) provide important information about the size, Hb concentration, and Hb weight of an average RBC.

Purpose

- To aid diagnosis and classification of anemias

Patient preparation

- Explain to the patient that this test helps determine if he has anemia.
- Tell the patient that a blood sample will be taken. Explain who will perform the venipuncture and when.
- Explain to the patient that he may feel slight discomfort from the needle puncture and the tourniquet.

Procedure and posttest care

- Perform a venipuncture and collect the sample in a 3- or 4.5-ml EDTA tube.
- Ensure subdermal bleeding has stopped before removing pressure.
- If a hematoma develops at the venipuncture site, apply warm soaks. If the hematoma is large, monitor pulses distal to the phlebotomy site.

Precautions

- Completely fill the collection tube and invert it gently several times to adequately mix the sample and the anticoagulant.
- Handle the sample gently to prevent hemolysis.

Reference values

The indices tested include mean corpuscular volume (MCV), mean corpuscular hemoglobin (MCH), and mean corpuscular hemoglobin concentration (MCHC).

MCV, the ratio of HCT (packed cell volume) to the RBC count, expresses the average size of the erythrocytes and

Comparative red cell indices in anemias

	NORMAL VALUES (Normocytic, normochromic)	IRON DEFICIENCY ANEMIA (Microcytic, hypochromic)	PERNICIOUS ANEMIA (Macrocytic, normochromic)
MCV	84 to 99 μm^3	60 to 80 μm^3	96 to 150 μm^3
MCH	26 to 32 pg/cell	5 to 25 pg/cell	33 to 53 pg/cell
MCHC	30 to 36 g/dl	20 to 30 g/dl	33 to 38 g/dl

Key:
MCV= Mean corpuscular volume
MCH= Mean corpuscular hemoglobin
MCHC= Mean corpuscular hemoglobin concentration

indicates whether they're undersized (microcytic), oversized (macrocytic), or normal (normocytic). MCH, the Hb-RBC ratio, gives the weight of Hb in an average red cell. MCHC, the ratio of Hb weight to HCT, defines the concentration of Hb in 100 ml of packed RBCs. It helps to distinguish normally colored (normochromic) RBCs from paler (hypochromic) RBCs.

The range of normal red cell indices is as follows:

- MCV: 84 to 99 μm^3
- MCH: 26 to 32 pg/cell
- MCHC: 30 to 36 g/dl.

Abnormal findings

Low MCV and MCHC indicate microcytic, hypochromic anemias caused by iron deficiency anemia, pyridoxine-responsive anemia, or thalassemia. A high MCV suggests macrocytic anemias caused by megaloblastic anemias, folic acid or vitamin B_{12} deficiency, inherited disorders of deoxyribonucleic acid synthesis, or reticulocytosis. Because MCV reflects the average volume of many cells, a value within the normal range can encompass RBCs of varying size, from microcytic to macrocytic. (See *Comparative red cell indices in anemias.*)

Interfering factors

- Failure to use the proper anticoagulant or to adequately mix the sample and the anticoagulant
- Hemolysis due to rough handling of the sample or use of a small-gauge needle for blood aspiration
- Hemoconcentration due to prolonged tourniquet constriction
- High white blood cell count (false-high RBC count in semiautomated and automated counters, invalidating MCV and MCHC results)
- Falsely elevated Hb values invalidate MCH and MCHC results
- Diseases that cause RBCs to agglutinate or form rouleaux (false-low RBC count)

ERYTHROCYTE SEDIMENTATION RATE

The erythrocyte sedimentation rate (ESR) measures the degree of erythrocyte settling in a blood sample during a specified time period. The ESR is a sensitive but nonspecific test that's commonly the earliest indicator of disease when other chemical or physical signs are normal. The ESR usually increases significantly in widespread inflammatory disorders; elevations may be prolonged in localized inflammation and malignant disease.

Purpose

- To monitor inflammatory or malignant disease
- To aid detection and diagnosis of occult disease, such as tuberculosis, tissue necrosis, or connective tissue disease

Patient preparation

- Explain to the patient that this test is used to evaluate the condition of red blood cells.
- Tell the patient that a blood sample will be taken. Explain who will perform the venipuncture and when.
- Explain to the patient that he may feel slight discomfort from the needle puncture and the tourniquet.
- Inform the patient that he need not restrict food and fluids.

Procedure and posttest care

- Perform a venipuncture and collect the sample in a 4.5-ml tube with EDTA added or a tube with sodium citrate added. (Check with the laboratory to determine its preference.)
- Ensure subdermal bleeding has stopped before removing pressure.
- If a hematoma develops at the venipuncture site, apply warm soaks. If the hematoma is large, monitor pulses distal to the phlebotomy site.

Precautions

- Completely fill the collection tube and invert it gently several times to thoroughly mix the sample and the anticoagulant.
- Because prolonged standing decreases the ESR, examine the sample for clots or clumps and send it to the laboratory immediately. It must be tested within 2 to 4 hours.
- Handle the sample gently to prevent hemolysis.

Reference values

The ESR normally ranges from 0 to 10 mm/hour (SI, 0 to 10 mm/hour) in males, 0 to 20 mm/ hour (SI, 0 to 20 mm/hour) in females. Rates gradually increase with age.

Abnormal findings

The ESR rises in pregnancy, anemia, acute or chronic inflammation, tuberculosis, paraproteinemias (especially multiple myeloma and Waldenström's macroglobulinemia), rheumatic fever, rheumatoid arthritis, and some cancers.

Polycythemia, sickle cell anemia, hyperviscosity, and low plasma fibrinogen or globulin levels tend to depress the ESR.

Interfering factors

- Failure to use the proper anticoagulant, to adequately mix the sample and the anticoagulant, or to send the sample to the laboratory immediately
- Use of a small-gauge needle for blood aspirations
- Hemolysis due to rough handling or excessive mixing of the sample
- Hemoconcentration due to prolonged tourniquet constriction

RETICULOCYTE COUNT

Reticulocytes are nonnucleated, immature red blood cells (RBCs) that remain in the peripheral blood for 24 to 48 hours while maturing. They're generally larger than mature RBCs. In the reticulocyte count test, reticulocytes in a whole blood sample are counted and expressed as a percentage of the total RBC count. Because the manual method of reticulocyte counting uses only a small sample, values may be imprecise and should be compared with RBC count or hematocrit.

Purpose

- To aid in distinguishing between hypoproliferative and hyperproliferative anemias
- To help assess blood loss, bone marrow response to anemia, and therapy for anemia

Patient preparation

- Explain to the patient that this test is used to detect anemia or to monitor its treatment.
- Tell the patient that a blood sample will be taken. Explain who will perform the venipuncture and when.
- Explain to the patient that he may feel slight discomfort from the needle puncture and the tourniquet.
- If the patient is an infant or child, explain to the parents that a small amount of blood will be taken from the finger or earlobe.
- Notify the laboratory and physician of medications the patient is taking that may affect test results; they may need to be restricted.
- Inform the patient that he need not restrict food and fluids.

Procedure and posttest care

- Perform a venipuncture and collect the sample in a 3- or 4.5-ml EDTA tube.
- Ensure subdermal bleeding has stopped before removing pressure.
- If a hematoma develops at the venipuncture site, apply warm soaks. If the hematoma is large, monitor pulses distal to the phlebotomy site.
- Instruct the patient that he may resume medications discontinued before the test as ordered.
- Monitor the patient with an abnormal reticulocyte count for trends or significant changes in repeated tests.

Precautions

- Completely fill the collection tube and invert it gently several times to mix the sample and the anticoagulant.
- Handle the sample gently.

Reference values

Reticulocytes compose 0.5% to 2.5% (SI, 0.005 to 0.025) of the total RBC count. In infants the normal reticulocyte count ranges from 2% to 6% (SI, 0.002 to 0.006) at birth, decreasing to adult levels in 1 to 2 weeks.

Abnormal findings

A low reticulocyte count indicates hypoproliferative bone marrow (hypoplastic anemia) or ineffective erythropoiesis (pernicious anemia).

A high reticulocyte count indicates a bone marrow response to anemia caused by hemolysis or blood loss. The reticulocyte count may also increase after therapy for iron deficiency anemia or pernicious anemia.

Interfering factors

- Failure to use the proper anticoagulant or to adequately mix the sample and the anticoagulant
- Prolonged tourniquet constriction

- Azathioprine, chloramphenicol, dactinomycin, and methotrexate (possible false-low)
- Corticotropin, antimalarials, antipyretics, furazolidone (in infants), levodopa (possible false-high)
- Sulfonamides (possible false-low or false-high)
- Recent blood transfusion
- Hemolysis caused by rough handling of the sample or use of a small-gauge needle for blood aspiration

OSMOTIC FRAGILITY

Osmotic fragility measures red blood cell (RBC) resistance to hemolysis when exposed to a series of increasingly dilute saline solutions. The sooner hemolysis occurs, the greater the osmotic fragility of the cells.

Purpose

- To aid diagnosis of hereditary spherocytosis
- To confirm morphologic RBC abnormalities

Patient preparation

- Explain to the patient that this test is used to identify the cause of anemia.
- Tell the patient that a blood sample will be taken. Explain who will perform the venipuncture and when.
- Explain to the patient that he may feel slight discomfort from the needle puncture and the tourniquet.
- Inform the patient that he need not restrict food and fluids.

Procedure and posttest care

- Perform a venipuncture, collecting the sample in a 4.5-ml heparinized tube.
- If a hematoma develops at the venipuncture site, apply warm soaks.

Precautions

- Because this test isn't routinely performed, notify the laboratory before drawing the sample. Reference laboratories have certain guidelines and testing dates that you'll need to follow.
- Completely fill the collection tube and invert it gently several times to mix the sample and anticoagulant thoroughly.
- Handle the sample gently to prevent accidental hemolysis.

Reference values

Osmotic fragility values (percentage of RBCs hemolyzed) that have been obtained photometrically are plotted against decreasing saline tonicity to produce an S-shaped curve with a slope characteristic of the disorder. Reference values differ with tonicities.

Abnormal findings

Low osmotic fragility (increased resistance to hemolysis) is characteristic of thalassemia, iron deficiency anemia, sickle cell anemia, and other red blood cell disorders in which target cells are found. Low osmotic fragility also occurs after splenectomy.

High osmotic fragility (increased tendency to hemolysis) occurs in hereditary spherocytosis; in spherocytosis associated with autoimmune hemolytic anemia, severe burns, or chemical poisoning; or in hemolytic disease of the newborn (erythroblastosis fetalis).

Interfering factors

- Failure to use the proper anticoagulant in the collection tube, to fill the tube completely, or to adequately mix the sample and the anticoagulant
- Hemolysis due to rough handling of the sample

- Presence of hemolytic organisms in the sample
- Conditions such as severe anemia will provide fewer RBCs for testing
- Recent blood transfusion

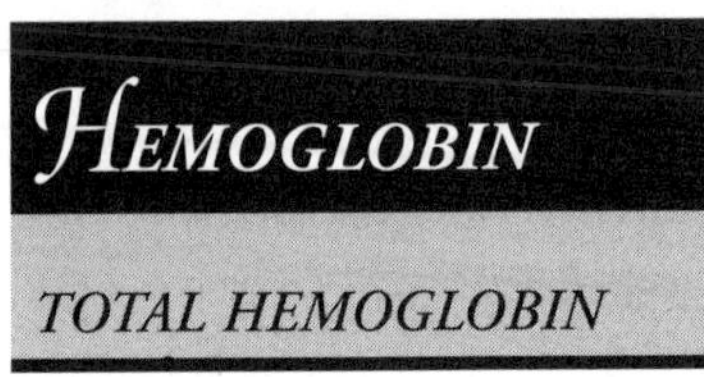

Total hemoglobin (Hb) is used to measure the amount of Hb found in a deciliter (dl, or 100 ml) of whole blood. It's usually part of a complete blood count. Hb concentration correlates closely with the red blood cell (RBC) count and affects the Hb-RBC ratio (MCH and MCHC).

Purpose

- To measure the severity of anemia or polycythemia and to monitor response to therapy
- To obtain data for calculating MCH and MCHC

Patient preparation

- Explain to the patient that this test is used to detect anemia or polycythemia, or to assess his response to treatment.
- Tell the patient that a blood sample will be taken. Explain who will perform the venipuncture and when.
- Explain to the patient that he may feel slight discomfort from the needle puncture and the tourniquet.
- If the patient is an infant or child, explain to the parents that a small amount of blood will be taken from the finger or earlobe.
- Inform the patient that he need not restrict food and fluids.

Procedure and posttest care

- For adults and older children, perform a venipuncture and collect the sample in a 3- or 4.5-ml tube with EDTA added.
- For younger children and infants, collect the sample by fingerstick or heel stick in a microcollection device with EDTA.
- If a hematoma develops at the venipuncture site, apply warm soaks. If the hematoma is large, monitor pulses distal to the venipuncture site.
- Ensure subdermal bleeding has stopped before removing pressure.

Precautions

- Completely fill the collection tube and invert it gently several times to thoroughly mix the sample and the anticoagulant.
- Handle the sample gently to prevent hemolysis.

Reference values

Hb concentration varies depending on the type of sample drawn and the patient's age and sex:

- neonates: 17 to 22 g/dL (SI, 170 to 220 g/L)
- 1 week: 15 to 20 g/dL (SI, 150 to 200 g/L)
- 1 month: 11 to 15 g/dL (SI, 110 to 150 g/L)
- children: 11 to 13 g/dL (SI, 110 to 130 g/L)
- adult males: 14 to 17.4 g/dL (SI, 140 to 174 g/L)
- males after middle age: 12.4 to 14.9 g/dL (SI, 124 to 149 g/L)
- adult females: 12 to 16 g/dl: (SI, 120 to 160 g/L)
- females after middle age: 11.7 to 13.8 g/dL (SI, 117 to 138 g/L)

Those who are more physically active or who live in high altitudes may have higher values.

Abnormal findings

Low Hb concentration may indicate anemia, recent hemorrhage, or fluid retention, causing hemodilution.

Elevated Hb suggests hemoconcentration from polycythemia or dehydration.

Interfering factors

- Failure to use the proper anticoagulant or to adequately mix the sample and the anticoagulant
- Hemolysis due to rough handling of the sample
- Hemoconcentration due to prolonged tourniquet constriction
- Very high white blood cell counts, lipemia, or RBCs that are resistant to lysis (false-high)

FETAL HEMOGLOBIN

Fetal hemoglobin (Hb), or Hb F, is a normal Hb produced in the red blood cells of a fetus and in smaller amounts in infants. It constitutes 50% to 90% of the Hb in a newborn; the remaining Hb consists of Hb A_1 and Hb A_2, the Hb in adults.

Under normal conditions, the body ceases to manufacture fetal Hb during the first years of life and begins to manufacture adult Hb. If this changeover doesn't occur and fetal Hb continues to constitute more than 5% of the Hb after age 6 months, an abnormality should be suspected, particularly thalassemia.

Purpose

- To diagnose thalassemia

Patient preparation

- Explain to the patient that this test is used to detect thalassemia disease.
- Tell the patient that a blood sample will be taken. Explain who will perform the venipuncture and when.
- Reassure the patient that drawing the sample will take less than 3 minutes.
- Explain to the patient that he may feel slight discomfort from the needle puncture and the tourniquet.
- If the patient is a child, explain to his parents that a small amount of blood will be taken from the finger or earlobe.
- Inform the patient or his parents that he need not restrict food and fluids.

Procedure and posttest care

- Perform a venipuncture and collect the sample of blood in a 4.5-ml EDTA tube.
- For a young child, collect capillary blood in a microcollection device.
- If a hematoma develops at the venipuncture site, apply warm soaks. If the hematoma is large, monitor pulses distal to the venipuncture site.
- Ensure subdermal bleeding has stopped before removing pressure.

Precautions

- Completely fill the collection tube and invert it gently several times to mix the sample and the anticoagulant thoroughly.
- Handle the sample gently to prevent hemolysis.

Reference values

Normal values for fetal Hb range as follows:

- age 0 to 30 days: 60% to 90% (SI, 0.60 to 0.90)
- age 1 to 23 months: 2% (SI, 0.02)
- age 24 months to adult: 0% to 2% (SI, 0 to 0.02).

Abnormal findings

In beta-thalassemia major, fetal Hb may be 30% or more of the total Hb. Slight increases in fetal Hb concentration appear in a variety of unrelated hematologic disorders, such as aplastic anemia, homozygous sickle cell disease, and myeloproliferative disorders. Fetal Hb commonly increases to as much as 5% during normal pregnancy.

Interfering factors

- Hemolysis due to rough handling of the sample
- Delay in analyzing the specimen for more than 2 to 3 hours (possible false-high)

HEMOGLOBIN ELECTROPHORESIS

Hemoglobin (Hb) electrophoresis is probably the most useful laboratory method for separating and measuring normal and some abnormal Hb. Through electrophoresis, different types of Hb are separated to form a series of distinctly pigmented bands in a medium. Results are then compared with those of a normal sample.

Hb A, A_2, S, and C are routinely checked, but the laboratory may change the medium or its pH to expand the range of this test.

Purpose

- To measure the amount of Hb A and to detect abnormal Hb
- To aid diagnosis of thalassemia

Patient preparation

- Explain to the patient that this test is used to evaluate Hb.
- Tell the patient that a blood sample will be taken. Explain who will perform the venipuncture and when.
- Explain to the patient that he may feel slight discomfort from the needle puncture and the tourniquet.
- If the patient is an infant or child, explain to the parents that a small amount of blood will be taken from the finger.
- Inform the patient that he need not restrict food and fluids.

Procedure and posttest care

- Perform a venipuncture and collect the sample in a 3- or 4.5-ml tube with EDTA added.
- For young children, collect capillary blood in a microcollection device.
- If a hematoma develops at the venipuncture site, apply warm soaks. If the hematoma is large, monitor pulses distal to the venipuncture site.
- Ensure subdermal bleeding has stopped before removing pressure.

Precautions

- Completely fill the collection tube and invert it gently several times to mix the sample and the anticoagulant.
- Don't shake the tube vigorously.

Reference values

In adults, Hb A accounts for 95% (SI, 0.95) of all Hb; Hb A_2, 1.5% to 3% (SI, 0.15 to 0.030); and Hb F < 2% (SI, < 0.02). In neonates, Hb F normally accounts for half the total. Hb S and Hb C are normally absent.

Abnormal findings

Hb electrophoresis allows identification of various types of Hb. Certain types may indicate a hemolytic disease. The chart on the opposite page shows some possible results and their associated conditions. (See *Variations of hemoglobin type and distribution.*)

Interfering factors

- Failure to fill the tube completely, to use the proper anticoagulant, or to adequately mix the sample and the anticoagulant

Variations of hemoglobin type and distribution

HEMOGLOBIN	PERCENTAGE OF TOTAL HEMOGLOBIN	CLINICAL IMPLICATIONS
Hb A	95% to 100% (SI, 0.95 to 1.0)	Normal
Hb A_2	4% to 5.8% (SI, 0.04 to 0.058) 1.5% to 3% (SI, 0.015 to 0.03) Under 1.5% (SI, < 0.015)	β-thalassemia minor Normal Hb H disease
Hb F	Under 1% (SI, < 0.01) 2% to 5% (SI, 0.02 to 0.05) 10% to 90% (SI, 0.10 to 0.9) 5% to 15% (SI, 0.05 to 0.15) 5% to 35% (SI, 0.05 to 0.35) 100% (SI, 1.0) 15% (SI, 0.15)	Normal β-thalassemia minor β-thalassemia major β-δ-thalassemia minor Heterozygous hereditary persistence of fetal Hb (HPFH) Homozygous HPFH Homozygous Hb S
Homozygous Hb S	70% to 98% (SI, 0.7 to 0.98)	Sickle cell disease
Homozygous Hb C	90% to 98% (SI, 0.9 to 0.98)	Hb C disease
Heterozygous Hb C	24% to 44% (SI, 0.24 to 0.44)	Hb C trait

- Hemolysis due to rough handling of the sample
- Blood transfusion within the past 4 months

SICKLE CELLS

The sickle cell test, also known as the hemoglobin (Hb) S test, is used to detect sickle cells, which are severely deformed, rigid erythrocytes that may slow blood flow. Sickle cell trait (characterized by heterozygous Hb S) is found almost exclusively in blacks: 0.2% of the blacks born in the United States have sickle cell disease.

Although the sickle cell test is useful as a rapid screening procedure, it may produce erroneous results. Hb electrophoresis should be performed to confirm the diagnosis if sickle cell disease is strongly suspected.

Purpose

- To identify sickle cell disease and sickle cell trait

Patient preparation

- Explain to the patient that this test is used to detect sickle cell disease.

- Tell the patient that a blood sample will be taken. Explain who will perform the venipuncture and when.
- Explain to the patient that he may feel slight discomfort from the needle puncture and the tourniquet.
- If the patient is an infant or child, explain to his parents that a small amount of blood will be taken from the finger or earlobe.
- Check the patient's history for a blood transfusion within the past 3 months.
- Inform the patient that he need not restrict food and fluids.

Procedure and posttest care

- Perform a venipuncture and collect the sample in a 3- or 4.5-ml EDTA tube.
- For young children, collect capillary blood in a microcollection device.
- If a hematoma develops at the venipuncture site, apply warm soaks. If the hematoma is large, monitor pulses distal to the phlebotomy site.
- Ensure subdermal bleeding has stopped before removing pressure.

Precautions

- Completely fill the collection tube and invert it gently several times to thoroughly mix the sample and the anticoagulant.
- Don't shake the tube vigorously.

Normal findings

Results of this test are reported as positive or negative. A negative result suggests the absence of Hb S.

Abnormal findings

A positive result may indicate the presence of sickle cells, but Hb electrophoresis is needed to further diagnose the sickling tendency of cells. Rarely, in the absence of Hb S, other abnormal Hb may cause sickling.

Interfering factors

- Failure to fill the tube completely, to use the proper anticoagulant in the collection tube, or to adequately mix the sample and the anticoagulant
- Hemolysis due to rough handling of the sample or use of a small-gauge needle for blood aspiration
- Hb concentration < 10%, elevated Hb S levels in infants under age 6 months, or transfusion within 3 months of the test (possible false-negative)

UNSTABLE HEMOGLOBIN

Unstable hemoglobin (Hb) is a rare, congenital defect caused by amino acid substitutions in the structure of Hb. It's called "unstable" because of the ease with which the Hb decomposes. The presence of unstable Hb may lead to the formation of small masses called Heinz bodies, which accumulate on red blood cell membranes. Although Heinz bodies are usually removed by the spleen or liver, they may cause mild to severe hemolysis. Unstable Hb is best detected by precipitation tests (heat stability or isopropanol solubility).

Purpose

- To detect unstable Hb

Patient preparation

- Explain to the patient that this test is used to detect abnormal Hb in the blood.
- Tell the patient that a blood sample will be taken. Explain who will perform the venipuncture and when.
- Explain to the patient that he may feel slight discomfort from the needle puncture and the tourniquet.

- Notify the laboratory and physician of medications the patient is taking that may affect test results; they may need to be restricted.
- Inform the patient that he need not restrict food and fluids.

Procedure and posttest care

- Perform a venipuncture and collect the sample in a 3- or 4.5-ml tube with EDTA added.
- If a hematoma develops at the venipuncture site, apply warm soaks. If the hematoma is large, monitor pulses distal to the venipuncture site.
- Ensure subdermal bleeding has stopped before removing pressure.
- Instruct the patient that he may resume medications discontinued before the test as ordered.

Precautions

- Completely fill the collection tube and invert it gently several times to mix the sample and the anticoagulant thoroughly.
- To avoid hemolysis, don't shake the tube vigorously.

Normal findings

When no unstable Hb appears in the sample, the heat stability test result is negative; the isopropanol solubility test result is reported as stable.

Abnormal findings

A positive heat stability test result or unstable solubility test result, especially with hemolysis, strongly suggests the presence of unstable Hb.

Interfering factors

- Failure to fill the tube completely, to use the proper anticoagulant, or to adequately mix the sample and the anticoagulant
- Hemoconcentration due to prolonged tourniquet constriction
- Hemolysis due to rough handling of the sample
- Hemolysis due to antimalarials, furazolidone (in infants), nitrofurantoin, phenacetin, procarbazine, sulfonamides (possible false-positive or unstable results)
- High levels of Hb F (possible false-positive isopropanol)
- Recent blood transfusion

HEINZ BODIES

Heinz bodies are particles of decomposed hemoglobin that precipitate from the cytoplasm of red blood cells (RBCs) and accumulate on RBC membranes. Although Heinz bodies are removed from RBCs by the spleen, they're a major cause of hemolytic anemias.

Heinz bodies can be detected in a whole blood sample using phase microscopy or supravital stains; when they don't form spontaneously, various oxidant drugs may be added to the sample to induce their formation.

Purpose

- To help detect causes of hemolytic anemia

Patient preparation

- Explain to the patient that this test is used to determine the cause of anemia.
- Tell the patient that a blood sample will be taken. Explain who will perform the venipuncture and when.
- Explain to the patient that he may feel slight discomfort from the needle puncture and the tourniquet.
- Notify the laboratory and physician of medications the patient is taking that may affect test results; they may need to be restricted.

- Inform the patient that he need not restrict food and fluids.

Procedure and posttest care

- Perform a venipuncture and collect the sample in a 3- or 4.5-ml tube with EDTA added.
- If a hematoma develops at the venipuncture site, apply warm soaks. If the hematoma is large, monitor pulses distal to the venipuncture site.
- Ensure subdermal bleeding has stopped before removing pressure.
- Instruct the patient that he may resume medications discontinued before the test as ordered.

Precautions

- Completely fill the sample collection tube.
- Invert the tube gently several times to mix the sample and the anticoagulant.

Normal findings

A negative test result indicates an absence of Heinz bodies.

Abnormal findings

The presence of Heinz bodies — a positive test result — may indicate an inherited RBC enzyme deficiency, the presence of unstable hemoglobin, thalassemia, or drug-induced RBC injury. Heinz bodies may also be present after splenectomy.

Interfering factors

- Failure to fill the collection tube completely, to use the appropriate anticoagulant, to adequately mix the sample and the anticoagulant, or to send the sample to the laboratory immediately
- Antimalarials, furazolidone (in infants), nitrofurantoin, phenacetin, procarbazine, sulfonamides (possible false-positive)
- Recent blood transfusion

IRON AND TOTAL IRON-BINDING CAPACITY

Iron is essential to the formation and function of hemoglobin as well as many other heme and nonheme compounds. After iron is absorbed by the intestine, it's distributed to various body compartments for synthesis, storage, and transport. Serum iron concentration is normally highest in the morning and declines progressively during the day; therefore, the sample should be drawn in the morning.

An iron assay is used to measure the amount of iron bound to transferrin in blood plasma. Total iron-binding capacity (TIBC) measures the amount of iron that would appear in plasma if all the transferrin were saturated with iron.

Serum iron and TIBC are of greater diagnostic usefulness when performed with the serum ferritin assay, but together these tests may not accurately reflect the state of other iron compartments, such as myoglobin iron and the labile iron pool. Bone marrow or liver biopsy, and iron absorption or excretion studies may yield more information.

Purpose

- To estimate total iron storage
- To aid diagnosis of hemochromatosis
- To help distinguish iron deficiency anemia from anemia of chronic disease (For information on another test used to differentiate anemias, see *Siderocyte stain.*)
- To help evaluate nutritional status

Patient preparation

- Explain to the patient that this test evaluates the body's capacity to store iron.

Siderocyte stain

Siderocytes are red blood cells (RBCs) containing particles of nonhemoglobin iron known as siderocytic granules. In neonates, siderocytic granules are normally present in normoblasts and reticulocytes during hemoglobin synthesis. However, the spleen removes most of these granules from normal RBCs, and they disappear rapidly with age.

In adults, an elevated siderocyte level usually indicates abnormal erythropoiesis, which may occur in congenital spherocytic anemia, chronic hemolytic anemias (such as the thalassemias), pernicious anemia, hemochromatosis, toxicities (such as lead poisoning), infection, or severe burns. Elevated levels may also follow splenectomy because the spleen normally removes siderocytic granules.

PERFORMING THE TEST

The siderocyte stain test measures the number of circulating siderocytes. Venous blood is drawn into a 3- or 4.5-ml EDTA tube or, for infants and children, collected in a Microtainer or a pipette and smeared directly on a 3″ × 5″ glass slide. When the blood smear is stained, siderocytic granules appear as purple-blue specks clustered around the periphery of mature erythrocytes. Cells containing these granules are counted as a percentage of total RBCs. The results aid differential diagnosis of the anemias and hemochromatosis and help detect toxicities.

INTERPRETING RESULTS

Normally, neonates have a slightly elevated siderocyte level that reaches the normal adult value of 0.5% (SI, 0.05) of total RBCs in 7 to 10 days. In patients with pernicious anemia, the siderocyte level is 8% to 14% (SI, 0.08 to 0.14); in chronic hemolytic anemia, 20% to 100% (SI, 0.20 to 1.00); in lead poisoning, 10% to 30% (SI, 0.10 to 0.30); and in hemochromatosis, 3% to 7% (SI, 0.03 to 0.07). A high siderocyte level calls for additional testing (including bone marrow examination) to determine the cause of abnormal erythropoiesis.

- Tell the patient that a blood sample will be taken. Explain who will perform the venipuncture and when.
- Explain to the patient that he may feel slight discomfort from the needle puncture and the tourniquet.
- Notify the laboratory and physician of medications the patient is taking that may affect test results; they may need to be restricted.
- Inform the patient that he need not restrict food and fluids.

Procedure and posttest care

- Perform a venipuncture and collect the sample in a 4.5-ml clot-activator.
- If a hematoma develops at the venipuncture site, apply warm soaks. If the hematoma is large, monitor pulses distal to the venipuncture site.
- Ensure subdermal bleeding has stopped before removing pressure.
- Instruct the patient that he may resume medications discontinued before the test as ordered.

Precautions

- Handle the sample gently to prevent hemolysis.
- Send the sample to the laboratory immediately.

Reference values

Normal serum iron and TIBC values are as follows:

- Serum iron
  - Males: 60 to 170 µg/dl (S1, 10.7 to 30.4 µmol/L)
  - Females: 50 to 130 µg/dl (S1, 9 to 23.3 µmol/L)
- TIBC
  - Males and females: 300 to 360 µg/dl (S1, 54 to 64 µmol/L)
- Saturation
  - Males and females: 20% to 50% (SI, 0.20 to 0.50).

Abnormal findings

In iron deficiency, serum iron levels decrease and TIBC increases, decreasing saturation. In cases of chronic inflammation (such as in rheumatoid arthritis), serum iron may be low in the presence of adequate body stores, but TIBC may remain unchanged or may decrease to preserve normal saturation. Iron overload may not alter serum levels until relatively late but, in general, serum iron increases and TIBC remains the same, which increases the saturation.

Interfering factors

- Hemolysis due to rough handling of the sample or failure to send the sample to the laboratory immediately
- Chloramphenicol and oral contraceptives (possible false-positive)
- Corticotropin (possible false-negative)
- Iron supplements (possible false-positive serum iron values but false-negative TIBC)

FERRITIN

Ferritin, a major iron-storage protein, normally appears in small quantities in serum. In healthy adults, serum ferritin levels are directly related to the amount of available iron stored in the body and can be measured accurately by radioimmunoassay.

Purpose

- To screen for iron deficiency and iron overload
- To measure iron storage
- To distinguish between iron deficiency (a condition of low iron storage) and chronic inflammation (a condition of normal storage)

Patient preparation

- Explain to the patient that this test is used to assess the available iron stored in the body.
- Tell the patient that a blood sample will be taken. Explain who will perform the venipuncture and when.
- Explain to the patient that he may feel slight discomfort from the needle puncture and the tourniquet.
- Review the patient's history for transfusion within the past 4 months.
- Inform the patient that he need not restrict food and fluids.

Procedure and posttest care

- Perform a venipuncture, collecting the sample in a 10-ml tube without additives.
- If a hematoma develops at the venipuncture site, apply warm soaks. If the hematoma is large, monitor pulses distal to the venipuncture site.
- Ensure subdermal bleeding has stopped before removing pressure.

Reference values

Normal serum ferritin values vary with age, as follows:

- neonates: 25 to 200 ng/ml (SI, 25 to 200 µg/L)
- age 1 month: 200 to 600 ng/ml (SI, 200 to 600 µg/L)

- age 2 to 5 months: 50 to 200 ng/ml (SI, 50 to 200 μg/L)
- age 6 months to 15 years: 7 to 140 mg/ml (SI, 7 to 140 μg/L)
- adult males: 20 to 300 ng/ml (SI, 20 to 300 μg/L)
- adult females: 20 to 120 ng/ml (SI, 20 to 120 μg/L).

Abnormal findings

High serum ferritin levels may indicate acute or chronic hepatic disease, iron overload, leukemia, acute or chronic infection or inflammation, Hodgkin's disease, or chronic hemolytic anemias. In these disorders, iron stores in the bone marrow may be normal or significantly increased. Serum ferritin levels are characteristically normal or slightly elevated in patients with chronic renal disease.

Low serum ferritin levels indicate chronic iron deficiency.

Interfering factor

- Recent blood transfusion (possible false-high)

METHEMOGLOBIN

Methemoglobin (MetHb, Hb M) is a structural hemoglobin (Hb) variant, which is formed when the heme portion of deoxygenated Hb is oxidized to a ferric state. When this occurs, the heme is incapable of combining with oxygen and transporting it to the tissues, and the patient becomes cyanotic.

Purpose

- To detect acquired methemoglobinemia, which is caused by excessive radiation or the toxic effects of chemicals or drugs
- To detect congenital methemoglobinemia

Patient preparation

- If possible, obtain a history of the patient's hematologic status and Hb disorder, conditions that produce nitrite, and exposure to sources of nitrites in drugs.
- Explain to the patient that this test is used to detect abnormal Hb in the blood.
- Tell the patient that a blood sample will be taken. Explain who will perform the venipuncture and when.
- Explain to the patient that he may feel slight discomfort from the needle puncture and the tourniquet.
- Notify the laboratory and physician of medications the patient is taking that may affect test results; they may need to be restricted.

Procedure and posttest care

- Perform a venipuncture and collect the sample in a 4.5-ml heparinized tube.
- If a hematoma develops at the venipuncture site, apply warm soaks.If the hematoma is large, monitor pulses distal to the venipuncture site.
- Ensure subdermal bleeding has stopped before removing pressure.

Precautions

- Completely fill the collection tube and invert it gently several times.
- To avoid hemolysis, don't shake the tube vigorously.
- Place the collection tube on ice and send it to the laboratory immediately.

Reference values

Normal MetHb levels are 0% to 1.5% (SI, 0 to 0.015) of total Hb.

Abnormal findings

Increased MetHb levels may indicate acquired or hereditary methemoglobinemia, or carbon monoxide poisoning. These levels can also be caused by use of certain drugs or exposure to certain substances.

Decreased MetHb levels may occur in pancreatitis.

Interfering factors

- Acetanilid, aniline dyes, nitroglycerin, benzocaine, chlorates, lidocaine, nitrates, nitrites, phenacetin, sulfonamides, radiation, primaquine, and resorcinol (possible increase)
- Nitrite toxicity in breast-feeding infants (increase due to conversion of inorganic nitrate to nitrite ion)

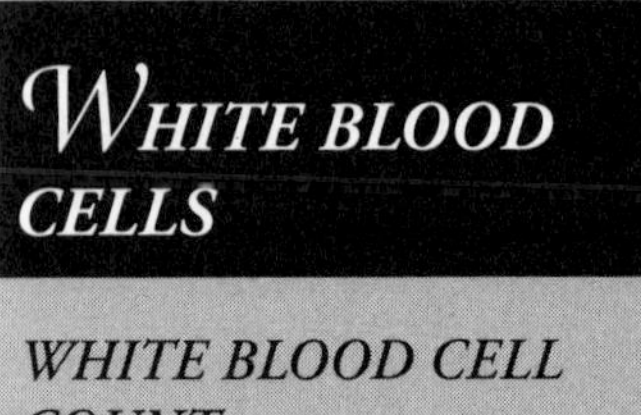

WHITE BLOOD CELLS

WHITE BLOOD CELL COUNT

A white blood cell (WBC) count, also called a leukocyte count, is part of a complete blood count. It indicates the number of white cells in a microliter (µl, or cubic millimeter) of whole blood.

WBC counts may vary by as much as 2,000 cells/µl (SI, 2×10^9/L) on any given day due to strenuous exercise, stress, or digestion. The WBC count may increase or decrease significantly in certain diseases, but is diagnostically useful only when the patient's white cell differential and clinical status are considered.

Purpose

- To determine infection or inflammation
- To determine the need for further tests, such as the WBC differential or bone marrow biopsy
- To monitor response to chemotherapy or radiation therapy

Patient preparation

- Explain to the patient that the test is used to detect an infection or inflammation.
- Tell the patient that a blood sample will be taken. Explain who will perform the venipuncture and when.
- Explain to the patient that he may feel slight discomfort from the needle puncture and the tourniquet.
- Inform the patient that he should avoid strenuous exercise for 24 hours before the test. Also tell him that he should avoid eating a heavy meal before the test.
- If the patient is being treated for an infection, advise him that this test will be repeated to monitor his progress.
- Notify the laboratory and physician of medications the patient is taking that may affect test results; they may need to be restricted.

Procedure and posttest care

- Perform a venipuncture and collect the sample in a 3- or 4.5-ml EDTA tube.
- If a hematoma develops at the venipuncture site, apply warm soaks. If the hematoma is large, monitor pulses distal to the venipuncture site.
- Ensure subdermal bleeding has stopped before removing pressure.
- Instruct the patient that he may resume his usual diet, activity, and medications discontinued before the test as ordered.
- A patient with severe leukopenia may have little or no resistance to infection and requires protective isolation.

Precautions

- Completely fill the sample collection tube.

■ Invert the sample gently several times to mix the sample and the anticoagulant.

Reference values

WBC count ranges from 4,000 to 10,000/µl (SI, 4 to 10 × 10^9/L).

Abnormal findings

An elevated WBC count (leukocytosis) often signals infection, such as an abscess, meningitis, appendicitis, or tonsillitis. A high count may also result from leukemia and tissue necrosis due to burns, myocardial infarction, or gangrene.

A low WBC count (leukopenia) indicates bone marrow depression that may result from viral infections or from toxic reactions, such as those following treatment with antineoplastics, ingestion of mercury or other heavy metals, or exposure to benzene or arsenicals. Leukopenia characteristically accompanies influenza, typhoid fever, measles, infectious hepatitis, mononucleosis, and rubella.

Interfering factors

■ Hemolysis due to rough handling of the sample

■ Exercise, stress, or digestion

■ Most antineoplastics; anti-infectives, such as metronidazole and flucytosine; anticonvulsants, such as phenytoin derivatives; thyroid hormone antagonists; and nonsteroidal anti-inflammatory drugs such as indomethacin (decrease)

WHITE BLOOD CELL DIFFERENTIAL

The white blood cell (WBC) differential is used to evaluate the distribution and morphology of WBCs, providing more specific information about a patient's immune system than the WBC count alone.

WBCs are classified as one of five major types of leukocytes — neutrophils, eosinophils, basophils, lymphocytes, and monocytes — and the percentage of each type is determined. The differential count is the percentage of each type of WBC in the blood. The total number of each type of WBC is obtained by multiplying the percentage of each type by the total WBC count.

High levels of these leukocytes are associated with various allergic diseases and reactions to parasites. An eosinophil count is sometimes ordered as a follow-up test when an elevated or depressed eosinophil level is reported.

Purpose

■ To evaluate the body's capacity to resist and overcome infection

■ To detect and identify various types of leukemia

■ To determine the stage and severity of an infection

■ To detect allergic reactions and parasitic infections, and assess their severity (eosinophil count)

■ To distinguish viral from bacterial infections

Patient preparation

■ Explain to the patient that this test is used to evaluate the immune system.

■ Notify the laboratory and physician of medications the patient is taking that may affect test results; they may need to be restricted.

■ Tell the patient that a blood sample will be taken. Explain who will perform the venipuncture and when.

■ Inform the patient that he need not restrict food and fluids, but should refrain from strenuous exercise for 24 hours before the test.

Interpreting WBC differential values

The differential count measures the types of white blood cells (WBCs) as a percentage of the total WBC count (the relative value). The absolute value is obtained by multiplying the relative value of each cell type by the total WBC count. The relative and absolute values must be considered to obtain an accurate diagnosis.

For example, consider a patient whose WBC count is 6,000/µl (SI, 6×10^9/L) and whose differential shows 30% (SI, 0.30) neutrophils and 70% (SI, 0.70) lymphocytes. His relative lymphocyte count seems to be quite high (lymphocytosis), but when this figure is multiplied by his WBC count (6,000 × 70% = 4,200 lymphocytes/µl), (SI, 6×10^9/L $\times$ 9.79 = 4.2×10^9/L lymphocytes), it's well within the normal range.

However, this patient's neutrophil count (30%) (SI, 0.30) is low; when this figure is multiplied by the WBC count (6,000 × 30% = 1,800 neutrophils/ml) (SI, 6×10^9/L $\times$ 0.30 = 1.8×10^9/L neutrophils), the result is a low absolute number, which may mean depressed bone marrow.

The normal percentages of WBC type in adults are:
Neutrophils: 54% to 75% (SI, 0.54 to 0.75)
Eosinophils: 1% to 4% (SI, 0.01 to 0.04)
Basophils: 0% to 1% (SI, 0 to 0.01)
Monocytes: 2% to 8% (SI, 0.02 to 0.08)
Lymphocytes: 25% to 40% (SI, 0.25 to 0.40)

- Explain to the patient that he may feel slight discomfort from the needle puncture and the tourniquet.

Procedure and posttest care

- Perform a venipuncture, collecting the sample in a 3- or 4.5-ml EDTA tube.
- If a hematoma develops at the venipuncture site, apply warm soaks. If the hematoma is large, monitor pulses distal to the venipuncture site.
- Ensure subdermal bleeding has stopped before removing pressure.

Precautions

- Completely fill the collection tube.
- Invert the sample gently several times to thoroughly mix the sample and the anticoagulant. To prevent hemolysis, don't shake the tube.

Reference values

For normal values for the five types of WBCs classified in the differential for adults and children, see *Interpreting WBC differential values*. For an accurate diagnosis, differential test results must always be interpreted in relation to the total WBC count.

Abnormal findings

Abnormal differential patterns provide evidence for a wide range of disease states and other conditions. (See *Influence of disease on blood cell count.*)

Interfering factors

- Failure to completely fill the collection tube, to use the proper anticoagulant, or to adequately mix the sample and the anticoagulant
- Hemolysis due to rough handling of the sample
- Methysergide, desipramine (increase or decrease eosinophil count), indo-

Influence of disease on blood cell count

White blood cell (WBC) differential aids diagnosis because some disorders affect only one WBC type. Below, each cell type is listed as well as the corresponding effect and its causes.

CELL TYPE	HOW AFFECTED
Neutrophils 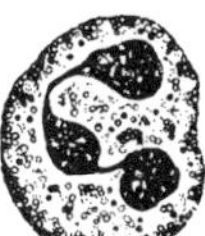	***Increased by:*** ◆ Infections, osteomyelitis, otitis media, saplingitis, septicemia, gonorrhea, endocarditis, smallpox, chickenpox, herpes, Rocky Mountain spotted fever ◆ Ischemic necrosis due to myocardial infarction, burns, carcinoma ◆ Metabolic disorders: diabetic acidosis, eclampsia, uremia, thyrotoxicosis ◆ Stress response due to acute hemorrhage, surgery, excessive exercise, emotional distress, third trimester of pregnancy, childbirth ◆ Inflammatory disease: rheumatic fever, rheumatoid arthritis, acute gout, vasculitis, myositis ***Decreased by:*** ◆ Bone marrow depression due to radiation or cytotoxic drugs ◆ Infections: typhoid, tularemia, brucellosis, hepatitis, influenza, measles, mumps, rubella, infectious mononucleosis ◆ Hypersplenism: hepatic disease and storage diseases ◆ Collagen vascular disease such as systemic lupus erythematosus (SLE) ◆ Folic acid or vitamin B_{12} deficiency
Eosinophils 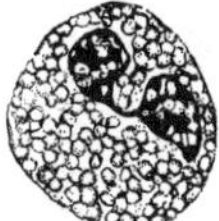	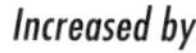 ***Increased by:*** ◆ Allergic disorders: asthma, hay fever, food or drug sensitivity, serum sickness, angioneurotic edema ◆ Parasitic infections: trichinosis, hookworm, roundworm, amebiasis ◆ Skin diseases: eczema, pemphigus, psoriasis, dermatitis, herpes ◆ Neoplastic diseases: chronic myelocytic leuemia, Hodgkin's disease, metastases and necrosis of solid tumors ***Decreased by:*** ◆ Stress response ◆ Cushing's syndrome
Basophils 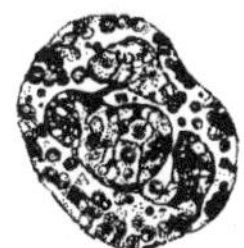	***Increased by:*** ◆ Chronic myelocytic leukemia, Hodgkin's disease, ulcerative colitis, chronic hypersensitivity states ***Decreased by:*** ◆ Hyperthyroidism ◆ Ovulation, pregnancy ◆ Stress

(continued)

Influence of disease on blood cell count *(continued)*

CELL TYPE	HOW AFFECTED
Lymphocytes 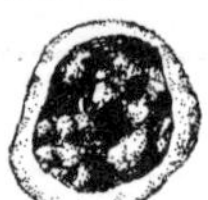	***Increased by:*** ◆ Infections: tuberculosis, hepatitis, infectious mononucleosis, mumps, rubella, cytomegalovirus ◆ Thyrotoxicosis, hypoadrenalism, ulcerative colitis, immune diseases, lymphocytic leukemia ***Decreased by:*** ◆ Severe debilitating illness, such as heart failure, renal failure, and advanced tuberculosis ◆ Defective lymphatic circulation, high levels of adrenal corticosteroids, immunodeficiency due to immunosuppressives
Monocytes 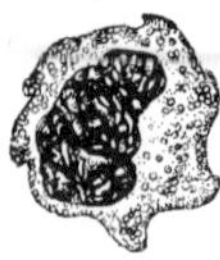	***Increased by:*** ◆ Infections: subacute bacterial endocarditis, tuberculosis, hepatitis, malaria ◆ Collagen vascular disease: SLE, rheumatoid arthritis ◆ Carcinomas ◆ Monocytic leukemia ◆ Lymphomas

methacin, procainamide (decrease eosinophil count), anticonvulsants, capreomycin, cephalosporins, D-penicillamine, gold compounds, isoniazid, nalidixic acid, novobiocin, para-aminosalicylic acid, paromomycin, penicillins, phenothiazines, rifampin, streptomycin, sulfonamides, and tetracyclines (increase count by provoking an allergic reaction)

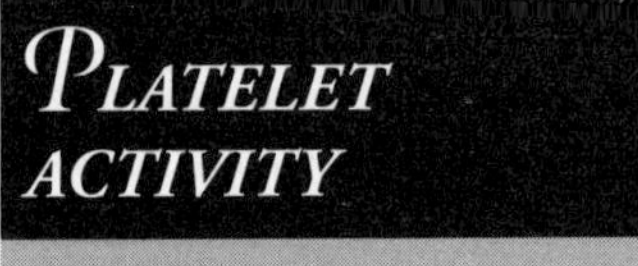

PLATELET ACTIVITY

BLEEDING TIME

Bleeding time is used to measure the duration of bleeding after a measured skin incision. Bleeding time may be measured by one of three methods: template, Ivy, or Duke. The template method is the most commonly used and the most accurate because the incision size is standardized. Bleeding time depends on the elasticity of the blood vessel wall and on the number and functional capacity of platelets.

Although the bleeding time test is usually performed on patients with a personal or family history of bleeding disorders, it's also useful — along with a platelet count — for preoperative screening. The test isn't usually recommended for patients with a platelet count of less than 75,000/µl (SI, 75 $\times 10^9$/L).

Purpose

- To assess overall hemostatic function (platelet response to injury and functional capacity of vasoconstriction)
- To detect congenital and acquired platelet function disorders

Patient preparation

- Explain to the patient that this test is used to measure the time required to form a clot and stop bleeding.
- Tell the patient who will be performing the test and when it will take place.
- Inform the patient that he need not restrict food and fluids.
- Inform the patient that he may feel some discomfort from the incisions, the antiseptic, and the tightness of the blood pressure cuff. Also inform the patient that depending on the method used, incisions or punctures may leave tiny scars that should be barely visible when healed.
- Notify the laboratory and physician of medications the patient is taking that may affect test results; they may need to be restricted.

Procedure and posttest care

- *Template method:* Wrap the pressure cuff around the upper arm and inflate the cuff to 40 mm Hg. Select an area on the forearm with no superficial veins and clean it with antiseptic. Allow the skin to dry completely before making the incision. Apply the appropriate template lengthwise to the forearm. Use the lancet to make two incisions 1 mm deep and 9 mm long. Start the stopwatch. Without touching the cuts, gently blot the drops of blood with filter paper every 30 seconds until the bleeding stops in both cuts. Average the time of the two cuts and record the result.
- *Ivy method:* After applying the pressure cuff and preparing the test site, make three small punctures with a disposable lancet. Start the stopwatch immediately. Taking care not to touch the punctures, blot each site with filter paper every 30 seconds until the bleeding stops. Average the bleeding time of the three punctures and record the result.
- *Duke method:* Drape the patient's shoulder with a towel. Clean the earlobe and let the skin air-dry. Make a puncture wound 2 to 4 mm deep on the earlobe with a disposable lancet. Start the stopwatch. Being careful not to touch the ear, blot the site with filter paper every 30 seconds until bleeding stops. Record bleeding time.
- In a patient with a bleeding tendency (hemophilia), maintain a pressure bandage over the incision for 24 to 48 hours to prevent further bleeding. Check the test area frequently; keep the edges of the cuts aligned to minimize scarring.
- In other patients, a piece of gauze held in place by an adhesive bandage is sufficient.
- Instruct the patient that he may resume medications discontinued before the test as ordered.

Precautions

- Be sure to maintain a cuff pressure of 40 mm Hg throughout the test.
- If the bleeding doesn't diminish after 15 minutes, discontinue the test.
- Apply direct pressure to the test site until bleeding ceases.

Reference values

The normal range of bleeding time is from 3 to 6 minutes (SI, 3 to 6 min) in the template method; from 3 to 6 minutes in the Ivy method; and from 1 to 3 minutes (SI, 1 to 3 min) in the Duke method.

Abnormal findings

Prolonged bleeding time may indicate the presence of disorders associated with thrombocytopenia, such as Hodgkin's disease, acute leukemia, disseminated intravascular coagulation, hemolytic disease of the neonate, Schönlein-Henoch purpura, severe hepatic disease (cirrhosis, for example), or severe deficiency of factors I, II, V, VII, VIII, IX, and XI. Prolonged bleeding time in a person with a normal platelet count suggests a platelet function disorder (thrombasthenia, thrombocytopathia) and requires further investigation with clot retraction, prothrombin consumption, and platelet aggregation tests.

Interfering factors

- Sulfonamides, thiazide diuretics, antineoplastics, anticoagulants, nonsteroidal anti-inflammatory drugs, vitamin E supplementation, aspirin and aspirin compounds, and some nonnarcotic analgesics (prolonged bleeding time)

PLATELET COUNT

Platelets, or thrombocytes, are the smallest formed elements in blood. They promote coagulation and the formation of a hemostatic plug in vascular injury.

Platelet count is one of the most important screening tests of platelet function. Accurate counts are vital.

Purpose

- To evaluate platelet production
- To assess effects of chemotherapy or radiation therapy on platelet production
- To diagnose and monitor severe thrombocytosis or thrombocytopenia
- To confirm a visual estimate of platelet number and morphology from a stained blood film

Patient preparation

- Explain to the patient that this test is used to determine if the patient's blood clots normally.
- Tell the patient that a blood sample will be taken. Explain who will perform the venipuncture and when.
- Inform the patient that he need not restrict food and fluids.
- Explain to the patient that he may feel slight discomfort from the needle puncture and the tourniquet.
- Notify the laboratory and physician of medications the patient is taking that may affect test results; they may need to be restricted.

Procedure and posttest care

- Perform a venipuncture and collect the sample in a 3- to 4.5-ml EDTA tube.
- If a hematoma develops at the venipuncture site, apply warm soaks. If the hematoma is large, monitor pulses distal to the venipuncture site.
- Ensure subdermal bleeding has stopped before removing pressure.

Precautions

- To prevent hemolysis, avoid excessive probing at the venipuncture site and handle the sample gently.
- Completely fill the collection tube and invert it gently several times to mix the sample and the anticoagulant thoroughly.

Reference values

Normal platelet counts range from 140,000 to 400,000/µl. (SI, 140 to 400 $\times$ 10^9/L) in adults and from 150,000 to 450,000/µl (SI, 150 to 450 $\times$ 10^9/L) in children.

Abnormal findings

A decreased platelet count (thrombocytopenia) can result from aplastic or hypoplastic bone marrow; infiltrative bone marrow disease such as leukemia, or disseminated infection; megakaryocytic hypoplasia; ineffective thrombopoiesis due to folic acid or vitamin B_{12} deficiency; pooling of platelets in an enlarged spleen; increased platelet destruction due to drugs or immune disorders; disseminated intravascular coagulation; Bernard-Soulier syndrome; or mechanical injury to platelets.

An increased platelet count (thrombocytosis) can result from hemorrhage, infectious disorders, iron deficiency anemia, recent surgery, pregnancy, splenectomy, or inflammatory disorders. In such cases, the platelet count returns to normal after the patient recovers from the primary disorder. However, the count remains elevated in primary thrombocythemia, myelofibrosis with myeloid metaplasia, polycythemia vera, and chronic myelogenous leukemia.

When the platelet count is abnormal, diagnosis usually requires further studies, such as complete blood count, bone marrow biopsy, direct antiglobulin test (direct Coombs' test), and serum protein electrophoresis.

Interfering factors

- Failure to use the proper anticoagulant or to mix the sample and anticoagulant promptly and adequately
- Hemolysis due to rough handling of the sample or excessive probing at the venipuncture site
- Heparin (decrease)
- Acetazolamide, acetohexamide, antineoplastics, brompheniramine maleate, carbamazepine, chloramphenicol, ethacrynic acid, furosemide, gold salts, hydroxychloroquine, indomethacin, isoniazid, mephenytoin, mefenamic acid, methazolamide, methimazole, methyldopa, oral diazoxide, oxyphenbutazone, penicillamine, penicillin, phenylbutazone, phenytoin, pyrimethamine, quinidine sulfate, quinine, salicylates, streptomycin, sulfonamides, thiazide and thiazide-like diuretics, and tricyclic antidepressants (possible decrease)
- High altitudes, persistent cold temperatures, strenuous exercise, or excitement (increase)

CAPILLARY FRAGILITY

Also called the tourniquet test, the positive-pressure test, and Rumpel-Leede test, the capillary fragility test is a nonspecific method for evaluating bleeding tendencies. A positive-pressure test, used to measure the capillaries' ability to remain intact under increased intracapillary pressure, is controlled by a blood pressure cuff around the patient's upper arm.

Purpose

- To assess the fragility of capillary walls
- To identify a platelet deficiency (thrombocytopenia)

Patient preparation

- Explain to the patient that this test is used to identify abnormal bleeding tendencies.
- Tell the patient who will be performing the procedure and when.

- Inform the patient that he need not restrict food and fluids.
- Explain to the patient that he may feel discomfort from the pressure of the blood pressure cuff.

Procedure and posttest care

- The patient's skin temperature and the room temperature should be normal to ensure accurate results.
- Select and mark a 2″ (5-cm) space on the patient's forearm. Ideally, the site should be free of petechiae; otherwise, record the number of petechiae present on the site before starting the test.
- Fasten the cuff around the arm and raise the pressure to a point midway between the systolic and diastolic blood pressures. Maintain this pressure for 5 minutes, then release the cuff.
- Count the number of petechiae that appear in the 2″ space.
- Record the test results.
- Encourage the patient to open and close his hand a few times to hasten return of blood to the forearm.

Precautions

- Don't repeat this test on the same arm within 1 week.
- This test is contraindicated in patients with disseminated intravascular coagulation (DIC) or other bleeding disorders, and in those with significant petechiae already present.

Reference values

A few petechiae may normally be present before the test. Less than 10 petechiae on the forearm 5 minutes (SI, 5 m) after the test is considered normal, or negative; more than 10 petechiae is considered a positive result. The following scale may also be used to report test results.

NUMBER OF PETECHIAE/5 CM	SCORE
11 to 20	2+
21 to 50	3+
over 50	4+

Abnormal findings

A positive finding (more than 10 petechiae, or a score of 2+ to 4+) indicates weakness of the capillary walls (vascular purpura) or a platelet defect. It may occur in such conditions as thrombocytopenia, thrombasthenia, purpura senilis, scurvy, DIC, von Willebrand's disease, vitamin K deficiency, dysproteinemia, and polycythemia vera and in severe deficiencies of factor VII, fibrinogen, or prothrombin. Conditions unrelated to bleeding defects, such as scarlet fever, measles, influenza, chronic renal disease, hypertension, and diabetes with coexistent vascular disease may also increase capillary fragility. An abnormal number of petechiae sometimes appear before menstruation and at other times in some healthy persons, especially in women over age 40.

Interfering factors

- Decreasing estrogen levels in postmenopausal women (possible increase)
- Glucocorticoids (possible decrease)
- Repeating the test on the same arm within 1 week, causing errors in counting the number of petechiae

PLATELET AGGREGATION

After vascular injury, platelets gather at the injury site and clump together to form an aggregate or plug that helps maintain hemostasis and promotes healing. The platelet aggregation test, an in vitro procedure, is used to measure the rate at which the platelets in a plasma sample form a clump after the addition of an aggregating reagent.

Purpose

- To assess platelet aggregation
- To detect congenital and acquired platelet bleeding disorders

Patient preparation

- Explain to the patient that this test is used to determine if blood clots properly.
- Tell the patient that the test requires a blood sample. Explain who will perform the venipuncture and when.
- Explain to the patient that he may feel slight discomfort from the needle puncture and the tourniquet.
- Instruct the patient to fast or to maintain a nonfat diet for 8 hours before the test because lipemia can affect the test results.
- Notify the laboratory and physician of medications the patient is taking that may affect test results; they may need to be restricted.

Procedure and posttest care

- Perform a venipuncture and collect the sample in a 4.5-ml siliconized tube.
- Completely fill the collection tube and invert it gently several times to mix the sample and the anticoagulant thoroughly.
- Apply pressure to the venipuncture site for 5 minutes or until bleeding stops.
- Instruct the patient that he may resume his usual diet and medications discontinued before the test as ordered.
- If a hematoma develops at the venipuncture site, apply warm soaks.

Precautions

- Because the list of medications known to alter the results of this test is long and continually growing, the patient should be as free of drugs as possible before the test.
- If the patient has taken aspirin within the past 14 days and the test can't be postponed, ask the laboratory to verify the presence of aspirin in the plasma. If test results are abnormal for such a sample, the use of aspirin must be discontinued and the test repeated in 2 weeks.
- Avoid excessive probing at the venipuncture site.
- Remove the tourniquet promptly to avoid bruising.
- Handle the sample gently to prevent hemolysis and keep it between 71.6° F and 98.6° F (22° C and 37° C) to prevent aggregation.

Reference values

Normal aggregation occurs in 3 to 5 minutes (SI, 3 to 5 m), but findings are temperature-dependent and vary with the laboratory. Aggregation curves obtained by using different reagents help to distinguish various qualitative platelet defects.

Abnormal findings

Abnormal findings may indicate von Willebrand's disease, Bernard-Soulier syndrome, storage pool disease, Glanzmann's thrombasthenia, polycythemia vera, severe liver disease, or uremia.

Interfering factors

- Failure to observe pretest restrictions
- Failure to use the proper anticoagulant or to adequately mix the sample and the anticoagulant
- Hemolysis due to rough handling of the sample or to excessive probing at the venipuncture site
- Aspirin and aspirin compounds, phenylbutazone, sulfinpyrazone, phenothiazines, anti-inflammatory drugs, antihistamines, and tricyclic antidepressants (decrease)

- Ingestion of large amounts of garlic (inhibits platelet aggregation)

COAGULATION

ACTIVATED PARTIAL THROMBOPLASTIN TIME

The activated partial thromboplastin time (APTT) (also now known as partial thromboplastin time or PTT) is used to evaluate all the clotting factors of the intrinsic pathway — except platelets — by measuring the time required for formation of a fibrin clot after the addition of calcium and phospholipid emulsion to a plasma sample. An activator, such as kaolin, is used to shorten clotting time.

Purpose

- To screen for deficiencies of the clotting factors in the intrinsic pathways
- To monitor response to heparin therapy

Patient preparation

- Explain to the patient that this test is used to determine if blood clots normally.
- Tell the patient that a blood sample will be taken. Explain who will perform the venipuncture and when.
- Explain to the patient that he may feel slight discomfort from the needle puncture and the tourniquet.
- When appropriate, tell the patient receiving heparin therapy that this test may be repeated at regular intervals to assess the response to treatment.
- Inform the patient that he need not restrict food and fluids.

Procedure and posttest care

- Perform a venipuncture and collect the sample in a 7-ml tube with sodium citrate added.
- If a hematoma develops at the venipuncture site, apply warm soaks. If the hematoma is large, monitor pulses distal to the venipuncture site.
- Ensure subdermal bleeding has stopped before removing pressure.

Precautions

- Completely fill the collection tube, invert it gently several times, and send it to the laboratory on ice.
- To prevent hemolysis, avoid excessive probing at the venipuncture site and handle the sample gently.
- For a patient on anticoagulant therapy, additional pressure may be needed at the venipuncture site to control bleeding.

Reference values

Normally, a fibrin clot forms 21 to 35 seconds (SI, 21 to 35 S) after adding reagents. For a patient on anticoagulant therapy, ask the attending physician to specify the reference values for the therapy being delivered.

Abnormal findings

Prolonged APTT may indicate a deficiency of certain plasma clotting factors, the presence of heparin, or the presence of fibrin split products, fibrinolysins, or circulating anticoagulants that are antibodies to specific clotting factors.

Interfering factors

- Failure to fill the collection tube completely, to use the proper anticoagulant, or to adequately mix the sample and the anticoagulant
- Hemolysis due to rough handling of the sample or to excessive probing at the venipuncture site

■ Failure to send the sample to the laboratory immediately or to place it on ice

PROTHROMBIN TIME

Prothrombin time (PT) measures the time required for a fibrin clot to form in a citrated plasma sample after addition of calcium ions and tissue thromboplastin (factor III).

Purpose
■ To evaluate extrinsic coagulation system (factors V, VII, and X, and prothrombin and fibrinogen)
■ To monitor response to oral anticoagulant therapy

Patient preparation
■ Explain to the patient that this test is used to determine if the blood clots normally.
■ Notify the laboratory and physician of medications the patient is taking that may affect test results; they may need to be restricted.
■ Tell the patient that a blood sample will be taken. Explain who will perform the venipuncture and when.
■ Explain to the patient that he may feel slight discomfort from the needle puncture and the tourniquet.
■ When appropriate, explain that this test is used to monitor the effects of oral anticoagulants; the test will be performed daily when therapy begins and will be repeated at longer intervals when medication levels stabilize.
■ Inform the patient that he need not restrict food and fluids.

Procedure and posttest care
■ Perform a venipuncture and collect the sample in a 3- to 4.5-ml siliconized tube.
■ If a hematoma develops at the venipuncture site, apply warm soaks. If the hematoma is large, monitor pulses distal to the venipuncture site.
■ Ensure subdermal bleeding has stopped before removing pressure.

Precautions
■ Completely fill the collection tube and invert it gently several times to mix the sample and the anticoagulant thoroughly. If the tube isn't filled to the correct volume, an excess of citrate appears in the sample.
■ To prevent hemolysis, avoid excessive probing during venipuncture and handle the sample gently.

Reference values
Normally, PT values range from 10 to 14 seconds (SI, 10 to 14 S). Values vary, however, depending on the source of tissue thromboplastin and the type of sensing devices used to measure clot formation. In a patient receiving oral anticoagulants, PT is usually maintained between 1 and 2½ times the normal control value.

Abnormal findings
Prolonged PT may indicate deficiencies in fibrinogen; prothrombin; factors V, VII, or X (specific assays can pinpoint such deficiencies); or vitamin K. It may also result from ongoing oral anticoagulant therapy. Prolonged PT that exceeds 2½ times the control value is commonly associated with abnormal bleeding.

Interfering factors
■ Failure to fill the collection tube completely (possible false-high)

- Failure to adequately mix the sample and the anticoagulant, or to send the sample to the laboratory promptly
- Hemolysis due to rough handling of the sample
- Salicylates, more than 1 g/day (increase)
- Fibrin or fibrin split products in the sample or plasma fibrinogen levels > 100 mg/dl (possible prolonged PT)
- Antihistamines, chloral hydrate, corticosteroids, cardiac glycosides, diuretics, glutethimide, griseofulvin, progestin-estrogen combinations, pyrazinamide, vitamin K, and xanthines, such as caffeine and theophylline (possible decrease)
- Corticotropin, anabolic steroids, cholestyramine resin, heparin I.V. (within 5 hours of sample collection), indomethacin, mefenamic acid, para-aminosalicylic acid, methimazole, oxyphenbutazone, phenylbutazone, phenytoin, propylthiouracil, quinidine, quinine, thyroid hormones, vitamin A, or alcohol in excess (prolonged PT)
- Antibiotics, barbiturates, hydroxyzine, sulfonamides, mineral oil, or clofibrate (possible increase or decrease)

ACTIVATED CLOTTING TIME

Activated clotting time, or automated coagulation time, measures whole blood clotting time. Activated clotting time is commonly performed during procedures that require extracorporeal circulation, such as cardiopulmonary bypass, ultrafiltration, hemodialysis, and extracorporeal membrane oxygenation (ECMO) and of the invasive procedures, such as cardiac catheterization and percutaneous transluminal coronary angioplasty.

Purpose

- To monitor the effect of heparin
- To monitor the effect of protamine sulfate in heparin neutralization
- To detect severe deficiencies in clotting factors (except factor VII)

Patient preparation

- Explain to the patient that this test is used to monitor the effect of heparin on the blood's ability to coagulate.
- Tell the patient that the test requires a blood sample, which is usually drawn from an existing vascular access site; therefore, no venipuncture will be needed.
- Explain who will perform the test and that the test is usually done at the bedside.
- Explain that two blood samples will be drawn. The first one will be discarded so that any heparin in the tubing doesn't interfere with the results.
- If the sample is drawn from a line with a continuous infusion, stop the infusion before drawing the sample.

Procedure and posttest care

- Withdraw 5 to 10 ml of blood from the line and discard it.
- Withdraw a clean sample of blood into the special tube containing celite provided with the activated clotting time unit.
- Activate the activated clotting time unit and wait for the signal to insert the tube.
- Flush the vascular access site according to your facility's policy.

Precaution

- Guard against contamination with heparin if drawn from an access site containing heparin.

Reference values

In a non-anticoagulated patient, normal activated clotting time is 107 seconds plus or minus 13 seconds (SI, 107 ± 13 s). During cardiopulmonary bypass, heparin is titrated to maintain an activated clotting time between 400 and 600 seconds (SI, 400 to 600 s). During ECMO, heparin is titrated to maintain the activated clotting time between 220 and 260 seconds (SI, 220 to 260 s).

Interfering factors

- Failure to fill the collection tube completely, to use the proper anticoagulant, to adequately mix the sample and the anticoagulant, or to send the sample to the laboratory immediately or place it on ice
- Hemolysis due to rough handling of the sample or to excessive probing at the venipuncture site
- Failure to draw at least 5 ml waste to avoid sample contamination when drawing the sample from a venous access device that's used for heparin infusion

ONE-STAGE FACTOR ASSAY: EXTRINSIC COAGULATION SYSTEM

When prothrombin time (PT) and partial thromboplastin time (PTT) are prolonged, a one-stage assay is used to detect a deficiency of factor II, factor V, or factor X. If PT is abnormal but PTT is normal, factor VII may be deficient.

Purpose

- To identify a specific factor deficiency in persons with prolonged PT or PTT
- To study patients with congenital or acquired coagulation defects
- To monitor the effects of blood component therapy in factor-deficient patients

Patient preparation

- Explain to the patient that this test is used to assess the function of the blood coagulation mechanism.
- Tell the patient that a blood sample will be taken. Explain who will perform the venipuncture and when.
- Explain to the patient that he may feel slight discomfort from the needle puncture and the tourniquet.
- When the patient is factor deficient and receiving blood component therapy, tell him that he may need a series of tests.
- Notify the laboratory and physician of medications the patient is taking that may affect test results; they may need to be restricted.
- Inform the patient that he need not restrict food and fluids.

Procedure and posttest care

- Perform a venipuncture and collect the sample in a 3- or 4.5-ml siliconized tube.
- Apply direct pressure to the venipuncture site until bleeding stops.
- If a hematoma develops at the venipuncture site, apply warm soaks.
- A patient with a bleeding disorder may require a pressure bandage to stop bleeding at the venipuncture site.

Precautions

- If the patient has a suspected coagulation defect, avoid excessive probing during venipuncture; don't leave the tourniquet on too long (it will cause bruising); and apply pressure to the puncture site for 5 minutes or until the bleeding stops.
- Completely fill the collection tube and invert it gently several times to mix the sample and the anticoagulant.
- Handle the sample gently to prevent hemolysis, and send it to the laboratory immediately or place it on ice.

Reference values

The reference ranges for most factors is 50% to 150% of normal (SI, 0.50 to 1.50)

Abnormal findings

Deficiency of factor X may also indicate disseminated intravascular coagulation (DIC). Factor V deficiency suggests severe hepatic disease, DIC, or fibrinogenolysis. Deficiencies of all four factors may be congenital; absence of factor II is lethal.

Interfering factors

- Failure to mix the sample and the anticoagulant adequately, or to send the sample to the laboratory immediately or place it on ice
- Hemolysis due to rough handling of the sample
- Oral anticoagulants (possible increase due to inhibition of vitamin K-dependent synthesis and activation of clotting factors II, VII, and X, which form in the liver)

ONE-STAGE FACTOR ASSAY: INTRINSIC COAGULATION SYSTEM

When prothrombin time (PT) is normal but partial thromboplastin time (PTT) is abnormal, a one-stage assay is used to identify a deficiency in the intrinsic coagulation system: factor VIII, factor IX, factor XI, or factor XII.

Purpose

- To identify a specific factor deficiency
- To study patients with congenital or acquired coagulation defects
- To monitor the effects of blood component therapy in factor-deficient patients

Patient preparation

- Explain to the patient that this test is used to assess the function of the blood coagulation mechanism.
- Tell the patient that a blood sample will be taken. Explain who will perform the venipuncture and when.
- Explain to the patient that he may feel slight discomfort from the needle puncture and the tourniquet.
- Notify the laboratory and physician of medications the patient is taking that may affect test results; they may need to be restricted.
- When the patient is factor deficient and receiving blood component therapy, tell him that a series of tests may be needed to monitor therapeutic progress.
- Inform the patient that he need not restrict food and fluids.

Procedure and posttest care

- Perform a venipuncture and collect the sample in a 3- or 4.5-ml siliconized tube.
- Apply direct pressure to the venipuncture site until bleeding subsides.
- If a hematoma develops at the venipuncture site, apply warm soaks. A patient with a bleeding disorder may require a pressure bandage to stop bleeding at the venipuncture site.
- Instruct the patient that he may resume medications discontinued before the test as ordered.

Precautions

- If a coagulation defect is suspected, avoid excessive probing during venipuncture, don't leave the tourniquet on too long (it will cause bruising), and apply pressure to the puncture site for 5 minutes or until the bleeding stops.
- Completely fill the collection tube and invert it gently several times to mix the sample and the anticoagulant thoroughly.

■ Handle the sample gently to prevent hemolysis and send it to the laboratory immediately or place it on ice.

Reference values

Reference ranges for most factors are 50% to 150% of normal activity (SI, 0.5 to 1.50).

Abnormal findings

Factor VIII deficiency may indicate hemophilia A, von Willebrand's disease, or a factor VIII inhibitor. An acquired deficiency of factor VIII may result from disseminated intravascular coagulation or fibrinolysis. Factor VIII antigen and ristocetin cofactor tests distinguish between hemophilia A (and its carrier state) and von Willebrand's disease.

Factor IX deficiency may suggest hemophilia B, or it may be acquired as a result of hepatic disease, a factor IX inhibitor, vitamin K deficiency, or coumarin therapy. Factor VIII and IX inhibitors occur after blood transfusions in patients deficient in either factor and are antibodies specific to each factor.

Factor XI deficiency may appear after the stress of trauma or surgery, or transiently in neonates. Factor XII deficiency may be inherited or acquired (such as nephrosis) and may also appear transiently in neonates.

Interfering factors

■ Failure to adequately mix the sample and the anticoagulant or to send the sample to the laboratory immediately
■ Hemolysis due to rough handling of the sample
■ Oral anticoagulants (decrease in factor IX)
■ Pregnancy (increase in factor VIII)

PLASMA THROMBIN TIME

Plasma thrombin time, or thrombin clotting time, measures how quickly a clot forms when a standard amount of bovine thrombin is added to a platelet-poor plasma sample from the patient and to a normal plasma control sample. After thrombin is added, the clotting time for each sample is compared and recorded. This test allows a quick but imprecise estimation of plasma fibrinogen levels, which are a function of clotting time. (See *Antithrombin III test,* page 120, for information about another test that helps determine the cause of coagulation disorders.)

Purpose

■ To detect fibrinogen deficiency or defect
■ To aid diagnosis of disseminated intravascular coagulation (DIC) and hepatic disease
■ To monitor the effectiveness of treatment with heparin or thrombolytic agents

Patient preparation

■ Explain to the patient that this test is used to determine if blood clots normally.
■ Notify the laboratory and physician of medications the patient is taking that may affect test results; they may need to be restricted.
■ Tell the patient that a blood sample will be taken. Explain who will perform the venipuncture and when.
■ Explain to the patient that he may feel slight discomfort from the needle puncture and the tourniquet.
■ Inform the patient that he need not restrict food and fluids.

Antithrombin III test

The antithrombin III test helps detect the cause of impaired coagulation, especially hypercoagulation, by measuring levels of antithrombin III (AT III), a protein that inactivates thrombin and inhibits coagulation. AT III may be evaluated by a functional clotting assay or synthetic substrates. Exogenous heparin is added to a fresh, citrated blood sample to accelerate activity, then excess thrombin (factor Xa) is added to the plasma. The amount of factor Xa not activated by AT III is quantitated and compared to a normal control. Reference values may vary for each laboratory, but should lie between 80% and 120% of normal.

Decreased AT III levels can indicate disseminated intravascular coagulation or thromboembolic, hypercoagulation, or hepatic disorders. Slightly decreased levels can result from oral contraceptives. Elevated levels can result from kidney transplantation and use of oral anticoagulants or anabolic steroids.

Procedure and posttest care

- Perform a venipuncture and collect the sample in a 3- to 4.5-ml siliconized tube.
- If a hematoma develops at the venipuncture site, apply warm soaks. If the hematoma is large, monitor pulses distal to the phlebotomy site.
- Ensure bleeding has stopped before removing pressure.

Precautions

- If the tube isn't filled to the correct volume, an excess of citrate appears in the sample. Completely fill the collection tube and invert it gently several times to mix the sample and the anticoagulant thoroughly.
- To prevent hemolysis, avoid excessive probing during venipuncture and rough handling of the sample.
- Immediately put the sample on ice and send it to the laboratory.

Reference values

Normal thrombin times range from 10 to 15 seconds (SI, 10 to 15 S). Test results are usually reported with a normal control value.

Abnormal findings

A prolonged thrombin time may indicate heparin therapy, hepatic disease, DIC, hypofibrinogenemia, or dysfibrinogenemia. Patients with prolonged thrombin times may require measurement of fibrinogen levels; in suspected DIC, the test for fibrin split products is also necessary.

Interfering factors

- Failure to use the proper anticoagulant, to adequately mix the sample and the anticoagulant, or to send the sample to the laboratory properly
- Hemolysis due to rough handling of the sample or to excessive probing at the venipuncture site
- Heparin, fibrinogen, or fibrin degradation products (possible increase)

PLASMA FIBRINOGEN

Fibrinogen (factor I) originates in the liver and is converted to fibrin by thrombin during clotting. Because fibrin is necessary for clot formation, fibrinogen deficiency can produce mild to severe bleeding disorders.

Purpose

- To aid the diagnosis of suspected clotting or bleeding disorders caused by fibrinogen abnormalities

Patient preparation

- Explain to the patient that this test is used to determine if blood clots normally.
- Tell the patient that a blood sample will be taken. Explain who will perform the venipuncture and when.
- Explain to the patient that he may feel slight discomfort from the needle puncture and the tourniquet.
- Notify the laboratory and physician of medications the patient is taking that may affect test results; they may need to be restricted.
- Inform the patient that he need not restrict food and fluids.

Procedure and posttest care

- Perform a venipuncture and collect the sample in a 3- or 4.5-ml tube with sodium citrate added.
- If a hematoma develops at the venipuncture site, apply warm soaks. If the hematoma is large, monitor pulses distal to the phlebotomy site.
- Ensure that subdermal bleeding has stopped before removing pressure.

Precautions

- This test is contraindicated in patients with active bleeding and acute infection or illness, and in those who have received blood transfusions within 4 weeks.
- Avoid excessive probing during venipuncture and handle the sample gently.
- Completely fill the collection tube, invert it gently several times, and send it to the laboratory immediately or place it on ice.

Reference values

Fibrinogen levels normally range from 200 to 400 mg/dl (SI, 2 to 4 g/L).

Abnormal findings

Depressed fibrinogen levels may indicate congenital afibrinogenemia; hypofibrinogenemia or dysfibrinogenemia; disseminated intravascular coagulation; fibrinolysis; severe hepatic disease; cancer of the prostate, pancreas, or lung; or bone marrow lesions. Obstetric complications or trauma may cause low levels.

Markedly decreased fibrinogen levels impede the accurate interpretation of coagulation tests that have a fibrin clot as an end point.

Elevated levels may indicate cancer of the stomach, breast, or kidney, or inflammatory disorders, such as pneumonia or membranoproliferative glomerulonephritis.

Prolonged PTT, prothrombin time and thrombin time may also indicate a fibrinogen deficiency.

Interfering factors

- Failure to fill the collection tube completely, to adequately mix the sample and anticoagulant, or to send the sample to the laboratory promptly
- Hemolysis due to excessive probing at the venipuncture site or to rough handling of the sample
- Heparin or oral contraceptives
- Third trimester of pregnancy and postoperative status (possible increase)

FIBRIN SPLIT PRODUCTS

After a fibrin clot forms in response to vascular injury, the clot is eventually degraded by plasmin, a fibrin-dissolving enzyme. The resulting fragments are known as fibrin split products (FSP), or fibrinogen degradation products. In the fibrin split products test, FSP are detected in the diluted serum that's left in a blood sample after clotting.

Purpose

- To detect FSP in the circulation
- To help determine the presence and the approximate severity of a hyperfibrinolytic state (such as disseminated intravascular coagulation [DIC]) that may result in primary fibrinogenolysis or hypercoagulability

Patient preparation

- Explain to the patient that this test is used to determine if blood clots normally.
- Tell the patient that a blood sample will be taken. Explain who will perform the venipuncture and when.
- Explain to the patient that he may feel slight discomfort from the needle puncture and the tourniquet.
- Notify the laboratory and physician of medications the patient is taking that may affect test results; they may need to be restricted.
- Inform the patient that he need not restrict food and fluids.

Procedure and posttest care

- Perform a venipuncture and draw 2 ml of blood into a plastic syringe.
- Transfer the sample to the tube provided by the laboratory, which contains a soybean trypsin inhibitor and bovine thrombin.
- If a hematoma develops at the venipuncture site, apply warm soaks. If the hematoma is large, monitor pulses distal to the phlebotomy site.
- Ensure subdermal bleeding has stopped before removing pressure.

Precautions

- Draw the sample before administering heparin to avoid false-positive test results.
- Gently invert the collection tube several times to mix the contents thoroughly.
- The blood clots within 2 seconds; after clotting, the sample must be sent immediately to the laboratory to be incubated at 98.6° F (37° C) for 30 minutes before testing proceeds.

Reference values

Serum contains < 10 µg/ml (SI, < 10 mg/L) of FSP. A quantitative assay shows levels of < 3 µg/ml (SI, < 3 mg/L).

Abnormal findings

FSP levels increase in primary fibrinolytic states due to increased levels of circulating profibrinolysin; in secondary states due to DIC and subsequent fibrinolysis; and in alcoholic cirrhosis, preeclampsia, abruptio placentae, congenital heart disease, sunstroke, burns, intrauterine death, pulmonary embolus, deep vein thrombosis (transient increase), and myocardial infarction (after 1 or 2 days). FSP levels usually exceed 100 µg/ml (SI, greater than 100 mg/L) in active renal disease or renal transplant rejection.

Interfering factors

- Pretest administration of heparin (false-high)
- Failure to fill the collection tube completely, to adequately mix the sample and additive, or to send the sample to the laboratory immediately
- Hemolysis due to rough handling of the sample
- Fibrinolytic drugs, such as urokinase, streptokinase, and tissue plasminogen activator, and large doses of barbiturates (increase)

PLASMA PLASMINOGEN

Plasma plasminogen testing is used to assess plasminogen levels in a plasma sample. During fibrinolysis, plasmin dissolves fibrin clots to prevent excessive coagulation and impaired blood flow. Plasmin doesn't circulate in active form, however, so it can't be directly measured. Its circulating precursor, plasminogen, can be measured and used to evaluate the fibrinolytic system.

Purpose

- To assess fibrinolysis
- To detect congenital and acquired fibrinolytic disorders

Patient preparation

- Explain to the patient that this test is used to evaluate blood clotting.
- Tell the patient that a blood sample will be taken. Explain who will perform the venipuncture and when.
- Explain to the patient that he may feel slight discomfort from the needle puncture and the tourniquet.
- Notify the laboratory and physician of medications the patient is taking that may affect test results; they may need to be restricted.
- Inform the patient that he need not restrict food and fluids.

Procedure and posttest care

- Perform a venipuncture and collect the sample in a 4.5-ml siliconized tube.
- If a hematoma develops at the venipuncture site, apply warm soaks. If the hematoma is large, monitor pulses distal to the venipuncture site.
- Ensure bleeding has stopped before removing pressure.
- Instruct the patient that he may resume medications discontinued before the test as ordered.

Precautions

- Collect the sample as quickly as possible to prevent stasis, which can slow blood flow, causing coagulation and plasminogen activation.
- To prevent hemolysis, avoid excessive probing during venipuncture and rough handling of the sample.
- Invert the tube gently several times and immediately send the sample to the laboratory. If testing must be delayed, plasma must be separated and frozen at –94° F (–67.8° C).

Reference values

Normal plasminogen levels range from 10 to 20 mg/dl (0.10 to 0.20 g/L) by immunologic methods.

Abnormal findings

Diminished plasminogen levels can result from disseminated intravascular coagulation, tumors, preeclampsia, and eclampsia, which accelerate plasminogen conversion to plasmin and increase fibrinolysis. Some liver diseases prevent formation of sufficient plasminogen, decreasing fibrinolysis.

Interfering factors

- Failure to use the proper collection tube, to adequately mix the sample and the citrate, to send the sample to the laboratory immediately, or to have the sample separated and frozen
- Hemolysis due to excessive probing during venipuncture or to rough handling of the sample
- Hemoconcentration due to prolonged tourniquet use before venipuncture (possible false-low)
- Oral contraceptives (possible slight increase)
- Thrombolytic drugs, such as streptokinase and urokinase (possible decrease)

PROTEIN C

Vitamin K-dependent, protein C is produced in the liver and circulates in the plasma. It acts as a potent anticoagulant by suppressing activated factors V and VIII. Deficiencies of protein C may be acquired or congenital.

If a deficiency of protein C is identified, further immunologic tests may be needed to determine the type of deficiency. Identifying the role of protein C deficiency in idiopathic venous thrombosis may help prevent thromboembolism.

Purpose

- To investigate the mechanism of idiopathic venous thrombosis.

Patient preparation

- Explain to the patient that this test evaluates blood clotting.
- Tell the patient that a blood sample will be taken. Explain who will perform the venipuncture and when.
- Explain to the patient that he may feel slight discomfort from the needle puncture and the tourniquet.
- Inform the patient that he need not restrict food and fluids.
- Notify the laboratory and physician of medications the patient is taking that may affect test results; they may need to be restricted.

Procedure and posttest care

- Perform a venipuncture. Collect a 3-ml sample in a siliconized vacuum specimen tube or in a special syringe with anticoagulant provided by the laboratory.
- If a hematoma develops at the venipuncture site, apply warm soaks. Apply direct pressure to the venipuncture site until bleeding stops.

Precautions

- Avoid excessive probing during venipuncture.
- Completely fill the collection tube and invert it several times to mix the sample and anticoagulant thoroughly; handle the sample gently.
- Send the sample to the laboratory immediately.

Reference values

The normal range is 70% to 140% (SI, 0.70 to 1.40).

Abnormal findings

Rare, homozygous protein C deficiency is characterized by rapidly fatal thrombosis in the perinatal period, a condition known as purpura fulminans.

The more common heterozygous deficiency is associated with genetic susceptibility to venous thromboembolism before age 30 and continuing throughout life. The patient may require long-term treatment with warfarin therapy or protein C supplements from plasma fractions.

Protein C deficiency is also seen in patients with liver cirrhosis and vitamin K deficiency, and in those taking warfarin.

Interfering factors

- Hemolysis due to excessive probing at the venipuncture site or to rough handling of the sample
- Anticoagulant therapy

EUGLOBULIN LYSIS TIME

Euglobulin lysis time measures the interval between clot formation and clot dissolution in plasma. A precipitated plasma extract is clotted with thrombin, and the time required for the clot to lyse is measured.

Purpose

- To assess the fibrinolytic system
- To help detect abnormal fibrinolytic states

Patient preparation

- Explain to the patient that this test is used to evaluate the blood clotting mechanism.
- Tell the patient that a blood sample will be taken. Explain who will perform the venipuncture and when.
- Explain to the patient that he may feel slight discomfort from the needle puncture and the tourniquet.
- Inform the patient that he need not restrict food and fluids.

Procedure and posttest care

- Perform a venipuncture. Collect a 4.5-ml sample in a tube with sodium citrate or in a chilled tube with 0.5 ml of sodium oxalate.
- Apply direct pressure to the venipuncture site until bleeding stops.
- If a hematoma develops at the venipuncture site, apply warm soaks.

Precautions

- When drawing the sample, be careful not to rub the area over the vein too vigorously, pump the fist excessively, or leave the tourniquet in place too long.
- Avoid excessive probing during venipuncture and handle the sample gently.
- If a tube with sodium citrate is used, mix the sample and anticoagulant thoroughly. If a chilled tube containing 0.5 ml sodium oxalate is used, mix the sample and preservative thoroughly, pack the sample in ice, and send it to the laboratory immediately.

Reference values

Lysis normally occurs 2 to 4 hours (SI, 2 to 4 h).

Abnormal findings

Clot lysis within 1 hour (SI, 1 h) indicates increased plasminogen activator activity. In pathologic fibrinolysis, lysis time may be as brief as 5 to 10 minutes (SI, 5 to 10 m).

Interfering factors

- Prolonged tourniquet constriction, vigorous vein preparation, or excessive pumping of the fist (decrease)
- Hemolysis due to excessive probing at the venipuncture site or to rough handling of the sample
- Failure to place the collection tube and sample on ice
- Thrombolytic therapy, dextran, and clofibrate (decrease)

D-DIMER

A D-dimer is an asymmetrical carbon compound fragment formed after thrombin converts fibrinogen to fibrin, factor XIIIa stabilizes it into a clot, and plasma acts on the cross-linked, or clotted, fibrin. The test is specific for fibrinolysis because it confirms the presence of fibrin split products.

Purpose

- To diagnose disseminated intravascular coagulation (DIC)
- To differentiate subarachnoid hemorrhage from a traumatic lumbar puncture in spinal fluid analysis

Patient preparation

- Obtain the patient's history of hematologic diseases, recent surgery, and the results of other tests performed.

■ Explain to the patient that the test is used to determine if the blood is clotting normally.
■ Tell the patient that the test requires a blood sample. Explain who will perform the venipuncture and when.
■ Explain to the patient that he may feel slight discomfort from the needle puncture and the tourniquet.

Procedure and posttest care

■ Perform a venipuncture and collect the sample in a 4.5-ml tube with sodium citrate added.
■ For a spinal fluid analysis, the sample is collected during a lumbar puncture and placed in a plastic vial. See "Cerebrospinal fluid analysis" in chapter 7 for details of the procedure.
■ Apply pressure to the venipuncture site for 5 minutes or until bleeding stops.
■ If a hematoma develops at the venipuncture site, apply warm soaks.

Precautions

■ Completely fill the collection tube, invert it gently several times, and send it to the laboratory immediately.
■ For a patient with coagulation problems, you may need to apply additional pressure at the venipuncture site to control bleeding.

Reference values

Normal D-dimer test results are negative or < 250 μg/L (SI, < 250 μg/L).

Abnormal findings

Increased D-dimer values may indicate DIC, pulmonary embolism, arterial or venous thrombosis, neoplastic disease, pregnancy (late and postpartum), surgery occurring up to 2 days before testing, subarachnoid hemorrhage (spinal fluid only), or secondary fibrinolysis.

Interfering factors

■ Failure to fill the collection tube completely or to send the sample to laboratory immediately
■ Hemolysis due to rough handling of the sample
■ High rheumatoid factor titers or increased CA-125 levels (possible false-positive)
■ Spinal fluid analysis in infants under age 6 months (possible false-negative)

INTERNATIONAL NORMALIZED RATIO

The international normalized ratio (INR) system is viewed as the best means of standardizing measurement of prothrombin time to monitor oral anticoagulant therapy. It isn't used as a screening test for coagulopathies.

Purpose

■ To evaluate effectiveness of oral anticoagulant therapy

Patient preparation

■ Explain to the patient that this test is used to determine the effectiveness of his oral anticoagulant therapy.
■ Tell the patient that a blood sample will be taken. Explain who will perform the venipuncture and when.
■ Explain to the patient that he may feel slight discomfort from the needle puncture and the tourniquet.

Procedure and posttest care

■ Perform a venipuncture and collect the sample in a 4.5-ml tube with sodium citrate added.
■ If a hematoma develops at the venipuncture site, apply warm soaks. If the hematoma is large, monitor pulses distal to the venipuncture site.

- Ensure subdermal bleeding has stopped before removing pressure.

Precautions

- Completely fill the collection tube; otherwise an excess of citrate appears in the sample.
- Gently invert the tube several times to thoroughly mix the sample and the anticoagulant.
- To prevent hemolysis, avoid excessive probing during venipuncture and handle the sample gently.
- Put the sample on ice and send it to the laboratory promptly.

Reference values

Normal INR for those receiving warfarin therapy is 2.0 to 3.0 (SI, 2.0 to 3.0). For those with mechanical prosthetic heart valves, an INR of 2.5 to 3.5 (SI, 2.5 to 3.5) is suggested.

Abnormal findings

Increased INR values may indicate disseminated intravascular coagulation, cirrhosis, hepatitis, vitamin K deficiency, salicylate intoxication, uncontrolled oral anticoagulation, or massive blood transfusion.

Interfering factors

- Failure to fill the collection tube completely, to adequately mix the sample and the anticoagulant, or to send the sample to the laboratory immediately
- Hemolysis due to excessive probing at the venipuncture site or to rough handling of the sample

2

Blood chemistry tests

ARTERIAL BLOOD GASES

ARTERIAL BLOOD GAS ANALYSIS

Arterial blood gas (ABG) analysis is used to measure the partial pressure of arterial oxygen (PaO_2), the partial pressure of arterial carbon dioxide ($PaCO_2$), and the pH of an arterial sample. Oxygen content (O_2CT), arterial oxygen saturation (SaO_2), and bicarbonate (HCO_3^-) values are also measured. A blood sample for ABG analysis may be drawn by percutaneous arterial puncture or from an arterial line.

Purpose

- To evaluate the efficiency of pulmonary gas exchange
- To assess the integrity of the ventilatory control system
- To determine the acid-base level of the blood
- To monitor respiratory therapy

Patient preparation

- Explain to the patient that this test is used to evaluate how well the lungs are delivering oxygen to blood and eliminating carbon dioxide.
- Tell the patient that the test requires a blood sample. Explain who will perform the arterial puncture and when, and which site—radial, brachial, or femoral artery—has been selected for the puncture.
- Inform the patient that he need not restrict food and fluids.
- Instruct the patient to breathe normally during the test, and warn him that he may experience a brief cramping or throbbing pain at the puncture site.

Procedure and posttest care

- Perform an arterial puncture or draw blood from an arterial line. Use a heparinized blood gas syringe to draw the sample. Eliminate air from the sample, place it on ice immediately, and transport it for analysis.
- After applying pressure to the puncture site for 3 to 5 minutes or until bleeding has stopped, tape a gauze pad firmly over it. (If the puncture site is on the arm, don't tape the entire circumference; this may restrict circulation.)
- If the patient is receiving anticoagulants or has a coagulopathy, apply pressure to the puncture site longer than 5 minutes if necessary.
- Monitor vital signs and observe for signs of circulatory impairment, such as swelling, discoloration, pain, numbness, and tingling in the bandaged arm or leg.
- Watch for bleeding from the puncture site.

Precautions

- Wait at least 20 minutes before drawing arterial blood when starting, changing, or discontinuing oxygen therapy; after initiating or changing settings of mechanical ventilation; or after extubation.
- Before sending the sample to the laboratory, note on the laboratory request whether the patient was breathing room air or receiving oxygen therapy when the sample was collected.
- If the patient was receiving oxygen therapy, note the flow rate and method of delivery. If he's on a ventilator, note the fraction of inspired oxygen, tidal volume mode, respiratory rate, and positive-end expiratory pressure.
- Note the patient's rectal temperature.

Reference values

Normal ABG values fall within the following ranges:

- PaO_2: 80 to 100 mm Hg (SI, 10.6 to 13.3 kPa)
- $PaCO_2$: 35 to 45 mm Hg (SI, 4.7 to 5.3 kPa)
- pH: 7.35 to 7.45 (SI, 7.35 to 7.45)
- O_2CT: 15% to 23% (SI, 0.15 to 0.23)
- SaO_2: 94% to 100% (SI, 0.94 to 1.00)
- HCO_3^-: 22 to 25 mEq/L (SI, 22 to 25 mmol/L).

Abnormal findings

Low PaO_2, O_2CT, and SaO_2 levels and a high $PaCO_2$ may result from conditions that impair respiratory function, such as respiratory muscle weakness or paralysis, respiratory center inhibition (from head injury, brain tumor, or drug abuse), and airway obstruction (possibly from mucus plugs or a tumor). Similarly, low readings may result from bronchiole obstruction caused by asthma or emphysema, from an abnormal ventilation-perfusion ratio due to partially blocked alveoli or pulmonary capillaries, or from alveoli that are damaged or filled with fluid because of disease, hemorrhage, or near-drowning.

When inspired air contains insufficient oxygen, PaO_2, O_2CT, and SaO_2 decrease, but $PaCO_2$ may be normal. Such findings are common in pneumothorax, impaired diffusion between alveoli and blood (due to interstitial fibrosis, for example), or an arteriovenous shunt that permits blood to bypass the lungs.

Low O_2CT — with normal PaO_2, SaO_2 and, possibly, $PaCO_2$ values — may result from severe anemia, decreased blood volume, and reduced hemoglobin oxygen-carrying capacity.

In addition to clarifying blood oxygen disorders, ABG values can give considerable information about acid-base disorders. (See *Acid-base disorders,* page 132.)

Interfering factors

- Failure to heparinize syringe, place sample in an iced bag, or send the sample to the laboratory immediately
- Exposing the sample to air (increase or decrease in PaO_2 and $PaCO_2$)
- Venous blood in the sample (possible decrease in PaO_2 and increase in $PaCO_2$)
- HCO_3^-, ethacrynic acid, hydrocortisone, metolazone, prednisone, and thiazides (possible increase in $PaCO_2$)
- Acetazolamide, methicillin, nitrofurantoin, and tetracycline (possible decrease in $PaCO_2$)
- Fever (possible false-high PaO_2 and $PaCO_2$)

TOTAL CARBON DIOXIDE CONTENT

When carbon dioxide (CO_2) pressure in red blood cells exceeds 40 mm Hg, CO_2 spills out of the cells and dissolves in plasma. There it may combine with water to form carbonic acid, which in turn may dissociate into hydrogen and bicarbonate ions.

The total CO_2 content test is used to measure the total concentration of all forms of CO_2 in serum, plasma, or whole blood samples. It's commonly ordered for patients with respiratory insufficiency and is usually included in an assessment of electrolyte balance. Test results are most significant when considered with pH and arterial blood gas values.

Purpose

- To help evaluate acid-base balance

Acid-base disorders

DISORDERS AND A.B.G. FINDINGS	POSSIBLE CAUSES
Respiratory acidosis (excess CO_2 retention) pH < 7.35 (SI, < 7.35) HCO_3^- > 26 mEq/L (SI, > 26 mmol/L) (if compensating) $Paco_2$ > 45 mm Hg (SI, > 5.3 kPa)	◆ Central nervous system depression from drugs, injury, or disease ◆ Asphyxia ◆ Hypoventilation due to pulmonary, cardiac, musculoskeletal, or neuromuscular disease ◆ Obesity ◆ Postoperative pain ◆ Abdominal distention
Respiratory alkalosis (excess CO_2 excretion) pH > 7.45 (SI, > 7.45) HCO_3^- < 22 mEq/L (SI, < 22 mmol/L) (if compensating) $Paco_2$ < 35 mm Hg (SI, < 4.7 kPa)	◆ Hyperventilation due to anxiety, pain, or improper ventilator settings ◆ Respiratory stimulation caused by drugs, disease, hypoxia, fever, or high room temperature ◆ Gram-negative bacteremia ◆ Compensation for metabolic acidosis (chronic renal failure)
Metabolic acidosis (HCO_3 loss, acid retention) pH < 7.35 (SI, < 7.35) HCO_3^- < 22 mEq/L < (SI, < 22 mmol/L) $Paco_2$ > 35 mm Hg (SI, > 4.7 kPa) (if compensating)	◆ HCO_3^- depletion due to renal disease, diarrhea, or small-bowel fistulas ◆ Excessive production of organic acids due to hepatic disease; endocrine disorders, including diabetes mellitus, hypoxia, shock, and drug intoxication ◆ Inadequate excretion of acids due to renal disease
Metabolic alkalosis (HCO_3^- retention, acid loss) pH > 7.45 (SI, > 7.45) HCO_3^- > 26 mEq/L (SI, > 26 mmol/L) $Paco_2$ > 45 mm Hg (SI, > 5.3 kPa)	◆ Loss of hydrochloric acid from prolonged vomiting or gastric suctioning ◆ Loss of potassium due to increased renal excretion (as in diuretic therapy) or steroid overdose ◆ Excessive alkali ingestion ◆ Compensation for chronic respiratory acidosis

SIGNS AND SYMPTOMS

◆ Diaphoresis, headache, tachycardia, confusion, restlessness, apprehension

◆ Rapid, deep breathing; paresthesia; light-headedness; twitching; anxiety; fear

◆ Rapid, deep breathing; fruity breath; fatigue; headache; lethargy; drowsiness; nausea; vomiting; coma (if severe)

◆ Slow, shallow breathing; hypertonic muscles; restlessness; twitching; confusion; irritability; apathy; tetany; seizures; coma (if severe)

Patient preparation

- Explain to the patient that this test is performed to measure the amount of CO_2 in the blood.
- Tell the patient that the test requires a blood sample. Explain who will perform the venipuncture and when.
- Explain to the patient that he may experience discomfort from the needle puncture and the tourniquet.
- Inform the patient that he need not restrict food and fluids.
- Notify the laboratory and physician of medications the patient is taking that may affect test results; they may need to be restricted.

Procedure and posttest care

- Perform a venipuncture.
- When CO_2 content is measured along with electrolytes, a 3- or 4-ml clot activator tube may be used.
- When this test is performed alone, a heparinized tube is appropriate.
- Apply direct pressure to the venipuncture site until the bleeding has stopped.
- If a hematoma develops at the venipuncture site, apply warm soaks.

Precautions

- Fill the tube completely to prevent diffusion of CO_2 into the vacuum.

Reference values

Normally, total CO_2 levels range from 22 to 26 mEq/L (SI, 22 to 26 mmol/L). Levels may vary, depending on sex and age.

Abnormal findings

High CO_2 levels may occur in metabolic alkalosis, respiratory acidosis, primary aldosteronism, and Cushing's syndrome. CO_2 levels may also increase after excessive loss of acids, such as severe vomiting and continuous gastric drainage.

Decreased CO_2 levels are common in metabolic acidosis. Decreased total CO_2 levels in metabolic acidosis also result from loss of bicarbonate. Levels may decrease in respiratory alkalosis.

Interfering factors

- Underfilling the collection tube allows CO_2 to escape, resulting in inaccurate levels
- Excessive use of corticotropin, cortisone, or thiazide diuretics; excessive ingestion of alkalis or licorice (increase)
- Salicylates, paraldehyde, methicillin, dimercaprol, ammonium chloride, and acetazolamide; ingestion of ethylene glycol or methyl alcohol (decrease)

ALVEOLAR-TO-ARTERIAL OXYGEN GRADIENT ($A\text{-}aDO_2$)

Using calculations based on the patient's laboratory values, the alveolar-to-arterial oxygen gradient ($A\text{-}aDO_2$) test can help identify the cause of hypoxemia and intrapulmonary shunting by providing an approximation of the partial pressure of oxygenation of the alveoli and arteries. It may help differentiate cause as ventilated alveoli but no perfusion, unventilated alveoli with perfusion, or collapse of both alveoli and capillaries.

Purpose

- To evaluate the efficiency of gas exchange
- To assess the integrity of the ventilatory control system
- To monitor respiratory therapy

Patient preparation

- Explain to the patient that this test is used to evaluate how well the lungs are delivering oxygen to blood and eliminating carbon dioxide.
- Tell the patient that the test requires a blood sample. Explain who will perform the arterial puncture and when.
- Inform the patient that he need not restrict food and fluids.
- Instruct the patient to breathe normally during the test, and warn him that he may experience cramping or throbbing pain at the puncture site.

Procedure and posttest care

- Perform an arterial puncture or draw blood from an arterial line using a heparinized blood gas syringe.
- Eliminate all air from the sample and place it on ice immediately.
- Apply pressure to the puncture for 3 to 5 minutes or until bleeding has stopped.
- Place a gauze pad over the site and tape it in place, but don't tape the entire circumference.
- Monitor vital signs and observe for signs of circulatory impairment, such as swelling, discoloration, pain numbness, and tingling in the bandaged arm or leg.
- Watch for bleeding from the puncture site.
- The arterial sample is analyzed for partial pressure of arterial oxygen (PaO_2) and partial pressure of arterial carbon dioxide ($PaCO_2$). Also examined are barometric pressure (P_B), water vapor pressure (PH_2O), and fractional concentration of inspired oxygen (FIO_2) (21% for room air). From these values, the alveolar oxygen tension (PAO_2), the arterial-to-oxygen ratio (a/A ratio), and the alveolar-to-arterial difference for PO_2 ($A\text{-}aDO_2$) are derived by solving the following mathematical formulas:

– $PAO_2 = FIO_2\,(P_B - PH_2O) - 1.25\,(PaCO_2)$
– a/A ratio = PaO_2 divided by PAO_2
– $A\text{-}aDO_2 = PAO_2 - PaO_2$

■ Based on the results of the formulas, appropriate interventions to correct patient problems are initiated.

Precautions

■ Before sending the sample to the laboratory, note on the laboratory request whether the patient was breathing room air or receiving oxygen therapy when the sample was collected.
■ If the patient was receiving oxygen therapy, note the flow rate and method of delivery. If he was on a ventilator, note the fraction of inspired oxygen, tidal volume, mode, respiratory rate, and positive-end expiratory pressure.
■ Note the patient's rectal temperature.

Reference values

Normal values on room air for A-aDO_2 at rest is < 10 mm Hg and at maximum exercise is 20 to 30 mm Hg

Abnormal findings

■ Increased values may be caused by mucus plugs, bronchospasm, or airway collapse (asthma, bronchitis, emphysema).
■ Hypoxemia results in increased A-aDO_2 and may be caused by arterial septal defects, pneumothorax, atelectasis, emboli, or edema.

Interfering factors

■ Failure to heparinize the syringe, place the sample in an iced bag or send the sample to the laboratory immediately
■ Exposing the sample to air (increase or decrease)
■ Age and increasing oxygen concentration (increase)

ARTERIAL-TO-ALVEOLAR OXYGEN RATIO (a/A RATIO)

Using calculations based on the patient's laboratory values, the arterial-to-alveolar oxygen ratio (a/A ratio) test can help identify the cause of hypoxemia and intrapulmonary shunting by providing an approximation of the partial pressure of oxygenation of the alveoli and arteries. It may help differentiate cause as ventilated alveoli but no perfusion, unventilated alveoli with perfusion, or collapse of both alveoli and capillaries.

Purpose

■ To evaluate the efficiency of gas exchange
■ To assess the integrity of the ventilatory control system
■ To monitor respiratory therapy

Patient preparation

■ Explain to the patient that this test is used to evaluate how well the lungs are delivering oxygen to blood and eliminating carbon dioxide.
■ Tell the patient that the test requires a blood sample. Explain who will perform the arterial puncture and when.
■ Inform the patient that he need not restrict food and fluids.
■ Instruct the patient to breathe normally during the test, and warn him that he may experience cramping or throbbing pain at the puncture site.

Procedure and posttest care

■ Perform an arterial puncture or draw blood from an arterial line using a heparinized blood gas syringe.
■ Eliminate all air from the sample and place it on ice immediately.

- Apply pressure to the puncture for 3 to 5 minutes or until bleeding has stopped.
- Place a gauze pad over the site and tape it in place, but don't tape the entire circumference.
- Monitor vital signs and observe for signs of circulatory impairment, such as swelling, discoloration, pain numbness, and tingling in the bandaged arm or leg.
- Watch for bleeding from the puncture site.
- The arterial sample is analyzed for partial pressure of arterial oxygen (PaO_2) and partial pressure of carbon dioxide ($PaCO_2$). Also examined are barometric pressure (PB), water vapor pressure (PH_2O), and fractional concentration of inspired oxygen (FIO_2) (21% for room air). From these values, the alveolar oxygen tension (PAO_2), the arterial-to-oxygen ratio (a/A ratio), and the alveolar-to-arterial difference for PO_2 (A-aDO_2) are derived by solving the following mathematical formulas:
  - $PaO_2 = FIO_2 (PB - PH_2O) - 1.25 (PaCO_2)$
  - a/A ratio = PaO_2 divided by PAO_2
  - A-aDO_2 = $PAO_2 - PaO_2$
- Based on the results of the formulas, appropriate interventions to correct patient problems are initiated.

Precautions

- Before sending the sample to the laboratory, note on the laboratory request whether the patient was breathing room air or receiving oxygen therapy when the sample was collected.
- If the patient was receiving oxygen therapy, note the flow rate and method of delivery. If he was on a ventilator, note the fraction of inspired oxygen, tidal volume, mode, respiratory rate, and positive-end expiratory pressure.
- Note the patient's rectal temperature.

Reference values

The normal value for a/A ratio is 75%.

Abnormal findings

- Increased values may be caused by mucus plugs, bronchospasm, or airway collapse (asthma, bronchitis, emphysema).
- Hypoxemia results in increased A-aDO_2 and may be caused by arterial septal defects, pneumothorax, atelectasis, emboli, or edema.

Interfering factors

- Failure to heparinize the syringe, place the sample in an iced bag or send the sample to the laboratory immediately
- Exposing the sample to air (increase or decrease)
- Age and increasing oxygen concentration (increase)

ELECTROLYTES

CALCIUM

About 99% of the body's calcium is found in the teeth. Approximately 1% of total calcium in the body circulates in the blood. Of this, about 50% is bound to plasma proteins and 40% is ionized, or free. Evaluation of serum calcium levels measures the total amount of calcium in the blood, and ionized calcium measures the fraction of serum calcium that's in the ionized form.

Purpose

- To evaluate endocrine function, calcium metabolism, and acid-base balance
- To guide therapy in patients with renal failure, renal transplant, endocrine disorders, malignancies, cardiac disease, and skeletal disorders

Patient preparation

- Explain to the patient that this test is used to determine blood calcium levels.
- Tell the patient that the test requires a blood sample. Explain who will perform the venipuncture and when.
- Explain to the patient that he may experience slight discomfort from the needle puncture and the tourniquet.
- Inform the patient that he need not restrict food and fluids.

Procedure and posttest care

- Perform a venipuncture (without a tourniquet if possible) and collect the sample in a 3- or 4-ml clot-activator tube.
- Apply direct pressure to the venipuncture site until bleeding stops.
- If a hematoma develops at the venipuncture site, apply warm soaks.

Reference values

Normally, total calcium levels range from 8.2 to 10.2 mg/dl (SI, 2.05 to 2.54 mmol/L) in adults and 8.6 to 11.2 mg/dl (SI, 2.15 to 2.79 mmol/L) in children. Ionized calcium levels are 4.65 to 5.28 mg/dl (SI, 1.1 to 1.25 mmol/L).

Abnormal findings

Abnormally high serum calcium levels (hypercalcemia) may occur in hyperparathyroidism and parathyroid tumors, Paget's disease of the bone, multiple myeloma, metastatic carcinoma, multiple fractures, and prolonged immobilization. Elevated levels may also result from inadequate excretion of calcium, such as adrenal insufficiency and renal disease; from excessive calcium ingestion; and from overuse of antacids such as calcium carbonate.

◆ **CLINICAL ALERT** *Observe the patient with hypercalcemia for deep bone pain, flank pain due to renal calculi, and muscle hypotonicity. Hypercalcemic crisis begins with nausea, vomiting, and dehydration, leading to stupor and coma, and can end in cardiac arrest.*

Low calcium levels (hypocalcemia) may result from hypoparathyroidism, total parathyroidectomy, and malabsorption. Decreased serum calcium levels may also occur with Cushing's syndrome, renal failure, acute pancreatitis, peritonitis, malnutrition with hypoalbuminemia, renal failure, and blood transfusions (due to citrate).

In the patient with hypocalcemia, be alert for circumoral and peripheral numbness and tingling, muscle twitching, Chvostek's sign (facial muscle spasm), tetany, muscle cramping, Trousseau's sign (carpopedal spasm), seizures, arrhythmias, laryngeal spasm, decreased cardiac output, prolonged bleeding time, fractures and prolonged Q interval.

Interfering factors

- Venous stasis due to prolonged tourniquet application (possible false-high)
- Excessive ingestion of vitamin D or its derivatives (dihydrotachysterol, calcitriol); use of androgens, calciferol-activated calcium salts, progestins-estrogens, and thiazide diuretics (increase)
- Acetazolamide, corticosteroids, mithramycin, chronic laxative use, excessive transfusions of citrated blood (possible increase or decrease)

CHLORIDE

The chloride test is used to measure serum levels of chloride, the major extracellular fluid anion. Chloride helps maintain osmotic pressure of blood and, therefore, helps regulate blood volume and arterial pressure. Chloride levels also affect acid-base balance. Chloride is absorbed from the intestines and excreted primarily by the kidneys.

Purpose

- To detect acid-base imbalance (acidosis or alkalosis) and to aid evaluation of fluid status and extracellular cation-anion balance

Patient preparation

- Explain to the patient that the test is used to evaluate the chloride content of blood.
- Tell the patient that the test requires a blood sample. Explain who will perform the venipuncture and when.
- Explain to the patient that he may experience slight discomfort from the needle puncture and the tourniquet.
- Inform the patient that he need not restrict food and fluids.
- Notify the laboratory and physician of medications the patient is taking that may affect test results; they may need to be restricted.

Procedure and posttest care

- Perform a venipuncture and collect the sample in a 3- to 4-ml clot-activator tube.
- Apply direct pressure to the venipuncture site until bleeding stops.
- If a hematoma develops at the venipuncture site, apply warm soaks.

Precautions

- Handle the sample gently to prevent hemolysis.

Reference values

Normally, serum chloride levels range from 100 to 108 mEq/L (SI, 100 to 108 mmol/L) in adults.

Abnormal findings

Chloride levels are inversely related to bicarbonate levels, reflecting acid-base balance. Excessive loss of gastric juices or other secretions containing chloride may cause hypochloremic metabolic alkalosis; excessive chloride retention or ingestion may lead to hyperchloremic metabolic acidosis.

Severe dehydration, complete renal shutdown, head injury (producing neurogenic hyperventilation), and primary aldosteronism (increase).

Low sodium and potassium levels due to prolonged vomiting, gastric suctioning, intestinal fistula, chronic renal failure, and Addison's disease (decrease). Heart failure or edema resulting in excess extracellular fluid can cause dilutional hypochloremia.

◆ **CLINICAL ALERT** *Observe the patient with hypochloremia for hypertonicity of muscles, tetany, depressed respirations and decreased blood pressure with dehydration. In the patient with hyperchloremia, be alert for signs of developing stupor, rapid deep breathing, and weakness that may lead to coma.*

Interfering factors

- Hemolysis due to rough handling of the sample
- Use of ammonium chloride, cholestyramine, boric acid, oxyphenbutazone, or phenylbutazone and excessive I.V. infusion of sodium chloride (possible increase)
- Use of thiazide diuretics, ethacrynic acid, furosemide, or bicarbonates and prolonged I.V. infusion of dextrose 5% in water (decrease)

MAGNESIUM

The magnesium test is used to measure serum levels of magnesium, an electrolyte that is not only vital to neuromuscular function. It also helps in intracellular metabolism, activates many essential enzymes, and affects the metabolism of nucleic acids and proteins. Magnesium also helps transport sodium and potassium across cell membranes, and influences intracellular calcium levels. Most magnesium is found in bone and intracellular fluid; a small amount is found in extracellular fluid. Magnesium is absorbed by the small intestine and excreted in the urine and stool.

Purpose

- To evaluate electrolyte status
- To assess neuromuscular and renal function

Patient preparation

- Explain to the patient that this test is used to determine the magnesium content of the blood.
- Instruct the patient not to use magnesium salts (such as milk of magnesia or Epsom salt) for at least 3 days before the test, but tell him that he need not restrict food and fluids.
- Tell the patient that the test requires a blood sample. Explain who will perform the venipuncture and when.
- Explain to the patient that he may experience slight discomfort from the needle puncture and the tourniquet.

Procedure and posttest care

- Perform a venipuncture without a tourniquet if possible and collect the sample in a 3- or 4-ml clot-activator tube.
- Apply pressure to the venipuncture site until bleeding stops.
- If a hematoma develops at the venipuncture site, apply warm soaks.

Precautions

- Handle the sample gently to prevent hemolysis.

Reference values

Serum magnesium levels range from 1.3 to 2.1 mg/dl (SI, 0.65 to 1.05 mmol/L)

Abnormal findings

Elevated serum magnesium levels (hypermagnesemia) most commonly occur in renal failure, when the kidneys excrete inadequate amounts of magnesium, and also by magnesium administration or ingestion. Adrenal insufficiency (Addison's disease) can also increase serum magnesium levels.

In suspected or confirmed hypermagnesemia, observe the patient for lethargy; flushing; diaphoresis; decreased blood pressure; slow, weak pulse; muscle weakness; diminished deep tendon reflexes; slow, shallow respiration, and electrocardiogram (ECG) changes (prolonged PR interval, wide QRS complex, elevated T waves, atrioventricular block, premature ventricular contractions).

Decreased serum magnesium levels (hypomagnesemia) most commonly result from chronic alcoholism. Other causes include malabsorption syndrome, diarrhea, faulty absorption after bowel resection, prolonged bowel or gastric aspiration, acute pancreatitis, primary aldosteronism, severe burns, hypercalcemic conditions (including hyperparathyroidism), malnutrition, and certain diuretic therapy.

In hypomagnesemia, watch for leg and foot cramps, hyperactive deep tendon reflexes, arrhythmias, muscle weakness, seizures, twitching, tetany, and tremors, ECG changes (PBCs and ventricular fibrillation).

Interfering factors

- Venous stasis due to tourniquet use
- Obtaining a sample above an I.V. site that's receiving a solution containing magnesium
- Excessive use of antacids or cathartics or excessive infusion of magnesium sulfate (increase)
- Prolonged I.V. infusions without magnesium; excessive use of diuretics (decrease)
- I.V. administration of calcium gluconate (possible false-low if measured using the Titan yellow method)
- Hemolysis (false-high)

PHOSPHATES

The phosphate test is used to measure serum levels of phosphates, the primary anion in intracellular fluid. Phosphates are essential in the storage and utilization of energy, calcium regulation, red blood cell function, acid-base balance, formation of bone, and the metabolism of carbohydrates, protein, and fat. The intestines absorb most phosphates from dietary sources; the kidneys excrete phosphates and serve as a regulatory mechanism. Abnormal concentrations of serum phosphates usually result from improper excretion rather than faulty ingestion or absorption from dietary sources.

Normally, calcium and phosphates have an inverse relationship; if one is increased, the other is decreased.

Purpose

- To aid diagnosis of renal disorders and acid-base imbalance
- To detect endocrine, skeletal, and calcium disorders

Patient preparation

- Explain to the patient that this test is used to measure phosphate levels in the blood.
- Tell the patient that the test requires a blood sample. Explain who will perform the venipuncture and when.
- Explain to the patient that he may experience slight discomfort from the needle puncture and the tourniquet.
- Inform the patient that he need not restrict food and fluids.
- Notify the laboratory and physician of medications the patient is taking that may affect test results; they may need to be restricted.

Procedure and posttest care

- Perform a venipuncture without using a tourniquet if possible, and collect the sample in 3- to 4-ml clot-activator tube.
- Apply pressure to the venipuncture site until bleeding stops.
- If a hematoma develops at the venipuncture site, apply warm soaks.

Precautions

- Handle the sample gently to prevent hemolysis.

Reference values

Normally, serum phosphate levels in adults range from 2.7 to 4.5 mg/dl (SI, 0.87 to 1.45 mmol/L). In children, the normal range is 4.5 to 6.7 mg/dl (SI, 1.45 to 1.78 mmol/L).

Abnormal findings

Decreased phosphate levels (hypophosphatemia) may result from malnutrition, malabsorption syndromes, hyperparathyroidism, renal tubular acidosis, and treatment of diabetic ketoacidosis. In children, hypophosphatemia can suppress normal growth. Symptoms of hypophosphatemia include anemia, prolonged bleeding, bone demineralization, decreased white blood cell count, and anorexia.

Increased levels (hyperphosphatemia) may result from skeletal disease, healing fractures, hypoparathyroidism, acromegaly, diabetic ketoacidosis, high intestinal obstruction, lactic acidosis (due to hepatic impairment) and renal failure. Hyperphosphatemia is seldom clinically significant, but it can alter bone metabolism in prolonged cases. Symptoms of hyperphosphatemia include tachycardia, muscular weakness, diarrhea, cramping, hyperreflexia.

Interfering factors

- Venous stasis due to tourniquet use
- Sample obtained above an I.V. site that's receiving a solution containing phosphate
- Excessive vitamin D intake or therapy with anabolic steroids or androgens (possible increase)
- Use of acetazolamide, insulin, epinephrine, or phosphate-binding antacids; excessive excretion due to prolonged vomiting or diarrhea; vitamin D deficiency; extended I.V. infusion of dextrose 5% in water (possible decrease)
- Hemolysis of the sample (false-high)

POTASSIUM

The potassium test is used to measure serum levels of potassium, the major intracellular cation. Potassium helps to maintain cellular osmotic equilibrium and to regulate muscle activity, enzyme activity, and acid-base balance. It also influences renal function.

The body has no efficient method for conserving potassium; the kidneys excrete nearly all ingested potassium, even when the body's supply is depleted. Potassium deficiency can develop rapidly and is quite common. Dietary intake of at least 40 mEq/day is essential.

Purpose

- To evaluate clinical signs of potassium excess (hyperkalemia) or potassium depletion (hypokalemia)
- To monitor renal function, acid-base balance, and glucose metabolism
- To evaluate neuromuscular and endocrine disorders
- To detect the origin of arrhythmias

Patient preparation

- Explain to the patient that this test is used to determine the potassium content of blood.
- Tell the patient that the test requires a blood sample. Explain who will perform the venipuncture and when.
- Explain to the patient that he may experience slight discomfort from the needle puncture and the tourniquet.
- Inform the patient that he need not restrict food and fluids.
- Notify the laboratory and physician of medications the patient is taking that may affect test results; they may need to be restricted.

Procedure and posttest care

- Perform a venipuncture and collect the sample in a 3- or 4-ml clot-activator tube.
- Apply direct pressure to the venipuncture site until bleeding stops.
- If a hematoma develops at the venipuncture site, apply warm soaks.

Precautions

- Draw the sample immediately after applying the tourniquet because a delay may increase the potassium level by allowing intracellular potassium to leak into the serum.

■ Handle the sample gently to avoid hemolysis.

Reference values

Normally, serum potassium levels range from 3.5 to 5 mEq/L (SI, 3.5 to 5 mmol/L).

Abnormal findings

Abnormally high serum potassium levels are common in conditions in which excess cellular potassium enters the blood, such as burn injuries, crush injuries, diabetic ketoacidosis, transfusions of large amounts of blood, and myocardial infarction. Hyperkalemia may also indicate reduced sodium excretion, possibly due to renal failure (preventing normal exchange of sodium and potassium) or Addison's disease (due to potassium buildup and sodium depletion).

◆ CLINICAL ALERT *Observe the patient with hyperkalemia for weakness, malaise, nausea, diarrhea, colicky pain, muscle irritability progressing to flaccid paralysis, oliguria, and bradycardia. The electrocardiogram (ECG) reveals flattened P waves, a prolonged PR interval; wide QRS complex; tall, tented T wave; and ST-segment depression. Cardiac arrest may occur without warning.*

Below-normal potassium values often result from aldosteronism or Cushing's syndrome, loss of body fluids (such as long-term diuretic therapy, vomiting, or diarrhea), and excessive licorice ingestion. Although serum values and clinical symptoms can indicate a potassium imbalance, an ECG allows a definitive diagnosis.

◆ CLINICAL ALERT *Observe the patient with hypokalemia for decreased reflexes; a rapid, weak, irregular pulse; mental confusion; hypotension; anorexia; muscle weakness; and paresthesia. ECG shows a flattened T wave, ST-segment depression, and U-wave elevation. In severe cases, ventricular fibrillation, respiratory paralysis, and cardiac arrest can develop.*

Interfering factors

■ Repeated clenching of the fist before venipuncture (possible increase)
■ Delay in drawing blood after applying a tourniquet or excessive hemolysis of the sample (increase)
■ Excessive or rapid potassium infusion, spironolactone or penicillin G potassium therapy, and renal toxicity from administration of amphotericin B, methicillin, or tetracycline (increase)
■ Insulin and glucose administration; diuretic therapy (especially with thiazides but not with triamterene, amiloride, or spironolactone); I.V. infusions without potassium (decrease)

SODIUM

The sodium test is used to measure serum levels of sodium in relation to the amount of water in the body. Sodium, the major extracellular cation, affects body water distribution, maintains osmotic pressure of extracellular fluid, and helps promote neuromuscular function. It also helps maintain acid-base balance and influences chloride and potassium levels.

Purpose

■ To evaluate fluid-electrolyte and acid-base balance and related neuromuscular, renal, and adrenal functions

Patient preparation

■ Explain to the patient that this test is used to determine the sodium content of blood.
■ Tell the patient that the test requires a blood sample. Explain who will perform the venipuncture and when.
■ Explain to the patient that he may experience slight discomfort from the needle puncture and the tourniquet.
■ Inform the patient that he need not restrict food and fluids.
■ Notify the laboratory and physician of medications the patient is taking that may affect test results; they may need to be restricted.

Procedure and posttest care

■ Perform a venipuncture and collect the sample in a 3- or 4-ml clot-activator tube.
■ Apply direct pressure to the venipuncture site until bleeding stops.
■ If a hematoma develops at the venipuncture site, apply warm soaks.

Precautions

■ Handle the sample gently to prevent hemolysis.

Reference values

Normally, serum sodium levels range from 135 to 145 mEq/L (SI, 135 to 145 mmol/L).

Abnormal findings

Sodium imbalance can result from a loss or gain of sodium or from a change in the patient's state of hydration. Increased serum sodium levels (hypernatremia) may be due to inadequate water intake, water loss in excess of sodium (such as diabetes insipidus, impaired renal function, prolonged hyperventilation and, occasionally, severe vomiting or diarrhea), and sodium retention (such as aldosteronism). Hypernatremia can also result from excessive sodium intake.

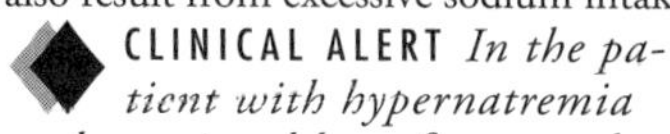

CLINICAL ALERT *In the patient with hypernatremia and associated loss of water, observe for signs of thirst, restlessness, dry and sticky mucous membranes, flushed skin, oliguria, and diminished reflexes. If increased total body sodium causes water retention, observe for hypertension, dyspnea, edema, and heart failure.*

Abnormally low serum sodium levels (hyponatremia) may result from inadequate sodium intake or excessive sodium loss due to profuse sweating, GI suctioning, diuretic therapy, diarrhea, vomiting, adrenal insufficiency, burns, and chronic renal insufficiency with acidosis. Urine sodium determinations are usually more sensitive to early changes in sodium balance and should be evaluated simultaneously with serum sodium findings.

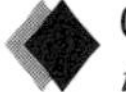

CLINICAL ALERT *In the patient with hyponatremia, watch for apprehension, lassitude, headache, decreased skin turgor, abdominal cramps, and tremors that may progress to seizures.*

Interfering factors

■ Hemolysis due to rough handling of the sample
■ Most diuretics (decrease by promoting sodium excretion)
■ Lithium, chlorpropamide, and vasopressin (decrease by inhibiting water excretion)
■ Corticosteroids (increase by promoting sodium retention)
■ Antihypertensives, such as methyldopa, hydralazine, and reserpine (possible increase due to sodium and water retention)

ANION GAP

Total concentrations of cations and anions are usually equal, making serum electrically neutral. Measuring the gap between measured cation and anion levels provides information about the level of anions (including sulfate, phosphate, organic acids such as ketone bodies and lactic acid, and proteins) that are not routinely measured in laboratory tests. In metabolic acidosis, measuring the anion gap helps to identify the type of acidosis and possible causes. Further tests are usually needed to determine the specific cause of metabolic acidosis.

Purpose

- To distinguish types of metabolic acidosis
- To monitor renal function and total parenteral nutrition

Patient preparation

- Explain to the patient that this test is used to determine the cause of acidosis.
- Tell the patient that the test requires a blood sample. Explain who will perform the venipuncture and when.
- Explain to the patient that he may experience slight discomfort from the needle puncture and the tourniquet.
- Inform the patient that he need not restrict food and fluids.
- Notify the lab and physician of medications the patient is taking that may affect test results; they may need to be restricted.

Procedure and posttest care

- Perform a venipuncture and collect the sample in a 3- or 4-ml clot-activator tube.
- Apply direct pressure to the venipuncture site until bleeding stops.
- If a hematoma develops at the venipuncture site, apply warm soaks.
- Instruct the patient to resume medications discontinued before the test as ordered.

Precautions

- Handle the sample gently to prevent hemolysis.

Reference values

Normally, the anion gap ranges from 8 to 14 mEq/L (SI, 8 to 14 mmol/L).

Abnormal findings

A normal anion gap does not rule out metabolic acidosis. It may occur in hyperchloremic acidoses, renal tubular acidosis, and severe bicarbonate-wasting conditions, such as biliary or pancreatic fistulas and poorly functioning ileal loops.

When acidosis results from loss of bicarbonate in the urine or other body fluids, the anion gap remains unchanged. This is known as *normal anion gap acidosis.*

An increased anion gap indicates an increase in one or more of the unmeasured anions (sulfate, phosphates, organic acids such as ketone bodies and lactic acid, and proteins). This may occur with acidoses that are characterized by excessive organic or inorganic acids, such as lactic acidosis or ketoacidosis.

When acidosis results from an accumulation of metabolic acids — as occurs in lactic acidosis, for example — the anion gap increases (> 14 mEq/L) with the increase in unmeasured anions. Metabolic acidosis caused by such an accumulation is known as *high anion gap acidosis.*

A decreased anion gap is rare but may occur with hypermagnesemia and paraproteinemic states, such as multiple myeloma and Waldenström's macroglobulinemia.

Interfering factors

- Hemolysis due to rough handling of the sample
- Diuretics, lithium, chlorpropamide, and vasopressin (possible decrease due to decreased serum sodium levels)
- Corticosteroids and antihypertensives (possible increase due to increased serum sodium levels)
- Salicylates, paraldehyde, methicillin, dimercaprol, ammonium chloride, acetazolamide, ethylene glycol, and methyl alcohol (possible increase due to decreased serum bicarbonate levels)
- Adrenocorticotrophic hormone, cortisone, mercurial or chlorthiazide diuretics, and excessive ingestion of alkalis or licorice (possible decrease due to increased serum bicarbonate levels)
- Ammonium chloride, cholestyramine, boric acid, oxyphenbutazone, phenylbutazone, and excessive I.V. infusion of sodium chloride (possible decrease due to increased serum chloride levels)
- Thiazide diuretics, ethacrynic acid, furosemide, bicarbonates, and prolonged I.V. infusion of dextrose 5% in water (possible increase due to decreased serum chloride levels)
- Iodine absorption from wounds packed with povidone-iodine or excessive use of magnesium-containing antacids, especially by patients with renal failure (possible false-low)

CARDIAC ENZYMES AND PROTEINS

B-TYPE NATRIURETIC PEPTIDE ASSAY

B-type natriuretic peptide (BNP) is a neurohormone produced predominantly by the heart ventricle. BNP is released from the heart in response to ventricle distension due to blood volume expansion or pressure overload.

Plasma BNP increases with the severity of heart failure. Studies have demonstrated that the heart is the major source of circulating BNP. It's an excellent hormonal marker of ventricular systolic and diastolic dysfunction.

Purpose

- To aid in the diagnosis of heart failure

Patient preparation

- Explain to the patient that this test is used to identify the presence and severity of heart failure.
- Tell the patient who will perform the venipuncture and when.
- Explain to the patient that he may experience some discomfort from the needle puncture and the tourniquet.
- Inform the patient that he need not restrict food and fluids.

Procedure and posttest care

- Perform a venipuncture and collect the sample in a 3.5-ml EDTA tube.
- Apply direct pressure to the venipuncture site until bleeding stops.
- If a hematoma develops at the venipuncture site, apply warm soaks.

Precautions

■ Handle the sample gently to prevent hemolysis.

Reference values

The normal value is < 100 pg/ml.

Abnormal findings

Blood concentrations greater than 100 pg/ml are an accurate predictor of heart failure.

Interfering factors

■ Hemolysis due to rough handling of the sample

CREATINE KINASE

Creatine kinase (CK) is an enzyme that catalyzes the creatine-creatinine metabolic pathway in muscle cells and brain tissue. Because of its intimate role in energy production, CK reflects normal tissue catabolism; increased serum levels indicate trauma to cells.

Fractionation and measurement of three distinct CK isoenzymes — CKBB (CK_1), CK-MB (CK_2), and CK-MM (CK_3) — have replaced the use of total CK levels to accurately localize the site of increased tissue destruction. CK-BB is most commonly found in brain tissue. CK-MM and CK-MB are found primarily in skeletal and heart muscle. In addition, subunits of CK-MB and CK-MM, called isoforms or isoenzymes, can be assayed to increase the test's sensitivity.

Purpose

■ To detect and diagnose acute myocardial infarction (MI) and reinfarction (CK-MB primarily used)

■ To evaluate possible causes of chest pain and to monitor the severity of myocardial ischemia after cardiac surgery, cardiac catheterization, and cardioversion (CK-MB primarily used)

■ To detect early dermatomyositis, and musculoskeletal disorders that aren't neurogenic in origin such as Duchenne muscular dystrophy (total CK primarily used)

Patient preparation

■ Explain to the patient that this test is used to assess myocardial and musculoskeletal function and that multiple blood samples are required to detect fluctuations in serum levels.

■ Tell the patient who will be performing the venipunctures and when.

■ Explain to the patient that he may experience slight discomfort from the needle puncture and the tourniquet.

■ If the patient is being evaluated for musculoskeletal disorders, advise him to avoid exercising for 24 hours before the test.

■ Notify the laboratory and physician of medications the patient is taking that may affect test results; they may need to be restricted.

Procedure and posttest care

■ Perform a venipuncture and collect the sample in a 4-ml tube without additives.

■ Apply direct pressure to the venipuncture site until bleeding stops.

■ If a hematoma develops at the venipuncture site, apply warm soaks.

■ Instruct the patient that he may resume exercise and medications discontinued before the test as ordered.

Precautions

■ Draw the sample before giving I.M. injections or 1 hour after giving them because muscle trauma increases total CK level.

■ Obtain the sample on schedule. Note on the laboratory request the time the sample was drawn and the hours elapsed since onset of chest pain.

■ Handle the sample gently to prevent hemolysis.

■ Send the sample to the laboratory immediately because CK activity diminishes significantly after 2 hours at room temperature.

Reference values

Total CK values determined by ultraviolet or kinetic measurement range from 55 to 170 U/L (SI, 0.94 to 2.89 μKat/L) for men and from 30 to 135 U/L (SI, 0.51 to 2.3 μKat/L) for women. CK levels may be significantly higher in muscular people. Infants up to age 1 have levels two to four times higher than adult levels, possibly reflecting birth trauma and striated muscle development. Normal ranges for isoenzyme levels are as follows: CK-BB, undetectable; CK-MB, < 5% (SI, < 0.05); CK-MM, 90% to 100% (SI, 0.90 to 1.00).

Abnormal findings

CK-MM makes up 99% of total CK normally present in serum. Detectable CK-BB isoenzyme may indicate, but doesn't confirm, a diagnosis of brain tissue injury, widespread malignant tumors, severe shock, or renal failure.

CK-MB levels > 5% of total CK indicate MI, especially if the lactate dehydrogenase isoenzyme ratio is > 1 (flipped LD). In acute MI and after cardiac surgery, CK-MB begins to increase within 2 to 4 hours, peaks within 12 to 24 hours, and usually returns to normal within 24 to 48 hours; persistent elevations and increasing levels indicate ongoing myocardial damage. Total CK follows roughly the same pattern, but increases slightly later. CK-MB levels may not increase in heart failure or during angina pectoris not accompanied by myocardial cell necrosis. Serious skeletal muscle injury that occurs in certain muscular dystrophies, polymyositis, and severe myoglobinuria may produce a mild CK-MB increase because a small amount of this isoenzyme is present in some skeletal muscles.

Increasing CK-MM values follow skeletal muscle damage from trauma, such as surgery and I.M. injections, and from diseases, such as dermatomyositis and muscular dystrophy (values may be 50 to 100 times normal). A moderate increase in CK-MM levels develops in patients with hypothyroidism; sharp increases occur with muscle activity caused by agitation, such as during an acute psychotic episode.

Total CK levels may be increased in patients with severe hypokalemia, carbon monoxide poisoning, malignant hyperthermia, and alcoholic cardiomyopathy. They may also be increased after seizures and, occasionally, in patients who have suffered pulmonary or cerebral infarctions. Troponin-I and cardiac troponin C are present in the contractile cells of cardiac myocardial tissue, and are released with injury to the myocardial tissue. Troponin levels increase within 1 hour of the infarction and may remain elevated for up to 14 days. (See *Serum protein and isoenzyme levels after MI,* page 148.)

Interfering factors

■ Hemolysis due to rough handling of the sample

■ Failure to send the sample to the laboratory immediately or to refrigerate the serum if testing will be delayed more than 2 hours (possible decrease in concentration)

■ Failure to draw the samples at the scheduled time (may miss peak levels)

■ Halothane and succinylcholine, alcohol, lithium, large doses of aminocaproic acid, I.M. injections, cardioversion, invasive diagnostic procedures, re-

Serum protein and isoenzyme levels after MI

Because they're released by damaged tissue, serum proteins and isoenzymes (catalytic proteins that vary in concentration in specific organs) can help identify the compromised organ and assess the extent of damage after myocardial infarction (MI). The serum protein and isoenzyme determinations listed below are most significant after MI.

ISOENZYMES

- Creatine kinase-MB (CK-MB): in the heart muscle and a small amount in skeletal muscle
- Lactate dehydrogenase 1 and 2 (LD_1, LD_2): in the heart, brain, kidneys, liver, skeletal muscles, and red blood cells

PROTEINS

- Troponin-I and troponin-T (the cardiac contractile proteins) have greater sensitivity than CK-MB in detecting myocardial injury.

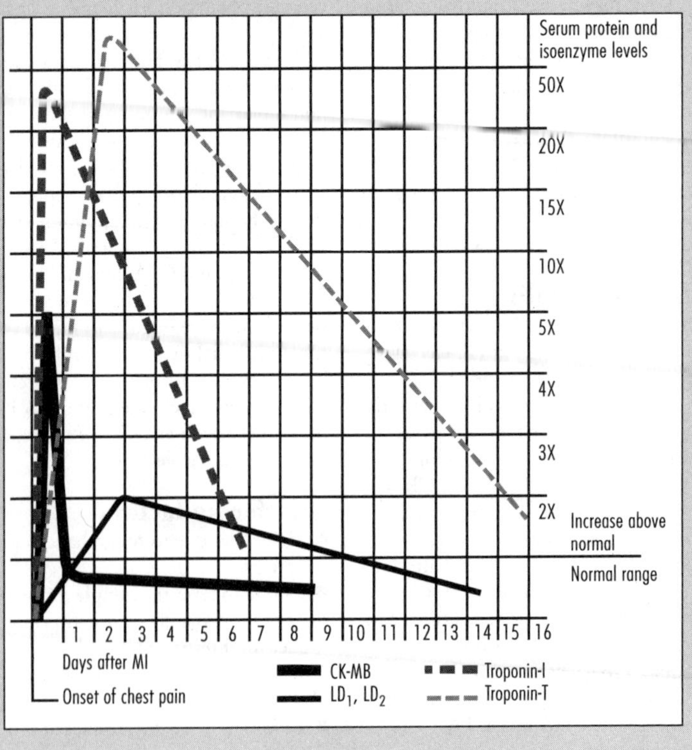

cent vigorous exercise or muscle massage, severe coughing, and trauma (increase in total CK)
- Surgery through skeletal muscle (increase in total CK)

LACTATE DEHYDROGENASE

Lactate dehydrogenase (LD) catalyzes the reversible conversion of muscle lactic acid into pyruvic acid, an essential step in the metabolic processes that ultimately produce cellular energy. Because LD is present in almost all body tissues, cellular damage increases total serum LD, limiting the diagnostic usefulness of LD.

Five tissue-specific isoenzymes can be identified and measured: LD_1 and LD_2 appear primarily in the heart, red blood cells (RBCs), and kidneys; LD_3 is primarily in the lungs; and LD_4 and LD_5 are in the liver, skin, and the skeletal muscles.

Purpose

- To aid differential diagnosis of myocardial infarction (MI), pulmonary infarction, anemias, and hepatic disease
- To support creatine kinase (CK) isoenzyme test results in diagnosing MI, or to provide diagnosis when CK-MB samples are drawn too late to display increase
- To monitor patient response to some forms of chemotherapy

Patient preparation

- Explain to the patient that this test is used primarily to detect tissue alterations.
- Tell the patient that the test requires a blood sample. Explain who will perform the venipuncture and when.
- Explain to the patient that he may experience slight discomfort from the needle puncture and the tourniquet.
- Inform the patient that he need not restrict food and fluids.
- If MI is suspected, tell the patient that the test will be repeated on the next two mornings to monitor progressive changes.

Procedure and posttest care

- Perform a venipuncture and collect the sample in a 4-ml clot-activator tube.
- Apply direct pressure to the venipuncture site until bleeding stops.
- If a hematoma develops at the venipuncture site, apply warm soaks.

Precautions

- Draw the samples on schedule to avoid missing peak levels and mark the collection time on the laboratory request.
- Handle the sample gently to prevent artifact blood sample hemolysis because RBCs contain LD_1.
- Send the sample to the laboratory immediately or, if transport is delayed, keep the sample at room temperature. Changes in temperature reportedly inactivate LD_5, thus altering isoenzyme patterns.

Reference values

Total LD levels normally range from 71 to 207 U/L (SI, 1.2 to 3.52 μKat/L). Normal distribution is as follows:

- LD_1: 14% to 26% (SI, 0.14 to 0.26) of total
- LD_2: 29% to 39% (SI, 0.29 to 0.39) of total
- LD_3: 20% to 26% (SI, 0.20 to 0.26) of total
- LD_4: 8% to 16% (SI, 0.08 to 0.16) of total
- LD_5: 6% to 16% (SI, 0.06 to 0.16) of total.

Abnormal findings

Because many common diseases increase total LD levels, isoenzyme electrophoresis is usually necessary for diagnosis. In some disorders, total LD may be within normal limits, but abnormal proportions of each enzyme indicate specific organ tissue damage. For instance, in acute MI, the concentration of LD_1 is greater than LD_2 within 12 to 48 hours after onset of symptoms; therefore the LD_1/LD_2 ratio is greater than 1. This reversal of normal isoenzyme pattern is typical of myocardial damage and is known as flipped LD.

Midzone fractions (LD_2, LD_3, LD_4) can be increased in granulocytic leukemia, lymphomas, and platelet disorders.

Interfering factors

- Hemolysis due to rough handling of the sample
- For diagnosis of acute MI, failure to draw the sample on schedule
- Failure to send the sample to the laboratory immediately (may obscure LD isoenzyme patterns)
- Failure to centrifuge the sample and separate the cells from the serum
- Recent surgery or pregnancy (possible increase)
- Prosthetic heart valve (possible increase due to chronic hemolysis)
- Anabolic steroids, anesthetics, alcohol, narcotics, and procainamide (increase)

MYOGLOBINS

Myoglobin, which is usually found in skeletal and cardiac muscle, functions as an oxygen-binding muscle protein. It's released into the bloodstream in ischemia, trauma, and inflammation of the muscle.

Purpose

- As a nonspecific test, to estimate damage to skeletal or cardiac muscle tissue
- To predict flareups of polymyositis
- Specifically, to determine if myocardial infarction (MI) has occurred

Patient preparation

- Explain the purpose of the test to the patient.
- Obtain a patient history, including disorders that may be associated with increased myoglobin levels.
- Tell the patient who will be performing the venipuncture and when.
- Explain to the patient that he may experience slight discomfort from the needle puncture and the tourniquet.
- Inform the patient that the results need to be correlated with other tests for a definitive diagnosis.

Procedure and posttest care

- Perform a venipuncture and collect the sample in a 4-ml tube with no additives.
- Apply direct pressure to the venipuncture site until bleeding stops.
- If a hematoma develops at the venipuncture site, apply warm soaks.

Precautions

- Expect to collect blood samples 4 to 8 hours after the onset of an acute MI.
- Handle the sample gently to avoid hemolysis.
- Send the sample to the laboratory immediately.

Reference values

Normal myoglobin values are 0 to 0.09 μg/ml (SI, 5 to 70 μ/L).

Abnormal findings

Besides MI, increased myoglobin levels may occur in acute alcohol intoxication, dermatomyositis, hypothermia (with prolonged shivering), muscular dystrophy, polymyositis, rhabomyelitis, severe burn injuries, trauma, severe renal failure, and systemic lupus erythematosus.

Interfering factors

- Hemolysis or radioactive scans performed within 1 week of the test
- Recent angina, cardioversion, or improper timing of the test (possible increase)
- I.M. injection (possible false-positive)

TROPONIN

Cardiac troponin I (cTnI) and cardiac troponin T (cTnT) are proteins in the striated cells that are extremely specific markers of cardiac damage. When injury occurs to the myocardial tissue, these proteins are released into the bloodstream. Elevations in troponin levels can be seen within 1 hour of myocardial infarction (MI) and will persist for a week or longer.

Purpose

- To detect and diagnose acute MI and reinfarction
- To evaluate possible causes of chest pain

Patient preparation

- Explain to the patient that this test helps assess myocardial injury and that multiple samples may be drawn to detect fluctuations in serum levels.
- Inform the patient he need not restrict foods and fluids.
- Tell the patient who will be performing the venipuncture and when.
- Explain to the patient that he may feel slight discomfort from the needle puncture and the tourniquet.

Procedure and posttest care

- Perform a venipuncture and collect the specimen in a 7-ml clot-activator tube.
- If a hematoma develops at the venipuncture site, apply warm soaks.

Precautions

- Obtain each specimen on schedule and note the date and collection time on each.

Reference values

Laboratory results may vary. Some laboratories may call a test positive if it shows any detectable levels, and others may give a range for abnormal results. Normally, cTnI levels are < 0.35 μg/L (SI, < 0.35 μg/L). cTnT levels are < 0.1 μg/L (SI, < 0.1 μg/L). cTnI levels > 2.0 μg/L (SI, > 2.0 μg/L) are suggestive of cardiac injury. Results of a qualitative cTnT rapid immunoassay that are > 0.1 μg/L (SI, > 0.1 μg/L) are considered positive for cardiac injury. As long as tissue injury continues, the troponin levels will remain high.

Abnormal findings

- Troponin levels rise rapidly and are detectable within 1 hour of myocardial cell injury. cTnI levels aren't detectable in people who don't have cardiac injury.

Interfering factors

- Sustained vigorous exercise (increase in absence of significant cardiac damage)
- Cardiotoxic drugs such as doxorubicin (increase)
- Renal disease, certain surgical procedures (possible increase)

C-REACTIVE PROTEIN

C-reactive protein (CRP) is a specific abnormal protein which appears in the blood during an inflammatory process. It's absent from the blood serum of healthy people. This nonspecific protein is mainly synthesized in the liver and is found in many body fluids (pleural, peritoneal, pericardial, synovial). It appears in the blood 18 to 24 hours after onset of tissue damage with levels that increase up to 1,000-fold and then decline rapidly when the inflammatory process regresses. CRP has been found to increase before rises in antibody titers and erythrocyte sedimentation rate (ESR) levels occur, and also decreases sooner than ESR levels.

Purpose

- To evaluate inflammatory disease course and severity in conditions where there is tissue necrosis (myocardial infarction [MI], malignancy, rheumatoid arthritis)
- To monitor acute inflammatory phases of rheumatoid arthritis and rheumatic fever so early treatment can be initiated
- To monitor response to treatment or determine if the acute phase is declining
- To help interpret the ESR
- To monitor the wound healing process of internal incisions, burns, and organ transplantation

Patient preparation

- Explain to the patient that this test is used to identify the presence of infection or to monitor treatment.
- Inform the patient that he needs to restrict all fluids except for water for 8 to 12 hours before the test.
- Tell the patient who will perform the venipuncture and when.
- Explain to the patient that he may experience slight discomfort from the needle puncture and the tourniquet.
- Notify the laboratory and physician of medications the patient is taking that may affect test results; they may need to be restricted.

Procedure and posttest care

- Perform a venipuncture and collect the sample in a 5-ml clot-activator tube.
- Apply direct pressure to the venipuncture site until bleeding stops.
- If a hematoma develops at the venipuncture site, apply warm soaks.
- Instruct the patient that he may resume his usual diet and medications discontinued before the test as ordered.

Precautions

- Keep the blood sample away from heat.

Reference values

Reference values usually aren't present. In adults, results may be reported as < 0.8 mg/dL (SI, < 8 mg/L).

Abnormal findings

- An elevated level may be present in rheumatoid arthritis, rheumatic fever, MI, cancer (active, widespread), acute bacterial and viral infections, inflammatory bowel disease
- Hodgkin's disease, systemic lupus erythematosus, postoperatively (declines after the fourth day).

Interfering factors

- Steroids and salicylates (false normal level)
- Oral contraceptives (false increase)
- Pregnancy (third trimester) and intrauterine contraceptive devices (increase)

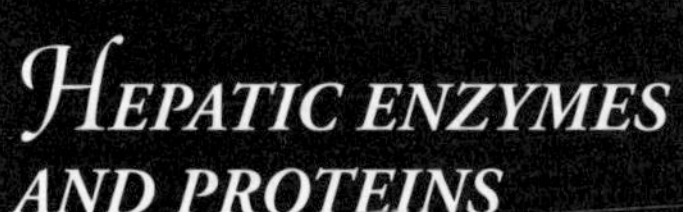

HEPATIC ENZYMES AND PROTEINS

ALPHA$_1$-ANTITRYPSIN

A protein produced by the liver, alpha$_1$-antitrypsin (also known as AAT or alpha$_1$-AT) is believed to inhibit the release of protease into body fluids by dying cells and is a major component of alpha$_1$-globulin. AAT is measured using radioimmunoassay or isoelectric focusing. Congenital absence or deficiency of AAT has been linked to high susceptibility to emphysema.

Purpose

- To screen for high-risk emphysema patients
- A nonspecific method of detecting inflammation, severe infection, and necrosis
- To test for congenital AAT deficiency

Patient preparation

- Explain to the patient that this test is used to diagnose respiratory or liver disease as well as inflammation, infection, or necrosis.
- Tell the patient to avoid smoking because irritants in tobacco stimulate leukocytes in the lungs to release protease.
- Tell the patient to avoid oral contraceptives and steroids for 24 hours before the test.
- Tell the patient to fast for at least 8 hours before the test.
- Tell the patient who will be performing the venipuncture and when.
- Explain to the patient that he may experience slight discomfort from the needle puncture and the tourniquet.

Procedure and posttest care

- Perform a venipuncture and collect the sample in a 4-ml tube without additives.
- Apply direct pressure to the venipuncture site until bleeding stops.

Precautions

- Handle the sample gently to avoid hemolysis.
- Send the sample to the laboratory promptly.
- If clinically indicated, patients with AAT levels lower than 125 mg/dl (SI, 1.25 g/L) should be phenotyped to confirm homozygous and heterozygous deficiencies. (Heterozygous patients don't appear to be at increased risk for early emphysema.)

Reference values

AAT levels vary by age, but the normal range is 110 to 200 mg/dl (SI, 1.10 to 2.0 g/L).

Abnormal findings

Decreased AAT levels may occur in early-onset emphysema and cirrhosis, nephrotic syndrome, malnutrition, congenital alpha$_1$-globulin deficiency and, transiently, in the neonate.

Increased AAT levels can occur in chronic inflammatory disorders, necrosis, pregnancy, acute pulmonary infections, hyaline membrane disease in infants, hepatitis, systemic lupus erythematosus, and rheumatoid arthritis.

Interfering factors

- Oral contraceptives and corticosteroid (possible false-high)
- Smoking or failure to fast for 8 hours before the test (possible false-high)

ASPARTATE AMINOTRANSFERASE

Aspartate aminotransferase (AST) is one of two enzymes that catalyze the conversion of the nitrogenous portion of an amino acid to an amino acid residue. It's essential to energy production in the Krebs cycle. AST is found in the cytoplasm and mitochondria of many cells, primarily in the liver, heart, skeletal muscles, kidneys, pancreas, and red blood cells. It's released into serum in proportion to cellular damage.

Purpose

- To aid detection and differential diagnosis of acute hepatic disease
- To monitor patient progress and prognosis in cardiac and hepatic diseases
- To aid diagnosis of myocardial infarction (MI) in correlation with creatine kinase and lactate dehydrogenase levels

Patient preparation

- Explain to the patient that this test is used to assess heart and liver function.
- Inform the patient that the test usually requires three venipunctures (one on admission and one each day for the next 2 days).
- Tell the patient that he need not restrict food and fluids.
- Reassure the patient that discomfort from the needle puncture and the tourniquet is transient.
- Notify the laboratory and physician of medications the patient is taking that may affect test results; they may need to be restricted.

Procedure and posttest care

- Perform a venipuncture and collect the sample in a 4-ml clot-activator tube.
- Apply direct pressure to the venipuncture site until bleeding stops.
- If a hematoma develops at the venipuncture, apply warm soaks.
- Instruct the patient that he may resume medications discontinued before the test as ordered.

Precautions

- To avoid missing peak AST levels, draw serum samples at the same time each day.
- Handle the sample gently to prevent hemolysis and send it to the laboratory immediately.

Reference values

AST levels range from 8 to 46 U/L (SI, 0.14 to 0.78 µKat/L) in males and from 7 to 34 U/L (SI, 0.12 to 0.58 µKat/L) in females. Normal values for infants are typically higher.

Abnormal findings

AST levels fluctuate in response to the extent of cellular necrosis, being transiently and minimally increased early in the disease process and extremely increased during the most acute phase. Depending on when the initial sample is drawn, AST levels may increase, indicating increasing disease severity and tissue damage, or decrease, indicating disease resolution and tissue repair.

Maximum elevations (more than 20 times normal) may indicate acute viral hepatitis, severe skeletal muscle trauma, extensive surgery, drug-induced hepatic injury, or severe passive liver congestion.

High levels (10 to 20 times normal) may indicate severe MI, severe infectious mononucleosis, or alcoholic cirrhosis. High levels also occur during the prodromal or resolving stages of conditions that cause maximum elevations.

Moderate to high levels (5 to 10 times normal) may indicate dermatomyositis, Duchenne muscular dystrophy, or chronic hepatitis. Moderate to high levels also occur during prodromal and resolving stages of diseases that cause high elevations.

Low to moderate levels (2 to 5 times normal) occur at some time during the preceding conditions or diseases or may indicate hemolytic anemia, metastatic hepatic tumors, acute pancreatitis, pulmonary emboli, delirium tremens, or fatty liver. AST levels rise slightly after the first few days of biliary duct obstruction.

Interfering factors

- Hemolysis due to rough handling of the sample
- Failure to draw the sample as scheduled (may miss peak)
- Chlorpropamide, opioids, methyldopa, erythromycin, sulfonamides, pyridoxine, dicumarol, and antitubercular agents; large doses of acetaminophen, salicylates, or vitamin A; and many other drugs known to affect the liver (increase)
- Strenuous exercise and muscle trauma due to I.M. injections (increase)

ALANINE AMINOTRANSFERASE

The alanine aminotransferase (ALT) test is used to measure serum levels of ALT, one of two enzymes that catalyze a reversible amino group transfer reaction in the Krebs cycle. ALT is necessary for tissue energy production. ALT is found primarily in the liver, with lesser amounts in the kidneys, heart, and skeletal muscles, and is a sensitive indicator of acute hepatocellular disease.

Purpose

- To detect and evaluate treatment of acute hepatic disease, especially hepatitis and cirrhosis without jaundice
- To distinguish between myocardial and hepatic tissue damage (used with aspartate aminotransferase)
- To assess hepatotoxicity of some drugs

Patient preparation

- Explain to the patient that this test is used to assess liver function.
- Tell the patient that the test requires a blood sample. Explain who will perform the venipuncture and when.
- Explain to the patient that he may experience slight discomfort from the needle puncture and the tourniquet.
- Inform the patient that he need not restrict food and fluids.
- Notify the laboratory and physician of medications the patient is taking that may affect test results; they may need to be restricted.

Procedure and posttest care

- Perform a venipuncture and collect the sample in a 4-ml tube without additives.
- Apply direct pressure to the venipuncture site until bleeding stops.
- If a hematoma develops at the venipuncture site, apply warm soaks.
- Instruct the patient that he may resume medications discontinued before the test as ordered.

Precautions

- Handle the sample gently to prevent hemolysis.
- ALT activity is stable in serum for up to 3 days at room temperature.

Reference values

Serum ALT levels range from 8 to 50 IU/L (SI, 0.14 to 0.85 μKat/L).

Abnormal findings

Very high ALT levels (up to 50 times normal) suggest viral or severe drug-induced hepatitis or other hepatic disease with extensive necrosis. Moderate to high levels may indicate infectious mononucleosis, chronic hepatitis, intrahepatic cholestasis or cholecystitis, early or improving acute viral hepatitis, or severe hepatic congestion due to heart failure.

Slight to moderate elevations of ALT may appear in any condition that produces acute hepatocellular injury, such as active cirrhosis and drug-induced or alcoholic hepatitis. Marginal elevations occasionally occur in acute myocardial infarction, reflecting secondary hepatic congestion or the release of small amounts of ALT from myocardial tissue.

Interfering factors

- Hemolysis due to rough handling of the sample
- Barbiturates, griseofulvin, isoniazid, nitrofurantoin, methyldopa, phenothiazines, phenytoin, salicylates, tetracycline, chlorpromazine, para-aminosalicylic acid, and other drugs that cause hepatic injury by competitively interfering with cellular metabolism (false-high)
- Narcotic analgesics, such as morphine, codeine, and meperidine (possible false-high due to increased intrabiliary pressure)
- Ingestion of lead or exposure to carbon tetrachloride (sharp increase due to direct injury to hepatic cells)

ALKALINE PHOSPHATASE

The alkaline phosphatase (ALP) test is used to measure serum levels of ALP, an enzyme that influences bone calcification as well as lipid and metabolite transport. ALP measurements reflect the combined activity of several ALP isoenzymes found in the liver, bones, kidneys, intestinal lining, and placenta. Bone and liver ALP are always present in adult serum, with liver ALP most prominent except during the third trimester of pregnancy (when the placenta originates about half of all ALP). The intestinal variant of ALP can be a normal component (in less than 10% of normal patterns; almost exclusively in the sera of blood groups B and O), or it can be an abnormal finding associated with hepatic disease.

Purpose

- To detect and identify skeletal diseases primarily characterized by marked osteoblastic activity
- To detect focal hepatic lesions causing biliary obstruction, such as a tumor or an abscess
- To assess response to vitamin D in the treatment of rickets
- To supplement information from other liver function studies and GI enzyme tests

Patient preparation

- Explain to the patient that this test is used to assess liver and bone function.
- Instruct the patient to fast for at least 8 hours before the test because fat intake stimulates intestinal ALP secretion.
- Tell the patient that this test requires a blood sample. Explain who will perform the venipuncture and when.
- Inform the patient that he may experience slight discomfort from the needle puncture and the tourniquet.

Procedure and posttest care

- Perform a venipuncture and collect the sample in a 4-ml clot-activator tube.
- Apply direct pressure to the venipuncture site until bleeding stops.

■ If a hematoma develops at the venipuncture site, apply warm soaks.
■ Instruct the patient that he may resume his usual diet.

Precautions
■ Handle the sample gently to prevent hemolysis.
■ Send the sample to the laboratory immediately; ALP activity increases at room temperature because of a rise in pH.

Reference values
Total ALP levels normally range from 30 to 85 IU/ml (SI, 42 to 128 U/L).

Abnormal findings
Although significant ALP elevations are possible with diseases that affect many organs, they usually indicate skeletal disease or extrahepatic or intrahepatic biliary obstruction causing cholestasis. Many acute hepatic diseases cause ALP elevations before they affect serum bilirubin levels.

Moderate increases in ALP levels may reflect acute biliary obstruction from hepatocellular inflammation in active cirrhosis, mononucleosis, and viral hepatitis. Moderate increases are also seen in osteomalacia and deficiency-induced rickets.

Sharp elevations in ALP levels may indicate complete biliary obstruction by malignant or infectious infiltrations or fibrosis, most common in Paget's disease and, occasionally, in biliary obstruction, extensive bone metastasis, and hyperparathyroidism. Metastatic bone tumors resulting from pancreatic cancer raise ALP levels without a concomitant rise in serum alanine aminotransferase levels.

Isoenzyme fractionation and additional enzyme tests (gamma glutamyl transferase, lactate dehydrogenase, 5′-nucleotidase, and leucine aminopeptidase) are sometimes performed when the cause of ALP elevations is in doubt. Rarely, low levels of serum ALP are associated with hypophosphatasia and protein or magnesium deficiency.

Interfering factors
■ Hemolysis due to rough handling of the sample
■ Failure to analyze the sample within 4 hours
■ Recent ingestion of vitamin D (possible increase due to effect on osteoblastic activity)
■ Recent infusion of albumin prepared from placental venous blood (marked increase)
■ Drugs that influence liver function or cause cholestasis, such as barbiturates, chlorpropamide, oral contraceptives, isoniazid, methyldopa, phenothiazines, phenytoin, and rifampin (possible mild increase)
■ Halothane sensitivity (possible drastic increase)
■ Clofibrate (decrease)
■ Healing long-bone fractures and third trimester of pregnancy (possible increase)
■ Age and sex (increase in infants, children, adolescents, and individuals over age 45)

LEUCINE AMINOPEPTIDASE

The leucine aminopeptidase (LAP) test is used to measure serum levels of LAP, an isoenzyme of alkaline phosphatase (ALP) that is widely distributed in body tissues. The greatest concentrations appear in the hepatobiliary tissues, pancreas, and small intestine. Serum levels of LAP parallel serum ALP levels in hepatic disease.

Purpose

- To provide information about suspected liver, pancreatic, and biliary diseases
- To differentiate skeletal disease from hepatobiliary or pancreatic disease
- To evaluate neonatal jaundice

Patient preparation

- Explain to the patient that this test is used to evaluate liver and pancreatic function.
- Tell the patient to fast for at least 8 hours before the test.
- Notify the laboratory and physician of medications the patient is taking that may affect test results; they may need to be restricted.
- Tell the patient that this test requires a blood sample. Explain who will perform the venipuncture and when.
- Explain to the patient that he may experience slight discomfort from the needle puncture and the tourniquet.

Procedure and posttest care

- Perform a venipuncture and collect the sample in a 4-ml clot-activator tube.
- Apply direct pressure to the venipuncture site until bleeding stops.
- Instruct the patient that he may resume his usual diet and medications discontinued before the test as ordered.

Precautions

- Handle the sample gently to avoid hemolysis.
- Transport the sample to the laboratory immediately.

Reference values

Normal values are 80 to 200 U/ml (SI, 80 to 200 kU/L) in men and 75 to 185 U/ml (SI, 75 to 185 kU/L) in women.

Abnormal findings

Elevated levels can occur in biliary obstruction, tumors, strictures, and atresia; advanced pregnancy; and therapy with drugs containing estrogen or progesterone.

Interfering factors

- Advanced pregnancy (false-high)
- Estrogen or progesterone (false-high)

GAMMA GLUTAMYL TRANSFERASE

Also called gamma glutamyl transpeptidase, gamma glutamyl transferase (GGT) participates in the transfer of amino acids across cellular membranes and, possibly, in glutathione metabolism. The highest concentrations of GGT exist in the renal tubules, but the enzyme also appears in the liver, biliary tract epithelium, pancreas, lymphocytes, brain, and testes. The GGT test is used to measure serum GGT levels.

Purpose

- To provide information about hepatobiliary diseases, to assess liver function, and to detect alcohol ingestion
- To distinguish between skeletal disease and hepatic disease when serum alkaline phosphatase level is elevated (a normal GGT level suggests that such elevation stems from skeletal disease)

Patient preparation

- Explain to the patient that this test is used to evaluate liver function.
- Tell the patient that the test requires a blood sample. Explain who will perform the venipuncture and when.
- Explain to the patient that he may experience slight discomfort from the needle puncture and the tourniquet.

■ Inform the patient that he need not restrict food and fluids.

Procedure and posttest care

■ Perform a venipuncture and collect the sample in a 4-ml tube without additives.
■ Apply direct pressure to the venipuncture site until bleeding stops.
■ If a hematoma develops, apply warm soaks.

Precautions

■ Handle the sample gently to prevent hemolysis.
■ GGT activity is stable in serum at room temperature for 2 days.

Reference values

Normal serum GTT levels range as follows:
■ males: age 16 and older, 6 to 38 U/L (SI, 0.10 to 0.63 μKat/L)
■ females: ages 16 to 45, 4 to 27 U/L (SI, 0.08 to 0.46 μKat/L); age 45 and older, 6 to 37 U/L (SI, 0.10 to 0.63 μKat/L)
■ children: 3 to 30 U/L (SI, 0.05 to 0.51 μKat/L).

Abnormal findings

Serum GGT levels rise in acute hepatic diseases because enzyme production increases in response to hepatocellular injury. Moderate increases occur in acute pancreatitis, renal disease, and prostatic metastases; postoperatively; and in some patients with epilepsy or brain tumors. Levels also increase after alcohol ingestion because of enzyme induction. The sharpest elevations occur in patients with obstructive jaundice and hepatic metastatic infiltrations.

GGT levels may also increase 5 to 10 days after acute myocardial infarction, either as a result of tissue granulation and healing or as an indication of the effects of cardiac insufficiency on the liver.

Interfering factors

■ Hemolysis due to rough handling of the sample
■ Clofibrate and oral contraceptives (decrease)
■ Aminoglycosides, barbiturates, phenytoin glutethimide, and methaqualone (increase)
■ Moderate intake of alcohol (increase for at least 60 hours)

5'-NUCLEOTIDASE

The enzyme 5′-nucleotidase (5′NT) is a phosphatase formed almost entirely in the hepatobiliary tract. Unlike alkaline phosphatase (ALP), it hydrolyzes nucleoside 5′-phosphate groups only. Measurement of serum 5′NT levels helps to determine whether ALP elevation is due to skeletal or hepatic disease. Because 5′NT remains normal in skeletal disease and pregnancy, it's more specific for assessing hepatic dysfunction than ALP or leucine aminopeptidase.

Purpose

■ To distinguish between hepatobiliary and skeletal disease when the source of increased ALP levels is uncertain
■ To help differentiate biliary obstruction from acute hepatocellular damage
■ To detect hepatic metastasis in the absence of jaundice

Patient preparation

■ Explain to the patient that this test is used to evaluate liver function.
■ Tell the patient that the test requires a blood sample. Explain who will perform the venipuncture and when.

■ Explain to the patient that he may experience slight discomfort from the needle puncture and the tourniquet.
■ Tell the patient that he need not restrict food and fluids.

Procedure and posttest care

■ Perform a venipuncture and collect the sample in a 4-ml tube without additives.
■ Apply direct pressure to the venipuncture site until bleeding stops.
■ If a hematoma develops at the venipuncture site, apply warm soaks.

Precautions

■ Handle the sample gently to prevent hemolysis.

Reference values

Serum 5′NT values for adults range from 2 to 17 U/L (SI, 0.034 to 0.29 μKat/L); values for children may be lower.

Abnormal findings

Extremely high levels of 5′NT occur in common bile duct obstruction by calculi or tumors in diseases that cause severe intrahepatic cholestasis, such as neoplastic infiltrations of the liver. Slight to moderate increases may reflect acute hepatocellular damage or active cirrhosis.

Interfering factors

■ Hemolysis due to rough handling of the sample
■ Cholestatic drugs, such as phenothiazines, morphine, meperidine, and codeine as well as aspirin, acetaminophen, and phenytoin (increase)

PANCREATIC ENZYMES

AMYLASE

An enzyme that is synthesized primarily in the pancreas and salivary glands, amylase (alpha-amylase or AML) helps to digest starch and glycogen in the mouth, stomach, and intestine. In cases of suspected acute pancreatic disease, measurement of serum or urine AML is the most important laboratory test.

Purpose

■ To diagnose acute pancreatitis
■ To distinguish between acute pancreatitis and other causes of abdominal pain that require immediate surgery
■ To evaluate possible pancreatic injury caused by abdominal trauma or surgery

Patient preparation

■ Explain to the patient that this test is used to assess pancreatic function.
■ Inform the patient that he need not fast before the test but must abstain from alcohol.
■ Tell the patient that this test requires a blood sample. Explain who will perform the venipuncture and when.
■ Inform the patient that he may experience slight discomfort from the needle puncture and the tourniquet.
■ Notify the laboratory and physician of medications the patient is taking that may affect test results; they may need to be restricted.

Procedure and posttest care

■ Perform a venipuncture and collect the sample in a 4-ml clot-activator tube.
■ Apply direct pressure to the venipuncture site until bleeding stops.

- If a hematoma develops at the venipuncture site, apply warm soaks.
- Instruct the patient that he may resume medications discontinued before the test as ordered.

Precautions

- If the patient has severe abdominal pain, draw the sample before diagnostic or therapeutic intervention. For accurate results, it's important to obtain an early sample.
- Handle the sample gently to prevent hemolysis.

Reference values

Normal serum amylase levels range from 25 to 85 U/L (SI, 0.39 to 1.45 μKat/L) for adults age 18 and older.

Abnormal findings

After the onset of acute pancreatitis, AML levels begin to rise within 2 hours, peak within 12 to 48 hours, and return to normal within 3 to 4 days. Determination of urine levels should follow normal serum AML results to rule out pancreatitis. Moderate serum elevations may accompany obstruction of the common bile duct, pancreatic duct, or ampulla of Vater; pancreatic injury from a perforated peptic ulcer; pancreatic cancer; and acute salivary gland disease. Impaired kidney function may increase serum levels.

Levels may be slightly elevated in a patient who is asymptomatic or responding unusually to therapy.

Decreased levels can occur in chronic pancreatitis, pancreatic cancer, cirrhosis, hepatitis, and toxemia of pregnancy.

Interfering factors

- Hemolysis due to rough handling of the sample
- Ingestion of ethyl alcohol (possible false-high)
- Aminosalicylic acid, asparaginase, azathioprine, corticosteroids, cyproheptadine, narcotic analgesics, oral contraceptives, rifampin, sulfasalazine, and thiazide or loop diuretics (possible false-high)
- Recent peripancreatic surgery, perforated ulcer or intestine, abscess, spasm of the sphincter of Oddi or, rarely, macroamylasemia (possible false-high)

LIPASE

Lipase is produced in the pancreas and secreted into the duodenum, where it converts triglycerides and other fats into fatty acids and glycerol. The destruction of pancreatic cells, which occurs in acute pancreatitis, causes large amounts of lipase to be released into the blood. The lipase test is used to measure serum lipase levels; it's most useful when performed with a serum or urine amylase test.

Purpose

- To aid diagnosis of acute pancreatitis

Patient preparation

- Explain to the patient that this test is used to evaluate pancreatic function.
- Instruct the patient to fast overnight before the test.
- Tell the patient that the test requires a blood sample. Explain who will perform the venipuncture and when.
- Inform the patient that he may experience slight discomfort from the needle puncture and the tourniquet.
- Notify the laboratory and physician of medications the patient is taking that may affect test results; they may need to be restricted.

Procedure and posttest care

- Perform a venipuncture and collect the sample in a 4-ml clot-activator tube.
- Apply direct pressure to the venipuncture site until bleeding stops.
- If a hematoma develops at the venipuncture site, apply warm soaks.
- Instruct the patient that he may resume medications discontinued before the test as ordered.

Precautions

- Handle the sample gently to prevent hemolysis.

Reference values

Serum lipase levels are normally < 160 U/L (SI, < 2.72 µKat/L)

Abnormal findings

High lipase levels suggest acute pancreatitis or pancreatic duct obstruction. After an acute attack, levels remain elevated for up to 14 days. Lipase levels may also increase in other pancreatic injuries, such as perforated peptic ulcer with chemical pancreatitis due to gastric juices, and in patients with high intestinal obstruction, pancreatic cancer, or renal disease with impaired excretion.

Interfering factors

- Hemolysis due to rough handling of the sample
- Cholinergics, codeine, meperidine, and morphine (false-high due to spasm of the sphincter of Oddi)

SPECIAL ENZYMES

ACID PHOSPHATASE

Acid phosphatase — a group of phosphatase enzymes most active at a pH of about 5.0 — is found primarily in the prostate gland and semen and, to a lesser extent, in the liver, spleen, red blood cells, bone marrow, and platelets. The acid phosphatase test is used to measure total acid phosphatase and the prostatic fraction in serum.

Purpose

- To detect prostate cancer
- To monitor response to therapy for prostate cancer; successful treatment decreases acid phosphatase levels

Patient preparation

- Explain to the patient that this test is used to evaluate prostate function.
- Tell the patient that the test requires a blood sample. Explain who will perform the venipuncture and when.
- Explain to the patient that he may experience slight discomfort from the needle puncture and the tourniquet.
- Inform the patient that he need not restrict food and fluids.
- Notify the laboratory and physician of medications the patient is taking that may affect test results; they may need to be restricted.

Procedure and posttest care

- Perform a venipuncture and collect the sample in a 4-ml tube without additives.
- Apply direct pressure to the venipuncture site until bleeding stops.
- If a hematoma develops at the venipuncture site, apply warm soaks.

■ Instruct the patient that he may resume medications discontinued before the test as ordered.

Precautions

■ Don't draw the sample within 48 hours of prostate manipulation (rectal examination).
■ Handle the sample gently to prevent hemolysis.
■ Send the sample to the laboratory immediately. Acid phosphatase levels decrease by 50% within 1 hour if the sample remains at room temperature without a preservative or if it isn't packed in ice.

Reference values

Serum values for total acid phosphatase depend on the assay method and range from 0 to 3.7 U/L (SI, 0 to 3.7 U/L).

Abnormal findings

High prostatic acid phosphatase levels generally indicate the presence of a tumor that has spread beyond the prostatic capsule. If the tumor has metastasized to bone, high acid phosphatase levels are accompanied by high alkaline phosphatase (ALP) levels, reflecting increased osteoblastic activity.

Acid phosphatase levels rise moderately in prostatic infarction, Paget's disease (some patients), Gaucher's disease and, occasionally, other conditions, such as multiple myeloma. False results may occur if ALP levels are high because acid phosphatase and ALP are similar, differing mainly in their optimum pH ranges.

Interfering factors

■ Hemolysis due to rough handling of the sample or improper sample storage
■ Delayed delivery of the sample to the laboratory (possible false-low or false-normal)
■ Fluorides, phosphates, and oxalates (possible false-low)
■ Clofibrate (possible false-high)
■ Prostate massage, catheterization, or rectal examination within 48 hours of the test

PROSTATE-SPECIFIC ANTIGEN

Prostate-specific antigen (PSA) appears in normal, benign hyperplastic, and malignant prostatic tissue as well as metastatic prostatic carcinoma. Serum PSA levels are used to monitor the spread or recurrence of prostate cancer and to evaluate the patient's response to treatment. Measurement of serum PSA levels along with a digital rectal examination is now recommended as a screening test for prostate cancer in men over age 50. It's also useful in assessing response to treatment in patients with stage B3 to D1 prostate cancer and in detecting tumor spread or recurrence.

Purpose

■ To screen for prostate cancer in men over age 50
■ To monitor the course of prostate cancer and aid evaluation of treatment

Patient preparation

■ Explain to the patient that this test is used to screen for prostate cancer or, if appropriate, to monitor the course of treatment.
■ Tell the patient that the test requires a blood sample. Explain who will perform the venipuncture and when.
■ Explain to the patient that he may experience slight discomfort from the needle puncture and the tourniquet.

■ Inform the patient that he need not restrict food and fluids.

Procedure and posttest care

■ Perform a venipuncture and collect the sample in a clot-activator tube.
■ Apply direct pressure to the venipuncture site until bleeding stops.
■ If a hematoma develops at the venipuncture site, apply warm soaks.

Precautions

■ Collect the sample either before digital prostate examination or at least 48 hours after examination to avoid falsely elevated PSA levels.
■ Handle the sample gently to prevent hemolysis.
■ Immediately put the sample on ice and send it to the laboratory.

Reference values

Normal values are as follows:
■ ages 40 to 50: 2 to 2.8 mg/ml (SI, 2 to 2.8 µg/L)
■ ages 51 to 60: 2.9 to 3.8 mg/ml (SI, 2.9 to 3.8 µg/L)
■ ages 61 to 70: 4 to 5.3 mg/ml (SI, 4 to 5.3 µg/L)
■ ages 71 and older: 5.6 to 7.2 mg/ml (SI, 5.6 to 7.2 µg/L).

Abnormal findings

About 80% of patients with prostate cancer have pretreatment PSA values > 4 ng/ml. However, PSA results alone don't confirm a diagnosis of prostate cancer. About 20% of patients with benign prostatic hyperplasia also have levels > 4 ng/ml. Further assessment and testing, including tissue biopsy, are needed to confirm cancer.

Interfering factors

■ Hemolysis due to rough handling of the sample
■ Excessive doses of chemotherapeutic drugs, such as cyclophosphamide, diethylstilbestrol, and methotrexate (possible increase or decrease)

PLASMA RENIN ACTIVITY

Renin secretion from the kidneys is the first stage of the renin-angiotensin-aldosterone cycle, which controls the body's sodium-potassium balance, fluid volume, and blood pressure. Renin is released into the renal veins in response to sodium depletion and blood loss. The plasma renin activity test is a screening procedure for renovascular hypertension but doesn't unequivocally confirm it.

Purpose

■ To screen for renal origin of hypertension
■ To help plan treatment of essential hypertension, a genetic disease commonly aggravated by excess sodium intake
■ To help identify hypertension linked to unilateral (sometimes bilateral) renovascular disease by renal vein catheterization
■ To help identify primary aldosteronism (Conn's syndrome) resulting from aldosterone-secreting adrenal adenoma
■ To confirm primary aldosteronism (sodium-depleted plasma renin test)

Patient preparation

■ Explain to the patient that this test is used to determine the cause of hypertension.
■ Notify the labortory and physician of medications the patient is taking that may affect test results; they may need to be restricted.
■ Tell the patient to maintain a normal sodium diet (3 g/day) during this period.

■ For the sodium-depleted plasma renin test, tell the patient that he'll receive furosemide (or, if he has angina or cerebrovascular insufficiency, chlorthiazide) and will follow a specific low-sodium diet for 3 days.
■ The patient shouldn't receive radioactive treatments for several days before the test.
■ Tell the patient that the test requires a blood sample. Explain who will perform the venipuncture and when.
■ Explain to the patient that he may experience slight discomfort from the needle puncture and the tourniquet. Collect a morning sample, if possible.
■ If a recumbent sample is ordered, instruct the patient to remain in bed at least 2 hours before the sample is obtained. (Posture influences renin secretion.) If an upright sample is ordered, instruct him to stand or sit upright for 2 hours before the test is performed.
■ If renal vein catheterization is ordered, make sure the patient has signed an informed consent form. Tell the patient that the procedure will be done in the X-ray department and that he'll receive a local anesthetic.

Procedure and posttest care

Peripheral vein sample
■ Perform a venipuncture and collect the sample in a 4-ml EDTA tube.
■ Note on the laboratory request if the patient was fasting and whether he was upright or in a supine position during sample collection.
■ Apply direct pressure to the venipuncture site until bleeding stops.
■ If a hematoma develops at the veniuncture site, apply warm soaks.
Renal vein catheterization
■ A catheter is advanced to the kidneys through the femoral vein under fluoroscopic control and samples are obtained from both renal veins and the vena cava.
■ After renal vein catheterization, apply pressure to the catheterization site for 10 to 20 minutes to prevent extravasation.
■ Monitor vital signs and check the catheterization site every 30 minutes for 2 hours and then every hour for 4 hours to ensure that the bleeding has stopped. Check distal pulse for signs of thrombus formation and arterial occlusion (cyanosis, loss of pulse, coolness of skin).
Both methods
■ Instruct the patient that he may resume his usual diet and medications discontinued before the test as ordered.

Precautions

■ Because renin is unstable, the sample must be drawn into a chilled syringe and collection tube, placed on ice, and sent to the laboratory immediately.
■ Completely fill the collection tube and invert it gently several times to mix the sample and the anticoagulant.

Reference values

Levels of plasma renin activity and aldosterone vary with dietary sodium intake as follows:
■ normal sodium diet: 1.1 to 4.1 ng/ml/hour (SI, 0.30 to 1.14 ng LS)
■ restricted sodium diet: 6.2 to 12.4 ng/ml/hour (SI, 1.72 to 3.44 ng LS).

Abnormal findings

Elevated renin levels may occur in essential hypertension (uncommon), malignant and renovascular hypertension, cirrhosis, hypokalemia, hypovolemia due to hemorrhage, renin-producing renal tumors (Bartter's syndrome), and adrenal hypofunction (Addison's disease). High renin levels may also be found in chronic renal failure with parenchymal disease, end-stage renal disease, and transplant rejection.

Decreased renin levels may indicate hypervolemia due to a high-sodium diet, salt-retaining steroids, primary aldosteronism, Cushing's syndrome, licorice ingestion syndrome, or essential hypertension with low renin levels.

High serum and urine aldosterone levels with low plasma renin activity help identify primary aldosteronism. In the sodium-depleted renin test, low plasma renin confirms this and differentiates it from secondary aldosteronism (characterized by increased renin).

Interfering factors

- Failure to observe pretest restrictions
- Improper patient positioning during the test
- Failure to use the proper anticoagulant in the collection tube, to completely fill it, or to adequately mix the sample and the anticoagulant (EDTA helps preserve angiotensin I; heparin doesn't.
- Failure to chill the collection tube, syringe, and sample or to send the sample to the laboratory immediately
- Salt intake, severe blood loss, ingestion of licorice, oral contraceptives, pregnancy, and therapy with diuretics, antihypertensives, or vasodilators (increase)
- Salt-retaining corticosteroid therapy and antidiuretic therapy (decrease)
- Radioisotope use within several days before the test

CHOLINESTERASE

The cholinesterase test is used to measure the amounts of two similar enzymes that hydrolyze acetylcholine: acetylcholinesterase and pseudocholinesterase. Acetylcholinesterase is present in nerve tissue, red cells of the spleen, and the gray matter of the brain. Pseudocholinesterase is produced primarily in the liver and appears in small amounts in the pancreas, intestines, heart, and white matter of the brain.

When poisoning by an organophosphate (used by the military in nerve gases and common in many insecticides) is suspected, either cholinesterase may be measured. For technical reasons, pseudocholinesterase is generally tested, although this analysis is less sensitive than the one for acetylcholinesterase.

In suspected poisoning by muscle relaxant, the patient lacks adequate pseudocholinesterase, which usually inactivates the muscle relaxant. In this case, measurement of pseudocholinesterase is required.

Purpose

- To evaluate before surgery or electroconvulsive therapy the patient's potential response to succinylcholine, which is hydrolyzed by cholinesterase
- To detect patients who may have adverse reactions to muscle relaxants
- To assess overexposure to insecticides containing organophosphate compounds
- To assess liver function and aid diagnosis of hepatic disease (a rare purpose)

Patient preparation

- Explain to the patient that this test is used to assess muscle function or the extent of poisoning.
- Tell the patient that the test requires a blood sample. Explain who will perform the venipuncture and when.
- Explain to the patient that he may experience slight discomfort from the needle puncture and the tourniquet.
- Inform the patient that he need not restrict food and fluids.
- Notify the laboratory and physician of medications the patient is taking that may affect test results; they may need to be restricted.

Procedure and posttest care

- Perform a venipuncture and collect the sample in a 7-ml clot-activator tube.
- Apply direct pressure to the venipuncture site until bleeding subsides.
- If a hematoma develops at the venipuncture site, apply warm soaks.
- Instruct the patient that he may resume his medications discontinued before the test as ordered.

Precautions

- Handle the sample gently to prevent hemolysis.
- If the sample can't be sent to the laboratory within 6 hours after being drawn, refrigerate it.

Reference values

Pseudocholinesterase levels range from 204 to 532 IU/dl (SI, 2.04 to 5.32 kU/L).

Abnormal findings

Severely decreased pseudocholinesterase levels suggest a congenital deficiency or organophosphate insecticide poisoning; levels near zero necessitate emergency treatment.

Pseudocholinesterase levels are usually normal in early extrahepatic obstruction and variably decreased in hepatocellular diseases, such as hepatitis and cirrhosis (especially cirrhosis with ascites and jaundice). Levels also drop in acute infections, chronic malnutrition, anemia, myocardial infarction, obstructive jaundice, and metastasis.

Interfering factors

- Hemolysis due to rough handling of the sample
- Pregnancy or recent surgery
- Cyclophosphamide, echothiophate iodide, monoamine oxidase inhibitors, succinylcholine, neostigmine, quinine, quinidine, chloroquine, caffeine, theophylline, epinephrine, ether, barbiturates, atropine, morphine, codeine, phenothiazines, vitamin K, and folic acid (possible false-low)

GLUCOSE-6-PHOSPHATE DEHYDROGENASE

An enzyme found in most body cells, glucose-6-phosphate dehydrogenase (G6PD) is involved in metabolizing glucose. The G6PD test is used to detect G6PD deficiency, a hereditary, sex-linked condition that impairs stability of the red cell membrane and allows red cells to be destroyed by strong oxidizing agents.

About 10% of Black males in the United States inherit a mild G6PD deficiency; some people of Mediterranean origin inherit a severe deficiency. In some White individuals, fava beans may produce hemolytic episodes. Although a deficiency of G6PD provides partial immunity to falciparum malaria, it precipitates an adverse reaction to antimalarials.

Purpose

- To detect hemolytic anemia caused by G6PD deficiency
- To aid differential diagnosis of hemolytic anemia

Patient preparation

- Explain to the patient that this test is used to detect an inherited enzyme deficiency that may affect red blood cells.
- Tell the patient that the test requires a blood sample. Explain who will perform the venipuncture and when.
- Explain to the patient that he may experience slight discomfort from the needle puncture and the tourniquet.

■ Inform the patient that he need not restrict food and fluids.
■ Check the patient's history and report recent blood transfusion or ingestion of aspirin, sulfonamides, phenacetin, nitrofurantoin, vitamin K derivatives, antimalarials, or fava beans, which cause hemolysis in people who are G6PD-deficient.

Procedure and posttest care

■ Perform a venipuncture and collect the sample in a 4-ml EDTA tube.
■ Apply direct pressure to the venipuncture site until bleeding stops.
■ If a hematoma develops at the venipuncture site, apply warm soaks.

Precautions

■ Completely fill the collection tube and invert it gently several times to mix the sample and the anticoagulant.
■ Handle the sample gently to prevent hemolysis.
■ Refrigerate the sample if you can't send it to the laboratory immediately.

Reference values

Serum values of G6PD vary with the measurement method used, but usually range from 4.3 to 11.8 U/G (SI, 0.28 to 0.76 mU/mol) of hemoglobin.

Abnormal findings

Fluorescent spot testing or staining for Heinz bodies or erythrocytes can test for G6PD deficiency. If results are positive, the kinetic quantitative assay for G6PD may be performed. Electrophoretic techniques assess genetic variants of deficiencies (which may cause lifelong, mild, or asymptomatic anemia). Some variants are symptomatic only when the patient experiences stress or illness or has been exposed to drugs or agents that elicit hemolytic episodes.

Interfering factors

■ Performing the test after a hemolytic episode or a blood transfusion (possible false-negative)
■ Failure to use the proper anticoagulant or to adequately mix the sample and the anticoagulant
■ Hemolysis due to rough handling of the sample
■ Aspirin, sulfonamides, nitrofurantoin, vitamin K derivatives, primaquine, and fava beans (decrease G6PD enzyme activity and precipitate hemolytic episode)

PYRUVATE KINASE

An erythrocyte enzyme, pyruvate kinase (PK) takes part in the anaerobic metabolism of glucose. An abnormally low PK level is an inherited autosomal recessive trait that may cause a red cell membrane defect associated with congenital hemolytic anemia. PK assay confirms PK deficiency when red cell enzyme deficiency is the suspected cause of anemia.

Purpose

■ To differentiate PK-deficient hemolytic anemia from other congenital hemolytic anemias or from acquired hemolytic anemia
■ To detect PK deficiency in asymptomatic, heterozygous inheritance

Patient preparation

■ Explain to the patient that this test is used to detect inherited enzyme deficiencies.
■ Tell the patient that the test requires a blood sample. Explain who will perform the venipuncture and when.

■ Explain to the patient that he may experience slight discomfort from the needle puncture and the tourniquet.
■ Inform the patient that he need not restrict food and fluids.
■ Check the patient's history for recent blood transfusion and note it on the laboratory request.

Procedure and posttest care

■ Perform a venipuncture and collect the sample in a 4-ml EDTA tube.
■ Apply direct pressure to the venipuncture site until bleeding stops.
■ If a hematoma develops at the venipuncture site, apply warm soaks.

Precautions

■ Completely fill the collection tube and invert it gently several times to mix the sample and the anticoagulant.
■ Handle the sample gently.
■ Refrigerate the sample if you can't send it to the laboratory immediately.

Reference values

Serum PK levels range from 9 to 22 U/g of hemoglobin (Hb); in the low substrate assay, they range from 1.7 to 6.8 U/g of Hb.

Abnormal findings

Low serum PK levels confirm a diagnosis of PK deficiency and allow differentiation between PK-deficient hemolytic anemia and other inherited disorders.

Interfering factors

■ Failure to use the proper anticoagulant or to adequately mix the sample and the anticoagulant
■ Hemolysis due to rough handling of the sample
■ Failure to remove white cells from sample (possible false results)
■ Recent blood transfusion or recent hemolytic event

HEXOSAMINIDASE A AND B

Hexosaminidase is a group of enzymes that are necessary for metabolism of gangliosides, water-soluble glycolipids found primarily in brain tissue. The hexosaminidase A and B test is used to measure the hexosaminidase A and B content of serum and amniotic fluid.

Deficiency of hexosaminidase A indicates Tay-Sachs disease, which affects people of eastern European Jewish ancestry about 100 times more often than the general population. Both parents must carry the defective gene to transmit Tay-Sachs disease to their children. Sandhoff's disease, which results from deficiency of both hexosaminidase A and B, is uncommon and not prevalent in any ethnic group.

Purpose

■ To confirm or rule out Tay-Sachs disease in neonates
■ To screen for Tay-Sachs carriers
■ To establish prenatal diagnosis of hexosaminidase A deficiency

Patient preparation

■ Explain to the patient that this test is used to identify carriers of Tay-Sachs disease.
■ Tell the patient that the test requires a blood sample. Explain who will perform the venipuncture and when.
■ Explain to the patient that he may experience slight discomfort from the needle puncture and the tourniquet.
■ Inform the patient that he need not restrict food and fluids.
■ When testing a neonate, explain to the parents that this test is used to detect Tay-Sachs disease. Tell them that blood will be drawn from the neonate's

arm, neck, or umbilical cord; that the procedure is safe and quickly performed; and that the neonate will have a small bandage on the venipuncture site. Inform them that no pretest restrictions of food or fluid are needed.

■ If the test is being performed prenatally, advise the patient of preparations for amniocentesis.

Procedure and posttest care

■ Perform a venipuncture, collect cord blood, or assist with amniocentesis, as appropriate. Collect the sample in a 7-ml clot-activator tube.

■ Apply direct pressure to the venipuncture site until bleeding stops.

■ If a hematoma develops at the venipuncture site, apply warm soaks.

■ When testing a neonate, follow laboratory procedure for collecting serum samples.

Precautions

■ Handle the sample gently to prevent hemolysis.

■ This test can't be done on a pregnant woman's serum (but her leukocytes or amniotic fluid may be tested, if necessary); if the father's blood test result is negative, Tay-Sachs disease won't be transmitted to the child.

■ If the test can't be performed immediately, freeze the sample.

Reference values

Total serum levels of hexosaminidase range from 5 to 12.9 U/L; hexosaminidase A accounts for 55% to 76% of the total.

Abnormal findings

Absence of hexosaminidase A indicates Tay-Sachs disease (total hexosaminidase levels can be normal). Absence of both hexosaminidase A and B indicates Sandhoff's disease, an uncommon, virulent variant of Tay-Sachs disease in which deterioration occurs more rapidly.

Interfering factors

■ Hemolysis due to rough handling of the sample

■ Oral contraceptives (false-high)

■ Rifampin and isoniazid (increase)

UROPORPHYRINOGEN I SYNTHASE

The uroporphyrinogen I synthase test is used to measure blood levels of uroporphyrinogen I synthase, an enzyme involved in heme biosynthesis. This enzyme is usually present in erythrocytes, fibroblasts, lymphocytes, hepatic cells, and amniotic fluid cells. A hereditary deficiency that can reduce uroporphyrinogen I synthase levels by 50% or more results in acute intermittent porphyria (AIP). This disorder can be latent indefinitely until certain factors (some sex hormones and drugs, a low-carbohydrate diet, or an infection) precipitate active disease.

Purpose

■ To aid diagnosis of latent or active AIP

■ To differentiate AIP from other types of porphyria

Patient preparation

■ Explain to the patient that this test is used to detect a red blood cell disorder.

■ Inform the patient that he'll need to fast for 12 to 14 hours before the test and to abstain from alcohol for 24 hours but that he may drink water.

■ Tell the patient that the test requires a blood sample. Explain who will perform the venipuncture and when.

■ Explain to the patient that he may experience slight discomfort from the needle puncture and the tourniquet.
■ If the patient's hematocrit is available, note on the laboratory request.
■ Notify the laboratory and physician of medications the patient is taking that may affect test results; they may need to be restricted.

Procedure and posttest care

■ Perform a venipuncture and collect the sample in a 10-ml heparizined tube.
■ Apply direct pressure to the venipuncture site until bleeding stops.
■ If a hematoma develops at the venipuncture site, apply warm soaks.
■ Instruct the patient that he may resume his usual diet and medications discontinued before the test as ordered.
■ If AIP is present, refer the patient for nutrition and genetic counseling. Advise him to avoid low-carbohydrate diets, alcohol, and drugs that may trigger an acute episode and to seek prompt care for all infections.

Precautions

■ Handle the sample gently to prevent hemolysis.
■ Place the sample on ice and send it to the laboratory immediately.

Reference values

Normal values for uroporphyrinogen I synthase are ≥ 7 nmol/sec/L.

Abnormal findings

Decreased uroporphyrinogen I synthase levels generally indicate latent or active AIP; symptoms differentiate these phases. Levels that are < 6 nmol/sec/L confirm AIP. Levels between 6 and 6.9 nmol/sec/L are indeterminate, in which case urine and stool tests for the porphyrin precursors aminolevulinic acid and porphobilinogen may be ordered to support the diagnosis.

Interfering factors

■ Failure to observe pretest restrictions or to freeze the sample (false-positive)
■ Hemolysis due to rough handling of the sample
■ Hemolytic and hepatic diseases (possible increase)
■ Alcohol and use of drugs, such as steroid hormones, estrogens, barbiturates, sulfonamides, phenytoin, griseofulvin, chlordiazepoxide, meprobamate, glutethimide, and ergot alkaloids (possible decrease)

GALACTOSE-1-PHOSPHATE URIDYL TRANSFERASE

Galactose-1-phosphate uridyl transferase is involved in the conversion of galactose to glucose during lactose metabolism. Deficiency may lead to galactosemia, a hereditary disorder marked by elevated serum galactose levels and decreased serum glucose levels. Unless detected and treated soon after birth, galactosemia can impair eye, brain, and liver development, causing irreversible cataracts, mental retardation, and cirrhosis.

The qualitative test, a simple screening test for deficiency of galactose-1-phosphate uridyl transferase, is required in some facilities for all neonates. Prenatal testing of amniotic fluid can also detect transferase deficiency but is seldom performed.

Purpose

■ To screen infants for galactosemia
■ To detect heterozygous carriers of galactosemia

Patient preparation

■ When testing a neonate, explain to the parents that the test screens for galactosemia, a potentially dangerous enzyme deficiency.

- If a blood sample wasn't taken from the umbilical cord at birth, tell the parents that a small amount of blood will be drawn from the infant's heel. Explain that the procedure is safe and quickly performed.
- When testing an adult, explain that this test is used to identify carriers of galactosemia, a genetic disorder that may be transmitted to offspring.
- Tell the patient that the test requires a blood sample. Explain who will perform the venipuncture and when.
- Explain to the patient that he may experience slight discomfort from the needle puncture and the tourniquet.
- Inform the patient that he need not restrict food and fluids.

Procedure and posttest care

- For a qualitative (screening) test, collect cord blood or blood from a heelstick on special filter paper, saturating all three circles.
- For a quantitative test, perform a venipuncture and collect a 4-ml sample in a heparinized or EDTA tube, depending on the laboratory method used.
- Indicate the patient's age on the laboratory request.
- Check the patient's history for a recent exchange transfusion. Note this on the laboratory request or postpone the test.
- Apply direct pressure to the venipuncture site until bleeding stops.
- If a hematoma develops at the venipuncture site, apply warm soaks.
- If test results indicate galactosemia, refer the parents for nutrition counseling, and provide a galactose- and lactose-free diet for their infant. A soybean- or meat-based formula may be substituted for formulas based on cow's milk.

Precautions

- Handle the sample gently to prevent hemolysis.
- Send the sample to the laboratory on wet ice.

Reference values

Normally, the qualitative test is negative. The normal range for the quantitative test is 18.5 to 28.5 U/g of hemoglobin (Hb); confirm the normal range with the laboratory in case a different method is used.

Abnormal findings

A positive qualitative test may indicate a transferase deficiency. A follow-up quantitative test should be performed as soon as possible. Quantitative test results showing < 5 U/g of Hb indicate galactosemia. Levels between 5 and 18.5 U/g of Hb may indicate a carrier state.

Interfering factors

- Hemolysis due to rough handling of the sample
- Failure to use the proper collection tube or to send the sample to the laboratory on wet ice (possible false-positive because heat inactivates transferase)
- Total exchange transfusion (transient false-negative because normal blood contains enzyme)

ANGIOTENSIN-CONVERTING ENZYME

The angiotensin-converting enzyme (ACE) test is used to measure serum levels of ACE, which is found in lung capillaries and, in lesser concentrations, blood vessels and kidney tissue. Its primary function is to help regulate arterial pressure by converting angiotensin I to angiotensin II. Measurement of ACE is of little use in diagnosing hypertension.

Purpose

- To aid diagnosis of sarcoidosis, especially pulmonary sarcoidosis
- To monitor response to therapy in sarcoidosis
- To help confirm Gaucher's disease or Hansen's disease

Patient preparation

- Explain to the patient that this test is used to diagnose sarcoidosis, Gaucher's disease, or Hansen's disease or, if appropriate, to check response to treatment for sarcoidosis.
- Tell the patient that the test requires a blood sample. Explain who will perform the venipuncture and when.
- Explain to the patient that he may experience slight discomfort from the needle puncture and the tourniquet.
- Inform the patient that he must fast for 12 hours before the test.
- Note the patient's age on the laboratory request. If he's under age 20, the test may have to be postponed because a person under age 20 has variable ACE levels.

Procedure and posttest care

- Perform a venipuncture and collect the sample in a 7-ml clot-activator tube.
- Apply direct pressure to the venipuncture site until bleeding stops.
- If a hematoma develops at the venipuncture site, apply warm soaks.

Precautions

- Avoid using a tube with EDTA because this can decrease ACE levels, altering test results.
- Handle the sample gently to prevent hemolysis.
- Send the sample to the laboratory immediately or freeze it and place it on dry ice until the test can be performed.

Reference values

In the colorimetric assay, normal values for serum ACE in patients age 20 and older range from 8 to 52 U/L (SI, 0.14 to 0.88 μKat/L).

Abnormal findings

Elevated serum ACE levels may indicate sarcoidosis, Gaucher's disease, or Hansen's disease but results must be correlated with the patient's clinical condition. In some patients, elevated ACE levels may result from hyperthyroidism, diabetic retinopathy, or hepatic disease.

Serum ACE levels decline as the patient responds to steroid or prednisone therapy for sarcoidosis.

Interfering factors

- Failure to fast before the test (may cause significant lipemia of the sample)
- Use of a collection tube with EDTA (possible decrease)
- Hemolysis due to excessive agitation of the sample
- Failure to send the sample to the laboratory at once or to freeze it and place it on dry ice (possible false-low due to ACE degradation)

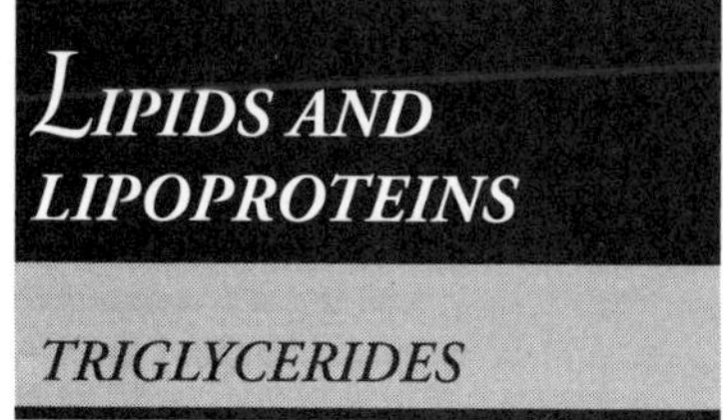

Serum triglyceride analysis provides quantitative analysis of triglycerides — the main storage form of lipids —

which constitute about 95% of fatty tissue. Although not in itself diagnostic, the triglyceride test permits early identification of hyperlipidemia and the risk of coronary artery disease (CAD).

Purpose

- To screen for hyperlipidemia or pancreatitis
- To help identify nephrotic syndrome and individuals with poorly controlled diabetes mellitus
- To determine the risk of CAD
- To calculate low-density lipoprotein cholesterol level using the Freidewald equation

Patient preparation

- Explain to the patient that this test is used to detect disorders of fat metabolism.
- Tell the patient that the test requires a blood sample. Explain who will perform the venipuncture and when.
- Explain to the patient that he may experience slight discomfort from the needle puncture and the tourniquet.
- Instruct the patient to fast for at least 12 hours before the test and to abstain from alcohol for 24 hours. Tell the patient that he can drink water.
- Notify the laboratory and physician of medications the patient is taking that may affect test results; they may need to be restricted.

Procedure and posttest care

- Perform a venipuncture and collect a sample in a 4-ml EDTA tube.
- Apply direct pressure to the venipuncture site until bleeding stops.
- If a hematoma develops at the venipuncture site, apply warm soaks.
- Instruct the patient that he may resume his usual diet and medications discontinued before the test as ordered.

Precautions

- Send the sample to the laboratory immediately.
- Avoid prolonged venous occlusion; remove the tourniquet within 1 minute of application.

Reference values

Triglyceride values vary with age and sex. There's some controversy about the most appropriate normal ranges, but values of 0.44 to 180 mg/dl (SI, 0.44 to 2.01 mmol/L) for adult men and 10 to 190 mg/dl (SI, 0.11 to 2.21 mmol/L) for adult women are widely accepted.

Abnormal findings

Increased or decreased serum triglyceride levels suggest a clinical abnormality; additional tests are required for a definitive diagnosis.

A mild to moderate increase in serum triglyceride levels indicates biliary obstruction, diabetes mellitus, nephrotic syndrome, endocrinopathies, or overconsumption of alcohol. Markedly increased levels without an identifiable cause reflect congenital hyperlipoproteinemia and necessitate lipoprotein phenotyping to confirm the diagnosis.

Decreased serum triglyceride levels are rare and occur mainly in malnutrition and abetalipoproteinemia.

Interfering factors

- Failure to observe pretest restrictions
- Use of glycol-lubricated collection tube
- Failure to send the sample to the laboratory immediately
- Antilipemics (decrease serum lipid levels)
- Cholestyramine and colestipol (decrease cholesterol levels but increase or have no effect on triglyceride levels)

- Corticosteroids (long-term use), oral contraceptives, estrogen, ethyl alcohol, furosemide, and miconazole (increase)
- Clofibrate, dextrothyroxine, gemfibrozil, and niacin (decrease cholesterol and triglyceride levels)
- Probucol (decreases cholesterol levels but has variable effect on triglyceride levels)

TOTAL CHOLESTEROL

The total cholesterol test, the quantitative analysis of serum cholesterol, is used to measure the circulating levels of free cholesterol and cholesterol esters; it reflects the level of the two forms in which this biochemical compound appears in the body. High serum cholesterol levels may be associated with an increased risk of coronary artery disease (CAD).

Purpose

- To assess the risk of CAD
- To evaluate fat metabolism
- To aid diagnosis of nephrotic syndrome, pancreatitis, hepatic disease, hypothyroidism, and hyperthyroidism
- To assess the efficacy of lipid-lowering drug therapy

Patient preparation

- Explain to the patient that this test is used to assess the body's fat metabolism.
- Tell the patient that the test requires a blood sample. Explain who will perform the venipuncture and when.
- Explain to the patient that he may experience slight discomfort from the needle puncture and the tourniquet.
- Instruct the patient not to eat or drink for 12 hours before the test, but that he may have water.
- Notify the laboratory and physician of medications the patient is taking that may affect test results; they may need to be restricted.

Procedure and posttest care

- Perform a venipuncture and collect the sample in a 4-ml tube containing EDTA.
- The patient should be in a sitting position for 5 minutes before the blood is drawn.
- Fingersticks can also be used for initial screening when using an automated analyzer.
- Apply direct pressure to the venipuncture site until bleeding stops.
- Instruct the patient that he may resume his usual diet and medications discontinued before the test as ordered.

Precautions

- Send the sample to the laboratory immediately.

Reference values

Total cholesterol concentrations vary with age and sex. Total cholesterol values are:

- adults: for men, desirable, < 205 mg/dl (SI, < 5.30 mmol/L); for women, < 190mg/dl (SI, < 4.90 mmol/L)
- children age 12 to 18: desirable < 170 mg/dl (SI, < 4.40 mmol/L).

Abnormal findings

Elevated serum cholesterol levels (hypercholesterolemia) may indicate a risk of CAD as well as incipient hepatitis, lipid disorders, bile duct blockage, nephrotic syndrome, obstructive jaundice, pancreatitis, and hypothyroidism.

Low serum cholesterol levels (hypocholesterolemia) are commonly associated with malnutrition, cellular necrosis of the liver, and hyperthyroidism. Abnormal cholesterol levels frequently necessitate further testing to pinpoint the cause.

Interfering factors

■ Failure to observe pretest restrictions
■ Failure to send the sample to the laboratory immediately
■ Cholestyramine, clofibrate, colestipol, dextrothyroxine, haloperidol, neomycin, niacin, and chlortetracycline (decrease)
■ Epinephrine, chlorpromazine, trifluoperazine, oral contraceptives, and trimethadione (increase)
■ Androgens (possible variable effect)

PHOSPHOLIPIDS

The phospholipid test is a quantitative analysis of phospholipids, the major form of lipids in cell membranes. Phospholipids are involved in cellular membrane composition and permeability and help control enzyme activity within the membrane. They aid transport of fatty acids and lipids across the intestinal barrier and from the liver and other fat depots to other body tissues. Phospholipids are essential for pulmonary gas exchange.

Purpose

■ To aid in the evaluation of fat metabolism
■ To aid diagnosis of hypothyroidism, diabetes mellitus, nephrotic syndrome, chronic pancreatitis, obstructive jaundice, and hypolipoproteinemia

Patient preparation

■ Explain to the patient that this test is used to determine how the body metabolizes fats.
■ Tell the patient that the test requires a blood sample. Explain who will perform the venipuncture and when.
■ Explain to the patient that he may experience slight discomfort from the needle puncture and the tourniquet.
■ Instruct the patient to abstain from drinking alcohol for 24 hours before the test and not to eat or drink anything after midnight before the test.
■ Notify the laboratory and physician of medications the patient is taking that may affect test results; they may need to be restricted.

Procedure and posttest care

■ Perform a venipuncture and collect the sample in a 10- to 15-ml tube without additives.
■ Apply direct pressure to the venipuncture site until bleeding stops.
■ If a hematoma develops at the venipuncture site, apply warm soaks.
■ Instruct the patient that he may resume diet and medications discontinued before the test as ordered.

Precautions

■ Send the sample to the laboratory immediately because spontaneous redistribution may occur among plasma lipids.

Reference values

Normal phospholipid levels range from 180 to 320 mg/dl (SI, 1.80 to 3.20 g/L). Although men usually have higher levels than women, values in pregnant women exceed those of men.

Abnormal findings

Elevated phospholipid levels may indicate hypothyroidism, diabetes mellitus, nephrotic syndrome, chronic pancreatitis, or obstructive jaundice. Decreased levels may indicate primary hypolipoproteinemia.

Interfering factors

■ Failure to observe pretest restrictions
■ Clofibrate and other antilipemics (possible decrease)

■ Estrogens, epinephrine, and some phenothiazines (increase)

LIPOPROTEIN-CHOLESTEROL FRACTIONATION

Cholesterol fractionation tests are used to isolate and measure the types of cholesterol in serum, low-density lipoproteins (LDLs) and high-density lipoproteins (HDLs). The HDL level is inversely related to the risk of coronary artery disease (CAD); the higher the HDL level, the lower the incidence of CAD. Conversely, the higher the LDL level, the higher the incidence of CAD.

Purpose

■ To assess the risk of CAD
■ To assess efficacy of lipid-lowering drug therapy

Patient preparation

■ Tell the patient that this test is used to determine the risk of CAD.
■ Tell the patient that the test requires a blood sample. Explain who will perform the venipuncture and when.
■ Explain to the patient that he may experience slight discomfort from the needle puncture and the tourniquet.
■ Instruct the patient to maintain his normal diet for 2 weeks before the test, to abstain from alcohol for 24 hours before the test, and to fast and avoid exercise for 12 to 14 hours before the test.
■ Notify the laboratory and physician of medications the patient is taking that may affect test results; they may need to be restricted.

Procedure and posttest care

■ Perform a venipuncture and collect the sample in a 7-ml tube with EDTA.
■ Apply direct pressure to the venipuncture site until bleeding stops.
■ If a hematoma develops at the venipuncture site, apply warm soaks.
■ Instruct the patient that he may resume diet and medications discontinued before the test as ordered.

Precautions

■ Send the sample to the laboratory immediately to avoid spontaneous redistribution among the lipoproteins.
■ If the sample can't be transported immediately, refrigerate it but don't freeze it.

Reference values

Normal lipoprotein values vary by age, sex, geographic area, and ethnic group; check the laboratory for reference values. HDL levels range from 37 to 70 mg/dl (SI, 0.96 to 1.8 mmol/L) for males and from 40 to 85 mg/dl for females (SI, 1.03 to 2.2 mmol/L). LDL levels are < 130 mg/dl (SI, < 3.36 mmol/K) in individuals who don't have CAD. Borderline high levels are > 160 mg/dl (SI, > 4.1 mmol/L).

The American College of Cardiology recommends an HDL ≥ 40 mg/dl with women maintaining an HDL cholesterol of at least 45 mg/dl. HDL levels > 60 mg/dl are considered heart healthy. LDL levels should optimally be < 100 mg/dl, with levels ≥ 160mg/dl considered high.

Abnormal findings

High LDL levels increase the risk of CAD. Elevated HDL levels generally reflect a healthy state but can also indicate chronic hepatitis, early-stage primary biliary cirrhosis, and alcohol consumption. Increased HDL levels can occur as a result of long-term aerobic and vigorous exercise. Rarely, a sharp rise (to as high as 100 mg/dl [SI,

2.58 mmol/L]) in a second type of HDL ($alpha_2$-HDL) may signal CAD.

Interfering factors

- Concurrent illness, especially if accompanied by fever, recent surgery, or myocardial infarction
- Collecting the sample in a heparinized tube (possible false-high due to activation of the enzyme lipase, which causes release of fatty acids from triglycerides)
- Failure to send the sample to the laboratory immediately
- Antilipemic medications, such as clofibrate, cholestyramine, colestipol, dextrothyroxine, niacin, probucol, and gemfibrozil (decrease)
- Oral contraceptives, disulfiram, alcohol, miconazole, and high doses of phenothiazines (possible increase)
- Estrogens (possible increase or decrease)
- The presence of bilirubin, hemoglobin, salycilates, iodine, and vitamins A and D may affect test results

LIPOPROTEIN PHENOTYPING

Lipoprotein phenotyping is used to determine levels of the four major lipoproteins: chylomicrons, very-low-density (prebeta) lipoproteins, low-density (beta) lipoproteins, and high-density (alpha) lipoproteins. (See *Familial hyperlipoproteinemias.*) Detecting altered lipoprotein patterns is essential in identifying hyperlipoproteinemia and hypolipoproteinemia.

Purpose

- To determine classification of hyperlipoproteinemia and hypolipoproteinemia

Patient preparation

- Explain to the patient that this test is used to determine how the body metabolizes fats.
- Tell the patient that the test requires a blood sample. Explain who will perform the venipuncture and when.
- Explain to the patient that he may experience slight discomfort from the needle puncture and the tourniquet.
- Instruct the patient to abstain from alcohol for 24 hours before the test and to fast after midnight before the test. Provide a low-fat meal the night before the test.
- Check the patient's drug history for use of heparin. As ordered, withhold antilipemics, such as cholestyramine, about 2 weeks before the test.
- Notify the laboratory if the patient is receiving treatment for another condition that might significantly alter lipoprotein metabolism, such as diabetes mellitus, nephrosis, or hypothyroidism.

Procedure and posttest care

- Perform a venipuncture and collect the sample in a 4-ml tube with EDTA.
- If a hematoma develops at the venipuncture site, apply warm soaks.
- Instruct the patient to resume his usual diet and medications discontinued before the test as ordered.

Precautions

- When drawing multiple samples, collect the sample for lipoprotein phenotyping first because venous obstruction for 2 minutes can affect test results.
- Fill the collection tube completely and invert it gently several times to mix the sample and anticoagulant thoroughly.
- Handle the sample gently to prevent hemolysis.

Familial hyperlipoproteinemias

TYPE	CAUSES AND INCIDENCE	CLINICAL SIGNS	LABORATORY FINDINGS
I	◆ Deficient lipoprotein lipase, resulting in increased chylomicrons ◆ May be induced by alcoholism ◆ Incidence: rare	◆ Eruptive xanthomas ◆ Lipemia retinalis ◆ Abdominal pain	◆ Increased chylomicron, total cholesterol, and triglyceride levels ◆ Normal or slightly increased very-low-density lipoproteins (VLDLs) ◆ Normal or decreased low-density lipoproteins (LDLs) and high-density lipoproteins ◆ Cholesterol-triglyceride ratio < 0.2
IIa	◆ Deficient cell receptor, resulting in increased LDL and excessive cholesterol synthesis ◆ May be induced by hypothyroidism ◆ Incidence: common	◆ Premature coronary artery disease (CAD) ◆ Arcus cornea ◆ Xanthelasma ◆ Tendinous and tuberous xanthomas	◆ Increased LDL ◆ Normal VLDL ◆ Cholesterol-triglyceride ratio > 2.0
IIb	◆ Deficient cell receptor, resulting in increased LDL and excessive cholesterol synthesis ◆ May be induced by dysgammaglobulinemia, hypothyroidism, uncontrolled diabetes mellitus, and nephrotic syndrome ◆ Incidence: common	◆ Premature CAD ◆ Obesity ◆ Possible xanthelasmas	◆ Increased LDL, VLDL, total cholesterol, and triglycerides
III	◆ Unknown cause, resulting in deficient VLDL-to-LDL conversion ◆ May be induced by hypothyroidism, uncontrolled diabetes mellitus, and paraproteinemia ◆ Incidence: rare	◆ Premature CAD ◆ Arcus cornea ◆ Eruptive tuberous xanthomas	◆ Increased total cholesterol, VLDL, and triglycerides ◆ Normal or decreased LDL ◆ Cholesterol-triglyceride ratio of VLDL > 0.4 ◆ Broad beta band observed on electrophoresis

(continued)

Familial hyperlipoproteinemias *(continued)*

TYPE	CAUSES AND INCIDENCE	CLINICAL SIGNS	LABORATORY FINDINGS
IV	♦ Unknown cause, resulting in decreased levels of lipoprotein lipase ♦ May be induced by uncontrolled diabetes mellitus, alcoholism, pregnancy, steroid or estrogen therapy, dysgammaglobulinemia, and hyperthyroidism ♦ Incidence: common	♦ Possible premature CAD ♦ Obesity ♦ Hypertension ♦ Peripheral neuropathy	♦ Increased VLDL and triglycerides ♦ Normal LDL ♦ Cholesterol-triglyceride ratio of VLDL < 0.25
V	♦ Unknown cause, resulting in defective triglyceride clearance ♦ May be induced by alcoholism, dysgammaglobulinemia, uncontrolled diabetes mellitus, nephrotic syndrome, pancreatitis, and steroid therapy ♦ Incidence: rare	♦ Premature CAD ♦ Abdominal pain ♦ Lipemia retinalis ♦ Eruptive xanthomas ♦ Hepatosplenomegaly	♦ Increased VLDL, total cholesterol, and triglyceride levels ♦ Chylomicrons present ♦ Cholesterol-triglyceride ratio < 0.6

Findings

The types of hyperlipoproteinemias and hypolipoproteinemias are identified by characteristic electrophoretic patterns.

Familial lipoprotein disorders are classified as either hyperlipoproteinemias or hypolipoproteinemias. There are six types of hyperlipoproteinemias: I, IIa, IIb, III, IV, and V. Types IIa, IIb, and IV are relatively common. All hypolipoproteinemias are rare, including hypobetalipoproteinemia, betalipoproteinemia, and alphalipoprotein deficiency.

Interfering factors

- Recent use of antilipemics (lower levels)
- Failure to observe pretest restrictions
- Hemolysis due to rough handling of the sample
- Administration of heparin (which activates the enzyme lipase, producing fatty acids from triglycerides) or collection of the sample in a heparinized tube (possible false-high)

PROTEINS AND PROTEIN METABOLITES

PROTEIN ELECTROPHORESIS

Protein electrophoresis is used to measure serum albumin and globulins, the major blood proteins, by separating the proteins into five distinct fractions: albumin and $alpha_1$, $alpha_2$, beta, and gamma proteins.

Purpose

- To aid diagnosis of hepatic disease, protein deficiency, renal disorders, and GI and neoplastic diseases

Patient preparation

- Explain to the patient that this test is used to determine the protein content of blood.
- Tell the patient that the test requires a blood sample. Explain who will perform the venipuncture and when.
- Explain to the patient that he may experience slight discomfort from the needle puncture and the tourniquet.
- Inform the patient that he need not restrict food and fluids.
- Notify the laboratory and physician of medications the patient is taking that may affect test results; they may need to be restricted.

Procedure and posttest care

- Perform a venipuncture and collect the sample in a 7-ml clot-activator tube.
- Apply direct pressure to the venipuncture site until bleeding stops.
- If a hematoma develops at the venipuncture site, apply warm soaks.

Precautions

- This test must be performed on a serum sample to avoid measuring the fibrinogen fraction.

Reference values

Normally, total serum protein levels range from 6.4 to 8.3 g/dl, (SI, 64 to 83 g/L) and the albumin fraction ranges from 3.5 to 5 g/dl (SI, 35 to 50 g/L). The $alpha_1$-globulin fraction ranges from 0.1 to 0.3 g/dl (SI, 1 to 3 g/L); $alpha_2$-globulin ranges from 0.6 to 1 g/dl (SI, 6 to 10 g/L). Beta globulin ranges from 0.7 to 1.1 g/dl (SI, 7 to 11 g/L); gamma globulin ranges from 0.8 to 1.6 g/dl (SI, 8 to 16 g/L).

Abnormal findings

For common abnormal findings, see *Clinical implications of abnormal protein levels,* page 182.

Interfering factors

- Pretest administration of a contrast agent, such as sulfobromophthalein (false-high total protein)
- Pregnancy or cytotoxic drugs (possible decrease in serum albumin)
- Use of plasma instead of serum

CERULOPLASMIN

The ceruloplasmin test is used to measure serum levels of ceruloplasmin, an $alpha_2$-globulin that binds about 95% of serum copper, usually in the liver. Ceruloplasmin is thought to regulate iron uptake by transferrin, making iron available to reticulocytes for heme synthesis.

Purpose

- To aid diagnosis of Wilson's disease, Menkes' kinky-hair syndrome, and copper deficiency

Clinical implications of abnormal protein levels

	Total proteins	Albumin	Globulins
INCREASED LEVELS	◆ Chronic inflammatory disease (such as rheumatoid arthritis or early-stage Laënnec's cirrhosis) ◆ Dehydration ◆ Diabetic ketoacidosis ◆ Fulminating and chronic infections ◆ Multiple myeloma ◆ Monocytic leukemia ◆ Vomiting, diarrhea	◆ Multiple myeloma	◆ Chronic syphilis ◆ Collagen diseases ◆ Diabetes mellitus ◆ Hodgkin's disease ◆ Multiple myeloma ◆ Rheumatoid arthritis ◆ Subacute bacterial endocarditis ◆ Systemic lupus erythematosus (SLE) ◆ Tuberculosis
DECREASED LEVELS	◆ Benzene and carbon tetrachloride poisoning ◆ Blood dyscrasias ◆ Essential hypertension ◆ GI disease ◆ Heart failure ◆ Hepatic dysfunction ◆ Hemorrhage ◆ Hodgkin's disease ◆ Hyperthyroidism ◆ Malabsorption ◆ Malnutrition ◆ Nephrosis ◆ Severe burns ◆ Surgical and traumatic shock ◆ Toxemia of pregnancy ◆ Uncontrolled diabetes mellitus	◆ Acute cholecystitis ◆ Collagen diseases ◆ Diarrhea ◆ Essential hypertension ◆ Hepatic disease ◆ Hodgkin's disease ◆ Hyperthyroidism ◆ Hypogammaglobulinemia ◆ Malnutrition ◆ Metastatic carcinoma ◆ Nephritis, nephrosis ◆ Peptic ulcer ◆ Plasma loss from burns ◆ Rheumatoid arthritis ◆ Sarcoidosis ◆ SLE	◆ Benzene and carbon tetrachloride poisoning ◆ Blood dyscrasias ◆ Essential hypertension ◆ GI disease ◆ Heart failure ◆ Hepatic dysfunction ◆ Hemorrhage ◆ Hodgkin's disease ◆ Hyperthyroidism ◆ Malabsorption ◆ Malnutrition ◆ Nephrosis ◆ Severe burns ◆ Surgical and traumatic shock ◆ Toxemia of pregnancy ◆ Uncontrolled diabetes mellitus

Patient preparation
- Explain to the patient that this test is used to determine the copper content of blood.
- Tell the patient that the test requires a blood sample. Explain who will perform the venipuncture and when.
- Explain to the patient that he may experience slight discomfort from the needle puncture and the tourniquet.
- Notify the laboratory and physician of medications the patient is taking that may affect test results; they may need to be restricted.

Procedure and posttest care
- Perform a venipuncture and collect the sample in a 7-ml clot-activator tube.
- Apply direct pressure to the venipuncture site until bleeding stops.
- If a hematoma develops at the venipuncture site, apply warm soaks.

Precautions
- Send the sample to the laboratory immediately.

Reference values
Serum ceruloplasmin levels normally range from 22.9 to 43.1 g/dl (SI, 0.22 to 0.43 g/L).

Abnormal findings
Low ceruloplasmin levels usually indicate Wilson's disease. Low levels may also occur in Menkes' kinky-hair syndrome, nephrotic syndrome, and hypocupremia caused by total parenteral nutrition. Elevated levels may indicate certain hepatic diseases and infections.

Interfering factors
- Estrogen, methadone, phenytoin, and pregnancy (possible increase)

HAPTOGLOBIN

The haptoglobin test is used to measure serum levels of haptoglobin, a glycoprotein produced in the liver. In acute intravascular hemolysis, haptoglobin concentration decreases rapidly and may remain low for 5 to 7 days, until the liver synthesizes more glycoprotein.

Purpose
- To serve as an index of hemolysis
- To distinguish between hemoglobin and myoglobin in plasma because haptoglobin doesn't bind with myoglobin
- To investigate hemolytic transfusion reactions
- To establish proof of paternity using genetic (phenotypic) variations in haptoglobin structure

Patient preparation
- Explain to the patient that this test is used to determine the condition of red blood cells.
- Tell the patient that the test requires a blood sample. Explain who will perform the venipuncture and when.
- Explain to the patient that he may experience slight discomfort from the needle puncture and the tourniquet.
- Inform the patient that he need not restrict food and fluids.
- Notify the laboratory and physician of medications the patient is taking that may affect test results; they may need to be restricted.

Procedure and posttest care
- Perform a venipuncture and collect the sample in a 7-ml clot-activator tube.
- Apply direct pressure to the venipuncture site until bleeding stops.
- If a hematoma develops at the venipuncture site, apply warm soaks.

Precautions

■ Handle the sample gently to prevent hemolysis.

Reference values

Normally, serum haptoglobin concentrations, measured in terms of the protein's hemoglobin-binding capacity, range from 40 to 180 mg/dl (SI, 0.4 to 1.8 g/L). Nephelometric procedures yield lower results.

Haptoglobin is absent in 90% of neonates, but in most cases, levels gradually increase to normal by age 4 months.

Abnormal findings

Markedly decreased serum haptoglobin levels are characteristic in acute and chronic hemolysis, severe hepatocellular disease, infectious mononucleosis, and transfusion reactions. Hepatocellular disease inhibits the synthesis of haptoglobin. In hemolytic transfusion reactions, haptoglobin levels begin decreasing after 6 to 8 hours and drop to 40% of pretransfusion levels after 24 hours.

If serum haptoglobin values are very low, watch for symptoms of hemolysis: chills, fever, back pain, flushing, distended neck veins, tachycardia, tachypnea, and hypotension.

In about 1% of the population, including 4% of blacks, haptoglobin is permanently absent; this disorder is known as congenital ahaptoglobinemia.

Strikingly elevated serum haptoglobin levels occur in diseases marked by chronic inflammatory reactions or tissue destruction, such as rheumatoid arthritis and malignant neoplasms.

Interfering factors

■ Hemolysis due to rough handling of the sample

■ Corticosteroids and androgens (possible increase; may mask hemolysis in patients with inflammatory disease)

TRANSFERRIN

A quantitative analysis of serum transferrin (siderophilin) levels is used to evaluate iron metabolism. Transferrin is a glycoprotein that is formed in the liver. It transports circulating iron obtained from dietary sources or the breakdown of red blood cells by reticuloendothelial cells to bone marrow for use in hemoglobin synthesis or to the liver, spleen, and bone marrow for storage. A serum iron level is usually obtained simultaneously.

Purpose

■ To determine the iron-transporting capacity of the blood

■ To evaluate iron metabolism in iron deficiency anemia

Patient preparation

■ Explain to the patient that this test is used to determine the cause of anemia.

■ Tell the patient that the test requires a blood sample. Explain who will perform the venipuncture and when.

■ Explain to the patient that he may experience slight discomfort from the needle puncture and the tourniquet.

■ Inform the patient that he need not restrict food and fluids.

■ Notify the laboratory and physician of medications the patient is taking that may affect test results; they may need to be restricted.

Procedure and posttest care

■ Perform a venipuncture and collect the sample in a 4-ml clot-activator tube.

■ Apply direct pressure to the venipuncture site until bleeding stops.

■ If a hematoma develops at the venipuncture site, apply warm soaks.

Precautions

- Handle the sample gently to prevent hemolysis.
- Send the sample to the laboratory immediately.

Reference values

Normal serum transferrin values range from 200 to 400 mg/dl (SI, 2 to 4 g/L).

Abnormal findings

Inadequate transferrin levels may lead to impaired hemoglobin synthesis and, possibly, anemia. Low serum levels may indicate inadequate production of transferrin due to hepatic damage or excessive protein loss from renal disease. Decreased transferrin levels may also result from acute or chronic infection and cancer.

Increased serum transferrin levels may indicate severe iron deficiency.

Interfering factors

- Hemolysis due to rough handling of the sample
- Oral contraceptives and late pregnancy (possible increase)

PLASMA AMINO ACID SCREENING

Plasma and amino acid screening is a qualitative screen for inborn errors of amino acid metabolism. Amino acids are the chief component of all proteins and polypeptides. The body contains at least 20 amino acids; 10 of these aren't formed in the body and must be acquired by diet. Certain congenital enzyme deficiencies interfere with normal metabolism of these amino acids, resulting in amino acid accumulation or deficiency.

Purpose

- To screen for inborn errors of amino acid metabolism

Patient preparation

- Explain to the parents that this test is used to determine how well their infant metabolizes amino acids.
- The infant must fast for 4 hours before the test.
- Tell the parents that a small amount of blood will be drawn from the infant's heel but that collecting the sample only takes a few minutes.

Procedure and posttest care

- Perform a heelstick and collect 0.1 ml of blood in a heparinized capillary tube.
- Apply direct pressure to the venipuncture site until bleeding stops.
- If a hematoma develops at the heelstick site, apply warm soaks.
- Tell the parents to resume their infant's usual diet.

Precautions

- Handle the sample gently to prevent hemolysis.

Normal findings

Chromatography shows a normal plasma amino acid pattern.

Abnormal findings

Excessive accumulation of amino acids typically produces overflow aminoacidurias. Congenital abnormalities of the amino acid transport system in the kidneys produce a second group of disorders called renal aminoacidurias. Comparisons of blood and urine chromatography can help distinguish between the two types of aminoacidurias. The plasma amino acid pattern is normal in renal aminoacidurias and abnormal in overflow aminoacidurias.

Interfering factors

- Failure to observe pretest restrictions
- Hemolysis due to rough handling of the sample

PHENYLALANINE SCREENING

The phenylalanine screening test, also called the Guthrie screening test, is used to screen infants for elevated serum phenylalanine levels, a possible indication of phenylketonuria (PKU). Phenylalanine is a naturally occurring amino acid essential to growth and nitrogen balance; an accumulation of this amino acid may indicate a serious enzyme deficiency. This test detects abnormal phenylalanine levels through the growth rate of *Bacillus subtilis,* an organism that needs phenylalanine to thrive. To ensure accurate results, the test must be performed after 3 full days (preferably 4 days) of milk or formula feeding.

Purpose

- To screen infants for possible PKU

Patient preparation

- Explain to the parents that the test is a routine screening measure for possible PKU and is required in many states.
- Tell the parents that a small amount of blood will be drawn from the infant's heel and that collecting the sample only takes a few minutes.

Procedure and posttest care

- Perform a heelstick, and collect three drops of blood — one in each circle — on the filter paper.
- Reassure the parents of a child who may have PKU that although this disease is a common cause of congenital mental deficiency, early detection and continuous treatment with a low-phenylalanine diet can prevent permanent mental retardation.

Precautions

- Note the infant's name and birth date and the date of the first milk or formula feeding on the laboratory request.
- Send the sample to the laboratory immediately.

Reference values

A negative test result indicates normal phenylalanine levels (< 2 mg/dl [SI, < 121 µmol/L]) and no appreciable danger of PKU.

Abnormal findings

At birth, a neonate with PKU usually has normal phenylalanine levels, but after milk or formula feeding begins, levels gradually increase because of a deficiency of the liver enzyme that converts phenylalanine to tyrosine. A positive test result suggests the *possibility* of PKU. A definitive diagnosis requires exact serum phenylalanine measurement and urine testing. A positive test result may also indicate hepatic disease, galactosemia, or delayed development of certain enzyme systems. (See *Confirming PKU.*)

Interfering factors

- Performing the test before the infant has received at least 3 full days of milk or formula feeding (false-negative)

Confirming PKU

If phenylalanine screening detects the possible presence of phenylketonuria (PKU), serum phenylalanine and tyrosine levels are measured to confirm the diagnosis. Phenylalanine hydroxylase is the enzyme that converts phenylalanine to tyrosine. If this enzyme is absent, increasing phenylalanine levels and falling tyrosine levels indicate PKU.

Samples are obtained by venipuncture (femoral or external jugular) and measured by fluorometry. Elevated serum phenylalanine levels (> 4 mg/dl [SI, > 242 µmol/L]) and low tyrosine levels — with urinary excretion of phenylpyruvic acid — confirm the diagnosis of PKU.

PLASMA AMMONIA

The plasma ammonia test measures plasma levels of ammonia, a nonprotein nitrogen compound that helps maintain acid-base balance. In such diseases as cirrhosis of the liver, ammonia can bypass the liver and accumulate in the blood. Plasma ammonia levels may help indicate the severity of hepatocellular damage.

Purpose

- To help monitor the progression of severe hepatic disease and the effectiveness of therapy
- To recognize impending or established hepatic coma

Patient preparation

- Explain to the patient (or to a family member if the patient is comatose) that this test is used to evaluate liver function.
- Tell the patient that the test requires a blood sample. Explain who will perform the venipuncture and when.
- Inform the patient that he may experience slight discomfort from the needle puncture and the tourniquet.
- Notify the laboratory and physician of medications the patient is taking that may affect test results; they may need to be restricted.

Procedure and posttest care

- Perform a venipuncture and collect the sample in a 10-ml heparinized tube.
- Apply direct prsesure to the venipuncture site until bleeding stops.
- If a hematoma develops at the venipuncture site, apply warm soaks.
- Watch for signs of impending or established hepatic coma if plasma ammonia levels are high.

Precautions

- Notify the laboratory before performing the venipuncture so that preliminary preparations can begin.
- Handle the sample gently to prevent hemolysis, pack it in ice, and send it to the laboratory immediately.
- Do *not* use a chilled container.

Reference values

Plasma ammonia levels in adults usually range from 15 to 45 µg/dl (SI, 11 to 32 µmol/L).

Abnormal findings

Elevated plasma ammonia levels are common in severe hepatic disease, such as cirrhosis and acute hepatic necrosis, and can lead to hepatic coma. Elevated levels may also occur in Reye's syndrome, severe heart failure, GI hemorrhage, and erythroblastosis fetalis.

Interfering factors

- Hemolysis due to rough handling of the sample
- Delay in testing
- Acetazolamide, thiazides, ammonium salts, and furosemide (increase)
- Parenteral nutrition or a portacaval shunt (possible increase)
- Lactulose, neomycin, and kanamycin (decrease)
- Smoking, poor venipuncture technique, and exposure to ammonia cleaners in the laboratory (possible increase)

BLOOD UREA NITROGEN

The blood urea nitrogen (BUN) test is used to measure the nitrogen fraction of urea, the chief end product of protein metabolism. Formed in the liver from ammonia and excreted by the kidneys, urea constitutes 40% to 50% of the blood's nonprotein nitrogen. The BUN level reflects protein intake and renal excretory capacity but is a less reliable indicator of uremia than the serum creatinine level.

Purpose

- To evaluate kidney function and aid diagnosis of renal disease
- To aid assessment of hydration

Patient preparation

- Tell the patient that this test is used to evaluate kidney function.
- Inform the patient that he need not restrict food and fluids, but should avoid a diet high in meat.
- Tell the patient that the test requires a blood sample. Explain who will perform the venipuncture and when.
- Explain to the patient that he may experience slight discomfort from the needle puncture and the tourniquet.
- Notify the laboratory and physician of medications the patient is taking that may affect test results; they may need to be restricted.

Procedure and posttest care

- Perform a venipuncture and collect the sample in a 3- to 4-ml clot-activator tube.
- Apply direct pressure to the venipuncture site until bleeding stops.
- If a hematoma develops at the venipuncture site, apply warm soaks.

Precautions

- Handle the sample gently to prevent hemolysis.

Reference values

BUN values normally range from 8 to 20 mg/dl (SI, 2.9 to 7.5 mmol/L), with slightly higher values in elderly patients.

Abnormal findings

Elevated BUN levels occur in renal disease, reduced renal blood flow (due to dehydration, for example), urinary tract obstruction, and increased protein catabolism (such as burn injuries).

Low BUN levels occur in severe hepatic damage, malnutrition, and overhydration.

Interfering factors

- Hemolysis due to rough handling of the sample
- Chloramphenicol (possible decrease)
- Aminoglycosides, amphotericin B, methicillin (increased due to nephrotoxicity)

CREATININE

Analysis of serum creatinine levels provides a more sensitive measure of renal damage than blood urea nitrogen levels. Creatinine is a nonprotein end product of creatine metabolism that appears in serum in amounts proportional to the body's muscle mass.

Purpose

- To assess glomerular filtration
- To screen for renal damage

Patient preparation

- Explain to the patient that this test is used to evaluate kidney function.
- Tell the patient that the test requires a blood sample. Explain who will perform the venipuncture and when.
- Explain to the patient that he may experience slight discomfort from the needle puncture and the tourniquet.
- Instruct the patient that he need not restrict food and fluids.
- Notify the laboratory and physician of medications the patient is taking that may affect test results; they may need to be restricted.

Procedure and posttest care

- Perform a venipuncture and collect the sample in a 3- or 4-ml clot-activator tube.
- Apply direct pressure to the venipuncture site until bleeding stops.
- If a hematoma develops at the venipuncture site, apply warm soaks.

Precautions

- Handle the sample gently.
- Send the sample to the laboratory immediately.

Reference values

Creatinine concentrations normally range from 0.8 to 1.2 mg/dl (SI, 62 to 115 μmol/L) in males and 0.6 to 0.9 mg/dl (SI, 53 to 97 μmol/L) in females.

Abnormal findings

Elevated serum creatinine levels generally indicate renal disease that has seriously damaged 50% or more of the nephrons. Elevated levels may also be associated with gigantism and acromegaly.

Interfering factors

- Ascorbic acid, barbiturates, and diuretics (possible increase)
- Exceptionally large muscle mass, such as that found in athletes (possible increase despite normal renal function)
- Hemolysis due to rough handling of the sample
- Sulfabromopthalein or phenosulfaphthalein (given within the previous 24 hours can elevate creatinine levels if the test is based on the Jaffé reaction)

URIC ACID

The uric acid test is used to measure serum levels of uric acid, the major end metabolite of purine. Disorders of purine metabolism, rapid destruction of nucleic acids, and conditions marked by impaired renal excretion characteristically raise serum uric acid levels.

Purpose

- To confirm diagnosis of gout
- To help detect renal dysfunction

Patient preparation

- Explain to the patient that this test is used to detect gout and kidney dysfunction.
- Tell the patient that the test requires a blood sample. Explain who will perform the venipuncture and when.
- Explain to the patient that he may experience slight discomfort from the needle puncture and the tourniquet.
- Instruct the patient to fast for 8 hours before the test.
- Notify the laboratory and physician of medications the patient is taking that may affect test results; they may need to be restricted.

Procedure and posttest care

- Perform a venipuncture and collect the sample in a 3- or 4-ml clot-activator tube.
- If a hematoma develops at the venipuncture site, apply warm soaks.

Precautions

- Handle the sample gently to prevent hemolysis.

Reference values

Uric acid concentrations in men normally range from 3.4 to 7 mg/dl (SI, 202 to 416 µmol/L); in women, normal levels range from 2.3 to 6 mg/dl (SI, 143 to 357 µmol/L).

Abnormal findings

Increased uric acid levels may indicate gout or impaired kidney function. Levels may also rise in heart failure, glycogen storage disease (type I, von Gierke's disease), infections, hemolytic and sickle cell anemia, polycythemia, neoplasms, and psoriasis.

Low uric acid levels may indicate defective tubular absorption (such as Fanconi's syndrome) or acute hepatic atrophy.

Interfering factors

- Failure to observe pretest restrictions
- Loop diuretics, ethambutol, vincristine, pyrazinamide, thiazides, and low doses of aspirin (possible increase)
- Acetaminophen, ascorbic acid, and levodopa (possible false-high if using colorimetric method)
- Aspirin in high doses (possible decrease)
- Starvation, high-purine diet, stress, and alcohol abuse (possible increase)

PIGMENTS

BILIRUBIN

The bilirubin test is used to measure serum levels of bilirubin, the predominant pigment in bile. Bilirubin is the major product of hemoglobin catabolism. Serum bilirubin measurements are especially significant in neonates because elevated unconjugated bilirubin can accumulate in the brain, causing irreparable damage.

Purpose

- To evaluate liver functions
- To aid differential diagnosis of jaundice and monitor its progress
- To aid diagnosis of biliary obstruction and hemolytic anemia
- To determine whether a neonate requires an exchange transfusion or phototherapy because of dangerously high unconjugated bilirubin levels

Patient preparation

- Explain to the patient that this test is used to evaluate liver function and the condition of red blood cells.

- Tell the patient that the test requires a blood sample. Explain who will perform the venipuncture and when.
- Explain to the patient that he may experience slight discomfort from the needle puncture and the tourniquet.
- Inform the adult patient that he need not restrict fluids, but should fast for at least 4 hours before the test. (Fasting isn't necessary for neonates.)
- If the patient is an infant, tell the parents that a small amount of blood will be drawn from his heel. Tell them who will be performing the heelstick and when.

Procedure and posttest care

- If the patient is an adult, perform a venipuncture and collect the sample in a 3- or 4-ml clot-activator tube.
- If the patient is an infant, perform a heelstick and fill the microcapillary tube to the designated level with blood.
- Apply direct pressure to the venipuncture site until bleeding stops.
- If a hematoma develops at the venipuncture or heelstick site, apply warm soaks.

Precautions

- Protect the sample from strong sunlight and ultraviolet light.
- Handle the sample gently and send it to the laboratory immediately.

Reference values

In adults, normal indirect serum bilirubin levels are 1.1 mg/dl (SI, 19 μmol/L), and direct serum bilirubin levels are < 0.5 mg/dl (SI, < 6.8 μmol/L). In neonates, total serum bilirubin levels are 2 to 12 mg/dl (SI, 34 to 205 μmol/L).

Abnormal findings

Elevated indirect serum bilirubin levels usually indicate hepatic damage. High levels of indirect bilirubin are also likely in severe hemolytic anemia. If hemolysis continues, both direct and indirect bilirubin levels may rise. Other causes of elevated indirect bilirubin levels include congenital enzyme deficiencies, such as Gilbert's disease.

Elevated direct serum bilirubin levels usually indicate biliary obstruction. If obstruction continues, both direct and indirect bilirubin levels may rise. In severe chronic hepatic damage, direct bilirubin concentrations may return to normal or near-normal levels, but indirect bilirubin levels remain elevated. In neonates, total bilirubin levels of 15 mg/dl (SI, 257 μmol/L) or more indicate the need for an exchange transfusion.

Interfering factors

- Exposure of the sample to direct sunlight or ultraviolet light (possible decrease)
- Hemolysis due to rough handling of the sample

FRACTIONATED ERYTHROCYTE PORPHYRINS

The fractionated erythrocyte porphyrin test is used to measure erythrocyte porphyrins (also called erythropoietic porphyrins): protoporphyrin, coproporphyrin, and uroporphyrin. Porphyrins are present in all protoplasm and are significant in energy storage and use. They are produced during heme biosynthesis and usually appear in small amounts in blood, urine, and stool. The production and excretion of porphyrins or their precursors increase in porphyria.

Purpose

- To aid diagnosis of congenital and acquired erythropoietic porphyrias
- To help confirm diagnosis of disorders affecting red blood cell (RBC) activity

Patient preparation

- Explain to the patient that this test is used to detect RBC disorders.
- Tell the patient that the test requires a blood sample. Explain who will perform the venipuncture and when.
- Explain to the patient that he may experience slight discomfort from the needle puncture and the tourniquet.

Procedure and posttest care

- Perform a venipuncture and collect the sample in a 5-ml or larger heparinized tube.
- Label the sample, place it on ice, and send it to the laboratory immediately.
- Apply direct pressure to the venipuncture site until bleeding stops.
- If a hematoma develops at the venipuncture site, apply warm soaks.

Precautions

- Handle the sample gently to prevent hemolysis.
- Send the sample to the laboratory promptly.

Reference values

Total porphyrin levels range from 16 to 60 µg/dl (SI, 0.25 to 1.062 µmol/L) of packed RBCs. Protoporphyrin levels range from 16 to 60 µg/dl (SI, 0.25 to 1.062 µmol/L). Coproporphyrin and uroporphyrin levels are normally < 2 µg/dl (SI, < 0.035 µmol/L)

Abnormal findings

Elevated total porphyrin levels suggest the need for further enzyme testing to identify the specific porphyria. Elevated protoporphyrin levels may indicate erythropoietic protoporphyria, infection, increased erythropoiesis, thalassemia, sideroblastic anemia, iron deficiency anemia, or lead poisoning.

Increased coproporphyrin levels may indicate congenital erythropoietic porphyria, erythropoietic protoporphyria or coproporphyria, or sideroblastic anemia.

Elevated uroporphyrin levels may indicate congenital erythropoietic porphyria or erythropoietic protoporphyria.

Interfering factors

- Hemolysis due to rough handling of the sample
- Exposure of the sample to direct sunlight or ultraviolet light

Carbohydrates

Fasting plasma glucose

The fasting plasma glucose (or fasting blood sugar) test is used to measure plasma glucose levels after a 12- to 14-hour fast. This test is commonly used to screen for diabetes mellitus, in which absence or deficiency of insulin allows persistently high glucose levels.

Purpose

- To screen for diabetes mellitus
- To monitor drug or diet therapy in patients with diabetes mellitus

Patient preparation

- Explain to the patient that this test is used to detect disorders of glucose metabolism and aids diagnosis of diabetes.
- Tell the patient that the test requires a blood sample. Explain who will perform the venipuncture and when.

- Explain to the patient that he may experience slight discomfort from the needle puncture and the tourniquet.
- Instruct the patient to fast for 12 to 14 hours before the test.
- Notify the laboratory and physician of medications the patient is taking that may affect test results; they may need to be restricted.
- Alert the patient to the symptoms of hypoglycemia (weakness, restlessness, nervousness, hunger, and sweating), and tell the patient to report such symptoms immediately.

Procedure and posttest care

- Perform a venipuncture and collect the sample in a 5-ml clot-activator tube.
- Apply direct pressure to the venipuncture site until bleeding stops.
- If a hematoma develops at the venipuncture site, apply warm soaks.
- Provide a balanced meal or a snack.
- Instruct the patient that he may resume medications discontinued before the test as ordered.

Precautions

- Send the sample to the laboratory immediately. If transport is delayed, refrigerate the sample.
- Note on the laboratory request when the patient last ate, the sample collection time, and when the last pretest dose of insulin or oral antidiabetic drug (if applicable) was given.

Reference values

The normal range for fasting plasma glucose varies according to the laboratory procedure. Generally, normal values after at least an 8-hour fast are 70 to 110 mg (SI, 3.9 to 6.1 mmol/L) of true glucose per deciliter of blood.

Abnormal findings

Confirmation of diabetes mellitus requires fasting plasma glucose levels of 126 mg/dl (SI, 7 mmol/L) or more obtained on two or more occasions. In patients with borderline or transient elevated levels, a 2-hour postprandial plasma glucose test or oral glucose tolerance test may be performed to confirm diagnosis.

Increased fasting plasma glucose levels can also result from pancreatitis, recent acute illness (such as myocardial infarction), Cushing's syndrome, acromegaly, and pheochromocytoma. Hyperglycemia may also stem from hyperlipoproteinemia (especially type III, IV, or V), chronic hepatic disease, nephrotic syndrome, brain tumor, sepsis, or gastrectomy with dumping syndrome and is typical in eclampsia, anoxia, and seizure disorder.

Low plasma glucose levels can result from hyperinsulinism, insulinoma, von Gierke's disease, functional and reactive hypoglycemia, myxedema, adrenal insufficiency, congenital adrenal hyperplasia, hypopituitarism, malabsorption syndrome, and some cases of hepatic insufficiency.

Interfering factors

- Failure to observe restrictions (possible increase)
- Recent illness, infection, or pregnancy (possible increase)
- Glycolysis due to failure to refrigerate the sample or to send it to the laboratory immediately (possible false-negative)
- Acetaminophen, if using the glucose oxidase or hexokinase method (possible false-positive)
- Chlorthalidone, thiazide diuretics, furosemide, triamterene, oral contraceptives, benzodiazepines, phenytoin, phenothiazines, lithium, epinephrine, arginine, phenolphthalein, dextrothyroxine, diazoxide, large doses of nicotinic acid, corticosteroids, and recent I.V. glucose infusions (increase)

- Ethacrynic acid (may cause hyperglycemia); large doses in patients with uremia (can cause hypoglycemia)
- Beta-adrenergic blockers, ethanol, clofibrate, insulin, oral antidiabetic agents, and monamine oxidase inhibitors (possible decrease)
- Strenuous exercise (decrease)

TWO-HOUR POSTPRANDIAL PLASMA GLUCOSE

Also called the 2-hour postprandial blood sugar test, the 2-hour postprandial plasma glucose procedure is a valuable screening tool for detecting diabetes mellitus. The test is performed when the patient demonstrates symptoms of diabetes (polydipsia and polyuria) or when results of the fasting plasma glucose test suggest diabetes.

Purpose

- To aid diagnosis of diabetes mellitus
- To monitor drug or diet therapy in patients with diabetes mellitus

Patient preparation

- Explain to the patient that this test is used to evaluate glucose metabolism and to detect diabetes.
- Tell the patient that the test requires a blood sample. Explain who will perform the venipuncture and when.
- Explain to the patient that he may experience slight discomfort from the needle puncture and the tourniquet.
- Tell the patient to eat a balanced meal or one containing 100 g of carbohydrates before the test and then fast for 2 hours. Instruct him to avoid smoking and strenuous exercise after the meal.
- Notify the laboratory and physician of medications the patient is taking that may affect test results; they may need to be restricted.

Procedure and posttest care

- Perform a venipuncture and collect the sample in a 5-ml clot-activator tube.
- If a hematoma develops at the venipuncture site, apply warm soaks.
- Instruct the patient that he may resume his usual diet, medications, and activity discontinued before the test as ordered.

Precautions

- Send the sample to the laboratory immediately or refrigerate it.
- Specify on the laboratory request when the patient last ate, the sample collection time, and when the last pretest dose of insulin or oral antidiabetic drug was given.
- If the sample is to be drawn by a technician, tell the patient the exact time the venipuncture must be performed.

Reference values

In the patient who doesn't have diabetes, postprandial glucose values are < 145 mg/dl (SI, < 8 mmol/L) by the glucose oxidase or hexokinase method; levels are slightly elevated in people over age 50. (See *Two-hour postprandial plasma glucose levels by age.*)

Abnormal findings

Two 2-hour postprandial blood glucose values of 200 mg/dl (SI, 11.1 mmol/L) or above indicate diabetes mellitus. High levels may also occur with pancreatitis, Cushing's syndrome, acromegaly, and pheochromocytoma. Hyperglycemia may also be caused by hyperlipoproteinemia (especially type III, IV, or V), chronic hepatic disease, nephrotic syndrome, brain tumor, sepsis, gastrectomy with dumping syndrome, eclampsia, anoxia, and seizure disorders.

Two-hour postprandial plasma glucose levels by age

The greatest difference in normal and diabetic insulin responses, and thus in plasma glucose concentration, occurs about 2 hours after a glucose challenge. Values of this test can fluctuate according to the patient's age. After age 50, for example, normal levels rise markedly and steadily, sometimes reaching 160 mg/dl (SI, 8.82 mmol/L) or higher. In a younger patient, glucose concentration > 145 mg/dl (SI, > 8 mmol/L) suggests incipient diabetes and requires further evaluation.

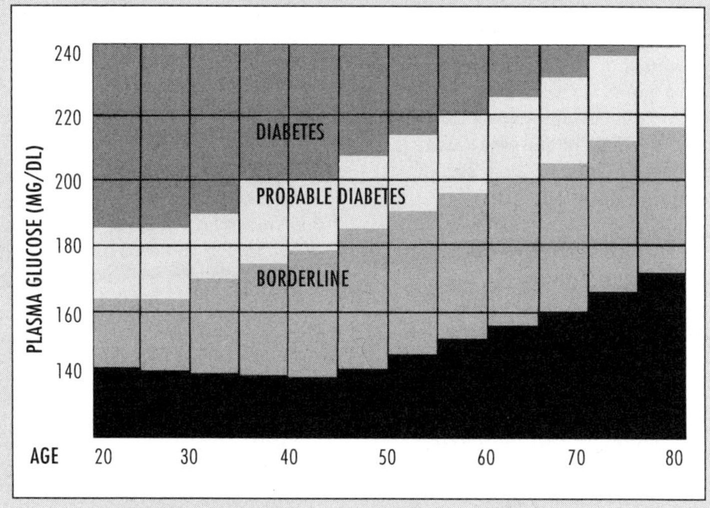

Low glucose levels occur in hyperinsulinism, insulinoma, von Gierke's disease, functional and reactive hypoglycemia, myxedema, adrenal insufficiency, congenital adrenal hyperplasia, hypopituitarism, malabsorption syndrome, and some cases of hepatic insufficiency.

Interfering factors

- Recent illness, infection, or pregnancy (possible increase)
- Acetaminophen, if using the glucose oxidase or hexokinase method (possible false-positive)
- Chlorthalidone, thiazide diuretics, furosemide, triamterene, oral contraceptives, benzodiazepines, phenytoin, phenothiazines, lithium, epinephrine, arginine, phenolphthalein, dextrothyroxine, diazoxide, large doses of nicotinic acid, corticosteroids, and recent I.V. glucose infusions (increase)
- Ethacrynic acid (possible increase); large doses in patients with uremia (possible decrease)
- Beta-adrenergic blockers, amphetamines, ethanol, clofibrate, insulin, oral antidiabetic drugs, and monoamine oxidase inhibitors (possible decrease)
- Strenuous exercise or stress (possible decrease)

■ Glycolysis caused by failure to refrigerate the sample or to send it to the laboratory immediately (possible decrease)

ORAL GLUCOSE TOLERANCE

The oral glucose tolerance test is the most sensitive method of evaluating borderline cases of diabetes mellitus. Plasma and urine glucose levels are monitored for 3 hours after ingestion of a challenge dose of glucose to assess insulin secretion and the body's ability to metabolize glucose.

The oral glucose tolerance test isn't generally used in patients with fasting plasma glucose values > 140 mg/dl (SI, > 7.7 mmol/L) or postprandial plasma glucose values > 200 mg/dl (SI, > 11 mmol/L).

Purpose

■ To confirm diabetes mellitus in selected patients

■ To aid diagnosis of hypoglycemia and malabsorption syndrome

Patient preparation

■ Explain to the patient that this test is used to evaluate glucose metabolism.

■ Instruct the patient to maintain a high-carbohydrate diet for 3 days and then to fast for 10 to 16 hours before the test as instructed by the physician.

■ Tell the patient not to smoke, drink coffee or alcohol, or exercise strenuously for 8 hours before or during the test.

■ Tell the patient that this test requires five blood samples and usually five urine samples. Explain who will perform the venipunctures and when and that the patient may experience transient discomfort from the needle punctures and the tourniquet.

■ Suggest to the patient that he bring a book or other quiet diversion with him to the test. The procedure usually takes 3 hours but can last as long as 6 hours.

■ Notify the laboratory and physician of medications the patient is taking that may affect test results; they may need to be restricted.

■ Alert the patient to the symptoms of hypoglycemia (weakness, restlessness, nervousness, hunger, and sweating), and tell the patient to report such symptoms immediately.

Procedure and posttest care

■ Between 7 a.m. and 9 a.m., perform a venipuncture to obtain a fasting blood sample. Draw this sample into a 7-ml clot-activator tube. A saline lock may be inserted and used to collect the multiple blood samples needed as per facility protocol.

■ Collect a urine sample at the same time if your facility includes this as part of the test.

■ After collecting these samples, administer the test load of oral glucose and record the time of ingestion. Encourage the patient to drink the entire glucose solution within 5 minutes.

■ Draw blood samples 30 minutes, 1 hour, 2 hours, and 3 hours after giving the loading dose using 7-ml clot-activator tube.

■ Collect urine samples at the same intervals.

■ Tell the patient to lie down if he feels faint from the numerous venipunctures.

■ Encourage the patient to drink water throughout the test to promote adequate urine excretion.

■ Apply direct pressure to the venipuncture site until bleeding stops.

■ If a hematoma develops at the venipuncture site, apply warm soaks.

■ Provide a balanced meal or a snack, but observe for a hypoglycemic reaction.

■ Instruct the patient that he may resume medications discontinued before the test as ordered.

Precautions

■ Send blood and urine samples to the laboratory immediately or refrigerate them.

■ Specify when the patient last ate and the blood and urine sample collection times.

■ As appropriate, record the time the patient received his last pretest dose of insulin or oral antidiabetic drug.

■ If the patient develops severe hypoglycemia, notify the physician. Draw a blood sample, record the time on the laboratory request, and discontinue the test. Have the patient drink a glass of orange juice with sugar added or administer glucose I.V. to reverse the reaction.

Reference values

Normal plasma glucose levels peak at 160 to 180 mg/dl (SI, 8.8 to 9.9 mmol/L) within 30 minutes to 1 hour after administration of an oral glucose test dose and return to fasting levels or lower within 2 to 3 hours. Urine glucose tests remain negative throughout.

Abnormal findings

Decreased glucose tolerance, in which levels peak sharply before falling slowly to fasting levels, may confirm diabetes mellitus or may result from Cushing's disease, hemochromatosis, pheochromocytoma, or central nervous system lesions.

Increased glucose tolerance, in which levels may peak at less than normal, may indicate insulinoma, malabsorption syndrome, adrenocortical insufficiency (Addison's disease), hypothyroidism, or hypopituitarism.

Interfering factors

■ Recent infection, fever, pregnancy, or acute illness, such as myocardial infarction (possible increase)

■ Failure to adhere to dietary and exercise restrictions may alter test results.

■ Carbohydrate deprivation before the test (may cause a diabetic response [abnormal increase with a delayed decrease] because the pancreas is unaccustomed to responding to high-carbohydrate load)

■ Chlorthalidone, thiazide diuretics, furosemide, triamterene, oral contraceptives, benzodiazepines, phenytoin, phenothiazines, lithium, epinephrine, phenolphthalein, caffeine, arginine, dextrothyroxine, diazoxide, corticosteroids, large doses of nicotinic acid, and recent I.V. glucose infusions (possible increase)

■ Beta-adrenergic blockers, amphetamines, ethanol, clofibrate, insulin, oral antidiabetic drugs, and monamine oxidase inhibitors (possible decrease)

■ Age 50 or older (decreasing carbohydrate tolerance, which causes increasing glucose tolerance to upper limits of about 1 mg/dl for every year over age 50)

β-*HYDROXYBUTYRATE*

The β-hydroxybutyrate test is used to measure serum levels of β-hydroxybutyric acid (beta-hydroxybutyrate), one of three ketone bodies. The other two ketone bodies are acetoacetate and acetone. An accumulation of all three ketone bodies is referred to as *ketosis;* excessive formation of ketone bodies in the blood is called *ketonemia.*

Purpose

■ To diagnose carbohydrate deprivation, which may result from starvation,

digestive disturbances, dietary imbalances, or frequent vomiting
■ To aid diagnosis of diabetes mellitus resulting from decreased utilization of carbohydrates
■ To aid diagnosis of glycogen storage diseases, specifically von Gierke's disease
■ To diagnose or monitor the treatment of metabolic disorders, such as diabetic ketoacidosis or lactic acidosis

Patient preparation

■ Explain to the patient that this test is used to evaluate ketones in the blood.
■ Tell the patient that the test requires a blood sample. Explain who will perform the venipuncture and when.
■ Explain to the patient that he may experience slight discomfort from the needle puncture and the tourniquet.
■ Inform the patient that he need not restrict food and fluids.

Procedure and posttest care

■ Perform a venipuncture and collect the sample in a 5-ml clot-activator tube.
■ Allow the sample to clot.
■ Centrifuge and remove the serum.
■ If an acetone level is requested, have this analysis performed first.
■ Serum β-hydroxybutyrate remains stable for at least 1 week at 25.6° to 46.4° F (–3.5° to 8° C). Plasma is also an acceptable sample for analysis of β-hydroxybutyrate.
■ Apply direct pressure to the venipuncture site until bleeding stops.
■ If a hematoma develops at the venipuncture site, apply warm soaks.

Precautions

■ Send the sample to the laboratory immediately.

Reference values

The normal value for serum or plasma β-hydroxybutyrate levels is < 0.4 mmol/L (SI, 0.4 mmol/L).

Abnormal findings

Elevated β-hydroxybutyrate levels may suggest worsening of ketosis. Reference values > 2 mmol/L (SI, > 2 mmol/L) should be reported to the patient's physician immediately.

Interfering factors

■ Presence of both lactate dehydrogenase at high concentrations and lactic acid at concentrations > 10 mmol/L (SI, > 10 mmol/L) (possible increase)
■ Increased sodium fluoride concentrations (possible decrease)
■ Fasting (increase with extended fasting time)

GLYCOSYLATED HEMOGLOBIN

Also called total fasting hemoglobin (Hb), the glycosylated Hb test is a tool for monitoring diabetes therapy. Measurement of glycosylated Hb levels provides information about the average blood glucose level during the preceding 2 to 3 months. This test requires only one venipuncture every 6 to 8 weeks and can, therefore, be used for evaluating long-term effectiveness of diabetes therapy.

Purpose

■ To assess control of diabetes mellitus

Patient preparation

■ Explain to the patient that this test is used to evaluate diabetes therapy.
■ Tell the patient that the test requires a blood sample. Explain who will perform the venipuncture and when.
■ Explain to the patient that he may experience slight discomfort from the needle puncture and the tourniquet.

■ Inform the patient that he need not restrict food and fluids, and instruct him to maintain his prescribed medication and diet regimens.

Procedure and posttest care

■ Perform a venipuncture and collect the sample in a 5-ml tube with EDTA added.
■ Apply direct pressure to the venipuncture site until bleeding stops.
■ If a hematoma develops at the venipuncture site, apply warm soaks.
■ Schedule the patient for an appointment in 6 to 8 weeks for appropriate follow-up testing.

Precautions

■ Completely fill the collection tube.
■ Invert the sample gently several times to mix the sample and anticoagulant adequately.

Reference values

Glycosylated Hb values are reported as a percentage of the total Hb within an erythrocyte. Glycosylated Hb accounts for 4% to 7%.

Abnormal findings

In diabetes, the patient has good control of blood glucose concentrations when the glycosylated Hb value is < 8%. A glycosylated Hb value > 10% indicates poor control.

Interfering factors

■ Failure to adequately mix the sample and the anticoagulant
■ Hemolytic anemia (decreased)
■ Hyperglycemia, thalassemia, chronic renal failure, those receiving dialysis, those that have a splenectomy, those with elevated triglycerides or Hb F levels (increased)

ORAL LACTOSE TOLERANCE

The oral lactose tolerance test is used to measure plasma glucose levels after ingestion of a challenge dose of lactose. It's used to screen for lactose intolerance due to lactase deficiency.

Absence or deficiency of lactase causes undigested lactose to remain in the intestinal lumen, producing such symptoms as abdominal cramps and watery diarrhea. True congenital lactase deficiency is rare. Usually, lactose intolerance is acquired because lactase levels generally decrease with age.

Purpose

■ To detect lactose intolerance

Patient preparation

■ Explain to the patient that this test is used to determine if his symptoms are due to an inability to digest lactose.
■ Instruct the patient to fast and to avoid strenuous activity for 8 hours before the test.
■ Inform the patient that this test requires four blood samples. Tell the patient who will be performing the venipunctures and when.
■ Explain to the patient that he may experience transient discomfort from the needle punctures and the tourniquet. Tell the patient that the entire procedure may take up to 2 hours.
■ Notify the laboratory and physician of medications the patient is taking that may affect test results; they may need to be restricted.

Procedure and posttest care

■ After the patient has fasted for 8 hours, perform a venipuncture and collect a blood sample in a 4-ml tube with sodium fluoride and potassium oxalate added.

■ Administer the test load of lactose: for an adult, 50 g of lactose dissolved in 400 ml of water; for a child, 50 g/m^2 of body surface area. Record the time of ingestion.

■ Draw a blood sample 30, 60, and 120 minutes after giving the loading dose. Use a 4-ml tube with sodium fluoride and potassium oxalate added.

■ If ordered, collect a stool sample 5 hours after giving the loading dose.

■ Apply direct pressure to the venipuncture site until bleeding stops.

■ If a hematoma develops at the venipuncture site, apply warm soaks.

■ Instruct the patient to resume his usual diet, medications, and activity discontinued before the test as ordered.

Precautions

■ Send blood and stool samples to the laboratory immediately or refrigerate them if transport is delayed.

■ Specify the collection time on the laboratory requests.

■ Watch for symptoms of lactose intolerance — abdominal cramps, nausea, bloating, flatulence, and watery diarrhea — caused by the loading dose.

Reference values

Normally, plasma glucose levels rise > 20 mg/dl (SI, > 1.1 mmol/L) over fasting levels within 15 to 60 minutes after ingestion of the lactose loading dose.

Abnormal findings

A rise in plasma glucose of < 20 mg/dl (SI, < 1.1 mmol/L) indicates lactose intolerance, as does stool acidity (pH of 5.5 or less) and high glucose content (> 1+ on the dipstick). Accompanying signs and symptoms provoked by the test also suggest, but don't confirm, the diagnosis because such symptoms may appear in patients with normal lactase activity after a loading dose of lactose. Small-bowel biopsy with lactase assay may be performed to confirm the diagnosis.

Interfering factors

■ Failure to follow diet and exercise restrictions

■ Thiazide diuretics, oral contraceptives, benzodiazepines, propranolol, and insulin (possible false-low)

■ Delayed emptying of stomach contents (possible decrease)

■ Glycolysis (possible false-negative)

LACTIC ACID AND PYRUVIC ACID

Lactic acid, present in blood as lactate ion, is derived primarily from muscle cells and erythrocytes. It's an intermediate product of carbohydrate metabolism and is usually metabolized by the liver. Blood lactate concentration depends on the rates of production and metabolism; levels may increase significantly during exercise.

Lactate and pyruvate together form a reversible reaction that's regulated by oxygen supply. When oxygen levels are deficient, pyruvate converts to lactate; when they're adequate, lactate converts to pyruvate. When the hepatic system fails to metabolize lactose sufficiently or when excess pyruvate converts to lactate, lactic acidosis may result. Measurement of blood lactate levels is recommended for all patients with symptoms of lactic acidosis such as Kussmaul's respiration.

Comparison of pyruvate and lactate levels provides reliable information about tissue oxidation, but measurement of pyruvate is technically difficult and infrequently performed.

Purpose

- To assess tissue oxidation
- To help determine the cause of lactic acidosis

Patient preparation

- Explain to the patient that this blood test is used to evaluate the oxygen level in tissues.
- Tell the patient that the test requires a blood sample. Explain who will perform the venipuncture and when.
- Explain to the patient that he may experience slight discomfort from the needle puncture and the tourniquet.
- Withhold food overnight and make sure the patient rests for at least 1 hour before the test.

Procedure and posttest care

- Perform a venipuncture and collect the sample in a 5-ml tube with sodium fluoride and potassium oxalate added.
- Apply direct pressure to the venipuncture site until bleeding stops.
- If a hematoma develops at the venipuncture site, apply warm soaks.
- Instruct the patient that he may resume his usual diet discontinued before the test as ordered.

Precautions

- Because venostasis may raise blood lactate levels, tell the patient that he must not clench his fist during the venipuncture.
- Avoid using a tourniquet; however, if one must be used, release it at least 2 minutes before collecting the sample so blood can circulate.
- Because lactate and pyruvate are extremely unstable, place the sample container in an ice-filled cup and send it to the laboratory immediately.

Reference values

Blood lactate values normally range from 0.93 to 1.65 mEq/L (SI, 0.93 to 1.65 mmol/L); pyruvate levels, from 0.08 to 0.16 mEq/L (SI, 0.08 to 0.16 mmol/L). The lactate-pyruvate ratio is normally < 10:1.

Abnormal findings

Elevated blood lactate levels associated with hypoxia may result from strenuous muscle exercise, shock, hemorrhage, septicemia, myocardial infarction, pulmonary embolism, and cardiac arrest. When no reason for diminished tissue perfusion is apparent, increased lactate levels may result from systemic disorders, such as diabetes mellitus, leukemias and lymphomas, hepatic disease, and renal failure, or from enzymatic defects, such as von Gierke's disease (glycogen storage disease) and fructose 1,6-diphosphatase deficiency.

Lactic acidosis can follow ingestion of large doses of acetaminophen and ethanol as well as I.V. infusion of epinephrine, glucagon, fructose, or sorbitol.

Interfering factors

- Failure to adhere to diet and activity restrictions may affect test results
- Failure to pack the sample in ice and to transport it to the laboratory immediately (possible increase)

Hormone tests

PITUITARY HORMONES

CORTICOTROPIN

The corticotropin test measures the plasma levels of corticotropin (also known as adrenocorticotropic hormone or ACTH) by radioimmunoassay. Corticotropin stimulates the adrenal cortex to secrete cortisol and, to a lesser degree, androgens and aldosterone. It also has some melanocyte-stimulating activity, increases the uptake of amino acids by muscle cells, promotes lipolysis by fat cells, stimulates pancreatic beta cells to secrete insulin, and may contribute to the release of growth hormone. Corticotropin levels vary diurnally, peaking between 6 a.m. and 8 a.m. and ebbing between 6 p.m. and 11 p.m.

The corticotropin test may be ordered for patients with signs of adrenal hypofunction (insufficiency) or hyperfunction (Cushing's syndrome). Corticotropin suppression or stimulation testing is usually necessary to confirm diagnosis. The instability and unavailability of corticotropin greatly limit this test's diagnostic significance and reliability.

Purpose

- To facilitate differential diagnosis of primary and secondary adrenal hypofunction
- To aid differential diagnosis of Cushing's syndrome

Patient preparation

- Explain to the patient that this test helps determine if his hormonal secretion is normal.
- Advise the patient that he must fast and limit his physical activity for 10 to 12 hours before the test.
- Tell the patient that the test requires a blood sample. Explain who will perform the venipuncture and when.
- Explain to the patient that he may experience slight discomfort from the needle puncture and the tourniquet.
- Check the patient's history for medications that may affect the accuracy of test results, as ordered. Withhold these medications for 48 hours or longer before the test. If they must be continued, note this on the laboratory request.
- Arrange with the dietary department to provide a low-carbohydrate diet for 2 days before the test. This requirement may vary, depending on the laboratory.

Procedure and posttest care

- For a patient with suspected adrenal hypofunction, perform the venipuncture for a baseline level between 6 a.m. and 8 a.m. (peak secretion).
- For a patient with suspected Cushing's syndrome, perform the venipuncture between 6 p.m. and 11 p.m. (low secretion).
- Collect the sample in a plastic tube (corticotropin may adhere to glass) with EDTA (ethylenediaminetetraacetic acid) added. The tube must be full because excess anticoagulant will affect results.
- Pack the sample in ice, and send it to the laboratory immediately, where plasma must be rapidly separated from blood cells at 39.2° F (4° C). The collection technique may vary, depending on the laboratory.
- Apply direct pressure to the venipuncture site until bleeding stops.
- If a hematoma develops at the venipuncture site, apply warm soaks.
- Instruct the patient that he may resume his usual diet and medications discontinued before the test as ordered.

Precautions

- Because proteolytic enzymes in plasma degrade corticotropin, a temperature of 39.2° F (4° C) is necessary to retard enzyme activity.
- Immediate transfer of the sample, packed in ice, to the laboratory is essential for reliable test results.

Reference values

Mayo Medical Laboratories sets baseline values at less than 120 pg/ml (SI, < 26.4 pmol/L at 6 a.m. to 8 a.m.), but these values may vary, depending on the laboratory.

Abnormal findings

A higher-than-normal corticotropin level may indicate primary adrenal hypofunction (Addison's disease), in which the pituitary gland attempts to compensate for the unresponsiveness of the target organ by releasing excessive corticotropin. The underlying cause of adrenocortical hypofunction may be idiopathic atrophy of the adrenal cortex or partial destruction of the gland by granuloma, neoplasm, amyloidosis, or inflammatory necrosis.

A low-normal corticotropin level suggests secondary adrenal hypofunction resulting from pituitary or hypothalamic dysfunction. The primary determinant may be panhypopituitarism, absence of corticotropin-releasing hormone in the hypothalamus, or chronic blunting of corticotropin levels by long-term corticosteroid therapy.

In suspected Cushing's syndrome, an elevated corticotropin level suggests Cushing's disease, in which pituitary dysfunction (due to adenoma) causes continuous hypersecretion of corticotropin and, consequently, continuously elevated cortisol levels without diurnal variations. Moderately elevated corticotropin levels suggest pituitary-dependent adrenal hyperplasia and nonadrenal tumors, such as oat cell carcinoma of the lungs.

A low-normal corticotropin level implies adrenal hyperfunction due to adrenocortical tumor or hyperplasia.

Interfering factors

- Failure to observe pretest restrictions
- Corticosteroids, including cortisone and its analogues (decrease)
- Drugs that increase endogenous cortisol secretion, such as estrogens, calcium gluconate, amphetamines, spironolactone, and ethanol (decrease)
- Lithium carbonate (decreases cortisol levels and may interfere with corticotropin secretion)
- Menstrual cycle and pregnancy
- Radioactive scan performed within 1 week before the test
- Acute stress (including hospitalization and surgery) and depression (increase)

RAPID CORTICOTROPIN

The rapid corticotropin test (also known as the rapid ACTH test or cosyntropin test) is gradually replacing the 8-hour corticotropin stimulation test as the most effective diagnostic tool for evaluating adrenal hypofunction. Using cosyntropin, the rapid corticotropin test provides faster results and causes fewer allergic reactions than the 8-hour test, which uses natural corticotropin from animal sources.

This test requires prior determination of baseline cortisol levels to evaluate the effect of cosyntropin administration on cortisol secretion. An unequivocally high morning cortisol level rules out adrenal hypofunction and makes further testing unnecessary.

Purpose

- To aid in identification of primary and secondary adrenal hypofunction

Patient preparation

- Explain to the patient that this test helps determine if his condition is due to a hormonal deficiency.
- Inform him that he may be required to fast for 10 to 12 hours before the test and must be relaxed and resting quietly for 30 minutes before the test.
- Tell him that the test takes at least 1 hour to perform.
- If the patient is an inpatient, withhold corticotropin and all steroid medications as ordered. If he's an outpatient, tell him to refrain from taking these drugs, if instructed by his physician. If the drugs must be continued, note this on the laboratory request.
- Explain to the patient that he may experience slight discomfort from the needle puncture and the tourniquet.

Procedure and posttest care

- Draw 5 ml of blood for a baseline value. Collect the sample in a 5-ml heparinized tube. Label this sample "preinjection," and send it to the laboratory.
- Inject 250 µg (0.25 mg) of cosyntropin I.V. or I.M. (I.V. administration provides more accurate results because ineffective absorption after I.M. administration may cause wide variations in response.) Direct I.V. injection should take about 2 minutes.
- Draw another 5 ml of blood at 30 and 60 minutes after the cosyntropin injection. Collect the samples in 5-ml heparinized tubes. Label the samples "30 minutes postinjection" and "60 minutes postinjection," and send them to the laboratory. Include the collection times on the laboratory request.
- Apply direct pressure to the venipuncture site until bleeding stops.
- If a hematoma develops at the venipuncture site, apply warm soaks.
- Observe the patient for signs of a rare allergic reaction to cosyntropin, such as hives, itching, and tachycardia.
- Instruct the patient that he may resume his normal diet and medications discontinued before the test.

Precautions

- Handle the samples gently to prevent hemolysis. They require no special precautions other than avoiding stasis.

Reference values

Normally, cortisol levels rise after 30 to 60 minutes to a peak of 18 mg/dl (SI, 500 mmol/L) or more 60 minutes after the cosyntropin injection. Generally, doubling the baseline value indicates a normal response.

Abnormal findings

A normal result excludes adrenal hypofunction (insufficiency). In patients with primary adrenal hypofunction (Addison's disease), cortisol levels remain low. Thus, the rapid corticotropin test provides an effective method of screening for adrenal hypofunction. If test results show subnormal increases in cortisol levels, prolonged stimulation of the adrenal cortex may be required to differentiate between primary and secondary adrenal hypofunction.

Interfering factors

- Failure to observe pretest restrictions
- Hemolysis due to rough handling of the sample
- Estrogens and amphetamines (increase in plasma cortisol)
- Smoking and obesity (possible increase in plasma cortisol)
- Lithium carbonate (decrease in plasma cortisol)
- Radioactive scan performed within 1 week before the test

GROWTH HORMONE

Human growth hormone (hGH), also called somatotropin, is a protein secreted by acidophils of the anterior pituitary gland. It's the primary regulator of human growth. Unlike other pituitary hormones, hGH has no easily defined feedback mechanism or single target gland — it affects many body tissues. Like insulin, hGH promotes protein synthesis and stimulates amino acid uptake by cells. Hyposecretion or hypersecretion of this hormone may induce pathologic states (such as dwarfism and gigantism, respectively).

This test is a quantitative analysis of plasma hGH levels and may be performed as part of an anterior pituitary stimulation or suppression test.

Purpose

- To aid differential diagnosis of dwarfism because growth retardation can result from pituitary or thyroid hypofunction
- To confirm diagnosis of acromegaly and gigantism in adults
- To aid diagnosis of pituitary and hypothalamic tumors
- To help evaluate hGH therapy

Patient preparation

- Explain to the patient, or his parents if the patient is a child, that this test measures hormone levels and helps determine the cause of abnormal growth.
- Instruct him to fast and limit physical activity for 10 to 12 hours before the test.
- Tell the patient that the test requires a blood sample. Explain who will perform the venipuncture and when.
- Explain to the patient that he may experience slight discomfort from the needle puncture and the tourniquet.
- Inform him that another sample may have to be drawn the next day for comparison.
- Withhold all medications that affect hGH levels such as pituitary-based steroids. If they must be continued, note this on the laboratory request.
- Make sure the patient is relaxed and recumbent for 30 minutes before the test because stress and physical activity elevate hGH levels.

Procedure and posttest care

- Between 6 a.m. and 8 a.m. on 2 consecutive days, or as ordered, perform a venipuncture and collect at least 7 ml of blood in a clot-activator tube.
- Apply direct pressure to the venipuncture site until bleeding stops.
- If a hematoma develops at the venipuncture site, apply warm soaks.
- Instruct the patient that he may resume his normal diet and medications discontinued before the test.

Precautions

- Handle the sample gently to prevent hemolysis.
- Send it to the laboratory immediately because hGH has a half-life of only 20 to 25 minutes.

Reference values

Normal hGH levels for males range from undetectable to 5 ng/ml (SI, 5 µg/L); for females, from undetectable to 10 ng/ml. Children's values may range from undetectable to 16 ng/ml (SI, 16 µg/L), and are usually higher.

Abnormal findings

Increased hGH levels may indicate a pituitary or hypothalamic tumor, frequently an adenoma, which causes gigantism in children and acromegaly in adults and adolescents. Some patients with diabetes mellitus have elevated hGH levels without acromegaly. Suppression testing is necessary to confirm diagnosis.

Pituitary infarction, metastatic disease, and tumors may decrease hGH levels. Dwarfism may be due to low hGH levels, although only 15% of all cases of growth failure relate to endocrine dysfunction. Confirmation of diagnosis requires stimulation testing with arginine or insulin.

Interfering factors

- Failure to observe pretest restrictions
- Hemolysis due to rough handling of the sample
- Arginine, beta-adrenergic blockers such as propranolol, and estrogens (increase)
- Amphetamines, bromocriptine, levodopa, dopamine, pituitary-based steroids, methyldopa, and histamine (increase)
- Insulin (induced hypoglycemia), glucagon, and nicotinic acid (increase)
- Phenothiazines (such as chlorpromazine) and corticosteroids (decrease)
- Radioactive scan performed within 1 week before the test

GROWTH HORMONE SUPPRESSION TEST

Also called glucose loading, the growth hormone suppression test evaluates excessive baseline levels of human growth hormone (hGH) from the anterior pituitary gland. Normally, a glucose load should suppress hGH secretion. In a patient with excessive hGH levels, failure of suppression indicates anterior pituitary dysfunction and confirms diagnosis of acromegaly and gigantism.

Purpose

- To assess elevated baseline levels of hGH
- To confirm diagnosis of gigantism in children and acromegaly in adults and adolescents

Patient preparation

- Explain to the patient, or his parents if the patient is a child, that this test helps determine the cause of his abnormal growth.
- Instruct him to fast and limit physical activity for 10 to 12 hours before the test.
- Tell him that two blood samples will be drawn. Warn him that he may experience nausea after drinking the glucose solution and some discomfort from the needle punctures and tourniquet.
- Withhold all steroids and other pituitary-based hormones. If they or other medications must be continued, note this on the laboratory request.
- Tell the patient to lie down and relax for 30 minutes before the test.

Procedure and posttest care

- Perform a venipuncture and collect 6 ml of blood (basal sample) in a 7-ml clot-activator tube.
- Administer 100 g of glucose solution by mouth. To prevent nausea, advise the patient to drink the glucose slowly.
- About 1 hour later, draw venous blood into a 7-ml clot-activator tube. Label the tubes appropriately, and send them to the laboratory immediately.
- Apply direct pressure to the venipuncture site until bleeding stops.
- If a hematoma develops at the venipuncture site, apply warm soaks.
- Instruct the patient that he may resume his normal diet and medications discontinued before the test.

Precautions

- Handle the samples gently to prevent hemolysis.
- Send each sample to the laboratory immediately because hGH has a half-life of only 20 to 25 minutes.

Reference values

Normally, glucose suppresses hGH to levels ranging from undetectable to 3 ng/ml (SI, 3 µg/L) in 30 minutes to 2 hours. In children, rebound stimulation may occur after 2 to 5 hours.

Abnormal findings

In a patient with active acromegaly, elevated baseline hGH levels (75 ng/ml [SI, 5 µg/L]) aren't suppressed to less than 5 ng/ml during the test. Unchanged or rising hGH levels in response to glucose loading indicate hGH hypersecretion and may confirm suspected acromegaly and gigantism. This response may be verified by repeating the test after a 1-day rest.

Interfering factors

- Failure to observe pretest restrictions
- Hemolysis due to rough handling of the sample
- Corticosteroids and phenothiazines such as chlorpromazine (possible decrease in hGH secretion)
- Arginine, levodopa, amphetamines, glucagon, niacin, and estrogens (possible increase in hGH secretion)
- Radioactive scan performed within 1 week before the test
- Physical activity

INSULIN TOLERANCE TEST

The insulin tolerance test measures serum levels of human growth hormone (hGH) and corticotropin after administration of a loading dose of insulin and is more reliable than direct measurement of hGH and corticotropin. Insulin-induced hypoglycemia stimulates hGH and corticotropin secretion. Failure of stimulation indicates anterior pituitary or adrenal hypofunction and helps confirm an hGH or a corticotropin insufficiency.

Purpose

- To aid diagnosis of hGH and corticotropin deficiency
- To identify pituitary dysfunction
- To aid differential diagnosis of primary and secondary adrenal hypofunction

Patient preparation

- Explain to the patient, or his parents if the patient is a child, that this test evaluates hormonal secretion.
- Instruct him to fast and restrict physical activity for 10 to 12 hours before the test.
- Explain that the test involves I.V. infusion of insulin and the collection of multiple blood samples.
- Warn him that he may experience an increased heart rate, diaphoresis, hunger, and anxiety after administration of insulin. Reassure him that these symptoms are transient, and that if they become severe, the test will be discontinued.
- Tell him to lie down and relax for 90 minutes before the test.

Procedure and posttest care

- Between 6 a.m. and 8 a.m., perform a venipuncture and collect three 5-ml samples of blood for basal levels: one in a *gray-top* tube (for blood glucose) and two in *green-top* tubes (for hGH and corticotropin).

■ Administer an I.V. bolus of U-100 regular insulin (0.15 U/kg, or as ordered) over 1 to 2 minutes.
■ Use an indwelling venous catheter to avoid repeated venipunctures. Collect additional blood samples 15, 30, 45, 60, 90, and 120 minutes after administration of insulin. At each interval, collect three samples: one in a tube with sodium fluoride and potassiam oxidate and two in heparizined tubes. Label the tubes appropriately, and send them to the laboratory immediately.
■ Apply direct pressure to the venipuncture site until bleeding stops.
■ If a hematoma develops at the I.V. or venipuncture site, apply warm soaks.
■ Instruct the patient that he may resume his normal diet, activities, and medications discontinued before the test.

Precautions

■ Be sure to have concentrated glucose solution readily available in the event that the patient has a severe hypoglycemic reaction to insulin.
■ Label the tubes appropriately, including the collection times on the laboratory request, and send all samples to the laboratory immediately.
■ Handle the samples gently to prevent hemolysis.

Reference values

Normally, blood glucose falls to 50% of the fasting level 20 to 30 minutes after insulin administration. This stimulates a 10- to 20-ng/dl (SI, 10 to 20 μg/L) increase in baseline values for hGH and corticotropin, with peak levels occurring 60 to 90 minutes after insulin administration.

Abnormal findings

Failure of stimulation or a blunted response suggests dysfunction of the hypothalamic-pituitary-adrenal axis. An hGH increase of less than 10 ng/dl (SI, < 10 μg/L) above baseline suggests hGH deficiency. A definitive diagnosis of hGH deficiency requires a supplementary stimulation test such as the arginine test. Additional testing is necessary to determine the site of the abnormality.

An increase in corticotropin levels of less than 10 ng/dl (SI, < 10 μg/L) above baseline suggests adrenal insufficiency. The metyrapone or corticotropin stimulation test then confirms the diagnosis and determines whether the insufficiency is primary or secondary.

Interfering factors

■ Failure to observe pretest restrictions of diet, medications, and physical activity
■ Hemolysis due to rough handling of the sample
■ Corticosteroids and pituitary-based drugs (increase in hGH)
■ Glucocorticoids and beta-adrenergic blockers (decrease in hGH)
■ Glucocorticoids, estrogens, calcium gluconate, amphetamines, methamphetamines, spironolactone, and ethanol (decrease in corticotropin)

ARGININE TEST

The arginine test, also known as the human growth hormone (hGH) stimulation test, measures hGH levels after I.V. administration of arginine, an amino acid that normally stimulates hGH secretion. It's commonly used to identify pituitary dysfunction in infants and children with growth retardation and to confirm hGH deficiency. This test may be performed concomitantly with an insulin tolerance test or after administration of other hGH stimulants, such as glucagon, vasopressin, and levodopa.

Purpose

- To aid diagnosis of pituitary tumors
- To confirm hGH deficiency in infants and children with low baseline levels

Patient preparation

- Explain to the patient, or his parents if the patient is a child, that this test identifies hGH deficiency.
- Instruct him to fast and limit physical activity for 10 to 12 hours before the test.
- Explain that this test requires I.V. infusion of a drug and collection of several blood samples. Tell him that the test takes at least 2 hours to perform.
- Wthhold all steroid medications, including pituitary-based hormones, as ordered. If they must be continued, record this on the laboratory request.
- Tell the patient to lie down and relax for at least 90 minutes before the test.

Procedure and posttest care

- Between 6 a.m. and 8 a.m., perform a venipuncture and collect 6 ml of blood (basal sample) in a clot-activator tube.
- Using an indwelling venous catheter avoids repeated venipunctures and minimizes stress and anxiety. Start I.V. infusion of arginine (0.5 g/kg of body weight) in normal saline solution, and continue for 30 minutes.
- Discontinue the I.V. infusion, and then draw a total of three 6-ml samples at 30-minute intervals. Collect each sample in a clot-activator tube, and label it appropriately.
- Apply direct pressure to the venipuncture site until bleeding stops.
- If a hematoma develops at the I.V. or venipuncture site, apply warm soaks.
- Instruct the patient that he may resume his normal diet, activities, and medications discontinued before the test as ordered.

Precautions

- Collect each sample at the scheduled time, and specify the collection time on the laboratory request.
- Send each sample to the laboratory immediately because hGH has a half-life of only 20 to 25 minutes.
- Handle the samples gently to prevent hemolysis.

Reference values

Arginine should raise hGH levels to more than 10 ng/ml (SI, > 10 µg/L) in men, more than 15 ng/ml (SI, > 15 µg/L) in women, and more than 48 ng/ml (SI, > 48 µg/L) in children. Such an increase may appear in the first sample collected 30 minutes after arginine infusion is discontinued or in the samples collected 60 and 90 minutes afterward.

Abnormal findings

Levels that are elevated during fasting or that rise during sleep help to rule out hGH deficiency. Failure of hGH levels to rise after arginine infusion indicates decreased anterior pituitary hGH reserve. In children, this deficiency causes dwarfism; in adults, it can indicate panhypopituitarism. When hGH levels fail to reach 10 ng/ml (SI, 10 µg/L), retesting is required at the same time of day as the original test.

Interfering factors

- Failure to observe pretest restrictions of diet, medications, and physical activity
- Hemolysis due to rough handling of the sample
- Radioactive scan performed within 1 week before the test

FOLLICLE-STIMULATING HORMONE

The follicle-stimulating hormone test of gonadal function, performed more often on women than on men, measures follicle-stimulating hormone (FSH) levels and is vital in infertility studies. Plasma levels fluctuate widely in females; to obtain a true baseline level, daily testing may be necessary for 3 to 5 days.

Purpose

- To aid in the diagnosis and treatment of infertility and disorders of menstruation such as amenorrhea
- To aid in the diagnosis of precocious puberty in girls (before age 9) and in boys (before age 10)
- To aid in the differential diagnosis of hypogonadism

Patient preparation

- Explain to the patient, or her parents if she's a minor, that this test helps determine if her hormonal secretion is normal.
- Tell the patient that the test requires a blood sample. Explain who will perform the venipuncture and when.
- Explain to the patient that she may experience discomfort from the needle puncture and the tourniquet.
- Withhold medications that may interfere with accurate determination of test results for 48 hours before the test, as ordered. If they must be continued (for example, for infertility treatment), note this on the laboratory request.
- Make sure the patient is relaxed and recumbent for 30 minutes before the test.

Procedure and posttest care

- Perform a venipuncture, preferably between 6 a.m. and 8 a.m., and collect the sample in a 7-ml clot-activator tube. Send the sample to the laboratory immediately.
- Apply direct pressure to the venipuncture site until bleeding stops.
- If a hematoma develops at the venipuncture site, apply warm soaks.
- Instruct the patient that she may resume her usual medications discontinued before the test as ordered.

Precautions

- Handle the sample gently to prevent hemolysis.
- If the patient is female, indicate the phase of her menstrual cycle on the laboratory request. If she's menopausal, note this on the laboratory request.

Reference values

Reference values vary greatly, depending on the patient's age, stage of sexual development, and — for a female — phase of her menstrual cycle. For menstruating females, approximate FSH values are as follows:

- Follicular phase: 5 to 20 mIU/ml (SI, 5 to 20 IU/L)
- Ovulatory phase: 15 to 30 mIU/ml (SI, 15 to 30 IU/L)
- Luteal phase: 5 to 15 mIU/ml (SI, 5 to 15 IU/L)

Approximate FSH values for men range from 5 to 20 mIU/ml (SI, 5 to 20 IU/L); for menopausal women, 50 to 100 mIU/ml (SI, 50 to 100 IU/L).

Abnormal findings

Decreased FSH levels may cause male or female infertility: aspermatogenesis in men and anovulation in women. Low FSH levels may indicate secondary hypogonadotropic states, which can result from anorexia nervosa, panhypopituitarism, or hypothalamic lesions.

High FSH levels in women may indicate ovarian failure associated with Turner's syndrome (primary hypogonadism) or Stein-Leventhal syndrome (polycystic ovary syndrome). Elevated levels may occur in patients with precocious puberty (idiopathic or with central nervous system lesions) and in postmenopausal women. In men, abnormally high FSH levels may indicate destruction of the testes (from mumps orchitis or X-ray exposure), testicular failure, seminoma, or male climacteric. Congenital absence of the gonads and early-stage acromegaly may cause FSH levels to rise in both sexes.

Interfering factors

- Failure to observe pretest restrictions of medications
- Hemolysis due to rough handling of the sample
- Ovarian steroid hormones, such as estrogen and progesterone, related compounds, and phenothiazines such as chlorpromazine (possible decrease through negative feedback by inhibiting FSH flow from the hypothalamus and pituitary gland)
- Radioactive scan performed within 1 week before the test

PLASMA LUTEINIZING HORMONE

The plasma luteinizing hormone (LH) test, usually ordered for anovulation and infertility studies on women, is a quantitative analysis of plasma LH or interstitial cell-stimulating hormone levels. In women, cyclic LH secretion (with follicle-stimulating hormone [FSH]) causes ovulation and transforms the ovarian follicle into the corpus luteum, which in turn secretes progesterone. (See *LH secretion peaks at ovulation.*) In males, continuous LH secretion stimulates the interstitial (Leydig) cells of the testes to release testosterone, which stimulates and maintains spermatogenesis (with FSH).

Purpose

- To detect ovulation
- To assess male or female infertility
- To evaluate amenorrhea
- To monitor therapy designed to induce ovulation

Patient preparation

- Explain to the patient that this test helps determine if her secretion of female hormones is normal.
- Because there's no evidence that plasma LH levels are affected by fasting, eating, or exercise, such pretest restrictions may be unnecessary.
- Tell the patient that this test requires a blood sample. Explain who will perform the venipuncture and when.
- Inform the patient that she may experience some discomfort from the needle puncture and tourniquet.
- Withhold drugs that may interfere with plasma LH levels, such as steroids (including estrogens and progesterone), for 48 hours before the test, as ordered. If they must be continued, note this on the laboratory request.

Procedure and posttest care

- Perform a venipuncture, and collect the sample in a 7-ml clot-activator tube.
- Apply direct pressure to the venipuncture site until bleeding stops.
- If a hematoma develops at the venipuncture site, apply warm soaks.
- Instuct the patient that she may resume medications discontinued before the test.

LH secretion peaks at ovulation

The menstrual cycle is divided into three distinct phases: the menstrual phase (days 1 to 5); the proliferative, or follicular, phase (days 6 to 13); and after ovulation on day 14, the secretory, or luteal, phase (days 15 to 28).

THE MENSTRUAL PHASE

This phase of the normal cycle is characterized by endometrial sloughing, corpus luteum degeneration, and new follicle growth. During this stage, the concentration of estrogen and progesterone is low, triggering increased follicle-stimulating hormone (FSH) and luteinizing hormone (LH) secretion.

THE FOLLICULAR PHASE

During the follicular phase, the follicle stimulated by FSH reaches full size and increases its secretion of estrogen. Simultaneously with increased estrogen, FSH decreases while LH increases slowly but steadily. During the late follicular phase, LH rises sharply and FSH rises slightly. At about the 14th day, within hours of this abrupt surge in LH, estrogen levels in the plasma drop and ovulation occurs. After ovulation, the concentration of LH and FSH falls rapidly.

THE SECRETORY PHASE

During the final, or luteal, phase, the follicle reorganizes as the corpus luteum secretes progesterone and estrogen. Within 7 or 8 days after ovulation, if fertilization hasn't occurred, the corpus luteum regresses and progesterone and estrogen levels decrease. The endometrium sloughs, and the menstrual cycle begins again.

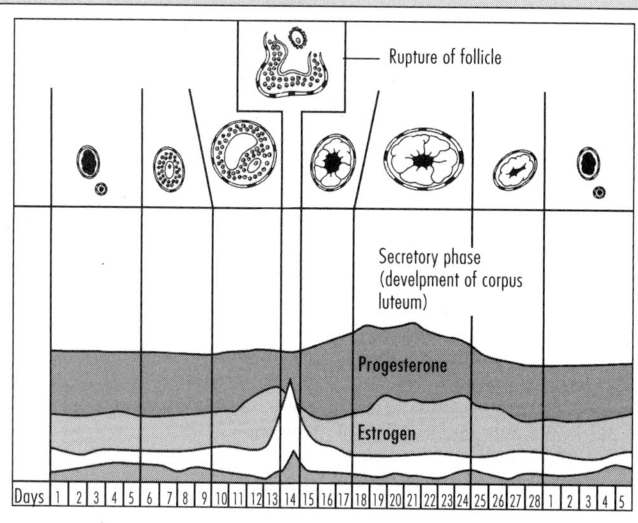

1. Menstrual phase (degeneration of corpus luteum)
2. Early follicular phase (development of follicle)
3. Late follicular phase (development of follicle)
4. Ovulation at midcycle (rupture of follicle)
5. Early luteal phase (development of corpus luteum)
6. Midluteal phase (development of corpus luteum)
7. Late luteal phase (development of corpus luteum)
8. Menstrual phase (degeneration of corpus luteum)

Precautions

- Handle the sample gently to prevent hemolysis.
- If the patient is a female, indicate the phase of her menstrual cycle on the laboratory request. Make a note if the patient is menopausal.

Reference values

Normal values may have a wide range, as follows:

- Adult females: follicular phase — 5 to 15 mIU/ml (SI, 5 to 15 IU/L); ovulatory phase — 30 to 60 mIU/ml (SI, 30 to 60 IU/L); luteal phase — 5 to 15 mIU/ml (SI, 5 to 15 IU/L)
- Postmenopausal females: 50 to 100 mIU/ml (SI, 50 to 100 IU/L)
- Adult males: 5 to 20 mIU/ml (SI, 5 to 20 IU/L)
- Children: 4 to 20 mIU/ml (SI, 4 to 20 IU/L).

Abnormal findings

In women, absence of a midcycle peak in plasma LH levels may indicate anovulation. Decreased or low-normal plasma LH levels may indicate hypogonadism; these findings are commonly associated with amenorrhea. High plasma LH levels may indicate congenital absence of ovaries or ovarian failure associated with Stein-Leventhal syndrome (polycystic ovary syndrome), Turner's syndrome (ovarian dysgenesis), menopause, or early-stage acromegaly. Infertility can result from primary or secondary gonadal dysfunction.

In men, low plasma LH values may indicate secondary gonadal dysfunction (of hypothalamic or pituitary origin); high values may indicate testicular failure (primary hypogonadism) or destruction or congenital absence of testes.

Interfering factors

- Failure to observe pretest restrictions of medication
- Hemolysis due to rough handling of the sample
- Steroids, including estrogens, progesterone, and testosterone (possible decrease)
- Radioactive scan performed within 1 week before the test

PROLACTIN

Prolactin is essential for the development of the mammary glands for lactation during pregnancy and for stimulating and maintaining lactation postpartum. Like human growth hormone, prolactin acts directly on tissues, and its levels rise in response to sleep and physical or emotional stress.

This radioimmunoassay is a quantitative analysis of serum prolactin levels, which normally rise 10- to 20-fold during pregnancy, corresponding to concomitant elevations in human placental lactogen levels. After delivery, prolactin secretion falls to basal levels in mothers who don't breast-feed. However, prolactin secretion increases during breastfeeding, apparently as a result of a stimulus triggered by suckling that curtails the release of prolactin-inhibiting factor by the hypothalamus. This in turn allows transient elevations of prolactin secretion by the pituitary gland.

This test is considered useful in patients suspected of having pituitary tumors, which are known to secrete prolactin in excessive amounts. Another test used to evaluate hypothalamic dysfunction is the thyrotropin-releasing hormone (TRH) stimulation test. (See *TRH stimulation test.*)

TRH stimulation test

The thyrotropin-releasing hormone (TRH) test evaluates hypothalamic dysfunction and pituitary tumors by stimulating the release of prolactin. The procedure is as follows: perform a venipuncture in the basal state to obtain a baseline prolactin level, and then place the patient in the supine position. Administer an I.V. bolus dose (500 µg) of synthetic TRH over 15 to 30 seconds. Take blood samples at 15- and 30-minute intervals to measure prolactin.

A baseline prolactin reading greater than 200 ng/ml (SI, 200 IU/L) indicates a pituitary tumor, but levels between 30 and 200 ng/ml (SI, 30 to 200 IU/L) are also consistent with this condition. Normally, patients show at least a twofold increase in prolactin after injection with TRH. If the prolactin level fails to rise, hypothalamic dysfunction or adenoma of the pituitary gland is likely.

Purpose

- To facilitate diagnosis of pituitary dysfunction, possibly due to pituitary adenoma
- To aid in the diagnosis of hypothalamic dysfunction regardless of cause
- To evaluate secondary amenorrhea and galactorrhea

Patient preparation

- Tell the patient that this test helps evaluate hormonal secretion.
- Advise her to restrict food and fluids and limit physical activity for 12 hours before the test. Encourage her to relax for about 30 minutes before the test.
- Tell the patient the test requires a blood sample. Explain who will perform the venipuncture and when.
- Explain to the patient that she may experience slight discomfort from the needle puncture and tourniquet.
- Withhold drugs that may interfere with test results, as ordered. If they must be continued, note this on the laboratory request.

Procedure and posttest care

- Perform a venipuncture at least 3 hours after the patient wakes; samples collected earlier are likely to show sleep-induced peak levels. Collect the sample in a 7-ml clot-activator tube.
- Apply direct pressure to the venipuncture site until bleeding stops.
- If a hematoma develops at the venipuncture site, apply warm soaks.
- Instruct the patient that she may resume her usual medications discontinued before the test.

Precautions

- Handle the sample gently to prevent hemolysis.
- Confirm slight elevations with repeat measurements on two other occasions.

Reference values

Normal values range from undetectable to 23 ng/ml (SI, 23 µg/L) in nonlactating females. Levels normally rise tenfold to twenty-fold during pregnancy and, after delivery, fall to basal levels in mothers who don't breast-feed. Prolactin secretion increases during breast-feeding.

Abnormal findings

Abnormally high prolactin levels (100 to 300 ng/ml) (SI, 100 to 300 IU/L) suggest autonomous prolactin production by a pituitary adenoma, especially when amenorrhea or galactorrhea is present (Forbes-Albright syndrome).

Rarely, hyperprolactinemia may also result from severe endocrine disorders such as hypothyroidism. Idiopathic hyperprolactinemia may be associated with anovulatory infertility. Confirm slight elevations with repeat measurements on two other occasions.

Decreased prolactin levels in a lactating mother cause failure of lactation and may be associated with postpartum pituitary infarction (Sheehan's syndrome). Abnormally low prolactin levels have also been found in some patients with empty-sella syndrome. In these patients, a flattened pituitary gland makes the pituitary fossa look empty.

Interfering factors

- Failure to take into account physiologic variations related to sleep or stress
- Ethanol, morphine, methyldopa, and estrogens (increase)
- Apomorphine, ergot alkaloids, and levodopa (decrease)
- Radioactive scan performed within 1 week before the test or recent surgery
- Breast stimulation
- Hemolysis due to rough handling of the sample

THYROID-STIMULATING HORMONE

Thyroid-stimulating hormone (TSH), or thyrotropin, promotes increases in the size, number, and activity of thyroid cells and stimulates the release of triiodothyronine and thyroxine. These hormones affect total body metabolism and are essential for normal growth and development.

This test measures serum TSH levels by radioimmunoassay. It can detect primary hypothyroidism and determine whether the hypothyroidism results from thyroid gland failure or from pituitary or hypothalamic dysfunction. Normal serum TSH levels rule out primary hypothyroidism. This test may not distinguish between low-normal and subnormal levels, especially in secondary hypothyroidism.

Purpose

- To confirm or rule out primary hypothyroidism and distinguish it from secondary hypothyroidism
- To monitor drug therapy in patients with primary hypothyroidism

Patient preparation

- Explain to the patient that this test helps assess thyroid gland function.
- Tell the patient that the test requires a blood sample. Explain who will perform the venipuncture and when.
- Explain to the patient that he may experience slight discomfort from the needle puncture and tourniquet.
- Withhold steroids, thyroid hormones, aspirin, and other medications that may influence test results, as ordered. If they must be continued, note this on the laboratory request.
- Keep the patient relaxed and recumbent for 30 minutes before the test.

Procedure and posttest care

- Between 6 a.m. and 8 a.m., perform a venipuncture, and collect the sample in a 5-ml clot-activator tube.
- Apply direct pressure to the venipuncture site until bleeding stops.
- If a hematoma develops at the venipuncture site, apply warm soaks.
- Instruct the patient that he may resume his usual medications discontinued before the test as ordered.

Precautions

- Handle the sample gently to prevent hemolysis.

TRH challenge test

The thyrotropin-releasing hormone (TRH) challenge test, which evaluates thyroid function and is the first direct test of pituitary reserve, is a reliable diagnostic tool in thyrotoxicosis (Graves' disease). The challenge test requires an injection of TRH.

One commonly accepted procedure is the following: After a venipuncture is performed to obtain a baseline thyroid-stimulating hormone (TSH) reading, synthetic TRH (protirelin) is administered by I.V. bolus in a dose of 200 to 500 µg. As many as five samples (5 ml each) are then drawn at 5, 10, 15, 20, and 60 minutes after the TRH injection to assess thyroid response. To facilitate blood collection, an indwelling catheter can be used to obtain the required samples.

A sudden spike above the baseline TSH reading indicates a normally functioning pituitary, but suggests hypothalamic dysfunction. If the TSH level fails to rise or remains undetectable, pituitary failure is likely. In thyrotoxicosis and thyroiditis, TSH levels fail to rise when challenged by TRH.

Reference values

Normal TSH values range from undetectable to 15 µIU/ml (SI, 15 mU/L).

Abnormal findings

TSH levels may be slightly elevated in euthyroid patients with thyroid cancer. Levels that exceed 20 µIU/ml (SI, 20 mU/L) suggest primary hypothyroidism or, possibly, endemic goiter.

Low or undetectable TSH levels may be normal, but occasionally indicate secondary hypothyroidism (with inadequate secretion of TSH or thyrotropin-releasing hormone [TRH]). Low TSH levels may also result from hyperthyroidism (Graves' disease) and thyroiditis; both are marked by hypersecretion of thyroid hormones, which suppresses TSH release. Provocative testing with TRH is necessary to confirm the diagnosis. (See *TRH challenge test.*)

Interfering factors

- Failure to observe pretest restrictions
- Hemolysis due to rough handling of the sample

NEONATAL THYROID-STIMULATING HORMONE

The neonatal thyroid-stimulating hormone (TSH) test is an immunoassay that confirms congenital hypothyroidism after an initial screening test detects low thyroxine (T_4) levels. Normally, TSH levels surge after birth, triggering a rise in thyroid hormone that's essential for neurologic development. In primary congenital hypothyroidism, the thyroid gland doesn't respond to TSH stimulation, resulting in diminished thyroid hormone levels and elevated TSH levels. Early detection and treatment of congenital hypothyroidism is critical to prevent mental retardation and cretinism.

Purpose

- To confirm diagnosis of congenital hypothyroidism

Patient preparation

- Explain to the infant's parents that this test helps confirm the diagnosis of congenital hypothyroidism. Emphasize the importance of detecting the disorder early so that prompt therapy can prevent irreversible brain damage.

Equipment

Filter paper sample

- Alcohol or povidone-iodine swabs, sterile lancet, specially marked filter paper, 2″ × 2″ sterile gauze pads, adhesive bandage, labels, gloves

Serum sample

- Venipuncture equipment

Procedure and posttest care

Filter paper sample

- Assemble the necessary equipment, wash your hands thoroughly, and put on gloves.
- Wipe the infant's heel with an alcohol or povidone-iodine swab, and then dry it thoroughly with a gauze pad.
- Perform a heelstick.
- Squeezing the infant's heel gently, fill the circles on the filter paper with blood. Make sure the blood saturates the paper.
- Gently apply pressure with a gauze pad to ensure hemostasis at the puncture site.
- Allow the filter paper to dry, label it appropriately, and send it to the laboratory.

Serum sample

- Perform a venipuncture, and collect the sample in a 3-ml clot-activator tube. Label the sample and send it to the laboratory immediately.
- Apply direct pressure to the venipuncture or heelstick site until bleeding stops.
- If a hematoma develops at the venipuncture site, apply warm soaks.

Precautions

- Handle the samples carefully to prevent hemolysis.

Reference values

At age 1 to 2 days, TSH levels are normally 25 to 30 μIU/ml (SI, 25 to 30 mU/L). Thereafter, levels are normally less than 25 μIU/ml (SI, < 25 mU/L).

Abnormal findings

Neonatal TSH levels must be interpreted in light of T_4 concentrations. Elevated TSH levels accompanied by decreased T_4 levels indicates primary congenital hypothyroidism (thyroid gland dysfunction). Low TSH and T_4 levels may be present in secondary congenital hypothyroidism (pituitary or hypothalamic dysfunction). Normal TSH levels accompanied by low T_4 levels may indicate hypothyroidism due to a congenital defect in T_4-binding globulin or transient congenital hypothyroidism due to prematurity or prenatal hypoxia. A complete thyroid workup must be done to confirm the cause of hypothyroidism before treatment can begin.

Interfering factors

- Failure to let a filter paper sample dry completely
- Hemolysis due to rough handling of the sample
- Corticosteroids, triiodothyronine, and T_4 (decrease)
- Lithium carbonate, potassium iodide, excessive topical resorcinol, and TSH injection (increase)

ANTIDIURETIC HORMONE

Antidiuretic hormone (ADH), also called vasopressin, promotes water reabsorption in response to increased osmolality (water deficiency with high concentration of sodium and other solutes). In response to decreased osmolality (water excess), reduced secretion of ADH allows increased excretion of water to maintain fluid balance. Along with aldosterone, ADH helps regulate sodium, potassium, and fluid balance. It also stimulates vascular smooth-muscle contraction, causing an increase in arterial blood pressure.

This relatively rare test, a quantitative analysis of serum ADH levels, may identify diabetes insipidus and other causes of severe homeostatic imbalance. It may be ordered as part of dehydration or hypertonic saline infusion testing, which determines the body's response to states of hyperosmolality.

Purpose

- To aid in the differential diagnosis of pituitary diabetes insipidus, nephrogenic diabetes insipidus (congenital or familial), and syndrome of inappropriate antidiuretic hormone (SIADH)

Patient preparation

- Explain to the patient that this test, used to measure hormonal secretion levels, may aid in identifying the cause of his symptoms.
- Instruct him to fast and limit physical activity for 10 to 12 hours before the test.
- Tell the patient that the test requires a blood sample. Explain who will perform the venipuncture and when.
- Explain to the patient that he may experience discomfort from the needle puncture and the tourniquet.
- Withhold medications that may cause SIADH before the test, as ordered. If they must be continued, note this on the laboratory request.
- Make sure the patient is relaxed and recumbent for 30 minutes before the test.

Procedure and posttest care

- Perform a venipuncture, and collect the sample in a plastic collection tube (without additives) or a chilled EDTA tube.
- Immediately send the sample to the laboratory, where serum must be separated from the clot within 10 minutes.
- Perform a serum osmolality test at the same time to facilitate interpretation of results.
- Apply direct pressure to the venipuncture site until bleeding stops.
- If a hematoma develops at the venipuncture site, apply warm soaks.
- Instruct the patient that he may resume his usual diet and medications discontinued before the test as ordered.

Precautions

- Make sure you use a syringe and collection tube made of plastic because the fragile ADH degrades on contact with glass.

Reference values

ADH values range from 1 to 5 pg/ml (SI, 1 to 5 mg/L). It may also be evaluated in light of serum osmolality; if serum osmolality is < 285 mOsm/kg, ADH is normally < 2 pg/ml (SI, 2 mg/L); if > 290 mOsm/kg, ADH may range from 2 to 12 pg/ml (SI, 2 to 12 mg/L).

Abnormal findings

Absent or below-normal ADH levels indicate pituitary diabetes insipidus, resulting from a neurohypophyseal or hypothalamic tumor, viral infection, metastatic disease, sarcoidosis, tuberculosis, Hand-Schüller-Christian disease, syphilis, neurosurgical procedures, or head trauma.

Normal ADH levels in the presence of signs of diabetes insipidus (such as polydipsia, polyuria, and hypotonic urine) may indicate the nephrogenic form of the disease, marked by renal tubular resistance to ADH; however, levels may rise if the pituitary gland tries to compensate.

Elevated ADH levels may also indicate SIADH, possibly as a result of bronchogenic carcinoma, acute porphyria, hypothyroidism, Addison's disease, cirrhosis of the liver, infectious hepatitis, severe hemorrhage, or circulatory shock.

Interfering factors

- Failure to observe pretest restrictions of diet, medications, or physical activity
- Morphine, anesthetics, estrogen, oxytocin, chlorpropamide, vincristine, carbamazepine, cyclophosphamide, tranquilizers, hypnotics, lithium carbonate, and chlorothiazide (increase)
- Stress, pain, and positive-pressure ventilation (increase)
- Alcohol and negative-pressure ventilation (decrease)
- Radioactive scan performed within 1 week before the test

ALPHA-SUBUNIT OF PITUITARY GLYCOPROTEIN HORMONES

Using radioimmunoassay, the alpha-subunit of pituitary glycoprotein hormone test measures the alpha-subunit of the pituitary glycoprotein hormones (alpha-PGH). These hormones—thyroid-stimulating hormone (TSH) and human chorionic gonadotropin—contain similar alpha-subunits but differ in their beta-subunits. Alpha-PGH measurement assesses total pituitary production of these hormones.

Purpose

- To aid diagnosis of recurrent pituitary tumors in patients who have undergone resection

Patient preparation

- Explain to the patient that this test helps assess pituitary function.
- Inform him that he need not fast.
- Tell the patient that the test requires a blood sample. Explain who will perform the venipuncture and when.
- Explain to the patient that he may experience discomfort from the needle puncture and the tourniquet.

Procedure and posttest care

- Perform a venipuncture, and collect the sample in a 5-ml clot-activator tube.
- Send the sample to the laboratory immediately.
- Apply direct pressure to the venipuncture site until bleeding stops.
- If a hematoma develops at the venipuncture site, apply warm soaks.

Precautions

- Handle the sample gently to prevent hemolysis.
- Indicate the patient's sex on the laboratory request.

Reference values

Normal alpha-PGH values are up to 1.2 ng/ml (SI, 1.2 µg/L).

Abnormal findings

Low levels of alpha-PGH appear in patients with inadequate pituitary hormone production. Hypopituitarism results in reduced follicle-stimulating hormone, luteinizing hormone, and TSH levels.

Elevated alpha-PGH levels indicate recurrent pituitary tumors or ineffective treatment.

Interfering factors

- Hemolysis due to rough handling of the sample

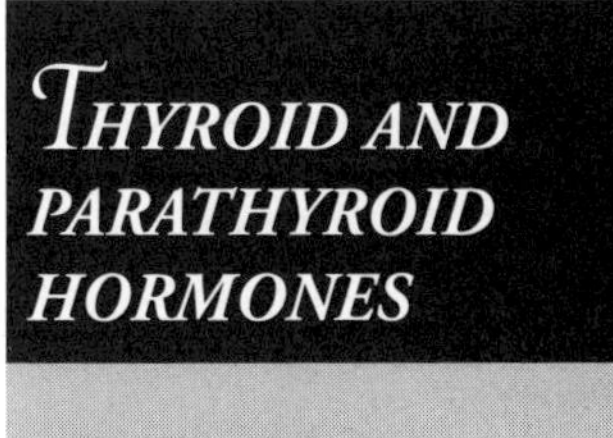

THYROID AND PARATHYROID HORMONES

THYROXINE

Thyroxine (T_4) is an amine secreted by the thyroid gland in response to thyroid-stimulating hormone (TSH) and, indirectly, thyrotropin-releasing hormone. The rate of secretion is normally regulated by a complex system of negative and positive feedback mechanisms.

Only a fraction of T_4 (about 0.05%) circulates freely in the blood; the rest binds strongly to plasma proteins, primarily thyroxine-binding globulin (TBG). This minute fraction is responsible for the clinical effects of thyroid hormone. TBG binds so tenaciously that T_4 survives in the plasma for a relatively long time, with a half-life of about 6 days. This immunoassay, one of the most common thyroid diagnostic tools, measures the total circulating T_4 level when TBG is normal. An alternative test is the Murphy-Pattee or T_4 (D), based on competitive protein binding.

Purpose

- To evaluate thyroid function
- To aid diagnosis of hyperthyroidism and hypothyroidism
- To monitor response to antithyroid medication in hyperthyroidism or to thyroid replacement therapy in hypothyroidism (TSH estimates are needed to confirm hypothyroidism.)

Patient preparation

- Explain to the patient that this test helps evaluate thyroid gland function.
- Inform him that he need not fast or restrict activity.
- Tell the patient that the test requires a blood sample. Explain who will perform the venipuncture and when.
- Withhold medications that may interfere with test results, as ordered. If they must be continued, note this on the laboratory request. If this test is being performed to monitor thyroid therapy, the patient should continue to receive daily thyroid supplements.

Procedure and posttest care

- Perform a venipuncture, and collect the sample in a 7-ml clot-activator tube.
- Send the sample to the laboratory immediately so that the serum can be separated.
- Apply direct pressure to the venipuncture site until bleeding stops.
- If a hematoma develops at the venipuncture site, apply warm soaks.
- Instruct the patient that he may resume his usual medications discontinued before the test as ordered.

Precautions

- Handle the sample gently to prevent hemolysis.

Reference values

Normally, total T_4 levels range from 5 to 13.5 µg/dl (SI, 60 to 165 mmol/L).

Abnormal findings

Abnormally elevated T_4 levels are consistent with primary and secondary hyperthyroidism, including excessive T_4 (levothyroxine) replacement therapy (factitious or iatrogenic hyperthyroidism). Subnormal levels suggest primary or secondary hypothyroidism or may be due to T_4 suppression by normal, elevated, or replacement levels of triiodothyronine (T_3). In doubtful cases of hypothyroidism, TSH levels may be indicated.

Normal T_4 levels don't guarantee euthyroidism; for example, normal readings occur in T_3 toxicosis. Overt signs of hyperthyroidism require further testing.

Interfering factors

- Hemolysis due to rough handling of the sample
- Hereditary factors and hepatic disease (possible increase or decrease in TBG)
- Protein-wasting disease (such as nephrotic syndrome) and androgens (possible decrease in TBG)
- Estrogens, progestins, levothyroxine, and methadone (increase)
- Free fatty acids, heparin, iodides, liothyronine sodium, lithium, methylthiouracil, phenylbutazone, phenytoin, propylthiouracil, salicylates (high doses), steroids, sulfonamides, and sulfonylureas (decrease)
- Clofibrate (possible increase or decrease)

TRIIODOTHYRONINE

Triiodothyronine (T_3) is highly specific radioimmunoassay that measures total (bound and free) serum content of T_3 to investigate clinical indications of thyroid dysfunction. Like thyroxine (T_4) secretion, T_3 secretion occurs in response to thyroid-stimulating hormone (TSH) and, secondarily, thyrotropin-releasing hormone.

Although T_3 is present in the bloodstream in minute quantities and is metabolically active for only a short time, its impact on body metabolism dominates that of T_4. Another significant difference between the two major thyroid hormones is that T_3 binds less firmly to thyroxine-binding globulin (TBG). Consequently, T_3 persists in the bloodstream for a short time; half disappears in about 1 day, whereas half of T_4 disappears in 6 days.

Purpose

- To aid diagnosis of T_3 toxicosis
- To aid diagnosis of hypothyroidism and hyperthyroidism
- To monitor clinical response to thyroid replacement therapy in hypothyroidism

Patient preparation

- Explain to the patient that this test helps to evaluate thyroid gland function and determine the cause of his symptoms.
- Withhold medications, such as steroids, propranolol, and cholestyramine, which may influence thyroid function, as ordered. If they must be continued, record this information on the laboratory request.
- Tell the patient that the test requires a blood sample. Explain who will perform the venipuncture and when.
- Explain to the patient that he may experience discomfort from the needle puncture and the tourniquet.

Procedure and posttest care

- Perform a venipuncture, and collect the sample in a 7-ml clot-activator tube.
- Send the sample to the laboratory as soon as possible to avoid stasis and to allow early separation of serum from the clotted blood.
- Apply direct pressure to the venipuncture site until bleeding stops.
- If a hematoma develops at the venipuncture site, apply warm soaks.

■ Instruct the patient that he may resume his usual medications discontinued before the test as ordered.

Precautions

■ Handle the sample gently to prevent hemolysis.

■ If the patient must receive thyroid preparations such as T_3 (liothyronine), note the administration time on the laboratory request. Otherwise, T_3 levels aren't reliable.

Reference values

Normal serum T_3 levels range from 80 to 200 ng/dl (SI, 1.2 to 3 nmol/L)

Abnormal findings

Serum T_3 and T_4 levels usually rise and fall in tandem. However, in T_3 toxicosis, T_3 levels rise while total and free T_4 levels remain normal. T_3 toxicosis occurs in patients with Graves' disease, toxic adenoma, or toxic nodular goiter. T_3 levels also surpass T_4 levels in patients receiving thyroid replacement therapy containing more T_3 than T_4. In iodine-deficient areas, the thyroid may produce larger amounts of the more cellularly active T_3 than of T_4 in an effort to maintain the euthyroid state.

Generally, T_3 levels appear to be a more accurate diagnostic indicator of hyperthyroidism. Although T_3 and T_4 levels are increased in about 90% of patients with hyperthyroidism, there's a disproportionate increase in T_3. In some patients with hypothyroidism, T_3 levels may fall within the normal range and not be diagnostically significant.

A rise in serum T_3 levels normally occurs during pregnancy. Low T_3 levels may appear in euthyroid patients with systemic illness (especially hepatic or renal disease), during severe acute illness, and after trauma or major surgery; in such patients, TSH levels are within normal limits. Low serum T_3 levels are found in some euthyroid patients with malnutrition.

Interfering factors

■ Hemolysis due to rough handling of the sample

■ Markedly increased or decreased TBG levels, regardless of cause

■ Failure to take into account medications that affect T_3 levels, such as steroids, clofibrate, cholestyramine, and propranolol

THYROXINE-BINDING GLOBULIN

The thyroxine-binding globulin test measures the serum level of thyroxine-binding globulin (TBG), the predominant protein carrier for circulating thyroxine (T_4).

Any condition that affects TBG levels and subsequent binding capacity also affects the amount of free T_4 (FT_4) in circulation. An underlying TBG abnormality renders tests for total triiodothyronine (T_3) and T_4 inaccurate but doesn't affect the accuracy of tests for free T_3 (FT_3) and FT_4.

Purpose

■ To evaluate abnormal thyrometabolic states that don't correlate with thyroid hormone (T_3 or T_4) values (for example, a patient with overt signs of hypothyroidism and a low FT_4 level with a high total T_4 level due to a marked increase of TBG secondary to oral contraceptives)

■ To identify TBG abnormalities

Patient preparation

- Explain to the patient that this test helps evaluate thyroid function.
- Tell the patient that the test requires a blood sample. Explain who will perform the venipuncture and when.
- Explain to the patient that he may experience discomfort from the needle puncture and the tourniquet.
- Withhold medications that may affect the accuracy of test results, such as estrogens, anabolic steroids, phenytoin, salicylates, or thyroid preparations, as ordered. If they must be continued, note this on the laboratory request. (They may be continued to determine if prescribed drugs are affecting TBG levels.)

Procedure and posttest care

- Perform a venipuncture, and collect the sample in a 7-ml clot activator tube.
- Apply direct pressure to the venipuncture site until bleeding stops.
- If a hematoma develops at the venipuncture site, apply warm soaks.
- Instruct the patient that he may resume his usual medications discontinued before the test as ordered.

Precautions

- Handle the sample gently to prevent hemolysis.

Reference values

Normal values for TBG by immunoassay range from 16 to 32 µg/dl (SI, 120 to 180 mg/ml).

Abnormal findings

Elevated TBG levels may indicate hypothyroidism or congenital (genetic) excess, some forms of hepatic disease, or acute intermittent porphyria. TBG levels normally rise during pregnancy and are high in neonates. Suppressed levels may indicate hyperthyroidism or congenital deficiency and can occur in active acromegaly, nephrotic syndrome, and malnutrition associated with hypoproteinemia, acute illness, or surgical stress.

Patients with TBG abnormalities require additional testing, such as the serum FT_3 and T_4 tests, to evaluate thyroid function more precisely.

Interfering factors

- Hemolysis due to rough handling of the sample
- Estrogens, including oral contraceptives, and phenothiazines such as perphenazine (increase)
- Androgens, prednisone, phenytoin, and high doses of salicylates (decrease)

T_3 UPTAKE

Also called triiodothyronine (T_3) uptake, the T_3 uptake test indirectly measures free thyroxine (FT_4) levels by demonstrating the availability of serum protein binding sites for thyroxine (T_4) The results of T_3 uptake are frequently combined with a T_4 radioimmunoassay or T_4 (D) (competitive protein-binding test) to determine the FT_4 index, a mathematical calculation thought to reflect FT_4 by correcting for thyroxine-binding globulin (TBG) abnormalities.

The T_3 uptake test has become less popular recently because rapid tests for T_3, T_4, and thyroid-stimulating hormone are readily available.

Purpose

- To aid diagnosis of hypothroidism and hyperthyroidism when TBG is normal
- To aid diagnosis of primary disorders of TBG levels

Patient preparation

- Explain to the patient that this test helps evaluate thyroid function.
- Tell the patient that the test requires a blood sample. Explain who will perform the venipuncture and when.
- Explain to the patient that he may experience discomfort from the needle puncture and the tourniquet.
- Tell him the laboratory requires several days to complete the analysis.
- Withhold medications, such as estrogens, androgens, phenytoin, salicylates, and thyroid preparations, that may interfere with test results, as ordered. If they must be continued, note this on the laboratory request.

Procedure and posttest care

- Perform a venipuncture, and collect the sample in a 7-ml clot-activator tube.
- Apply direct pressure to the venipuncture site until bleeding stops.
- If a hematoma develops at the venipuncture site, apply warm soaks.
- Instruct the patient that he may resume his usual medications discontinued before the test as ordered.

Precautions

- Handle the sample gently to prevent hemolysis.

Reference values

Normal T_3 uptake values are 25% to 35%.

Abnormal findings

A high T_3 uptake percentage in the presence of elevated T_4 levels indicates hyperthyroidism (implying few TBG free binding sites and high FT_4 levels). A low uptake percentage, together with low T_4 levels, indicates hypothyroidism (implying more TBG free binding sites and low FT_4 levels). Thus, in primary thyroid disease, T_4 and T_3 uptake vary in the same direction; availability of binding sites varies inversely.

Discordant variance in T_4 and T_3 uptake suggests abnormality of TBG. For example, a high T_3 uptake percentage and a low or normal FT_4 level suggest decreased TBG levels. Such decreased levels may result from protein loss (as in nephrotic syndrome), decreased production (due to androgen excess or genetic or idiopathic causes), or competition for T_4 binding sites by certain drugs (salicylates, phenylbutazone, and phenytoin). Conversely, a low T_3 uptake percentage and a high or normal FT_4 level suggest increased TBG levels. Such increased levels may be due to exogenous or endogenous estrogen (pregnancy) or result from idiopathic causes. Thus, in primary disorders of TBG levels, measured T_4 and free sites change in the same direction.

Interfering factors

- Radioisotope scans performed before sample collection
- Anabolic steroids, heparin, phenytoin, salicylates (high dose), thyroid preparations, and warfarin (possible increase in TBG and thyroxine-binding protein electrophoresis)
- Antithyroid agents, clofibrate, estrogen, oral contraceptives, and thiazide diuretics (decrease uptake)

FREE THYROXINE AND FREE TRIIODOTHYRONINE

The free thyroxine (FT_4) and free triiodothyronine (FT_3) tests, commonly done simultaneously, measure serum levels of FT_4 and FT_3, the minute portions of T_4 and T_3 not bound to thyroxine-binding globulin (TBG) and other serum proteins. These unbound hormones are responsible for the thyroid's effects on cellular metabolism. Measurement of free hormone levels is the best indicator of thyroid function.

Because of disagreement as to whether FT_4 or FT_3 is the better indicator, laboratories commonly measure both. The disadvantages of these tests include a cumbersome and difficult laboratory method, inaccessibility, and cost. This test may be useful in the 5% of patients in whom the standard T_3 or T_4 tests fail to produce diagnostic results.

Purpose

- To measure the metabolically active form of the thyroid hormones
- To aid diagnosis of hyperthyroidism and hypothyroidism when TBG levels are abnormal

Patient preparation

- Explain to the patient that this special test helps evaluate thyroid function.
- Tell the patient that the test requires a blood sample. Explain who will perform the venipuncture and when.
- Explain to the patient that he may experience discomfort from the needle puncture and the tourniquet.

Procedure and posttest care

- Perform a venipuncture, and collect the sample in a 7-ml clot-activator tube.
- Apply direct pressure to the venipuncture site until bleeding stops.
- If a hematoma develops at the venipuncture site, apply warm soaks.

Precautions

- Handle the sample gently to prevent hemolysis.

Reference values

Normal range for FT_4 is 0.9 to 2.3 ng/dl (SI, 10 to 30 nmol/L); for FT_3, 0.2 to 0.6 ng/dl (SI, 0.003 to 0.009 nmol/L). Values vary, depending on the laboratory.

Abnormal findings

Elevated FT_4 and FT_3 levels indicate hyperthyroidism, unless peripheral resistance to thyroid hormone is present. T_3 toxicosis, a distinct form of hyperthyroidism, yields high FT_3 levels with normal or low FT_4 values. Low FT_4 levels usually indicate hypothyroidism, except in patients receiving replacement therapy with T_3. Patients receiving thyroid therapy may have varying levels of FT_4 and FT_3, depending on the preparation used and the time of sample collection.

Interfering factors

- Hemolysis due to rough handling of the sample
- Thyroid therapy, depending on dosage (possible increase)

SCREENING TEST FOR CONGENITAL HYPOTHYROIDISM

The screening test for congenital hypothyroidism measures serum thyroxine (T_4) levels in the neonate to detect congenital hypothyroidism. Characterized by low or absent levels of T_4, congenital hypothyroidism affects roughly 1 in 5,000 neonates, occurring in girls three times more often than in boys. This disorder can result from thyroid dysgenesis or hypoplasia, congenital goiter, or maternal use of thyroid inhibitors during pregnancy. If untreated, it can lead to irreversible brain damage by age 3 months.

Because clinical signs are few, in the past, most cases of congenital hypothyroidism went undetected until cretinism became apparent or death followed respiratory distress. Recently, radioimmunoassays for T_4 and thyroid-stimulating hormone (TSH) have been used effectively to screen neonates for congenital hypothyroidism. This test is now mandatory in some states.

Purpose

■ To screen neonates for congenital hypothyroidism

Patient preparation

■ Explain to the parents that although hypothyroidism is uncommon in infants, this screening test detects the disorder early enough to begin therapy before irreversible brain damage occurs.
■ Tell the parents that the test will be performed before the infant is discharged from the facility and again 4 to 6 weeks later.
■ Emphasize the importance of the screening and the need for following the test protocol.
■ Because false-positive findings can result from variations in the test procedure or from a congenital thyroxine-binding globulin (TBG) defect, inform the parents that a second test may be done before the infant is discharged.

Equipment

Gloves, alcohol or povidone-iodine swabs, sterile lancet, specially marked filter paper, 2″ × 2″ sterile gauze pads, small adhesive bandage strip, labels for infant's and mother's names, physician's name, room number, and date

Procedure and posttest care

■ After assembling the necessary equipment and washing your hands, put on gloves.
■ Wipe the infant's heel with an alcohol or a povidone-iodine swab, and then dry it thoroughly with a gauze pad.
■ Perform a heelstick.
■ Squeezing the heel gently, fill the circles on the filter paper with blood. Make sure the blood saturates the paper. Apply gentle pressure with a gauze pad to ensure hemostasis at the puncture site.
■ When the filter paper is dry, label it appropriately and send it to the laboratory.
■ Heelsticks heal readily and require no special care.
■ If results of the screening test indicate congenital hypothyroidism, tell the parents that additional testing is necessary to determine the cause of the disorder.
■ If the sample isn't processed in the facility's laboratory, make sure the parents are notified when test results are available.

Reference values

Immediately after birth, neonatal T_4 levels are considerably higher than normal adult levels. By the end of the first week, T_4 values decrease markedly:
■ 1 to 5 days: 4.9 µg/dl (SI, 58.8 nmol /L)
■ 6 to 8 days: 4 µg/dl (SI, 48 nmol/L)
■ 9 to 11 days: 3.5 µg/dl (SI, 42 nmol /L)
■ 12 to 120 days: 3 µg/dl (SI, 36 nmol/L).

Abnormal findings

Low serum T_4 levels in the neonate require TSH testing for clarification of the diagnosis. Decreased T_4 levels accompanied by elevated TSH readings (> 25 µU/ml [SI, 300 nmol/L]) indicate primary congenital hypothyroidism (thyroid gland dysfunction). If T_4 and TSH levels are depressed, secondary congenital hypothyroidism (resulting from pituitary or hypothalamic dysfunction) should be suspected.

If T_4 levels are subnormal in the presence of normal TSH readings, further testing is required. Serum TBG levels must be analyzed to identify infants with hypothyroidism resulting from congenital defects in TBG. This low T_4–normal TSH pattern also occurs in a transient form of congenital hypothyroidism, which may accompany prematurity, or prenatal hypoxia.

A complete thyroid workup, including serum T_3, TBG, and free T_4 levels, is necessary for unequivocal diagnosis of congenital hypothyroidism before treatment begins.

Interfering factors

- Failure to allow filter paper to dry completely

PLASMA CALCITONIN

The plasma calcitonin test is a radioimmunoassay that measures plasma levels of calcitonin (thyrocalcitonin). The exact role of calcitonin in normal human physiology hasn't been fully defined. However, calcitonin is known to act as an antagonist to parathyroid hormone and to lower serum calcium levels.

The usual clinical indication for this test is suspected medullary carcinoma of the thyroid, which causes hypersecretion of calcitonin (without associated hypocalcemia). Equivocal results require provocative testing with I.V. pentagastrin or calcium to rule out disease.

Purpose

- To aid diagnosis of thyroid medullary carcinoma and ectopic calcitonin-producing tumors (rare)

Patient preparation

- Explain to the patient that this test helps evaluate thyroid function.
- Instruct him to fast overnight because food may interfere with calcium homeostasis and, subsequently, calcitonin levels.
- Tell the patient that the test requires a blood sample. Explain who will perform the venipuncture and when.
- Explain to the patient that he may experience discomfort from the needle puncture and the tourniquet.
- Tell him that the laboratory requires several days to complete the analysis.

Procedure and posttest care

- Perform a venipuncture, and collect the sample in a 7-ml heparinized tube.
- Apply direct pressure to the venipuncture site until bleeding stops.
- If a hematoma develops at the venipuncture site, apply warm soaks.
- Instruct the patient that he may resume his normal diet.

Precautions

- Handle the sample gently to prevent hemolysis.
- Send the sample to the laboratory immediately.

Reference values

Serum calcitonin levels (basal) normally are 40 pg/ml (SI, 40 ng/L) for males and 20 pg/ml (SI, 20 ng/L) for females.

Reference values after 4-hour calcium infusion are:

- Males: 190 pg/ml (SI, 190 ng/L)
- Females: 130 pg/ml (SI, 130 ng/L).

Values after testing with pentagastrin infusion are:

- Males: 110 pg/ml (SI, 110 ng/L)
- Females: 30 pg/ml (SI, 30 ng/L).

Abnormal findings

Elevated serum calcitonin levels in the absence of hypocalcemia usually indicate medullary carcinoma of the thyroid. Transmitted as an autosomal dominant trait, thyroid medullary carcinoma may occur as part of multiple endocrine neoplasia. Occasionally, increased calcitonin levels may be due to ectopic calcitonin production by oat cell carcinoma of the lung or by breast carcinoma.

Interfering factors

- Failure to fast overnight before the test
- Hemolysis due to rough handling of the sample

PARATHYROID HORMONE

Parathyroid hormone (PTH) regulates plasma concentration of calcium and phosphorus. The overall effect of PTH is to raise plasma levels of calcium while lowering phosphorus levels.

Circulating PTH exists in three distinct molecular forms: the intact PTH molecule, which originates in the parathyroid glands, and two smaller circulating forms, N-terminal fragments and C-terminal fragments. Two radioimmunoassays are available to detect intact PTH and the N- and C-terminal fragments. Both tests can be used to confirm diagnosis of hyperparathyroidism and hypoparathyroidism.

Each test has other specific applications as well. The C-terminal PTH assay is more useful in diagnosing chronic disturbances in PTH metabolism, such as secondary and tertiary hyperparathyroidism; it also better differentiates ectopic from primary hyperparathyroidism. The assay for intact PTH and the N-terminal fragment (both forms are measured concomitantly) more accurately reflects acute changes in PTH metabolism and thus is useful in monitoring a patient's response to PTH therapy.

The clinical and diagnostic effects of PTH excess or deficiency are directly related to the effects of PTH on bone and the renal tubules and to its interaction with ionized calcium and biologically active vitamin D. Therefore, measuring serum calcium, phosphorus, and creatinine levels with serum PTH is helpful when trying to understand the causes and effects of pathologic parathyroid function. Suppression or stimulation tests may help confirm findings.

Purpose

- To aid the differential diagnosis of parathyroid disorders

Patient preparation

- Explain to the patient that this test helps evaluate parathyroid function.
- Instruct him to observe an overnight fast because food may affect PTH levels and interfere with the test results.
- Tell the patient that the test requires a blood sample. Explain who will perform the venipuncture and when.
- Explain to the patient that he may experience discomfort from the needle puncture and the tourniquet, collecting the sample takes only a few minutes.

Procedure and posttest care

- Perform a venipuncture, and collect 3 ml of blood into two separate 7-ml clot-activator tubes.
- Apply direct pressure to the venipuncture site until bleeding stops.
- If a hematoma develops at the venipuncture site, apply warm soaks.
- Instruct the patient that he may resume his normal diet.

Precautions

- Handle the sample gently to prevent hemolysis.
- Send the sample to the laboratory immediately so the serum can be separated and frozen for assay.

Clinical implications of abnormal parathyroid secretion

CONDITIONS	CAUSES	P.T.H. LEVELS	IONIZED CALCIUM LEVELS
Primary hyperparathyroidism	◆ Parathyroid adenoma or carcinoma	High	High to Normal
Secondary hyperparathyroidism	◆ Chronic renal disease ◆ Severe vitamin D deficiency ◆ Calcium malabsorption ◆ Pregnancy and lactation	High	Low
Tertiary hyperparathyroidism	◆ Progressive secondary hyperparathyroidism	High	High to Normal
Hypoparathyroidism	◆ Accidental removal of the parathyroid glands ◆ Autoimmune disease	Low	Low
Malignant tumors	◆ Squamous cell carcinoma of the lung ◆ Renal, pancreatic, or ovarian carcinoma	High to Normal	High

KEY:
High ● Normal ● Low ○

Reference values

Normal serum PTH levels vary, depending on the laboratory, and must be interpreted in association with serum calcium levels. Typical values for intact PTH range from 10 to 50 pg/ml (SI, 1.1 to 5.3 pmol/L); N-terminal fraction is 8 to 24 pg/ml (SI, 0.8 to 2.5 pmol/L); C-terminal fraction, 0 to 340 pg/ml (SI, 0. to 35.8 pmol/L).

Abnormal findings

Measured concomitantly with serum calcium levels, abnormally elevated PTH values may indicate primary, secondary, or tertiary hyperparathyroidism. Abnormally low PTH levels may result from hypoparathyroidism and from certain malignant diseases. (See *Clinical implications of abnormal parathyroid secretion*.)

Interfering factors

- Failure to fast overnight before the test
- Hemolysis due to rough handling of the sample

Adrenal and Renal Hormones

Aldosterone

The aldosterone test measures serum aldosterone levels by quantitative analysis and radioimmunoassay. Aldosterone regulates ion transport across cell membranes to promote reabsorption of sodium and chloride in exchange for potassium and hydrogen ions. Consequently, it helps to maintain blood pressure and volume and to regulate fluid and electrolyte balance.

This test identifies aldosteronism and, when supported by plasma renin levels, distinguishes between the primary and secondary forms of this disorder.

Purpose

- To aid diagnosis of primary and secondary aldosteronism, adrenal hyperplasia, hypoaldosteronism, and salt-losing syndrome

Patient preparation

- Explain to the patient that this test helps determine if symptoms are due to improper hormonal secretion.
- Tell the patient that the test requires a blood sample. Explain who will perform the venipuncture and when.
- Explain to the patient that he may experience discomfort from the needle puncture and the tourniquet.
- Instruct him to maintain a low-carbohydrate, normal-sodium diet (135 mEq or 3 g/day) for at least 2 weeks or, preferably, for 30 days before the test.
- Withhold all drugs that alter fluid, sodium, and potassium balance — especially diuretics, antihypertensives, steroids, oral contraceptives, and estrogens — for at least 2 weeks or, preferably, for 30 days before the test, as ordered.
- Withhold all renin inhibitors for 1 week before the test, as ordered. If they must be continued, note this on the laboratory request.
- Tell the patient to avoid licorice for at least 2 weeks before the test because it produces an aldosterone-like effect.

Procedure and posttest care

- Perform a venipuncture while the patient is still supine after a night's rest.
- Collect the sample in a 7-ml clot-activator tube, and send it to the laboratory immediately.
- Draw another sample 4 hours later, while the patient is standing and after he has been up and about, to evaluate the effect of postural change.
- Collect the second sample in a 7-ml clot-activator tube, and send it to the laboratory immediately.
- Apply direct pressure to the venipuncture site until bleeding stops.
- If a hematoma develops at the venipuncture site, apply warm soaks.
- Instruct the patient that he may resume his usual diet and medications discontinued before the test as ordered.

Precautions

- Handle the sample gently to prevent hemolysis.
- Record on the laboratory request whether the patient was in supine or standing during the venipuncture.
- If the patient is a premenopausal female, specify the phase of her menstrual cycle because aldosterone levels may fluctuate during the menstrual cycle.
- Send the sample to the laboratory immediately.

Reference values

Laboratory values vary with time of day and posture — upright postures have higher values. In upright individuals, normal is 7 to 30 ng/dl (SI, 190 to 832 pmol/L). In supine individuals, values are 3 to 16 ng/dl (SI, 80 to 440 pmol/L).

Abnormal findings

Excessive aldosterone secretion may indicate a primary or secondary disease. Primary aldosteronism (Conn's syndrome) may result from adrenocortical adenoma or carcinoma or from bilateral adrenal hyperplasia. Secondary aldosteronism can result from renovascular hypertension, heart failure, cirrhosis of the liver, nephrotic syndrome, idiopathic cyclic edema, and the third trimester of pregnancy.

Low serum aldosterone levels may indicate primary hypoaldosteronism, salt-losing syndrome, eclampsia, or Addison's disease.

Interfering factors

- Failure to observe pretest restrictions of diet, medications, or physical activity
- Hemolysis due to rough handling of the sample
- Some antihypertensives, such as methyldopa, that promote sodium and water retention (possible decrease)
- Diuretics (possible increase)
- Some corticosteroids, such as fludrocortisone, that mimic mineralocorticoid activity (possible decrease)
- Radioactive scan performed within 1 week before the test

PLASMA CORTISOL

Cortisol — the principal glucocorticoid secreted by the zona fasciculata of the adrenal cortex — helps metabolize nutrients, mediate physiologic stress, and regulate the immune system. Cortisol secretion normally follows a diurnal pattern: Levels rise during the early morning hours and peak around 8 a.m. and then decline to very low levels in the evening and during the early phase of sleep. Intense heat or cold, infection, trauma, exercise, obesity, and debilitating disease influence cortisol secretion.

This radioimmunoassay, a quantitative analysis of plasma cortisol levels, is usually ordered for patients with signs of adrenal dysfunction. Dynamic tests, suppression tests for hyperfunction, and stimulation tests for hypofunction are generally required for confirmation of diagnosis.

Purpose

- To aid in the diagnosis of Cushing's disease, Cushing's syndrome, Addison's disease, and secondary adrenal insufficiency

Patient preparation

- Explain to the patient that this test helps determine if his symptoms are due to improper hormonal secretion.
- Instruct him to maintain a normal salt diet (2 to 3 g/day) for 3 days before the test and to fast and limit physical activity for 10 to 12 hours before the test.
- Tell the patient that the test requires a blood sample. Explain who will perform the venipuncture and when.
- Explain to the patient that he may experience discomfort from the needle puncture and the tourniquet.
- Withhold all medications that may interfere with plasma cortisol levels, such as estrogens, androgens, and phenytoin, for 48 hours before the test, as ordered. If the patient is receiving replacement therapy and is dependent on exogenous steroids for survival, note this on the laboratory request as well as other medications that must be continued.

■ Make sure the patient is relaxed and recumbent for at least 30 minutes before the test.

Procedure and posttest care

■ Perform a venipuncture between 6 a.m. and 8 a.m.
■ Collect the sample in a 7-ml heparinized tube, label it appropriately, and send it to the laboratory immediately.
■ For diurnal variation testing, draw another sample between 4 p.m. and 6 p.m.
■ Collect the second sample in a 7-ml heparinized tube, label it appropriately, and send it to the laboratory immediately.
■ Apply direct pressure to the venipuncture site until bleeding stops.
■ If a hematoma develops at the venipuncture site, apply warm soaks.
■ Instruct the patient that he may resume his normal diet and medications discontinued before the test.

Precautions

■ Handle the sample gently to prevent hemolysis.
■ Record the collection time on the laboratory request.

Reference values

Normally, plasma cortisol levels range from 9 to 35 µg/dl (SI, 250 to 690 nmol/L)in the morning and from 3 to 12 µg/dl (SI, 80 to 330 nmol/L) in the afternoon. The afternoon level is usually half the morning level.

Abnormal findings

Increased plasma cortisol levels may indicate adrenocortical hyperfunction in Cushing's disease (a rare disease due to basophilic adenoma of the pituitary gland) or Cushing's syndrome (glucocorticoid excess from any cause). In most patients with Cushing's syndrome, the adrenal cortex secretes independently of a natural rhythm. Thus, absence of diurnal variation in cortisol secretion is a significant finding in almost all patients with Cushing's syndrome; in these patients, little difference in values is found between morning and afternoon samples. Diurnal variations may also be absent in otherwise healthy people who are under considerable emotional or physical stress.

Decreased cortisol levels may indicate primary adrenal hypofunction (Addison's disease), most often due to idiopathic glandular atrophy (a presumed autoimmune process). Tuberculosis, fungal invasion, and hemorrhage can cause adrenocortical destruction. Low cortisol levels resulting from secondary adrenal insufficiency may occur in conditions of impaired corticotropin secretion, such as hypophysectomy, postpartum pituitary necrosis, craniopharyngioma, and chromophobe adenoma.

Interfering factors

■ Failure to observe restrictions of diet, medications, or physical activity
■ Hemolysis due to rough handling of the sample
■ Pregnancy or use of oral contraceptives because of increase in cortisol-binding plasma proteins (false-high)
■ Obesity, stress, and severe hepatic or renal disease (possible increase)
■ Androgens and phenytoin due to decrease in cortisol-binding plasma proteins (possible decrease)
■ Radioactive scan performed within 1 week before the test

PLASMA CATECHOLAMINES

The plasma catecholamines test, a quantitative (total or fractionated) analysis of plasma catecholamines, has clinical importance in patients with hypertension and signs of adrenal medullary tumor as well as in those with neural tumors that affect endocrine function. Elevated plasma catecholamine levels necessitate supportive confirmation by urinalysis.

Major catecholamines include the hormones epinephrine, norepinephrine, and dopamine. When secreted into the bloodstream, catecholamines produced in the adrenal medulla prepare the body for the fight-or-flight reaction. They increase heart rate and contractility, constrict blood vessels and redistribute circulating blood toward the skeletal and coronary muscles, mobilize carbohydrate and lipid reserves, and sharpen alertness. Excessive catecholamine secretion by tumors causes hypertension, weight loss, episodic sweating, headache, palpitations, and anxiety.

Plasma levels commonly fluctuate in response to temperature, stress, postural change, diet, smoking, anoxia, volume depletion, renal failure, obesity, and many drugs.

Purpose

- To rule out pheochromocytoma (adrenal medullary or extra-adrenal) in patients with hypertension
- To help identify neuroblastoma, ganglioneuroblastoma, and ganglioneuroma
- To distinguish between adrenal medullary tumors and other catecholamine-producing tumors through fractional analysis (Urinalysis for catecholamine degradation products is recommended to support diagnosis.)
- To aid diagnosis of autonomic nervous system dysfunction such as idiopathic orthostatic hypotension

Patient preparation

- Explain to the patient that this test helps determine if hypertension or other symptoms are related to improper hormonal secretion. As ordered, instruct him to refrain from using self-prescribed medications, especially cold and allergy remedies that may contain sympathomimetics, for 2 weeks before the test.
- Tell him to exclude amine-rich foods and beverages, such as bananas, avocados, cheese, coffee, tea, cocoa, beer, and Chianti, from his diet for 48 hours; to maintain vitamin C intake, which is necessary for formation of catecholamines; to abstain from smoking for 24 hours; and to fast for 10 to 12 hours before the test.
- Tell the patient that the test requires one or two blood samples. Explain who will perform the venipuncture and when.
- Explain to the patient that he may experience discomfort from the needle puncture and the tourniquet.
- If the patient is in your facility, withhold medications that affect catecholamine levels, such as amphetamines, phenothiazines (chlorpromazine), sympathomimetics, and tricyclic antidepressants, as ordered.
- Insert an indwelling venous catheter (heparin lock) 24 hours before the test because the stress of the venipuncture itself may significantly raise catecholamine levels.
- Make sure the patient is relaxed and recumbent for 45 to 60 minutes before the test.
- If necessary, provide blankets to keep him warm; low temperatures stimulate catecholamine secretion.

Procedure and posttest care

- Perform a venipuncture between 6 a.m. and 8 a.m.

■ Collect the sample in a 10-ml chilled tube containing EDTA (sodium metabisulfite solution), which can be obtained from the laboratory on request.
■ If a second sample is requested, have the patient stand for 10 minutes, and draw the sample into another tube exactly like the first.
■ If a heparin lock is used, it may be necessary to discard the first 1 or 2 ml of blood. Check with the laboratory for the preferred procedure.
■ Apply direct pressure to the venipuncture site until bleeding stops.
■ If a hematoma develops at the venipuncture site, apply warm soaks.
■ Instruct the patient that he may resume his normal diet and medications discontinued before the test as ordered.

Precautions

■ After collecting each sample, roll the tube slowly between your palms to distribute the EDTA without agitating the blood.
■ Pack the tube in crushed ice to minimize deactivation of catecholamines, and send it to the laboratory immediately.
■ Indicate on the laboratory request whether the patient was in a supine position or standing during the venipuncture and the time the sample was drawn.

Reference values

In fractional analysis, catecholamine levels range as follows:
■ supine: epinephrine, undetectable to 110 pg/ml (SI, undetectable to 600 pmol/L); norepinephrine, 70 to 750 pg/ml (SI, 413 to 4,432 pmol/L)
■ standing: epinephrine, undetectable to 140 pg/ml (SI, undetectable to 764 pmol/L); norepinephrine, 200 to 1,700 pg/ml (SI, 1,182 to 10,047 pmol/L)

Abnormal findings

High catecholamine levels may indicate pheochromocytoma, neuroblastoma, ganglioneuroblastoma, or ganglioneuroma. Elevations are possible, but don't directly confirm thyroid disorders, hypoglycemia, and cardiac disease. Electroconvulsive therapy, shock resulting from hemorrhage, endotoxins, and anaphylaxis also raise catecholamine levels.

In the patient with normal or low baseline catecholamine levels, failure to show an increase in the sample taken after standing suggests autonomic nervous system dysfunction.

Fractional analysis helps identify the cause of elevated catecholamine levels. For example, adrenal medullary tumors secrete epinephrine, whereas ganglioneuromas, ganglioblastomas, and neuroblastomas secrete norepinephrine.

Interfering factors

■ Failure to observe pretest restrictions
■ Epinephrine, levodopa, amphetamines, phenothiazines, sympathomimetics, decongestants, and tricyclic antidepressants (increase)
■ Reserpine (decrease)
■ Radioactive scan performed within 1 week before the test

ANDROSTENEDIONE

The androstenedione test helps identify disorders related to altered hormone levels, such as female virilization syndromes and polycystic ovary (Stein-Leventhal) syndrome. Androstenedione is a precursor of cortisol, aldosterone, estrogen, and testosterone. Tumors of the ovaries or adrenal glands can secrete excessive amounts of androstenedione, which then converts to testosterone, resulting in virilizing symptoms, such as hirsutism and sterility.

Increased androstenedione production may induce premature sexual development in children. It may produce renewed ovarian stimulation, endometriosis, bleeding, and polycystic ovaries in postmenopausal women. In obese women, increased levels of estrogen can lead to menstrual irregularities. In men, overproduction of androstenedione may cause feminizing signs such as gynecomastia.

Purpose

- To help determine the cause of gonadal dysfunction, menstrual or menopausal irregularities, virilizing symptoms, and premature sexual development

Patient preparation

- Explain to the patient that this test determines the cause of her symptoms.
- Tell the patient that the test requires a blood sample. Explain who will perform the venipuncture and when.
- Explain to the patient that she may experience discomfort from the needle puncture and the tourniquet.
- If appropriate, explain that the test should be done 1 week before or after her menstrual period and that it may be repeated.
- Withhold steroid and pituitary-based hormones, as ordered. If they must be continued, note this on the laboratory request.

Procedure and posttest care

- Perform a venipuncture, and collect a serum sample in a 7-ml clot-activator tube or collect a plasma sample in a *green-top* tube. (If a plasma sample is taken, refrigerate it or place it on ice.)
- Label the sample appropriately, and send it to the laboratory immediately.
- Apply direct pressure to the venipuncture site until bleeding stops.
- If a hematoma develops at the venipuncture site, apply warm soaks.
- Instruct the patient that she may resume her usual medications discontinued before the test.

Precautions

- Handle the sample gently to prevent hemolysis.
- Refrigerate plasma samples or place them on ice.
- Record the patient's age, sex, and (if appropriate) phase of her menstrual cycle on the laboratory request.

Reference values

Normal values by radioimmunoassay are:

- females: 85 to 275 ng/dl (SI, 3.0 to 9.6 nmol/L)
- males: 75 to 205 ng/dl (SI, 2.6 to 7.2 nmol/L).

Abnormal findings

Elevated androstenedione levels are associated with polycystic ovary (Stein-Leventhal) syndrome; Cushing's syndrome; ovarian, testicular, and adrenocortical tumors; ectopic corticotropin-producing tumors; late-onset congenital adrenal hyperplasia; and ovarian stromal hyperplasia. Elevated levels result in increased estrone levels, causing premature sexual development in children; menstrual irregularities in premenopausal women; bleeding, endometriosis, and polycystic ovaries in postmenopausal women; and feminizing signs, such as gynecomastia, in men. Decreased levels occur in hypogonadism.

Interfering factors

- Hemolysis due to rough handling of the sample
- Steroids and pituitary hormones (possible increase)

ERYTHROPOIETIN

The erythropoietin test of renal hormone production measures erythropoietin (EPO) by immunoassay. It's used to evaluate anemia, polycythemia, and kidney tumors. It's also used to evaluate abuse of commercially prepared EPO by athletes who believe that the drug enhances performance.

Purpose

- To aid diagnosis of anemia and polycythemia
- To aid diagnosis of kidney tumors
- To detect EPO abuse by athletes

Patient preparation

- Explain to the patient that this test determines if hormonal secretion is causing changes in his red blood cells (RBCs).
- Instruct him to fast for 8 to 10 hours before the test.
- Tell the patient that the test requires a blood sample. Explain who will perform the venipuncture and when.
- Explain to the patient that he may experience discomfort from the needle puncture and the tourniquet.
- Keep the patient relaxed and recumbent for 30 minutes before the test.

Procedure and posttest care

- Perform a venipuncture, and collect the sample in a 5-ml clot-activator tube.
- If requested, a hematocrit may be drawn at the same time by collecting an additional sample in a 2-ml tube with EDTA added.
- Apply direct pressure to the venipuncture site until bleeding stops.
- If a hematoma develops at the venipuncture site, apply warm soaks.

Precautions

- Handle the sample gently to prevent hemolysis.

Reference values

The reference range for EPO is 5 to 36 mU/ml (SI, 5 to 36 IU/L).

Abnormal findings

Low levels of EPO appear in patients with anemia who have inadequate or absent hormone production. Congenital absence of EPO can occur. Severe renal disease may decrease EPO production.

Elevated EPO levels occur in anemias as a compensatory mechanism in the reestablishment of homeostasis. Inappropriate elevations (when the hematocrit is normal to high) are seen in polycythemia and EPO-secreting tumors.

Some athletes use EPO to enhance performance. The increased RBC volume conveys additional oxygen-carrying capacity to the blood. Adverse reactions include clotting abnormalities, headache, seizures, hypertension, nausea, vomiting, diarrhea, and rash.

Interfering factors

- Failure to collect a sample in the fasting state
- Hemolysis due to rough handling of the sample

PLASMA ATRIAL NATRIURETIC FACTOR

The plasma atrial natriuretic factor is a radioimmunoassay that measures the plasma level of atrial natriuretic factor (ANF), also known as atrial natriuretic peptides or atriopeptins. An extremely potent natriuretic agent and vasodilator,

ANF rapidly produces diuresis and increases the glomerular filtration rate. ANF's role in regulating extracellular fluid volume, blood pressure, and sodium metabolism appears critical.

Patients with overt heart failure have highly elevated plasma levels of ANF. Patients with cardiovascular disease and elevated cardiac filling pressure but without heart failure also have markedly elevated ANF levels. ANF may provide a marker for early asymptomatic left ventricular dysfunction and increased cardiac volume.

Purpose

- To confirm heart failure
- To identify asymptomatic cardiac volume overload

Patient preparation

- As appropriate, explain the purpose of the test to the patient.
- Inform him that he must fast for 12 hours before the test.
- Tell the patient that the test requires a blood sample. Explain who will perform the venipuncture and when.
- Explain to the patient that he may experience discomfort from the needle puncture and the tourniquet.
- Explain that the test results will be available within 4 days.
- Check the patient's history for medications that can influence test results.
- Withhold beta-adrenergic blockers, calcium antagonists, diuretics, vasodilators, and cardiac glycosides for 24 hours before collection, as ordered.

Procedure and posttest care

- Perform a venipuncture, and collect the sample in a prechilled potassium-EDTA tube.
- After chilled centrifugation, the EDTA plasma should be promptly frozen and sent to the laboratory.
- Apply direct pressure to the venipuncture site until bleeding stops.
- If a hematoma develops at the venipuncture site, apply warm soaks.
- Instruct the patient that he may resume his normal diet and medications discontinued before the test.

Precautions

- Handle the sample gently to prevent hemolysis.

Reference values

Normal ANF levels range from 20 to 77 pg/ml.

Abnormal findings

Markedly elevated levels of ANF occur in patients with frank heart failure and significantly elevated cardiac filling pressure.

Interfering factors

- Cardiovascular drugs, including beta-adrenergic blockers, calcium antagonists, diuretics, vasodilators, and cardiac glycosides

PANCREATIC AND GASTRIC HORMONES

INSULIN

The insulin test, a radioimmunoassay, is a quantitative analysis of serum insulin levels. Insulin is usually measured concomitantly with glucose levels because glucose is the primary stimulus for insulin release.

Insulin regulates the metabolism and transport or mobilization of carbohydrates, amino acids, proteins, and lipids.

Stimulated by increased plasma levels of glucose, insulin secretion reaches peak levels after meals, when metabolism and food storage are greatest.

Purpose

■ To aid diagnosis of hyperinsulinemia as well as hypoglycemia resulting from a tumor or hyperplasia of pancreatic islet cells, glucocorticoid deficiency, or severe hepatic disease

■ To aid diagnosis of diabetes mellitus and insulin-resistant states

Patient preparation

■ Explain to the patient that this test helps determine if the pancreas is functioning normally.

■ Instruct the patient to fast for 10 to 12 hours before the test.

■ Tell the patient that the test requires a blood sample. Explain who will perform the venipuncture and when.

■ Explain to the patient that he may experience discomfort from the needle puncture and the tourniquet.

■ Explain that questionable results may require a repeat test or a simultaneous glucose tolerance test, which requires that the patient drink a glucose solution.

■ Withhold corticotropin, corticosteroids (including oral contraceptives), thyroid supplements, epinephrine, and other medications that may interfere with test results, as ordered. If they must be continued, note this on the laboratory request.

■ Make sure the patient is relaxed and recumbent for 30 minutes before the test.

Procedure and posttest care

■ Perform a venipuncture, and collect one sample for insulin level in a 7-ml tube with EDTA.

■ Collect a sample for glucose level in a tube with sodium fluoride and potassium oxalate.

■ Apply direct pressure to the veni puncture site until bleeding stops.

■ If a hematoma develops at the venipuncture site, apply warm soaks.

■ Instruct the patient that he may resume his normal diet and medications discontinued before the test as ordered.

Precautions

■ Pack the insulin sample in ice, and send it, along with the glucose sample, to the laboratory immediately.

■ In the patient with an insulinoma, fasting for this test may precipitate dangerously severe hypoglycemia. Keep an ampule of dextrose 50% available to counteract possible hypoglycemia.

■ Handle the samples gently to prevent hemolysis.

Reference values

Serum insulin levels normally range from 0 to 35 μU/ml (SI, 144 to 243 pmol/L).

Abnormal findings

Insulin levels are interpreted in light of the prevailing glucose concentration. A normal insulin level may be inappropriate for the glucose results. High insulin and low glucose levels after a significant fast suggest the presence of an insulinoma. Prolonged fasting or stimulation testing may be required to confirm the diagnosis. In insulin-resistant diabetes mellitus, insulin levels are elevated; in non–insulin-resistant diabetes, they're low.

Interfering factors

■ Failure to observe pretest restrictions

■ Agitation and stress

■ Hemolysis due to rough handling of the sample

- Failure to pack the insulin sample in ice and send it to the laboratory promptly
- Corticotropin, corticosteroids (including oral contraceptives), thyroid hormones, and epinephrine (possible increase)
- Use of insulin by non-insulin-dependent patients (possible increase)
- High levels of insulin antibodies in patients with insulin-dependent diabetes mellitus

GASTRIN

Gastrin is a polypeptide hormone produced and stored primarily in the antrum of the stomach and to a lesser degree in the islets of Langerhans. Its main function is to facilitate food digestion by triggering gastric acid secretion. It also stimulates the release of pancreatic enzymes and the gastric enzyme pepsin, increases gastric and intestinal motility, and stimulates bile flow from the liver. Abnormal secretion of gastrin can result from tumors (gastrinomas) and pathologic disorders that affect the stomach, pancreas and, less commonly, the esophagus and small bowel.

This radioimmunoassay, a quantitative analysis of gastrin levels, is especially useful in patients suspected of having gastrinomas (Zollinger-Ellison syndrome). In doubtful situations, provocative testing may be necessary.

Purpose

- To confirm a diagnosis of gastrinoma, the gastrin-secreting tumor in Zollinger-Ellison syndrome
- To aid differential diagnosis of gastric and duodenal ulcers and pernicious anemia (Gastrin estimation has limited value in patients with duodenal ulcers.)

Patient preparation

- Explain to the patient that this test helps determine the cause of GI symptoms.
- Instruct him to abstain from alcohol for at least 24 hours before the test and to fast and avoid caffeinated drinks for 12 hours before the test, although he may drink water.
- Tell the patient that the test requires a blood sample. Explain who will perform the venipuncture and when.
- Explain to the patient that he may experience discomfort from the needle puncture and the tourniquet.
- Withhold all drugs that may interfere with test results, especially insulin and anticholinergics, such as atropine and belladonna, as ordered. If they must be continued, note this on the laboratory request.
- Tell the patient to lie down and relax for at least 30 minutes before the test.

Procedure and posttest care

- Perform a venipuncture, and collect the sample in a 10- to 15-ml clot-activator tube.
- Apply direct pressure to the venipuncture site until bleeding stops.
- If a hematoma develops at the venipuncture site, apply warm soaks.
- Instruct the patient that he may resume his normal diet and medications discontinued before the test as ordered.

Precautions

- Handle the sample gently to avoid hemolysis.
- To prevent destruction of serum gastrin by proteolytic enzymes, immediately send the sample to the laboratory to have the serum separated and frozen.

Reference values

Normal serum gastrin levels are 50 to 150 pg/ml (SI, 50 to 150 ng/L).

Abnormal findings

Strikingly high serum gastrin levels (> 1,000 pg/ml [SI, > 1,000 ng/L]) confirm Zollinger-Ellison syndrome. (Levels as high as 450,000 pg/ml [SI, 450,000 ng/L] have been reported.)

Increased serum levels of gastrin may occur in a few patients with duodenal ulceration (< 1%) and in patients with achlorhydria (with or without pernicious anemia) or extensive stomach carcinoma (because of hyposecretion of gastric juices and hydrochloric acid).

Interfering factors

- Failure to observe restrictions of diet, medications, or physical activity
- Hemolysis due to rough handling of the sample
- Amino acids (especially glycine), calcium carbonate, acetylcholine, calcium chloride, and ethanol (increase)
- Anticholinergics, such as atropine, as well as hydrochloric acid and secretin, a strongly basic polypeptide (decrease)
- Insulin-induced hypoglycemia (increase)

PLASMA GLUCAGON

The plasma glucagon test is a quantitative analysis of plasma glucagon by radioimmunoassay. Glucagon, a polypeptide hormone, is secreted by alpha cells of the islets of Langerhans in the pancreas. It acts primarily on the liver to promote glucose production and control glucose secretion.

Purpose

- To aid diagnosis of glucagonoma and hypoglycemia due to chronic pancreatitis or idiopathic glucagon deficiency

Patient preparation

- Explain to the patient that this test helps to evaluate pancreatic function.
- Instruct the patient to fast for 10 to 12 hours before the test.
- Tell the patient that the test requires a blood sample. Explain who will perform the venipuncture and when.
- Explain to the patient that he may experience discomfort from the needle puncture and the tourniquet.
- Withhold insulin, catecholamines, and other drugs that could influence the test results, as ordered. If they must be continued, note this on the laboratory request.
- Have the patient lie down and relax for 30 minutes before the test.

Procedure and posttest care

- Perform a venipuncture, and collect the sample in a chilled, 10-ml EDTA tube.
- Apply direct pressure to the venipuncture site until bleeding stops.
- If a hematoma develops at the venipuncture site, apply warm soaks.
- Instruct the patient that he may resume his normal diet and medications discontinued before the test.

Precautions

- Place the sample on ice, and send it to the laboratory immediately.
- Handle the sample gently to prevent hemolysis.

Reference values

Fasting glucagon levels are normally less than 60 pg/ml (SI, < 60 ng/L).

Abnormal findings

Elevated fasting glucagon levels (900 to 7,800 pg/ml [SI, 900 to 7,800 ng/L]) can occur in glucagonoma, diabetes mellitus, acute pancreatitis, and pheochromocytoma.

Abnormally low glucagon levels are associated with idiopathic glucagon deficiency and hypoglycemia due to chronic pancreatitis.

Interfering factors

- Failure to observe pretest restrictions
- Hemolysis due to rough handling of the sample
- Failure to pack the sample in ice and send it to the laboratory immediately
- Exercise, stress, prolonged fasting, insulin, or catecholamines (increase)
- Radioactive scans and tests performed within 48 hours of the test

C-PEPTIDE

Connecting peptide (C-peptide) is a biologically inactive chain formed during the proteolytic conversion of proinsulin to insulin in the pancreatic beta cells. It has no insulin effect either biologically or immunologically. Circulating insulin is measured by immunologic assay. As insulin is released into the bloodstream, the C-peptide chain splits off from the hormone.

Purpose

- To determine the cause of hypoglycemia
- To indirectly measure insulin secretion in the presence of circulating insulin antibodies
- To detect residual tissue after total pancreatectomy for carcinoma
- To determine beta-cell function in patients with diabetes mellitus

Patient preparation

- Explain to the patient that this test helps to evaluate pancreatic function and determine the cause of hypoglycemia.
- Instruct the patient to fast for 8 to 12 hours before the test, except for water.
- Tell the patient that the test requires a blood sample. Explain who will perform the venipuncture and when.
- Explain to the patient that he may experience discomfort from the needle puncture and the tourniquet.
- If the patient is scheduled for radioisotope testing, it should take place after blood is drawn for C-peptide levels. Blood glucose levels are usually drawn at the same time as C-peptide levels.
- If the C-peptide stimulation test is done, I.V. glucagon is administered as ordered after a baseline value blood sample is drawn.
- Withhold drugs that may interfere with test results, as ordered. If they must be continued, note this on the laboratory request.

Procedure and posttest care

- Perform a venipuncture, and collect a 1-ml sample in a chilled clot-activator tube.
- Collect a sample for glucose level in a tube with sodium fluoride and potassium oxalate, if ordered.
- Apply direct pressure to the venipuncture site until bleeding stops.
- If a hematoma develops at the venipuncture site, apply warm soaks.
- The blood is separated and frozen to be tested later.
- Instruct the patient that he may resume his normal diet and medications discontinued before the test as ordered.

Precautions

- Pack the sample in ice, and send it, along with the glucose sample, to the laboratory immediately.
- Handle the samples gently to prevent hemolysis.

Reference values

Serum C-peptide levels generally parallel those of insulin. Normal fasting values range between 0.78 and 1.89 ng/ml (SI, 0.26 to 0.63 mmol/L). An insulin: C-peptide ratio may be performed to differentiate insulinoma from factitious hypoglycemia. A ratio of 1.0 or less indicates increased, endogenous insulin secretion; a ratio of 1.0 or more indicates exogenous insulin.

Abnormal findings

- Endogenous hyperinsulinism (insulinemia), oral hypoglycemic drug ingestion, pancreas or B-cell transplant, renal failure, or type 2 diabetes mellitus (elevated levels)
- Factitious hypoglycemia (surreptitious insulin administration), radical pancreatectomy, or type 1 diabetes (decreased)

Interfering factors

- Failure to follow pretest restrictions
- Hemolysis due to rough handling of the sample
- Failure to pack the sample in ice and send it to the laboratory

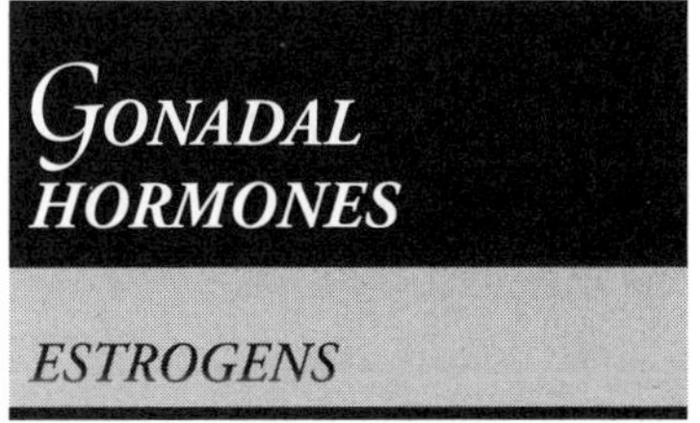

GONADAL HORMONES

ESTROGENS

Estrogens (and progesterone) are secreted by the ovaries. They're responsible for the development of secondary female sexual characteristics and for normal menstruation. Levels are usually undetectable in children. These hormones are secreted by ovarian follicular cells during the first half of the menstrual cycle and by the corpus luteum during the luteal phase and during pregnancy. In menopause, estrogen secretion drops to a constant, low level.

This radioimmunoassay measures serum levels of estradiol, estrone, and estriol (the only estrogens that appear in serum in measurable amounts) and has diagnostic significance in evaluating female gonadal dysfunction. (See *Predicting premature labor,* page 244.) Tests of hypothalamic-pituitary function may be required to confirm the diagnosis.

Purpose

- To determine sexual maturation and fertility
- To aid diagnosis of gonadal dysfunction, such as precocious or delayed puberty, menstrual disorders (especially amenorrhea), and infertility
- To determine fetal well-being
- To aid diagnosis of tumors known to secrete estrogen

Patient preparation

- Explain to the patient that this test helps determine if secretion of female hormones is normal and that the test may be repeated during the various phases of the menstrual cycle.
- Tell her that she need not restrict food or fluids.
- Tell the patient that the test requires a blood sample. Explain who will perform the venipuncture and when.
- Explain to the patient that she may experience discomfort from the needle puncture and the tourniquet.
- Withhold all steroid and pituitary-based hormones, as ordered. If they must be continued, note this on the laboratory request.

Procedure and posttest care

Procedure and posttest care may vary slightly, depending on whether plasma or serum is being measured.

Predicting premature labor

A simple salivary test can now help determine whether a pregnant woman is at risk for premature labor, a complication that's detrimental to the health of the premature infant. The test, known as the SalEst test, measures salivary levels of estriol, an estrogen that increases 1,000-fold during pregnancy. For women determined to be at risk, the SalEst test is 98% accurate in ruling out premature labor and delivery.

The test is performed on women between 22 and 36 weeks' gestation, using their saliva and the SalEst test kit. Estriol has been found to increase 2 to 3 weeks before the spontaneous onset of labor and delivery. A positive test indicates that the patient is at risk for premature labor. With this knowledge and evaluation by a physician, precautions can be instituted to decrease the risk of preterm labor and maintain fetal viability.

- Perform a venipuncture, and collect the sample in a 10-ml clot-activator tube.
- If the patient is premenopausal, indicate the phase of her menstrual cycle on the laboratory request.
- Apply direct pressure to the venipuncture site until bleeding stops.
- If a hematoma develops at the venipuncture site, apply warm soaks.
- Instruct the patient that she may resume her usual medications discontinued before the test.

Precautions

- Handle the sample gently to prevent hemolysis.
- Send the sample to the laboratory immediately.

Reference values

Normal serum estrogen levels for premenopausal women vary widely during the menstrual cycle, ranging from 26 to 149 pg/ml (SI, 90 to 550 pmol/L). The range for postmenopausal women is 0 to 34 pg/ml (SI, 0 to 125 pmol/L).

Serum estrogen levels in men range from 12 to 34 pg/ml (SI, 40 to 125 pmol/L). In children under age 6, the normal level of serum estrogen is 3 to 10 pg/ml (SI, 10 to 36 pmol/L). Estriol is secreted in large amounts by the placenta during pregnancy. Levels range from 2 ng/ml (SI, 7 nmol/L) by 30 weeks' gestation to 30 ng/ml (SI, 105 nmol/L) by week 40.

Abnormal findings

Decreased estrogen levels may indicate primary hypogonadism, or ovarian failure, as in Turner's syndrome or ovarian agenesis; secondary hypogonadism, such as in hypopituitarism; or menopause.

Abnormally high estrogen levels may occur with estrogen-producing tumors, in precocious puberty, and in severe hepatic disease, such as cirrhosis, that prevents clearance of plasma estrogens. High levels may also result from congenital adrenal hyperplasia (increased conversion of androgens to estrogen).

Interfering factors

- Hemolysis due to rough handling of the sample
- Pregnancy and pretest use of estrogens such as oral contraceptives (possible increase)
- Clomiphene, an estrogen antagonist (possible decrease)
- Steroids and pituitary-based hormones such as dexamethasone

PLASMA PROGESTERONE

Progesterone, an ovarian steroid hormone secreted by the corpus luteum, causes thickening and secretory development of the endometrium in preparation for implantation of the fertilized ovum. Progesterone levels, therefore, peak during the midluteal phase of the menstrual cycle. If implantation doesn't occur, progesterone (and estrogen) levels drop sharply and menstruation begins about 2 days later.

During pregnancy, the placenta releases about 10 times the normal monthly amount of progesterone to maintain the pregnancy. Increased secretion begins toward the end of the first trimester and continues until delivery. Progesterone prevents abortion by decreasing uterine contractions. Along with estrogen, progesterone helps prepare the breasts for lactation.

This radioimmunoassay is a quantitative analysis of plasma progesterone levels and provides reliable information about corpus luteum function in fertility studies and placental function in pregnancy. Serial determinations are recommended. Although plasma levels provide accurate information, progesterone can also be monitored by measuring urine pregnanediol, a catabolite of progesterone.

Purpose

- To assess corpus luteum function as part of infertility studies
- To evaluate placental function during pregnancy
- To aid in confirming ovulation; test results support basal body temperature readings

Patient preparation

- Explain to the patient that this test helps determine if her female sex hormone secretion is normal.
- Inform her that she need not restrict food or fluids.
- Tell the patient that the test requires a blood sample. Explain who will perform the venipuncture and when.
- Explain to the patient that she may experience discomfort from the needle puncture and the tourniquet.
- Inform her that the test may be repeated at specific times coinciding with phases of her menstrual cycle or with each prenatal visit.
- Check the patient's history to determine if she's taking drugs that may interfere with test results, including progesterone and estrogen. Note your findings on the laboratory request.

Procedure and posttest care

- Perform a venipuncture, and collect the sample in a 7-ml heparinized tube.
- Apply direct pressure to the venipuncture site until bleeding stops.
- If a hematoma develops at the venipuncture site, apply warm soaks.

Precautions

- Handle the sample gently to prevent hemolysis.
- Completely fill the collection tube; then invert it gently at least 10 times to mix the sample and anticoagulant adequately.
- Indicate the date of the patient's last menstrual period and the phase of her cycle on the laboratory request. If the patient is pregnant, also indicate the month of gestation.
- Send the sample to the laboratory immediately.

Reference values

During menstruation, normal progesterone values are:

- Follicular phase: < 150 ng/dl (SI, < 5 nmol/L)
- Luteal phase: 300 to 1,200 ng/dl (SI, 10 to 40 nmol/L).

During pregnancy, normal progesterone values are:

- First trimester: 1,500 to 5,000 ng/dl (SI, 50 to 160 nmol/L)
- Second and third trimester: 8,000 to 20,000 ng/dl (SI, 250 to 650 nmol/L).

Normal values in menopausal women are 10 to 22 ng/dl (SI, < 2 nmol/L).

Abnormal findings

Elevated progesterone levels may indicate ovulation, luteinizing tumors, ovarian cysts that produce progesterone, or adrenocortical hyperplasias and tumors that produce progesterone along with other steroidal hormones.

Low progesterone levels are associated with amenorrhea due to several causes (such as panhypopituitarism and gonadal dysfunction), eclampsia, threatened abortion, and fetal death.

Interfering factors

- Hemolysis due to rough handling of the sample
- Progesterone or estrogen therapy
- Radioactive scans performed within 1 week of the test

TESTOSTERONE

The principal androgen secreted by the interstitial cells of the testes (Leydig cells), testosterone induces puberty in the male and maintains male secondary sex characteristics. Prepubertal levels of testosterone are low. Increased testosterone secretion during puberty stimulates growth of the seminiferous tubules and sperm production; it also contributes to the enlargement of external genitalia, accessory sex organs (such as prostate glands), and voluntary muscles and to the growth of facial, pubic, and axillary hair.

Testosterone production begins to increase at onset of puberty and continues to rise during adulthood. Production begins to taper off at about age 40 and eventually drops to about one-fifth the peak level by age 80. In women, the adrenal glands and ovaries secrete small amounts of testosterone.

This competitive protein-binding test measures plasma or serum testosterone levels. When combined with measurement of plasma gonadotropin levels (follicle-stimulating hormone and luteinizing hormone), it's a reliable aid in the evaluation of gonadal dysfunction in men and women.

Purpose

- To facilitate differential diagnosis of male sexual precocity in boys under age 10 (True precocious puberty must be distinguished from pseudoprecocious puberty.)
- To aid differential diagnosis of hypogonadism (Primary hypogonadism must be distinguished from secondary hypogonadism.)
- To evaluate male infertility or other sexual dysfunction
- To evaluate hirsutism and virilization in women

Patient preparation

- Explain to the patient that this test helps determine if male sex hormone secretion is adequate.
- Inform him that he need not restrict food or fluids.
- Tell the patient that the test requires a blood sample. Explain who will perform the venipuncture and when.
- Explain to the patient that he may experience discomfort from the needle

puncture and the tourniquet, but that collecting the sample takes only a few minutes.

Procedure and posttest care

- Perform a venipuncture, and collect the serum sample in a 7-ml clot-activator tube.
- If plasma is to be collected, use a heparinized tube.
- Indicate the patient's age, sex, and history of hormone therapy on the laboratory request.
- Apply direct pressure to the venipuncture site until bleeding stops.
- If a hematoma develops at the venipuncture site, apply warm soaks.

Precautions

- Handle the sample gently to prevent hemolysis, and send it to the laboratory promptly.
- The sample is stable and requires no refrigeration or preservative for up to 1 week. Frozen samples are stable for at least 6 months.

Reference values

Normal testosterone levels are (laboratory values vary slightly):

- males: 300 to 1,200 ng/dl (SI, 10.4 to 41.6 nmol/L)
- females: 20 to 80 ng/dl (SI, 0.7 to 2.8 nmol/L)
- prepubertal children: values lower than adult levels.

Abnormal findings

Elevated testosterone levels in prepubertal boys may indicate true sexual precocity due to excessive gonadotropin secretion or pseudoprecocious puberty due to male hormone production by a testicular tumor. They can also indicate congenital adrenal hyperplasia, which results in precocious puberty in boys (from ages 2 to 3) and pseudohermaphroditism and milder virilization in girls.

Increased testosterone levels can occur with a benign adrenal tumor or cancer, hyperthyroidism, and incipient puberty. In women with ovarian tumors or polycystic ovary syndrome, testosterone levels may rise, leading to hirsutism.

Low testosterone levels can indicate primary hypogonadism (as in Klinefelter's syndrome) or secondary hypogonadism (hypogonadotropic eunuchoidism) from hypothalamic-pituitary dysfunction. Low levels can also follow orchiectomy, testicular or prostate cancer, delayed male puberty, estrogen therapy, and cirrhosis of the liver.

Interfering factors

- Hemolysis due to rough handling of the sample
- Exogenous sources of estrogens and androgens, thyroid and growth hormones, and other pituitary-based hormones
- Estrogens (decrease free testosterone levels by increasing sex hormone-binding globulin, which binds testosterone)
- Androgens (possible increase)

PLACENTAL HORMONES

HUMAN CHORIONIC GONADOTROPIN

Human chorionic gonadotropin (hCG) is a glycoprotein hormone produced in the placenta. If conception occurs, a specific assay for hCG — commonly called the beta-subunit assay — may detect this hormone in the blood 9 days after ovulation. This interval coincides with the implantation of the fertilized ovum into the uterine wall. Although the precise function of hCG is still unclear, it appears that hCG, with progesterone, maintains the corpus luteum during early pregnancy.

Production of hCG increases steadily during the first trimester, peaking around 10 weeks' gestation. Levels then fall to less than 10% of first-trimester peak levels during the remainder of the pregnancy. About 2 weeks after delivery, the hormone may no longer be detectable.

This serum immunoassay, a quantitative analysis of hCG beta-subunit level, is more sensitive (and costlier) than the routine pregnancy test using a urine sample.

Purpose

- To detect early pregnancy
- To determine adequacy of hormonal production in high-risk pregnancies (for example, habitual abortion)
- To aid diagnosis of trophoblastic tumors, such as hydatidiform moles and choriocarcinoma, and tumors that ectopically secrete hCG
- To monitor treatment for induction of ovulation and conception

Patient preparation

- Explain to the patient that this test determines if she's pregnant. If detection of pregnancy isn't the diagnostic objective, offer the appropriate explanation.
- Inform her that she need not restrict food or fluids.
- Tell the patient that the test requires a blood sample. Explain who will perform the venipuncture and when.
- Explain to the patient that she may experience discomfort from the needle puncture and the tourniquet.

Procedure and posttest care

- Perform a venipuncture, and collect the sample in a 7-ml clot-activator tube.
- Apply direct pressure to the venipuncture site until bleeding stops.
- If a hematoma develops at the venipuncture site, apply warm soaks.

Precautions

- Handle the sample gently to prevent hemolysis.
- Send the sample to the laboratory immediately.

Reference values

Normally, hCG levels are less than 4 IU/L. During pregnancy, hCG levels vary widely, depending partly on the number of days after the last normal menstrual period.

Abnormal findings

Elevated hCG beta-subunit levels indicate pregnancy; significantly higher concentrations are present in a multiple pregnancy. Increased levels may also suggest hydatidiform mole, trophoblastic neoplasms of the placenta, and nontrophoblastic carcinomas that secrete hCG (including gastric, pancreatic, and ovarian adenocarcinomas). Low hCG beta-subunit levels can occur in ectopic pregnancy or pregnancy of less than 9 days. Beta-subunit levels can't differentiate between pregnancy and tumor recurrence because they're high in both conditions.

Interfering factors

- Hemolysis due to rough handling of the sample
- Heparin anticoagulants and EDTA (decrease; ask laboratory whether test will be performed on plasma or serum)

HUMAN PLACENTAL LACTOGEN

A polypeptide hormone, human placental lactogen (hPL) — also known as human chorionic somatomammotropin — displays lactogenic and somatotropic (growth hormone) properties in a pregnant female. In combination with prolactin, hPL prepares the breasts for lactation. It also indirectly provides energy for maternal metabolism and fetal nutrition. It facilitates protein synthesis and mobilization essential to fetal growth. Secretion is autonomous, beginning at about 5 weeks' gestation and declining rapidly after delivery. According to some evidence, this hormone may not be essential for a successful pregnancy.

This radioimmunoassay measures plasma hPL levels, which are roughly proportional to placental mass. Such assays may be required in high-risk pregnancies (patients with diabetes mellitus or hypertension) and suspected placental tissue dysfunction. Because values vary widely during the latter half of pregnancy, serial determinations over several days provide the most reliable test results.

Purpose

- To assess placental function and fetal well-being (combined with measurement of estriol levels)
- To aid diagnosis of hydatidiform moles and choriocarcinoma (human chorionic gonadotropin levels may be more useful in diagnosing these conditions)
- To aid diagnosis and monitor treatment of nontrophoblastic tumors that ectopically secrete hPL

Patient preparation

- Explain to the patient that this test helps assess placental function and fetal well-being. If assessing fetal well-being isn't the diagnostic objective, offer an appropriate explanation.
- Tell the patient that the test requires a blood sample. Explain who will perform the venipuncture and when.
- Explain to the patient that she may experience discomfort from the needle puncture and the tourniquet.
- Inform the pregnant patient that this test may be repeated during her pregnancy.

Procedure and posttest care

- Perform a venipuncture, and collect the sample in a 7-ml clot-activator tube.
- Apply direct pressure to the venipuncture site until bleeding stops.
- If a hematoma develops at the venipuncture site, apply warm soaks.

Precautions

- Handle the sample gently to prevent hemolysis
- Send the sample to the laboratory immediately.

Reference values

For pregnant women, normal hPL levels vary with gestational phase and slowly increase throughout pregnancy, reaching 8.6 µg/ml at term. At term, patients with diabetes may have mean levels of 9 to 11 µg/ml. Normal levels for males and nonpregnant females are less than 0.5 µg/ml.

Abnormal findings

For reliable interpretation, hPL levels must be correlated with gestational age; for example, after 30 weeks' gestation, levels below 4 µg/ml may indicate placental dysfunction. Low hPL concentrations are also characteristically associated with postmaturity syndrome, intrauterine growth retardation, preeclampsia, and eclampsia. Declining concentrations may help differentiate incomplete abortion from threatened abortion.

Be aware that low hPL concentrations don't confirm fetal distress. Conversely, concentrations over 4 μg/ml after 30 weeks' gestation don't guarantee fetal well-being because elevated levels have been reported after fetal death.

An hPL value above 6 μg/ml after 30 weeks' gestation may suggest an unusually large placenta, commonly occurring in patients with diabetes mellitus, multiple pregnancy, and Rh isoimmunization. The usefulness of this test in predicting fetal death in a patient with diabetes mellitus and in managing Rh isoimmunization during pregnancy is limited.

Below-normal concentrations of hPL may be associated with trophoblastic neoplastic disease, such as hydatidiform mole and choriocarcinoma. Abnormal concentrations of hPL have been found in the sera of patients with other neoplastic disorders, including bronchogenic carcinoma, hepatoma, lymphoma, and pheochromocytoma. In these patients, hPL levels are used as tumor markers for evaluating chemotherapy, monitoring tumor growth and recurrence, and detecting residual tissue after excision.

Interfering factors

- Hemolysis due to rough handling of the sample

4

Vitamin and trace element tests

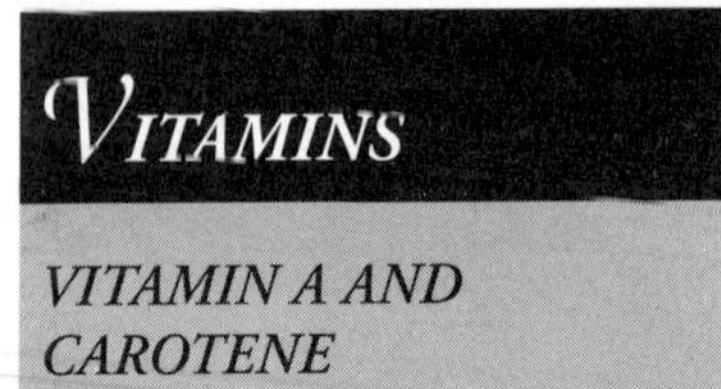

The vitamin A and carotene test measures serum levels of vitamin A (retinol) and its precursor, carotene. A fat-soluble vitamin normally supplied by diet, vitamin A is important for reproduction, vision (especially night vision), and epithelial tissue and bone growth. Vitamin A is found mostly in fruits, vegetables, eggs, poultry, meat, and fish. Carotene is present in leafy green vegetables and in yellow fruits and vegetables.

In this serum test, the color reactions produced by vitamin A and related compounds with various reagents provide quantitative and qualitative information.

Purpose

- To investigate suspected vitamin A deficiency or toxicity
- To aid diagnosis of visual disturbances, especially night blindness and xerophthalmia
- To aid diagnosis of skin diseases, such as keratosis follicularis or ichthyosis
- To screen for malabsorption

Patient preparation

- Explain to the patient that this test measures the vitamin A level in the blood.
- Instruct the patient to fast overnight, but that he need not restrict water intake.
- Tell the patient that the test requires a blood sample. Explain who will perform the venipuncture and when.
- Explain to the patient that he may experience discomfort from the needle puncture and the tourniquet.

Procedure and posttest care

- Perform a venipuncture, and collect the sample in a chilled 7-ml siliconized tube.
- Apply direct pressure to the venipuncture site until bleeding stops.
- If a hematoma develops at the venipuncture site, apply warm soaks.
- Instruct the patient that he may resume his normal diet discontinued before the test.

Precautions

- Protect the sample from light because vitamin A characteristically absorbs light.
- Handle the sample gently, and send it to the laboratory immediately.
- Keep the specimen on ice.

Reference values

Normal serum levels for carotene are 10 to 85 µg/dl (SI, 0.19 to 1.58 µmol/L) and vitamin A are 30 to 80 µg/dl (SI, 1.05 to 2.8 µmol/L).

Abnormal findings

Low serum levels of vitamin A (hypovitaminosis A) may indicate impaired fat absorption, as in celiac disease, infectious hepatitis, cystic fibrosis of the pancreas, or obstructive jaundice. Low levels are also associated with protein-calorie malnutrition (marasmic kwashiorkor). Similar decreases in vitamin A levels may also result from chronic nephritis.

Elevated vitamin A levels (hypervitaminosis A) usually indicate chronically excessive intake of vitamin A supplements or of foods high in vitamin A. Increased levels are also associated with hyperlipemia and hypercholesterolemia of uncontrolled diabetes mellitus.

Decreased serum carotene levels may indicate impaired fat absorption or, rarely, insufficient dietary intake of carotene. Carotene levels may also be suppressed during pregnancy. Elevated carotene levels indicate grossly excessive dietary intake.

Interfering factors

- Failure to observe overnight fast
- Hemolysis due to rough handling of the sample
- Mineral oil, neomycin, and cholestyramine (possible decrease)
- Glucocorticoids and oral contraceptives (possible increase)

VITAMIN B_2

The serum vitamin B_2 test evaluates serum levels of vitamin B_2 (riboflavin), a vitamin essential for growth and tissue function. The serum test is considered more reliable than the urine test, which can produce artificially high values in patients after surgery or prolonged fasting.

Purpose

- To detect vitamin B_2 deficiency

Patient preparation

- Explain to the patient that this test evaluates vitamin B_2 levels.
- Instruct the patient to maintain a normal diet before the test.
- Tell the patient that the test requires a blood sample. Explain who will perform the venipuncture and when.
- Explain to the patient that he may experience discomfort from the needle puncture and the tourniquet.

Procedure and posttest care

- Perform a venipuncture, and collect the sample in a 4.5-ml siliconized tube.
- Apply direct pressure to the venipuncture site until bleeding stops.
- If a hematoma develops at the venipuncture site, apply warm soaks.
- Inform the patient with vitamin B_2 deficiency that good dietary sources of vitamin B_2 are milk products, organ meats (liver and kidneys), fish, green leafy vegetables, legumes, and fortified breads and cereals.

Precautions

- Handle the sample gently to prevent hemolysis.
- Send the sample to the laboratory immediately.
- Don't refrigerate or freeze the sample.

Reference values

Normal test results are 3 to 15 µg/dl; 2 to 3 µg/dl is considered marginally low, and less than 2 µg/dl is considered significantly diminished.

Abnormal findings

Marginally low test results (less than 3 µg/dl) indicate vitamin B_2 deficiency. Such deficiency can result from insufficient dietary intake of vitamin B_2, malabsorption syndrome, or conditions that increase metabolic demands such as stress.

Interfering factors

- Hemolysis due to rough handling of the sample

VITAMIN B_{12}

The vitamin B_{12} radioisotope assay of competitive binding is a quantitative analysis of serum levels of vitamin B_{12}

Cobalt: Critical trace element

A trace element found mainly in the liver, cobalt is an essential component of vitamin B_{12} and therefore is a critical factor in hematopoiesis. A balanced diet supplies sufficient cobalt to maintain hematopoiesis, primarily through foods containing vitamin B_{12}.

However, excessive ingestion of cobalt may have toxic effects. Toxicity has occurred, for example, in individuals who consumed large quantities of beer containing cobalt as a stabilizer, resulting in heart failure from cardiomyopathy. Because quantitative analysis of cobalt alone is difficult because of the minute amount found in the body, cobalt is often measured by bioassay as part of vitamin B_{12} testing.

Normal cobalt concentration in human plasma is 60 to 80 pg/ml.

(also called cyanocobalamin, antipernicious anemia factor, or extrinsic factor). This test is usually performed concurrently with measurement of serum folic acid levels.

A water-soluble vitamin containing cobalt, vitamin B_{12} is essential to hematopoiesis, deoxyribonucleic acid synthesis and growth, myelin synthesis, and central nervous system (CNS) integrity. This vitamin is found almost exclusively in animal products, such as meat, shellfish, milk, and eggs. (See *Cobalt: Critical trace element.*)

Purpose

- To aid differential diagnosis of megaloblastic anemia, which may be due to a deficiency of vitamin B_{12} or folic acid
- To aid differential diagnosis of CNS disorders that are affecting peripheral and spinal myelinated nerves

Patient preparation

- Explain to the patient that this test determines the amount of vitamin B_{12} in the blood.
- Instruct the patient to fast overnight before the test.
- Tell the patient that the test requires a blood sample. Explain who will perform the venipuncture and when.
- Explain to the patient that he may experience discomfort from the needle puncture and the tourniquet.
- Check the patient's history for drugs that may alter test results, and note these on the laboratory request.

Procedure and posttest care

- Perform a venipuncture, and collect the sample in a 4.5-ml siliconized tube.
- Apply direct pressure to the venipuncture site until bleeding stops.
- If a hematoma develops at the venipuncture site, apply warm soaks.
- Instruct the patient that he may resume his normal diet discontinued before the test.

Precautions

- Handle the sample gently to prevent hemolysis.
- Send the sample to the laboratory immediately.

Reference values

Normally, serum vitamin B_{12} values range from 200 to 900 pg/ml (SI, 148 to 664 pmol/L).

Abnormal findings

Decreased serum levels may indicate inadequate dietary intake, especially if the patient is a strict vegetarian. Low levels are also associated with malabsorption syndromes such as celiac disease; isolated malabsorption of vitamin B_{12}; hypermetabolic states such as hyperthyroidism; pregnancy; and CNS damage (for example, posterolateral sclerosis or funicular degeneration).

Elevated levels of serum vitamin B_{12} may result from excessive dietary intake; hepatic disease, such as cirrhosis or acute or chronic hepatitis; and myeloproliferative disorders such as myelocytic leukemia.

Interfering factors

- Failure to fast overnight and administration of substances that decrease vitamin B_{12} absorption
- Neomycin, metformin, anticonvulsants, and ethanol (possible decrease)
- Oral contraceptives (increase)

VITAMIN C

Vitamin C chemical assay measures plasma levels of vitamin C (ascorbic acid), a water-soluble vitamin required for collagen synthesis and cartilage and bone maintenance. Vitamin C also promotes iron absorption, influences folic acid metabolism, and may be necessary for withstanding the stresses of injury and infection.

This vitamin is present in generous amounts in citrus fruits, berries, tomatoes, raw cabbage, green peppers, green leafy vegetables, and fortified juices. Severe vitamin C deficiency, or scurvy, causes capillary fragility, joint abnormalities, and multisystemic symptoms.

Purpose

- To aid diagnosis of scurvy, scurvylike conditions, and metabolic disorders, such as malnutrition and malabsorption syndromes

Patient preparation

- Explain to the patient that this test detects the amount of vitamin C in the blood.
- Instruct the patient to fast overnight before the test.
- Tell the patient that the test requires a blood sample. Explain who will perform the venipuncture and when.
- Explain to the patient that he may experience discomfort from the needle puncture and the tourniquet.

Procedure and posttest care

- Perform a venipuncture, and collect the sample in a 4.5-ml heparinized tube.
- Apply direct pressure to the venipuncture site until bleeding stops.
- If a hematoma develops at the venipuncture site, apply warm soaks.
- Instruct the patient that he may resume his normal diet discontinued before the test.

Precautions

- Avoid rough handling or excessive agitation of the sample to prevent hemolysis.
- Send the sample to the laboratory immediately.

Reference values

Normal plasma vitamin C levels range from 0.2 to 2 mg/dl (SI, 11 to 114 µmol/L).

Abnormal findings

Values less than 0.3 mg/dl (16.5 µmol/L) indicate significant deficiency. Vitamin C levels diminish during pregnancy to a low point immediately postpartum. Depressed levels occur with infection, fever, and anemia. Severe deficiencies result in scurvy.

High plasma levels can indicate increased ingestion of vitamin C. Excess vitamin C is converted to oxalate, which is excreted in the urine. Excessive concentration of oxalate can produce urinary calculi.

Interfering factors

- Failure to observe pretest dietary restrictions
- Hemolysis due to rough handling of the sample
- Failure to promptly send the sample to the laboratory

VITAMIN D_3

Vitamin D_3 (cholecalciferol), the major form of vitamin D, is endogenously produced in the skin by the sun's ultraviolet rays and occurs naturally in fish liver oils, egg yolks, liver, and butter.

This test, a competitive protein-binding assay, determines serum levels of 25-hydroxycholecalciferol after chromatography has separated it from other vitamin D metabolites and contaminants. It's commonly combined with measurement of serum calcium and alkaline phosphatase levels.

Purpose

- To evaluate skeletal disease, such as rickets and osteomalacia
- To aid diagnosis of hypercalcemia
- To detect vitamin D toxicity
- To monitor therapy with vitamin D_3

Patient preparation

- Explain to the patient that this test measures vitamin D in the body.
- Tell the patient to restrict food or fluids for 8 to 12 hours before the test.
- Tell the patient that the test requires a blood sample. Explain who will perform the venipuncture and when.
- Explain to the patient that he may experience discomfort from the needle puncture and the tourniquet.
- Check for drugs that alter test results (corticosteroids or anticonvulsants). If they must be continued, note this on the laboratory request.

Procedure and posttest care

- Perform a venipuncture, and collect the sample in a 4.5-ml siliconized tube.
- Apply direct pressure to the venipuncture site until bleeding stops.
- If a hematoma develops at the venipuncture site, apply warm soaks.

Precautions

- Handle the sample carefully to prevent hemolysis.

Reference values

The range for serum 25-hydroxycholecalciferol values is from 10 to 60 ng/ml (SI, 25 to 150 nmol/L).

Abnormal findings

Low or undetectable levels may result from vitamin D deficiency, which can cause rickets or osteomalacia. Such deficiency may stem from poor diet, decreased exposure to the sun, or impaired absorption of vitamin D (secondary to hepatobiliary disease, pancreatitis, celiac disease, cystic fibrosis, or gastric or small-bowel resection). Low levels may also be related to various hepatic, parathyroid, and renal diseases that directly affect vitamin D metabolism.

Elevated levels (over 100 ng/ml [SI, > 250 nmol/L]) may indicate toxicity due to excessive self-medication or prolonged therapy. Elevated levels associated with hypercalcemia may be due to hypersensitivity to vitamin D, as in sarcoidosis.

Interfering factors

- Hemolysis due to rough handling of the sample
- Anticonvulsants, isoniazid, mineral oil, corticosteroids, aluminum hydroxide, cholestyramine, and colestipol (possible decrease)

FOLIC ACID

The folic acid test is a quantitative analysis of serum folic acid levels (also called pteroylglutamic acid, folacin, or folate) by radioisotope assay of competitive binding. It's commonly performed concomitantly with measurement of serum vitamin B_{12} levels. Like vitamin B_{12}, folic acid is a water-soluble vitamin that influences hematopoiesis, deoxyribonucleic acid synthesis, and overall body growth.

Normally, diet supplies folic acid in liver, kidney, yeast, fruits, leafy vegetables, fortified breads and cereals, eggs, and milk. Inadequate dietary intake may cause a deficiency, especially during pregnancy. Because of folic acid's vital role in hematopoiesis, the usual indication for this test is a suspected hematologic abnormality.

Purpose

- To aid differential diagnosis of megaloblastic anemia, which may result from folic acid or vitamin B_{12} deficiency
- To assess folate stores in pregnancy

Patient preparation

- Explain to the patient that this test determines the folic acid level in the blood.
- Instruct the patient to fast overnight before the test.
- Tell the patient that the test requires a blood sample. Explain who will perform the venipuncture and when.
- Explain to the patient that he may experience discomfort from the needle puncture and the tourniquet.
- Check the patient's history for drugs that may affect test results, such as phenytoin or pyrimethamine.

Procedure and posttest care

- Perform a venipuncture, and collect the sample in a 4.5-ml tube without additives.
- Apply direct pressure to the venipuncture site until bleeding stops.
- If a hematoma develops at the venipuncture site, apply warm soaks.
- Instruct the patient that he may resume his normal diet.

Precautions

- Handle the sample gently to prevent hemolysis.
- Protect it from light.
- Send the sample to the laboratory immediately.

Reference values

Normally, serum folic acid values are 1.8 to 9 ng/ml (SI, 4 to 20 nmol/L).

Abnormal findings

Low serum levels may indicate hematologic abnormalities, such as anemia (especially megaloblastic anemia), leukopenia, and thrombocytopenia. The Schilling test is usually performed to rule out vitamin B_{12} deficiency, which also causes megaloblastic anemia. Decreased folic acid levels can also result from hypermetabolic states (such as hyperthyroidism), inadequate dietary intake, small-bowel malabsorption syndrome, hepatic or renal diseases, chronic alcoholism, or pregnancy.

Serum levels greater than normal may indicate excessive dietary intake of folic acid or folic acid supplements. Even when taken in large doses, this vitamin is nontoxic.

Interfering factors

- Hemolysis due to rough handling of the sample
- Alcohol; phenytoin; pyrimethamine; anticonvulsants, such as primidone; antineoplastics; antimalarials; and oral contraceptives (possible decrease)

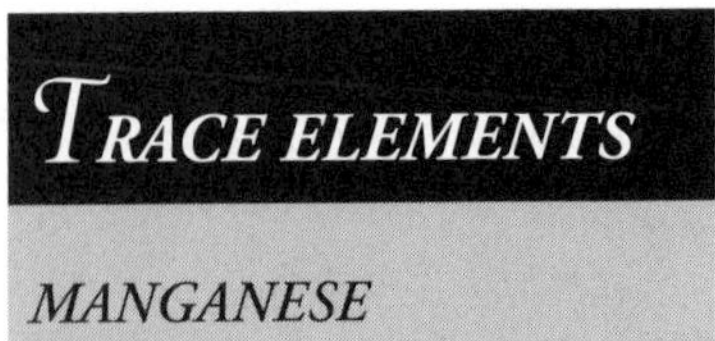

TRACE ELEMENTS

MANGANESE

The manganese test, an analysis by atomic absorption spectroscopy, measures serum levels of manganese, a trace element. Although its function is only partially understood, manganese is known to activate several enzymes—including cholinesterase and arginase—that are essential to metabolism. Dietary sources of manganese include unrefined cereals, green leafy vegetables, and nuts.

Manganese toxicity may result from the inhalation of manganese dust or fumes—a hazard in the steel and dry-cell battery industries—or from ingestion of contaminated water.

Purpose

- To detect manganese toxicity

Patient preparation

- Explain to the patient that this test determines the level of manganese in the blood.
- Inform the patient that he need not restrict food or fluids.
- Tell the patient that the test requires a blood sample. Explain who will perform the venipuncture and when.
- Explain to the patient that he may experience discomfort from the needle puncture and the tourniquet.
- Check the patient's history for medications that may influence serum manganese levels, such as estrogens and glucocorticoids.

Procedure and posttest care

- Perform a venipuncture, and collect the sample in a metal-free collection tube. Laboratories will supply a special kit for this test on request.
- Apply direct pressure to the venipuncture site until bleeding stops.
- If a hematoma develops at the venipuncture site, apply warm soaks.

Precautions

- Handle the sample gently to prevent hemolysis.
- Send the sample to the laboratory immediately.

Reference values

Normally, serum manganese values range from 0.4 to 1.4 µg/ml.

Abnormal findings

Significantly elevated serum levels indicate manganese toxicity, which requires prompt medical attention to prevent central nervous system deterioration. Depressed serum manganese levels may indicate deficient dietary intake, although deficiency hasn't been linked to disease.

Interfering factors

- Failure to use a metal-free collection tube
- Hemolysis due to rough handling of the sample
- High dietary intake of calcium and phosphorus (possible decrease due to interference with intestinal absorption of manganese)
- Estrogen (increase)

■ Glucocorticoids (increase or decrease due to altered distribution of manganese in the body)

ZINC

The zinc test, an analysis by atomic absorption spectroscopy, measures serum zinc levels. An important trace element, zinc is an integral component of more than 80 enzymes and proteins and plays a critical role in enzyme catalytic reactions.

Zinc occurs naturally in water and in most foods; high concentrations are found in meat, seafood, dairy products, whole grains, nuts, and legumes. Zinc deficiency can seriously impair body metabolism, growth, and development.

Purpose

■ To detect zinc deficiency or toxicity

Patient preparation

■ Explain to the patient that this test determines the concentration of zinc in the blood.
■ Inform the patient that he need not restrict food or fluids.
■ Tell the patient that the test requires a blood sample. Explain who will perform the venipuncture and when.
■ Explain to the patient that he may experience discomfort from the needle puncture and the tourniquet.

Procedure and posttest care

■ Perform a venipuncture, and collect a 7- to 10-ml sample in a zinc-free collection tube.
■ Apply direct pressure to the venipuncture site until bleeding stops.
■ If a hematoma develops at the venipuncture site, apply warm soaks.

Precautions

■ Handle the sample gently to prevent hemolysis.
■ Send the sample to the laboratory immediately. Reliable analysis must begin before platelet disintegration can alter test results.

Reference values

Normally, plasma zinc values range from 70 to 120 μg/dl (SI, 10.7 to 18.4 μmol/L).

Abnormal findings

Decreased serum zinc levels may indicate an acquired deficiency (from insufficient dietary intake or due to an underlying disease) or a hereditary deficiency. Markedly depressed levels are common in leukemia and may be related to impaired zinc-dependent enzyme systems. Low serum zinc levels are commonly associated with alcoholic cirrhosis of the liver, myocardial infarction, ileitis, chronic renal failure, rheumatoid arthritis, and anemia (such as hemolytic or sickle cell anemia).

Elevated and potentially toxic serum zinc levels may result from accidental ingestion or industrial exposure.

Interfering factors

■ Failure to use a metal-free collection tube
■ Hemolysis due to rough handling of the sample
■ Delayed transport to the laboratory
■ Time of day and time of last meal (possible increase or decrease)
■ Zinc-chelating agents, such as penicillinase, and corticosteroids (decrease)
■ Estrogens; penicillamine; antineoplastics, such as cisplatin; antimetabolites; and diuretics (possible decrease)

Immunologic tests

IMMUNO-HEMATOLOGY

ABO BLOOD TYPING

ABO blood typing classifies blood according to the presence of major antigens A and B on red blood cell (RBC) surfaces and according to serum antibodies anti-A and anti-B. ABO blood typing using forward and reverse methods is required before transfusion to prevent a lethal reaction.

In forward typing, the patient's RBCs are mixed with anti-A serum, then with anti-B serum; the presence or absence of agglutination determines the blood group. In reverse typing, the results of the forward method are verified by mixing the patient's serum with known group A and group B cells. Blood group determination is confirmed when the results of forward and reverse typing match perfectly.

Purpose

- To establish blood group according to the ABO system
- To check compatibility of donor and recipient blood before transfusion

Patient preparation

- Tell the patient that this test determines his blood group.
- If the patient is scheduled for a transfusion, explain that after his blood group is known, it can be matched with the right donor blood.
- Inform the patient that he need not restrict food or fluids.
- Tell the patient that the test requires a blood sample. Explain who will perform the venipuncture and when.
- Explain to the patient that he may experience discomfort from the needle puncture and the tourniquet.
- Check the patient's history for recent administration of blood, dextran, or I.V. contrast media.

Procedure and posttest care

- Perform a venipuncture, and collect the sample in a 10-ml tube without additives.
- Apply direct pressure to the venipuncture site until bleeding stops.
- If a hematoma develops at the venipuncture site, apply warm soaks.

Precautions

- Label the sample with the patient's name, the hospital or blood bank number, the date, and the phlebotomist's initials.
- Handle the sample gently to prevent hemolysis, and send it to the laboratory immediately with a properly completed laboratory request.

Findings

In forward typing, if agglutination occurs when the patient's RBCs are mixed with anti-A serum, the A antigen is present and the blood is typed A. If agglutination occurs when the patient's RBCs are mixed with anti-B serum, the B antigen is present and the blood is typed B. If agglutination occurs in both mixes, A and B antigens are present and the blood is typed AB. If it doesn't occur in either mix, no antigens are present and the blood is typed O.

In reverse typing, if agglutination occurs when B cells are mixed with the patient's serum, anti-B is present and the blood is typed A. If agglutination occurs when A cells are mixed, anti-A is present and the blood is typed B. If agglutination occurs when A and B cells are mixed, anti-A and anti-B are present and the blood is typed O. If agglutination doesn't occur when A and B cells are mixed, neither anti-A nor anti-B is present and the blood is typed AB.

◆ CLINICAL ALERT *Donor blood may be transfused only when ABO compatibility has been confirmed with the recipient's blood. The transfusion of blood containing either A or B antigens to a recipient whose RBCs lack these antigens can cause a potentially fatal reaction.*

Interfering factors

- Recent administration of dextran or I.V. contrast media, causing cellular aggregation resembling antibody-mediated agglutination
- Hemolysis due to rough handling of the sample
- Blood transfusion or pregnancy in the past 3 months (possibility of lingering antibodies)

RH TYPING

The Rhesus (Rh) system classifies blood by the presence or absence of antigen D, formerly known as Rh_o, on the surface of red blood cells (RBCs). In Rh typing, a patient's RBCs are mixed with serum containing anti-Rh_o(D) antibodies and are observed for agglutination. If agglutination occurs, the Rh_o(D) antigen is present and the patient's blood is typed Rh-positive; if agglutination doesn't occur, the antigen is absent and the patient's blood is typed Rh-negative.

Prospective blood donors are fully tested to exclude the D^u variant, a weak variant of the D antigen, before being classified as having Rh-negative blood. People who have this antigen are considered Rh-positive donors, but are generally transfused as Rh-negative recipients.

Purpose

- To establish blood type according to the Rh system
- To help determine the donor's compatibility before transfusion
- To determine if the patient will require an Rh_o(D) immune globulin injection

Patient preparation

- Explain to the patient that the test determines or verifies blood group to ensure safe transfusion.
- Inform the patient that he need not restrict food or fluids.
- Tell the patient that the test requires a blood sample. Explain who will perform the venipuncture and when.
- Explain to the patient that he may experience discomfort from the needle puncture and the tourniquet.
- Check the patient's history for recent administration of dextran, I.V. contrast media, or drugs that may alter results.

Procedure and posttest care

- Perform a venipuncture, and collect the sample in a 7-ml tube with EDTA.
- Apply direct pressure to the venipuncture site until bleeding stops.
- If a hematoma develops at the venipuncture site, apply warm soaks.
- If necessary, give the pregnant patient a card identifying that she may need to receive Rh_o(D).

Precautions

- Label the sample with the patient's name, the hospital or blood bank number, the date, and the phlebotomist's initials.
- Handle the sample gently and send it to the laboratory immediately.

- If a transfusion is ordered, a transfusion request form must accompany the sample to the laboratory.

Findings

Classified as Rh-positive or Rh-negative, donor blood may be transfused only if it's compatible with the recipient's blood.

If an Rh-negative woman delivers an Rh-positive baby or aborts a fetus whose Rh type is unknown, she should receive an $Rh_o(D)$ injection within 72 hours to prevent hemolytic disease of the neonate in future births.

Interfering factors

- Recent administration of dextran or I.V. contrast media (cellular aggregation resembling antibody-mediated agglutination)
- Methyldopa, cephalosporins, and levodopa (possible false-positive for the D^u antigen due to positive direct antiglobulin [Coombs'] test)

FETAL-MATERNAL ERYTHROCYTE DISTRIBUTION

Some transfer of red blood cells (RBCs) from the fetal to the maternal circulation occurs during most spontaneous or elective abortions and most normal deliveries. Usually, the amount of blood transferred is minimal and has no clinical significance. However, transfer of significant amounts of blood from an Rh-positive fetus to an Rh-negative mother can result in maternal immunization to the D antigen and the development of anti-D antibodies in the maternal circulation.

During a subsequent pregnancy, the maternal immunization subjects an Rh-positive fetus to potentially fatal hemolysis and erythroblastosis. This test measures the number of fetal RBCs in the maternal circulation.

Purpose

- To detect and measure fetal-maternal blood transfer
- To determine the amount of $Rh_o(D)$ immune globulin needed to prevent maternal immunization to the D antigen

Patient preparation

- Explain to the patient that this test determines the amount of fetal blood transferred to the maternal circulation and helps determine the appropriate treatment, if necessary.
- Inform the patient that she need not restrict food or fluids.
- Tell the patient that the test requires a blood sample. Explain who will perform the venipuncture and when.
- Explain to the patient that she may experience slight discomfort from the needle puncture and the tourniquet.
- Check the patient's history for recent administration of dextran, I.V. contrast media, or drugs that may alter results.

Procedure and posttest care

- Perform a venipuncture, and collect the sample in a 7-ml tube with EDTA.
- Apply direct pressure to the venipuncture site until bleeding stops.
- If a hematoma develops at the venipuncture site, apply warm soaks.

Precautions

- Label the sample with the patient's name, the hospital or blood bank number, the date, and the phlebotomist's initials.
- Send the sample to the laboratory immediately with a properly completed laboratory request.

Normal findings

Normal maternal whole blood contains no fetal RBCs.

Abnormal findings

An elevated fetal RBC volume in the maternal circulation necessitates administration of more than one dose of Rh_o(D) immune globulin. The number of vials needed is determined by dividing the calculated fetomaternal hemorrhage by 30 (a single vial of Rh_o(D) immune globulin provides protection against a 30-ml fetomaternal hemorrhage).

Administration of Rh_o(D) immune globulin to an unsensitized Rh-negative mother as soon as possible (no later than 72 hours) after the birth of an Rh-positive infant or after a spontaneous or elective abortion prevents complications in subsequent pregnancies. Most clinicians are now administering Rh_o(D) immune globulin prophylactically at 28 weeks' gestation to women who are Rh-negative but have no detectable Rh antibodies.

The following patients should be screened for Rh isoimmunization or irregular antibodies: all Rh-negative mothers during their first prenatal visit and at 28 weeks' gestation and all Rh-positive mothers with histories of transfusion, a jaundiced infant, stillbirth, cesarean delivery, or induced or spontaneous abortion.

Interfering factors

- Delay of testing for more than 72 hours after sample collection

CROSSMATCHING

Crossmatching (also known as compatibility testing) establishes compatibility or incompatibility of a donor's and a recipient's blood. It's the best antibody detection test available for avoiding lethal transfusion reactions. After the donor's and the recipient's ABO and Rh-factor type are determined, major crossmatching determines compatibility between the donor's red blood cells (RBCs) and the recipient's serum. Minor crossmatching determines compatibility between the donor's serum and the recipient's RBCs. Because the antibody-screening test is routinely performed on all blood donors, minor crossmatching is often omitted.

Because a complete crossmatch may take from 45 minutes to 2 hours, an incomplete (10-minute) crossmatch may be performed in an emergency such as severe blood loss due to trauma. In an emergency, transfusion can begin with limited amounts of group O packed RBCs while crossmatching is completed. Incomplete typing and crossmatching increase the risk of complications. After crossmatching, compatible units of blood are labeled and a compatibility record is completed.

◆ **CLINICAL ALERT** *The most carefully performed crossmatch may not detect all the possible sources of patient-donor incompatibility.*

Purpose

- To serve as the final check for compatibility between a donor's and a recipient's blood

Patient preparation

- Explain to the patient that this test ensures that the blood he receives matches his own to prevent a transfusion reaction.
- Inform the patient that he need not restict food or fluids.

- Tell the patient that the test requires a blood sample. Explain who will perform the venipuncture and when.
- Explain to the patient that he may experience discomfort from the needle puncture and the tourniquet.
- Check the patient's history for recent administration of blood, dextran, or I.V. contrast media.

Procedure and posttest care

- Perform a venipuncture, and collect the sample in a 10-ml tube without additives or EDTA. ABO typing, Rh typing, and crossmatching are all done together.
- Apply direct pressure to the venipuncture site until bleeding stops.
- If a hematoma develops at the venipuncture site, apply warm soaks.

Precautions

- Handle the sample gently to prevent hemolysis, which can mask hemolysis of the donor's RBCs.
- Label the sample with the patient's name, the hospital or blood bank number, the date, and the phlebotomist's initials.
- Indicate on the laboratory request the amount and type of blood component needed.
- Send the sample to the laboratory immediately.
- If more than 72 hours have elapsed since an earlier transfusion, previously crossmatched donor blood must be recrossmatched with a new recipient serum sample to detect newly acquired incompatibilities before transfusion.
- If the patient is scheduled for surgery and has received blood during the past 3 months, his blood needs to be crossmatched again if his surgery is rescheduled to detect recently acquired incompatibilities.

Normal findings

Absence of agglutination indicates compatibility between the donor's and the recipient's blood, which means that the transfusion of donor blood can proceed. Note that this doesn't guarantee a safe transfusion.

Abnormal findings

A positive crossmatch indicates incompatibility between the donor's blood and the recipient's blood, which means that the donor's blood can't be transfused to the recipient. The sign of a positive crossmatch is agglutination, or clumping, when the donor's RBCs and the recipient's serum are correctly mixed and incubated. Agglutination indicates an undesirable antigen-antibody reaction. The donor's blood must be withheld and the crossmatch continued to determine the cause of the incompatibility and identify the antibody.

Interfering factors

- Recent administration of dextran or I.V. contrast media (causing cellular aggregation resembling antibody-mediated agglutination)
- Previous blood transfusion (possibility of new antibodies to donor blood)
- Hemolysis due to rough handling of the sample
- Delay of testing for more than 72 hours after sample collection

DIRECT ANTIGLOBULIN

The direct antiglobulin test (or direct Coombs' test) detects immunoglobulins (antibodies) on the surface of red blood cells (RBCs). These immunoglobulins coat RBCs when they become sensitized to an antigen such as the Rh factor.

In this test, antiglobulin (Coombs') serum added to saline-washed RBCs results in agglutination if immunoglobulins or complement is present. This test is "direct" because it requires only one step — the addition of Coombs' serum to washed cells.

Purpose

- To diagnose hemolytic disease of the neonate (HDN)
- To investigate hemolytic transfusion reactions
- To aid differential diagnosis of hemolytic anemias, which may be congenital or may result from an autoimmune reaction or use of certain drugs

Patient preparation

- If the patient is a neonate, explain to the parents that this test helps diagnose HDN.
- If the patient is suspected of having hemolytic anemia, explain that the test determines whether the condition results from an abnormality in the body's immune system, the use of certain drugs, or some unknown cause.
- Inform the adult patient that he need not restrict food or fluids.
- Tell the patient (or a neonate's parents) that the test requires a blood sample. Explain who will perform the venipuncture and when.
- Explain to the patient that he may experience slight discomfort from the needle puncture and the tourniquet.
- Withhold medications that may interfere with test results, including quinidine, methyldopa, cephalosporins, sulfonamides, chlorpromazine, diphenylhydantoin, ethosuximide, hydralazine, levodopa, mefenamic acid, melphalan, penicillin, procainamide, rifampin, streptomycin, tetracyclines, and isoniazid, as ordered.

Procedure and posttest care

- For an adult, perform a venipuncture, and collect the sample in two 5-ml tubes with EDTA.
- For a neonate, draw 5 ml of cord blood into a tube with EDTA or additives, as ordered, after the cord is clamped and cut.
- Apply direct pressure to the venipuncture site until bleeding stops.
- If a hematoma develops at the venipuncture site, apply warm soaks.
- Instruct the patient that he may resume his usual medications discontinued before the test as ordered.
- Tell the patient or the parents of the neonate with HDN that further tests will be necessary to monitor anemia.

Precautions

- Handle the sample gently to prevent hemolysis.
- Label the sample with the patient's full name, the facility or blood bank number, the date, and the phlebotomist's initials.
- Send the sample to the laboratory immediately.

Normal findings

A negative test, in which neither antibodies nor complement appears on the RBCs, is normal.

Abnormal findings

A positive test on umbilical cord blood indicates that maternal antibodies have crossed the placenta and coated fetal RBCs, causing HDN. Transfusion of compatible blood lacking the antigens to these maternal antibodies may be necessary to prevent anemia.

In other patients, a positive test result may indicate hemolytic anemia and help differentiate between autoimmune and secondary hemolytic anemia, which can be drug-induced or associated with an underlying disease. A positive test can also indicate sepsis.

A weakly positive test may suggest a transfusion reaction in which the patient's antibodies react with transfused RBCs containing the corresponding antigen.

Interfering factors

- Hemolysis due to rough handling of the sample
- Quinidine, methyldopa, cephalosporins, sulfonamides, chlorpromazine, diphenylhydantoin, dipyrone, ethosuximide, hydralazine, levodopa, mefenamic acid, melphalan, penicillin, procainamide, rifampin, streptomycin, tetracyclines, and isoniazid (positive test results, possibly due to immune hemolysis)

ANTIBODY SCREENING

Also called the indirect Coombs' test, the antibody screening test detects unexpected circulating antibodies in the patient's serum. After incubating the serum with group O red blood cells (RBCs), which are unaffected by anti-A or anti-B antibodies, an antiglobulin (Coombs') serum is added. Agglutination occurs if the patient's serum contains an antibody to one or more antigens on the red cells.

The antibody screening test detects 95% to 99% of the circulating antibodies. After this screening procedure detects them, the antibody identification test can determine the specific identity of the antibodies present.

Purpose

- To detect unexpected circulating antibodies to RBC antigens in the recipient's or donor's serum before transfusion
- To determine the presence of anti-D antibody in maternal blood
- To evaluate the need for Rh_0(D) immune globulin
- To aid diagnosis of acquired hemolytic anemia

Patient preparation

- Explain to the prospective blood recipient that the antibody screening test helps evaluate the possibility of a transfusion reaction or to determine if fetal antibodies are in her blood and if treatment is needed, as appropriate.
- If the test is being performed because the patient is anemic, explain to him that it helps identify the specific type of anemia.
- Inform the patient that he need not restrict food or fluids.
- Tell the patient that the test requires a blood sample. Explain who will perform the venipuncture and when.
- Explain to the patient that he may experience discomfort from the needle puncture and the tourniquet.
- Check the patient's history for recent administration of blood, dextran, or I.V. contrast media.

Procedure and posttest care

- Perform a venipuncture, and collect the sample in two 10-ml tubes. If the antibody screen is positive, antibody identification is performed on the blood.
- Apply direct pressure to the venipuncture site until bleeding stops.
- If a hematoma develops at the venipuncture site, apply warm soaks.

Precautions

- Handle the sample gently to prevent hemolysis.
- Label the sample with the patient's name, the hospital or blood bank number, the date, and the phlebotomist's initials. Be sure to include on the labo-

ratory request the patient's diagnosis and pregnancy status, history of transfusions, and current drug therapy.

- Send the sample to the laboratory immediately.

Normal findings

Normally, agglutination doesn't occur, indicating that the patient's serum contains no circulating antibodies other than anti-A or anti-B.

Abnormal findings

A positive result indicates the presence of unexpected circulating antibodies to RBC antigens. Such a reaction demonstrates donor and recipient incompatibility.

A positive result in a pregnant patient with Rh-negative blood may indicate the presence of antibodies to the Rh factor from an earlier transfusion with incompatible blood or from a previous pregnancy with an Rh-positive fetus.

A positive result indicates that the fetus may develop hemolytic disease of the neonate. As a result, repeated testing throughout the pregnancy is necessary to evaluate progressive development of circulating antibody levels.

Interfering factors

- Previous administration of dextran or I.V. contrast media (causing aggregation resembling agglutination)
- Hemolysis due to rough handling of the sample
- Blood transfusion or pregnancy within the past 3 months (possible presence of antibodies)

LEUKOAGGLUTININS

This test detects leukoagglutinins (also known as white blood cell [WBC] antibodies or HLA antibodies) antibodies that react with WBCs and may cause a transfusion reaction. These antibodies usually develop after exposure to foreign WBCs through transfusions, pregnancies, and allografts.

If a blood recipient has these antibodies, a febrile nonhemolytic reaction may occur 1 to 4 hours after the start of whole blood, red blood cell, platelet, or granulocyte transfusion. This nonhemolytic reaction (marked by fever and severe chills, sometimes with nausea, headache, and transient hypertension) must be distinguished from a true hemolytic reaction before further transfusion can proceed.

The technique used to detect leukoagglutinins is the microlymphocytotoxicity test. In this test, the recipient serum is tested against donor lymphocytes or against a panel of lymphocytes of known HLA phenotype. The antibodies in the recipient serum bind to the corresponding antigen present in the lymphocytes and cause cell membrane injury when the complement is added to the test system. Cell injury is detected by examining the lymphocytes under a microscope. If the lymphocytes don't absorb the added dye, the test is negative. If the lymphocytes show dye uptake, the test is positive.

Purpose

- To detect leukoagglutinins in blood recipients who develop transfusion reactions, thus differentiating between hemolytic and febrile nonhemolytic transfusion reactions

- To detect leukoagglutinins in blood donors after transfusion of donor blood causes a reaction

Patient preparation

- Explain to the patient that this test helps determine the cause of his transfusion reaction.
- Tell the patient that the test requires a blood sample. Explain who will perform the venipuncture and when.
- Explain to the patient that he may experience discomfort from the needle puncture and the tourniquet.
- Check the patient's history for recent administration of blood, dextran, or I.V. contrast media and note this on the laboratory request.

Procedure and posttest care

- Perform a venipuncture, and collect a sample in a 10-ml clot-activator tube. The laboratory requires 3 to 4 ml of serum for testing.
- Apply direct pressure to the venipuncture site until bleeding stops.
- If a hematoma develops at the venipuncture site, apply warm soaks.
- If a transfusion recipient has a positive leukoagglutinin test, continued transfusions require premedication with acetaminophen 1 to 2 hours before the transfusion, specially prepared leukocyte-poor blood, or use of leukocyte removal blood filters to prevent further reactions.

Precautions

- Label the sample with the patient's name, the hospital or blood bank number, the date, and the phlebotomist's initials.
- Be sure to include on the laboratory request the patient's suspected diagnosis and history of blood transfusions, pregnancies, and drug therapy.
- Note that tests for these antibodies aren't useful in deciding which patients should receive leukocyte-poor blood components; the decision must be based on clinical experience.

Normal findings

Normally, test results are negative. Agglutination doesn't occur because the serum contains no antibodies.

Abnormal findings

A positive result in a transfusion recipient indicates the presence of leukoagglutinins in his blood, identifying his transfusion reaction as a febrile nonhemolytic reaction to these antibodies.

Recipients who test positive for HLA antibodies may need HLA-matched platelets to control bleeding episodes caused by a thrombocytopenia.

Interfering factors

None known

GENERAL CELLULAR FUNCTION

T- AND B-LYMPHOCYTE ASSAYS

Lymphocytes — key cells in the immune system — have the capacity to recognize antigens through special receptors found on their surfaces.

Cell separation is used to isolate lymphocytes from other cellular blood elements. This procedure recovers about 80% of the lymphocytes, but doesn't differentiate between T cells and B cells. The percentage of T cells and B cells is determined by attaching a label or marker and using different identification techniques.

Null cells possess Fc receptors but no other detectable surface markers and have no diagnostic significance. The number of null cells is usually determined by subtracting the sum of T cells and B cells from total lymphocytes.

Purpose

- To aid diagnosis of primary and secondary immunodeficiency diseases
- To distinguish benign from malignant lymphocytic proliferative diseases
- To monitor response to therapy

Patient preparation

- Explain to the patient that this test measures certain white blood cells.
- Tell the patient that the test requires a blood sample. Explain who will perform the venipuncture and when.
- Explain to the patient that he may experience discomfort from the needle puncture and the tourniquet.

Procedure and posttest care

- Perform a venipuncture, and collect the sample in a 7-ml heparinized tube.
- Because many patients with T-cell and B-cell changes have a compromised immune system, keep the venipuncture site clean and dry. Assess site for changes and report promptly.
- Apply direct pressure to the venipuncture site until bleeding stops.
- If a hematoma develops at the venipuncture site, apply warm soaks.

Precautions

- Completely fill the collection tube, and invert it gently several times to adequately mix the sample and anticoagulant.
- Send the sample to the laboratory immediately to ensure viable lymphocytes.
- If antilymphocyte antibodies are suspected, as in autoimmune disease, notify the laboratory.

Reference values

T-cell and B-cell assays are being standardized, and values may differ from one laboratory to another, depending on test technique.

- Percentage of total lymphocytes:
  - T cells: 68% to 75%
  - B cells: 10% to 20%
  - Null cells: 5% to 20%
- Total lymphocyte count: 1,500 to 3,000/µl
- T-cell count: 1,400 to 2,700/µl
- B-cell count: 270 to 640/µl

These counts are higher in children.

Normal T-cell and B-cell counts don't necessarily ensure a competent immune system. In autoimmune diseases, such as systemic lupus erythematosus and rheumatoid arthritis, T cells and B cells, although present in normal numbers, may not be functionally competent.

Abnormal findings

An abnormal T-cell or B-cell count suggests but doesn't confirm specific diseases. The B-cell count is elevated in chronic lymphocytic leukemia, multiple myeloma, Waldenström's macroglobulinemia, and DiGeorge syndrome.

B cells decrease in acute lymphocytic leukemia and in certain congenital or acquired immunoglobulin deficiency diseases. In other immunoglobulin deficiency diseases, especially if only one immunoglobulin class is deficient, the B-cell count remains normal.

The T-cell count rises occasionally in infectious mononucleosis; it rises more often in multiple myeloma and acute lymphocytic leukemia.

The T-cell count decreases in congenital T-cell deficiency diseases, such as DiGeorge, Nezelof, and Wiskott-Aldrich syndromes, and in certain B-cell proliferative disorders, such as chronic lymphocytic leukemia,

Waldenström's macroglobulinemia, and acquired immunodeficiency syndrome.

Interfering factors

- Exposing the sample to temperature extremes, or failure to use the proper collection tube, to mix the sample adequately, or to send the sample to the laboratory
- Changes in health status, from the effects of stress, surgery, chemotherapy, steroid or immunosuppressive therapy, or radiography (possible rapid change in T- and B-cell counts)
- Immunoglobulins such as autologous antilymphocyte antibodies that sometimes occur in autoimmune disease (possible change in results)

LYMPHOCYTE TRANSFORMATION

Transformation tests evaluate lymphocyte competency without injection of antigens into the patient's skin. These in vitro tests eliminate the risk of adverse effects, but can still accurately assess the ability of lymphocytes to proliferate and to recognize and respond to antigens.

The mitogen assay evaluates the mitotic response of T lymphocytes and B lymphocytes to a foreign antigen. The antigen assay uses specific substances, such as purified protein derivative, *Candida*, mumps, tetanus toxoid, and streptokinase, to stimulate lymphocyte transformation. The mixed lymphocyte culture (MLC) assay is useful in matching transplant recipients and donors and in testing immunocompetence. (See *Lymphocyte marker assays.*)

The neutrophils' ability to engulf and destroy bacteria and foreign particles can also be determined. (See *Neutrophil function tests,* page 274.)

Purpose

- To assess and monitor genetic and acquired immunodeficiency states
- To provide histocompatibility typing of tissue transplant recipients and donors
- To detect if a patient has been exposed to various pathogens such as those that cause malaria, hepatitis, and mycoplasmal pneumonia

Patient preparation

- Explain to the patient that this test evaluates lymphocyte function, which is crucial to the immune system.
- Inform the patient that the test monitors his response to therapy, if appropriate.
- For histocompatibility typing, explain that this test helps determine the best match for a transplant.
- Inform the patient that he need not restrict food or fluids.
- Tell the patient that the test requires a blood sample. Explain who will perform the venipuncture and when.
- Explain to the patient that he may experience discomfort from the needle puncture and the tourniquet.
- If a radioisotope scan is scheduled, make sure the serum sample for this test is drawn first.

Procedure and posttest care

- Perform a venipuncture. If the patient is an adult, collect the sample in a 7-ml heparinized tube; for a child, use a 5-ml heparinized tube.
- Because many of these patients may have a compromised immune system, take special care to keep the venipuncture site clean and dry.
- Apply direct pressure to the venipuncture site until bleeding stops.

Lymphocyte marker assays

A normal immune response requires a balance between the regulatory activities of several interacting cell types, most notably T-helper and T-suppressor cells. By using highly specific monoclonal antibodies, levels of lymphocyte differentiation can be defined, and normal and malignant cell populations can be analyzed. Direct and indirect immunofluorescence, microcytotoxicity, and immunoperoxidase immunoassay techniques are used most frequently: They use an anticoagulated blood sample combined with monoclonal antibodies that react with specific T- and B-cell markers. The chart below lists some commonly ordered lymphocyte marker assays and their indications.

LYMPHOCYTE MARKER	PURPOSE
Pan T-cell marker (CD3)	◆ To measure mature T cells in immune dysfunction
T-helper/inducer subset marker (CD4)	◆ To identify and characterize the proportion of T-helper cells in autoimmune or immunoregulatory disorders ◆ To detect immunodeficiency disorders such as acquired immunodeficiency syndrome ◆ To differentiate T-cell acute lymphoblastic leukemia from T-cell lymphomas and other lymphoproliferative disorders
T-suppressor/cytotoxic subset marker (CD8)	◆ To identify and characterize the proportion of T-suppressor cells in autoimmune and immunoregulatory disorders ◆ To characterize lymphoproliferative disorders
T-cell/E-Rosette receptor (CD2)	◆ To differentiate lymphoproliferative disorders of T-cell origin, such as T-cell lymphocytic leukemia and lymphoblastic lymphoma, from those of non-T-cell origin
Pan-B (B-1) marker (CD20)	◆ To differentiate lymphoproliferative disorders of B-cell origin, such as B-cell chronic lymphocytic leukemia, from those of T-cell origin
Pan-B (BA-1) marker (CD19)	◆ To identify B-cell lymphoproliferative disorders such as B-cell chronic lymphocytic leukemia
CALLA (common acute lymphocytic leukemia antigen) marker, CD10	◆ To identify bone marrow regeneration ◆ To identify non-T-cell acute lymphocytic leukemia
Lymphocyte subset panel (CD3/CD4/CD8/CD19)	◆ To evaluate immunodeficiencies ◆ To identify immunoregulation associated with autoimmune disorders ◆ To characterize lymphoid neoplasms
Lymphocytic leukemia marker panel (CD3/CD4/CD8/CD19/CD10)	◆ To characterize lymphocytic leukemias as T, B, non-T, or non-B, regardless of the stage of differentiation of the malignant cells

Neutrophil function tests

Neutrophil function tests may reveal the inability of neutrophils to kill a target bacterial or to migrate to the bacterial site (chemotaxis). The killing ability can be evaluated by the nitroblue tetrazolium (NBT) test, which relies on neutrophil generation of bactericidal enzymes and toxins during killing. This action results in increased oxygen consumption and glucose metabolism, which reduces colorless NBT to blue formazan. The reduced dye is then extracted with pyridine and measured photometrically; the level of reduction indicates phagocytic activity.

Neutrophil killing activity can also be evaluated by noting the neutrophil's chemiluminescence, its ability to emit light. After a neutrophil phagocytizes a microorganism, oxygen-containing substances form within phagocytic vacuoles. As the cell is stimulated, it emits light in proportion to the amount of oxygen-containing substances that are formed, providing an indirect measurement of phagocytosis.

Chemotaxis can be assessed in vitro by placing bacteria in the lower half of a two-part chamber and phagocytic neutrophils in the upper half. After incubation, migrating cells are counted microscopically and compared with standard values.

- If a hematoma develops at the venipuncture site, apply warm soaks.

Precautions

- Completely fill the collection tube, and invert it gently several times to mix the sample and anticoagulant.
- Send the sample to the laboratory immediately.
- Don't refrigerate or freeze the specimen.

Reference values

Results depend on the mitogens used. Reference ranges accompany test results. In general, a positive test is normal; a negative test indicates deficiency.

Abnormal findings

In the mitogen and antigen assays, a low stimulation index or unresponsiveness indicates a depressed or defective immune system. Serial testing can be performed to monitor the effectiveness of therapy in a patient with an immunodeficiency disease.

In the MLC test, the stimulation index is a measure of compatibility. A high index indicates poor compatibility. Conversely, a low stimulation index indicates good compatibility.

A high stimulation index, in response to the relevant pathogen, can also demonstrate exposure to malaria, hepatitis, mycoplasmal pneumonia, periodontal disease, and certain viral infections in patients who no longer have detectable serum antibodies.

Interfering factors

- Pregnancy or use of oral contraceptives, depressing lymphocyte response to phytohemagglutinin (low stimulation index)
- Chemotherapy (unless pretherapy baseline values are available for comparison)
- Radioisotope scan within 1 week before the test
- Failure to send the sample to the laboratory immediately

TERMINAL DEOXYNUCLEOTIDYL TRANSFERASE

Using indirect immunofluorescence, the terminal deoxynucleotidyl transferase test measures levels of terminal deoxynucleotidyl transferase (TdT). The TdT test differentiates certain types of leukemias and lymphomas marked by primitive cells that can't be identified by histology alone.

Purpose

- To help differentiate acute lymphocytic leukemia (ALL) from acute nonlymphocytic leukemia
- To help differentiate lymphoblastic lymphomas from malignant lymphomas
- To monitor response to therapy, help determine the patient's prognosis, or obtain early diagnosis of a relapse

Patient preparation

- Explain to the patient that this test detects an enzyme that can help classify tissue origin.

For a blood test:

- Tell the patient to fast for 12 to 14 hours before the test.
- Tell the patient that the test requires a blood sample. Explain who will perform the venipuncture and when.
- Explain to the patient that he may experience discomfort from the needle puncture and the tourniquet.

For bone marrow aspiration:

- Describe the procedure to the patient and answer his questions.
- Inform the patient that he need not restrict food or fluids.
- Tell the patient who will perform the biopsy and where, and that it usually takes 5 to 10 minutes.
- Make sure the patient or a responsible family member has signed an informed consent form.
- Administer a mild sedative 1 hour before the test, as ordered.
- Check the patient's history for hypersensitivity to the local anesthetic.
- After checking with the physician, tell the patient which bone will be the biopsy site.
- Inform the patient that he'll receive a local anesthetic, but will feel pressure on insertion of the biopsy needle and a brief, pulling pain when the marrow is withdrawn.

Procedure and posttest care

- If a blood test is scheduled, perform a venipuncture, and collect the sample in one 10-ml heparinized blood tube and one tube with EDTA.
- If assisting with bone marrow aspiration, inject 1 ml of bone marrow into a 7-ml heparinized tube and dilute it with 5 ml of normal saline solution, or submit four air-dried marrow smears.
- Send the sample to the laboratory immediately.
- Because the patient may have a compromised immune system, take special care to keep the venipuncture site clean and dry.
- Because a patient with leukemia may bleed excessively, apply pressure to the venipuncture site until bleeding stops.
- If a hematoma develops at the venipuncture site, apply warm soaks.
- Check the bone marrow aspiration site for bleeding and inflammation, and observe the patient for signs of hemorrhage and infection.

Precautions

- Before performing the venipuncture, contact the laboratory to ensure that it can process the sample and to find out how much blood to draw.

- Because the patient with leukemia is more susceptible to infection, clean the skin thoroughly before performing the venipuncture.
- Send the sample to the laboratory immediately.

Reference values

TdT is present in less than 2% of marrow cells and is undetectable in normal peripheral blood.

Abnormal findings

Positive cells are present in more than 90% of patients with ALL, in 33% of patients with chronic myelogenous leukemia in blast crisis, and in 5% of patients with nonlymphocytic leukemias. TdT-positive cells are absent in patients with ALL who are in remission.

Interfering factors

- Failure to obtain a representative sample during bone marrow aspiration
- Performing bone marrow aspiration on a child because of presence of TdT-positive bone marrow during proliferation of prelymphocytes (possible false-positive)
- Bone marrow regeneration, idiopathic thrombocytopenic purpura, and neuroblastoma, causing TdT-positive bone marrow (possible false-positive)
- Failure to send the sample to the laboratory immediately

GENERAL HUMORAL FUNCTION

QUANTITATIVE IMMUNOGLOBULINS G, A, AND M

Immunoglobulins, proteins that can function as specific antibodies in response to antigen stimulation, are responsible for the humoral aspects of immunity. Deviations from normal immunoglobulin percentages are characteristic in many immune disorders, including cancer, hepatic disorders, rheumatoid arthritis, and systemic lupus erythematosus.

Immunoelectrophoresis identifies immunoglobulin (Ig) G, IgA, and IgM in a serum sample; the level of each is measured by radial immunodiffusion or nephelometry. Some laboratories detect immunoglobulin by indirect immuno fluorescence and radioimmunoassay.

Purpose

- To diagnose paraproteinemias, such as multiple myeloma and Waldenström's macroglobulinemia
- To detect hypogammaglobulinemia and hypergammaglobulinemia as well as nonimmunologic diseases, such as cirrhosis and hepatitis, that are associated with abnormally high immunoglobulin levels
- To assess the effectiveness of chemotherapy and radiation therapy

Patient preparation

- Explain to the patient that this test measures antibody levels.

- If appropriate, tell the patient that the test evaluates the effectiveness of treatment.
- Instruct the patient to restrict food and fluids, except for water, for 12 to 14 hours before the test.
- Tell the patient that the test requires a blood sample. Explain who will perform the venipuncture and when.
- Explain to the patient that he may experience discomfort from the needle puncture and the tourniquet.
- Check the patient's history for drugs that may affect test results.
- Be aware that alcohol or narcotic abuse may affect results.

Procedure and posttest care

- Perform a venipuncture, and collect the sample in a 7-ml clot-activator tube.
- Advise the patient with abnormally low immunoglobulin levels (especially of IgG or IgM) to protect himself against bacterial infection. When caring for such a patient, watch for signs of infection, such as fever, chills, rash, and skin ulcers.
- Instruct the patient with abnormally high immunoglobulin levels and symptoms of monoclonal gammopathies to report bone pain and tenderness. Such a patient has numerous antibody-producing malignant plasma cells in bone marrow, which hamper production of other blood components. Watch for signs of hypercalcemia, renal failure, and spontaneous pathologic fractures.
- Apply direct pressure to the venipuncture site until bleeding stops.
- If a hematoma develops at the venipuncture site, apply warm soaks.
- Instruct the patient that he may resume his usual diet and medications discontinued before the test as ordered.

Precautions

- Send the sample to the laboratory immediately to prevent immunoglobulin deterioration.

Reference values

When using nephelometry, serum immunoglobulin levels for adults range as follows:

- IgG: 800 to 1800 mg/dl (SI, 8 to 18 g/L)
- IgA: 100 to 400 mg/dl (SI, 1 to 4 g/L)
- IgM: 55 to 150 mg/dl (SI, 0.55 to 1.5 g/L).

Abnormal findings

The accompanying chart shows IgG, IgA, and IgM levels in various disorders. (See *Serum immunoglobulin levels in various disorders,* page 278.) In congenital and acquired hypogammaglobulinemias, myelomas, and macroglobulinemia, the findings confirm the diagnosis. In hepatic and autoimmune diseases, leukemias, and lymphomas, such findings are less important, but they can support the diagnosis based on other tests, such as biopsies and white blood cell differential, and on the physical examination.

Interfering factors

- Radiation therapy or chemotherapy (possible decrease due to suppressive effects on bone marrow)
- Aminophenazone, anticonvulsants, asparaginase, hydralazine, hydantoin derivatives, oral contraceptives, and phenylbutazone (possible increase)
- Methotrexate and severe hypersensitivity to bacille Calmette-Guérin vaccine (possible decrease)
- Dextrans and methylprednisolone (decrease in IgM levels)
- Dextrans and high doses of methylprednisolone and phenytoin (decrease in IgG and IgA levels)
- Methadone (increase in IgA levels)

Serum immunoglobulin levels in various disorders

DISORDER	IgG	IgA	IgM
Immunoglobulin disorders			
Lymphoid aplasia	D	D	D
Agammaglobulinemia	D	D	D
Type I dysgammaglobulinemia (selective immunoglobulin [Ig] G and IgA deficiency)	D	D	N or I
Type II dysgammaglobulinemia (absent IgA and IgM)	N	D	D
IgA globulinemia	N	D	N
Ataxia-telangiectasia	N	D	N
Multiple myeloma, macroglobulinemia, lymphomas			
Heavy chain disease (Franklin's disease)	D	D	D
IgG myeloma	I	D	D
IgA myeloma	D	I	D
Macroglobulinemia	D	D	I
Acute lymphocytic leukemia	N	D	N
Chronic lymphocytic leukemia	D	D	D
Acute myelocytic leukemia	N	N	N
Chronic myelocytic leukemia	N	D	N
Hodgkin's disease	N	N	N
Hepatic disorders			
Hepatitis	I	I	I
Laënnec's cirrhosis	I	I	N
Biliary cirrhosis	N	N	I
Hepatoma	N	N	D
Other disorders			
Rheumatoid arthritis	I	I	I
Systemic lupus erythematosus	I	I	I
Nephrotic syndrome	D	D	N
Trypanosomiasis	N	N	I
Pulmonary tuberculosis	I	N	N

KEY: N = normal; I = increased; D = decreased

IMMUNE COMPLEX ASSAYS

When immune complexes are produced faster than they can be cleared by the lymphoreticular system, immune complex disease, such as postinfectious syndromes, serum sickness, drug sensitivity, rheumatoid arthritis, and systemic lupus erythematosus (SLE), may occur.

Histologic examination of tissue obtained by biopsy and the use of fluorescence or peroxidase staining with antibodies specific for immunologic types generally detect immune complexes. However, tissue biopsies can't provide information about titers of complexes still in circulation; therefore, serum assays, which detect circulating immune complexes indirectly, may be required. Because of the inherent variability of these complexes, several serum test methods may be appropriate.

Most immune complex assays haven't been standardized, so more than one test may be required to achieve accurate results.

Purpose

- To demonstrate circulating immune complexes in serum
- To monitor response to therapy
- To estimate severity of disease

Patient preparation

- Explain to the patient that these tests help evaluate his immune system.
- Inform the patient that the test will be repeated to monitor his response to therapy, if appropriate.
- Inform the patient that he need not restrict food or fluids.
- Tell the patient that the test requires a blood sample. Explain who will perform the venipuncture and when.
- Explain to the patient that he may experience discomfort from the needle puncture and the tourniquet.
- If the patient is scheduled for C1q assay (a component of C1), check his history for recent heparin therapy and report such therapy to the laboratory.

Procedure and posttest care

- Perform a venipuncture, and collect the sample in a 7-ml clot-activator tube.
- Because many patients with immune complexes have a compromised immune system, keep the venipuncture site clean and dry.
- Apply direct pressure to the venipuncture site until bleeding stops.
- If a hematoma develops at the venipuncture site, apply warm soaks.

Precautions

- Send the sample to the laboratory immediately to prevent deterioration of immune complexes.

Normal findings

Normally, immune complexes aren't detectable in serum.

Abnormal findings

The presence of detectable immune complexes in serum has etiologic importance in many autoimmune diseases, such as SLE and rheumatoid arthritis. For definitive diagnosis, the presence of these complexes must be considered with the results of other studies. For example, in SLE, immune complexes are associated with high titers of antinuclear antibodies and circulating antinative deoxyribonucleic acid antibodies.

Because of their filtering function, renal glomeruli seem most vulnerable to immune complex deposition, although blood vessel walls and choroid plexuses (vascular folds in the ventricles of the brain) can be affected. Renal biopsy to detect immune complexes can provide conclusive evidence for immune complex (type III) glomerulonephritis, differentiating it from other types of glomerulonephritis.

Interfering factors

- Failure to send the sample to the laboratory immediately
- Presence of cryoglobulins in the serum
- Inability to standardize rheumatoid factor inhibition tests and platelet aggregation assays

RAJI CELL ASSAY

Raji cell assay, which is performed to detect the presence of circulating immune complexes, studies the Raji lymphoblastoid cell line. Identifying these cells, which have receptors for immunoglobulin G complement, helps to evaluate autoimmune disease.

Purpose

- To detect circulating immune complexes
- To aid the study of autoimmune disease

Patient preparation

- Explain to the patient the purpose of the test, as appropriate.
- Tell the patient that the test requires a blood sample. Explain who will perform the venipuncture and when.
- Explain to the patient that he may experience discomfort from the needle puncture and the tourniquet.

Procedure and posttest care

- Perform a venipuncture, collect a sample in a clot-activator tube, and promptly send it to the laboratory.
- Apply direct pressure to the venipuncture site until bleeding stops.
- If a hematoma develops at the venipuncture site, apply warm soaks.

Precautions

- Handle the sample gently to prevent hemolysis.

Reference values

Normally Raji cells aren't present.

Abnormal findings

A positive Raji cell assay can detect immune complexes, including those found in viral, microbial, and parasitic infections; metastasis; autoimmune disorders; and drug reactions. This test may also detect immune complexes associated with celiac disease, cirrhosis of the liver, Crohn's disease, cryoglobulinemia, dermatitis herpetiformis, sickle cell anemia, and ulcerative colitis.

Interfering factors

- Hemolysis due to rough handling of the sample

COMPLEMENT ASSAYS

Complement is a collective term for a system of at least 15 serum proteins designed to destroy foreign cells and help remove foreign materials. Complement deficiency can increase susceptibility to infection and predispose patients to other diseases. Complement assays are indicated in patients with known or suspected immunomediated disease or repeatedly abnormal response to infection. Various laboratory methods are used to evaluate and measure total complement and its components; hemolytic assay, laser nephelometry, and radial immunodiffusion are the most common.

Although complement assays provide valuable information about the patient's immune system, the results must be considered in light of serum immunoglobulin and autoantibody tests for a definitive diagnosis of immunomediated disease or abnormal response to infection.

Purpose

■ To help detect immunomediated disease and genetic complement deficiency
■ To monitor effectiveness of therapy

Patient preparation

■ Explain to the patient that this test measures a group of proteins that fight infection.
■ Inform the patient that he need not restrict food or fluids.
■ Tell the patient that the test requires a blood sample. Explain who will perform the venipuncture and when.
■ Explain to the patient that he may experience discomfort from the needle puncture and the tourniquet.
■ If the patient is scheduled for C1q assay, check his history for recent heparin therapy. Report such therapy to the laboratory.

Procedure and posttest care

■ Perform a venipuncture, and collect the sample in a 7-ml tube without additives.
■ Because many patients with complement defects have a compromised immune system, keep the venipuncture site clean and dry.
■ Apply direct pressure to the venipuncture site until bleeding stops.
■ If a hematoma develops at the venipuncture site, apply warm soaks.

Precautions

■ Handle the sample gently to prevent hemolysis.
■ Send it to the laboratory immediately because complement is heat labile and deteriorates rapidly.

Reference values

Normal values for complement range as follows:
■ total complement: 25 to 110 U/ml (SI, 0.25 to 1.1 g/L)
■ C3: 70 to 150 mg/dl (SI, 0.7 to 1.5 g/L)
■ C4: 15 to 45 mg/dl (SI, 0.15 to 0.45 g/L).

Abnormal findings

Complement abnormalities may be genetic or acquired; acquired abnormalities are most common. Depressed total complement levels (which are clinically more significant than elevations) may result from excessive formation of antigen-antibody complexes, insufficient synthesis of complement, inhibitor formation, or increased complement catabolism and are characteristic in such conditions as systemic lupus erythematosus (SLE), acute poststreptococcal glomerulonephritis, and acute serum sickness. Low levels may also occur in some patients with advanced cirrhosis of the liver, multiple myeloma, hypogammaglobulinemia, or rapidly rejecting allografts.

Elevated total complement may occur in obstructive jaundice, thyroiditis, acute rheumatic fever, rheumatoid arthritis, acute myocardial infarction, ulcerative colitis, and diabetes.

C1 esterase inhibitor deficiency is characteristic in hereditary angioedema, the most common genetic abnormality associated with complement; C3 deficiency is characteristic in recurrent pyogenic infection and disease activation in SLE; C4 deficiency is characteristic in SLE and rheumatoid arthritis. C4 is increased in autoimmune hemolytic anemia.

Interfering factors

- Hemolysis due to rough handling of the sample
- Failure to send the sample to the laboratory immediately
- Recent heparin therapy

RADIOALLERGOSORBENT TEST

The radioallergosorbent test (RAST) measures immunoglobulin (Ig) E antibodies in serum by radioimmunoassay and identifies specific allergens that cause rash, asthma, hay fever, drug reactions, and other atopic complaints. RAST is easier to perform and more specific than skin testing; it's also less painful for and less dangerous to the patient. Careful selection of specific allergens, based on the patient's history, is crucial for effective testing.

Although skin testing is still the preferred means of diagnosing IgE-mediated hypersensitivities, RAST may be more useful when a skin disorder makes accurate reading of skin tests difficult, when a patient requires continual antihistamine therapy, or when skin tests are negative but the patient's history supports IgE-mediated hypersensitivity.

Purpose

- To identify allergens to which the patient has an immediate (IgE-mediated) hypersensitivity
- To monitor the patient's response to therapy

Patient preparation

- Explain to the patient that this test may detect the cause of allergy or monitor the effectiveness of allergy treatment.
- Inform the patient that he need not restrict food or fluids.
- Tell the patient that the test requires a blood sample. Explain who will perform the venipuncture and when.
- Explain to the patient that he may experience discomfort from the needle puncture and the tourniquet.
- If the patient is scheduled for a radioactive scan, make sure the blood sample is collected before the scan.

Procedure and posttest care

- Perform a venipuncture, and collect the sample in a 7-ml clot-activator tube. Generally, 1 ml of serum is sufficient for five allergen assays.
- Note on the laboratory request the specific allergens to be tested.
- Apply direct pressure to the venipuncture site until bleeding stops.
- If a hematoma develops at the venipuncture site, apply warm soaks.

Reference values

RAST results are interpreted in relation to a control or reference serum that differs among laboratories.

Abnormal findings

Elevated serum IgE levels suggest hypersensitivity to the specific allergen or allergens used.

Interfering factors

- Radioactive scan within 1 week before sample collection

HAM TEST

The Ham test, or acidified serum lysis test, is performed to determine the cause of undiagnosed hemolytic anemia, hemoglobinuria, and bone marrow aplasia. This test determines the stability of the red blood cell (RBC) membrane. It helps establish a diagnosis of paroxysmal nocturnal hemoglobinuria (PNH), a rare hematologic disease.

Purpose
- To help establish a diagnosis of PNH

Patient preparation
- Explain to the patient that this test helps determine the cause of his anemia or other signs.
- Inform the patient that he need not restrict food or fluids.
- Tell the patient that the test requires a blood sample. Explain who will perform the venipuncture and when.
- Explain to the patient that he may experience discomfort from the needle puncture and the tourniquet.

Procedure and posttest care
- Because the blood sample must be defibrinated immediately, laboratory personnel perform the venipuncture and collect the sample.
- Apply direct pressure to the venipuncture site until bleeding stops.
- If a hematoma develops at the venipuncture site, apply warm soaks.

Normal findings
Normally, RBCs don't undergo hemolysis. Test results should be negative.

Abnormal findings
Hemolysis of RBCs indicates PNH.

Interfering factors
- Blood containing large numbers of spherocytes (possible false-positive)
- Blood from patients with congenital dyserythropoietic anemia (false-positive)

HUMAN LEUKOCYTE ANTIGEN

The human leukocyte antigen (HLA) test identifies a group of antigens present on the surface of all nucleated cells, but most easily detected on lymphocytes. There are four types of HLA: HLA-A, HLA-B, HLA-C, and HLA-D. These antigens are essential to immunity and determine the degree of histocompatibility between transplant recipients and donors. Numerous antigenic determinants (more than 60, for instance, at the HLA-B locus) are present for each site; one set of each antigen is inherited from each parent.

A high incidence of specific HLA types has been linked to specific diseases, such as rheumatoid arthritis and multiple sclerosis, but these findings have little diagnostic significance.

Purpose
- To provide histocompatibility typing of transplant recipients and donors
- To aid genetic counseling
- To aid paternity testing

Patient preparation
- Explain to the patient that this test detects antigens on white blood cells.
- Inform the patient that he need not restrict food or fluids.
- Tell the patient that the test requires a blood sample. Explain who will perform the venipuncture and when.

- Explain to the patient that he may experience slight discomfort from the needle puncture and the tourniquet.
- Check the patient's history for recent blood transfusions. HLA testing may need to be postponed if he has recently undergone a transfusion.

Procedure and posttest care

- Perform a venipuncture, and collect the sample in a tube containing anticoagulant acid citrate dextrose solution.
- Apply direct pressure to the venipuncture site until bleeding stops.
- If a hematoma develops at the venipuncture site, apply warm soaks.

Precautions

- Handle the sample gently to prevent hemolysis.

Normal findings

In HLA-A, HLA-B, and HLA-C testing, lymphocytes that react with the test antiserum undergo lysis; they're detected by phase microscopy. In HLA-D testing, leukocyte incompatibility is marked by blast formation, deoxyribonucleic acid synthesis, and proliferation.

Abnormal findings

Incompatible HLA-A, HLA-B, HLA-C, and HLA-D groups may cause unsuccessful tissue transplantation.

Many diseases have a strong association with certain types of HLAs. For example, HLA-DR5 is associated with Hashimoto's thyroiditis. B8 and Dw3 are associated with Graves' disease, whereas B8 alone is associated with chronic autoimmune hepatitis, celiac disease, and myasthenia gravis. Dw3 alone is associated with Addison's disease, Sjögren's syndrome, dermatitis herpetiformis, and systemic lupus erythematosus.

In paternity testing, a putative father who presents a phenotype (two haplotypes: one from the father and one from the mother) with no haplotype or antigen pair identical to one of the child's is excluded as the father. A putative father with one haplotype identical to one of the child's may be the father; the probability varies with the incidence of the haplotype in the population.

Interfering factors

- Hemolysis due to rough handling of the sample
- HLA from blood transfusion within 72 hours before sample collection

AUTOANTIBODIES

ANTINUCLEAR ANTIBODIES

In such conditions as systemic lupus erythematosus (SLE), scleroderma, and certain infections, the body's immune system may perceive portions of its own cell nuclei as foreign and may produce antinuclear antibodies (ANAs). Specific ANAs include antibodies to deoxyribonucleic acid (DNA), nucleoprotein, histones, nuclear ribonucleoprotein, and other nuclear constituents.

Because they don't penetrate living cells, ANAs are harmless, but sometimes form antigen-antibody complexes that cause tissue damage (as in SLE). Because of multiorgan involvement, test results aren't diagnostic and can only partially confirm clinical evidence. (See *Comparative incidence of antinuclear antibodies.*)

Comparative incidence of antinuclear antibodies

CONDITION	INCIDENCE OF POSITIVE ANTINUCLEAR ANTIBODIES
Systemic lupus erythematosus (SLE)	95% to 100%
Lupoid hepatitis	95% to 100%
Felty's syndrome	95% to 100%
Progressive systemic sclerosis (scleroderma)	75% to 80%
Drugs associated with SLE-like syndrome (hydralazine, procainamide, isoniazid)	Approximately 50%
Sjögren's syndrome	40% to 75%
Rheumatoid arthritis	25% to 60%
Healthy family member of patient with SLE	Approximately 25%
Chronic discoid lupus erythematosus	15% to 50%
Juvenile arthritis	15% to 30%
Polyarteritis nodosa	15% to 25%
Miscellaneous disorders	10% to 50%
Dermatomyositis, polymyositis	10% to 30%
Rheumatic fever	Approximately 5%

Purpose

- To screen for SLE (failure to detect ANAs essentially rules out active SLE)
- To monitor the effectiveness of immunosuppressive therapy for SLE

Patient preparation

- Explain to the patient that this test evaluates the immune system and that further testing is usually required for diagnosis.
- Inform the patient that the test will be repeated to monitor his response to therapy, if appropriate.
- Inform the patient that he need not restrict food or fluids.
- Tell the patient that the test requires a blood sample. Explain who will perform the venipuncture and when.
- Explain to the patient that he may experience discomfort from the needle puncture and the tourniquet.
- Check the patient's history for drugs that may affect test results, such as isoniazid and procainamide. Note findings on the laboratory request.

Procedure and posttest care

- Perform a venipuncture, and collect the sample in a 7-ml tube without additives.
- Because a patient with an autoimmune disease has a compromised immune system, observe the venipuncture site for signs of infection, and report changes to the physician immediately.
- Keep a clean, dry bandage over the site for at least 24 hours.
- Apply direct pressure to the venipuncture site until bleeding stops.
- If a hematoma develops at the venipuncture site, apply warm soaks.

Reference values

Test results are reported as positive (with pattern and serum titer noted) or negative.

Abnormal findings

Although this test is a sensitive indicator of ANAs, it isn't specific for SLE. Low titers may occur in patients with viral diseases, chronic hepatic disease, collagen vascular disease, and autoimmune diseases and in some healthy adults; the incidence increases with age. The higher the titer, the more specific the test is for SLE (titer often exceeds 1:256).

The pattern of nuclear fluorescence helps identify the type of immune disease present. A peripheral pattern is almost exclusively associated with SLE because it indicates the presence of anti-DNA antibodies; sometimes anti-DNA antibodies are measured by radioimmunoassay if ANA titers are high or a peripheral pattern is observed. A homogeneous, or diffuse, pattern is also associated with SLE as well as with related connective tissue disorders; a nucleolar pattern, with scleroderma; and a speckled, irregular pattern, with infectious mononucleosis and mixed connective tissue disorders (for example, SLE and scleroderma).

A single serum sample, especially one collected from a patient with collagen vascular disease, may contain antibodies to several parts of the cell's nucleus. In addition, as serum dilution increases, the fluorescent pattern may change because different antibodies are reactive at different titers.

Interfering factors

- Most commonly isoniazid, hydralazine, and procainamide, but also para-aminosalicylic acid, chlorpromazine, clofibrate, phenytoin, griseofulvin, ethosuximide, gold salts, methyldopa, oral contraceptives, penicillin, propylthiouracil, phenylbutazone, methysergide, streptomycin, sulfonamides, tetracyclines, mephenytoin, quinidine, primidone, reserpine, and trimethadione (possible production of a syndrome resembling SLE)

EXTRACTABLE NUCLEAR ANTIGEN ANTIBODIES

Extractable nuclear antigen (ENA) is a complex of at least four antigens. One of them — ribonucleoprotein (RNP) — is susceptible to degradation by ribonuclease. The second — Smith (Sm) antigen — is an acidic nuclear protein that resists ribonuclease degradation. The third and fourth antigens that are sometimes included in this group — Sjögren's syndrome A (SS-A) antigen and Sjögren's syndrome B (SS-B) antigen — form a precipitate when an antibody is present.

Antibodies to these antigens are associated with certain autoimmune disorders. Tests to detect ENA antibodies help differentiate autoimmune disorders with similar signs and symptoms.

Purpose

- To aid differential diagnosis of autoimmune disease
- To distinguish between anti-RNP and anti-Sm antibodies
- To screen for anti-RNP antibodies (common in mixed connective tissue disease)
- To screen for anti-Sm antibodies (common in systemic lupus erythematosus [SLE])
- To support diagnosis of collagen vascular autoimmune diseases

Patient preparation

- Explain to the patient that this test detects certain antibodies and that test results help determine diagnosis and treatment.
- Explain that the test assesses the effectiveness of treatment, when appropriate.
- Inform the patient that he need not restrict food or fluids.
- Tell the patient that the test requires a blood sample. Explain who will perform the venipuncture and when.
- Explain to the patient that he may experience discomfort from the needle puncture and the tourniquet.

Procedure and posttest care

- Perform a venipuncture, and collect the sample in a 7-ml tube without additives.
- Because a patient with an autoimmune disease has a compromised immune system, check the venipuncture site for infection, and report changes promptly.
- Keep a clean, dry bandage over the site for at least 24 hours.
- Apply direct pressure to the venipuncture site until bleeding stops.
- If a hematoma develops at the venipuncture site, apply warm soaks.

Precautions

- Send the sample to the laboratory immediately.

Reference values

Serum should be negative for anti-RNP, anti-Sm, and SS-B antibodies.

Abnormal findings

Anti-RNP antibodies are elevated in SLE (35% to 40% of patients) and in mixed connective tissue disease. Anti-Sm antibodies are specific for SLE. Anti-SS-A and anti-SS-B antibodies are elevated in Sjögren's syndrome (40% to 45% of patients). Anti-SS-B antibodies are also elevated in SLE.

Interfering factors

- Failure to send the sample to the laboratory immediately

ANTIMITOCHONDRIAL ANTIBODIES

Usually performed with the test for anti-smooth-muscle antibodies, the Antimitochondrial antibodies test detects antimitochondrial antibodies in serum by indirect immunofluorescence. These autoantibodies are present in several hepatic diseases. Their role in disease pathogenesis is unknown, and there's no evidence that they cause hepatic damage. Most commonly, they're associated with primary biliary cirrhosis and, sometimes, chronic active hepatitis and drug-induced jaundice. Antimitochondrial antibodies are also associated with autoimmune diseases, such as systemic lupus erythematosus, rheumatoid arthritis, pernicious anemia, and idiopathic Addison's disease.

Purpose

- To aid diagnosis of primary biliary cirrhosis
- To distinguish between extrahepatic jaundice and biliary cirrhosis

Patient preparation

- Explain to the patient that this test evaluates liver function.
- Inform the patient that he need not restrict food or fluids.
- Tell the patient that the test requires a blood sample. Explain who will perform the venipuncture and when.

■ Explain to the patient that he may experience discomfort from the needle puncture and the tourniquet.
■ Check the patient's medication history for oxyphenisatin use, and report it to the laboratory because it may produce antimitochondrial antibodies.

Procedure and posttest care

■ Perform a venipuncture, and collect the sample in a 7-ml tube with no additives.
■ Because patients with hepatic disease may bleed excessively, apply pressure to the venipuncture site until bleeding stops.
■ If a hematoma develops at the venipuncture site, apply warm soaks.

Normal findings

Serum is normally negative for antimitochondrial antibodies. Positive results are titered.

Abnormal findings

Although antimitochondrial antibodies appear in 79% to 94% of patients with primary biliary cirrhosis, this test alone doesn't confirm the diagnosis. Further tests, such as serum alkaline phosphatase, serum bilirubin, aspartate aminotransferase, alanine aminotransferase and, possibly, liver biopsy or cholangiography, may also be necessary. The autoantibodies also appear in some patients with chronic active hepatitis, drug-induced jaundice, and cryptogenic cirrhosis. Antimitochondrial antibodies seldom appear in patients with extrahepatic biliary obstruction, and a positive test helps rule out this condition.

Interfering factors

■ Confusion of antimitochondrial antibodies with heterophil antibodies, cardiolipin antibodies to syphilis, ribosomal antibodies, and microsomal hepatic or renal autoantibodies
■ Oxyphenisatin (possible false-positive results)

ANTI-SMOOTH-MUSCLE ANTIBODIES

Using indirect immunofluorescence, the anti-smooth-muscle antibodies test measures the relative concentration of anti-smooth-muscle antibodies in serum; it's usually performed with the test for antimitochondrial antibodies.

Anti-smooth-muscle antibodies appear in several hepatic diseases, especially chronic active hepatitis and, less often, primary biliary cirrhosis. Although anti-smooth-muscle antibodies are most commonly associated with hepatic diseases, their etiologic role is unknown, and there's no evidence that they cause hepatic damage.

Purpose

■ To aid diagnosis of active chronic hepatitis and primary biliary cirrhosis

Patient preparation

■ Explain to the patient that this test helps evaluate liver function.
■ Inform the patient that he need not restrict food or fluids.
■ Tell the patient that the test requires a blood sample. Explain who will perform the venipuncture and when.
■ Explain to the patient that he may experience slight discomfort from the needle puncture and the tourniquet.

Procedure and posttest care

■ Perform a venipuncture, and collect the sample in a 7-ml tube without additives.

- Because patients with hepatic disease may bleed excessively, apply pressure to the venipuncture site until bleeding stops.
- If a hematoma develops at the venipuncture site, apply warm soaks.

Reference values

A normal titer of anti-smooth-muscle antibodies is negative. Positive results are titered.

Abnormal findings

The test for anti-smooth-muscle antibodies isn't specific; these antibodies appear in a number of patients with chronic active hepatitis and in fewer patients with primary biliary cirrhosis.

Anti-smooth-muscle antibodies may also be present in patients with infectious mononucleosis, acute viral hepatitis, malignant tumor of the liver, and intrinsic asthma.

Interfering factors

- None significant

ANTITHYROID ANTIBODIES

In autoimmune disorders — such as Hashimoto's thyroiditis and Graves' disease (hyperthyroidism) — thyroglobulin, the major colloidal storage compound, is released into the blood. Antithyroglobulin antibodies are produced to attack this foreign substance; the ensuing autoimmune response damages the thyroid gland.

Purpose

- To detect circulating antithyroglobulin antibodies when clinical evidence indicates Hashimoto's thyroiditis, Graves' disease, or other thyroid diseases

Patient preparation

- Explain to the patient that this test evaluates thyroid function.
- Inform the patient that he need not restrict food or fluids.
- Tell the patient that the test requires a blood sample. Explain who will perform the venipuncture and when.
- Explain to the patient that he may experience discomfort from the needle puncture and the tourniquet.

Procedure and posttest care

- Perform a venipuncture, and collect the sample in a 7-ml tube without additives.
- Apply direct pressure to the venipuncture site until bleeding stops.
- If a hematoma develops at the venipuncture site, apply warm soaks.

Reference values

The normal titer is less than 1:100 for antithyroglobulin and antimicrosomal antibodies.

Abnormal findings

The presence of antithyroglobulin or antimicrosomal antibodies in serum can indicate subclinical autoimmune thyroid disease, Graves' disease, or idiopathic myxedema. Titers of 1:400 or greater strongly suggest Hashimoto's thyroiditis. Antithyroglobulin antibodies may also occur in some patients with other autoimmune disorders, such as systemic lupus erythematosus, rheumatoid arthritis, and autoimmune hemolytic anemia.

Interfering factors

- None significant

THYROID-STIMULATING IMMUNOGLOBULIN

Thyroid-stimulating immunoglobulin (TSI), formerly called long-acting thyroid stimulator, appears in the blood of most patients with Graves' disease. It stimulates the thyroid gland to produce and excrete excessive amounts of thyroid hormone.

Reportedly, 90% of people with Graves' disease have elevated TSI levels. Positive results of this test strongly suggest Graves' disease, despite normal routine thyroid tests in patients still suspected of having Graves' disease or progressive exophthalmos.

Purpose

- To aid evaluation of suspected thyroid disease
- To aid diagnosis of suspected thyrotoxicosis, especially in patients with exophthalmos
- To monitor treatment of thyrotoxicosis

Patient preparation

- Explain to the patient that this test evaluates thyroid function, as appropriate.
- Tell the patient that the test requires a blood sample. Explain who will perform the venipuncture and when.
- Explain to the patient that he may experience discomfort from the needle puncture and the tourniquet.

Procedure and posttest care

- Perform a venipuncture, and collect the sample in a 5-ml clot-activator tube.
- Apply direct pressure to the venipuncture site until bleeding stops.
- If a hematoma develops at the venipuncture site, apply warm soaks.
- If the patient had a radioactive iodine scan with 48 hours of the test, note this on the laboratory request.

Precautions

- Handle the sample gently to prevent hemolysis, and send it to the laboratory promptly.

Reference values

TSI doesn't normally appear in serum. However, it's considered normal at levels equal to or greater than 1.3 index.

Abnormal findings

Increased TSI levels are associated with exophthalmos, Graves' disease (thyrotoxicosis), and recurrence of hyperthyroidism.

Interfering factors

- Hemolysis due to rough handling of the sample
- Administration of radioactive iodine within 48 hours of the test

CARDIOLIPIN ANTIBODIES

The cardiolipin antibodies test measures serum concentrations of immunoglobulin (Ig) G and IgM antibodies in relation to the phospholipid cardiolipin. These antibodies appear in some lupus erythematosus (LE) patients whose serum also contains a coagulation inhibitor (lupus anticoagulant). They also appear in some patients who don't fulfill all the diagnostic criteria for LE, but who experience recurrent episodes of spontaneous thrombosis, fetal loss, or thrombocytopenia. Serum concentrations of cardiolipin antibodies are measured by enzyme-linked immunosorbent assay.

Purpose

■ To aid diagnosis of cardiolipin antibody syndrome in patients with or without LE who experience recurrent episodes of spontaneous thrombosis, fetal loss, or thrombocytopenia

Patient preparation

■ Tell the patient that this test helps diagnose cardiolipin antibody syndrome and LE.
■ Inform the patient that he need not restrict food or fluids.
■ Tell the patient that the test requires a blood sample. Explain who will perform the venipuncture and when.
■ Explain to the patient that he may experience discomfort from the needle puncture and the tourniquet.

Procedure and posttest care

■ Perform a venipuncture, and collect the sample in a 5-ml tube without additives.
■ Apply direct pressure to the venipuncture site until bleeding stops.
■ If a hematoma develops at the venipuncture site, apply warm soaks.

Precautions

■ Handle the sample gently to prevent hemolysis, and send it to the laboratory immediately.

Reference values

Cardiolipin antibody results are reported as negative or positive. A positive result is titered.

Abnormal findings

A positive result along with a history of recurrent spontaneous thrombosis, fetal loss, or thrombocytopenia suggests cardiolipin antibody syndrome. Treatment may involve anticoagulant or platelet inhibitor therapy.

Interfering factors

■ Hemolysis due to rough handling of the sample
■ Failure to send the sample to the laboratory immediately

RHEUMATOID FACTOR

The rheumatoid factor (RF) test is the most useful immunologic test for confirming rheumatoid arthritis (RA). In this disease, "renegade" immunoglobulin (Ig) G antibodies, produced by lymphocytes in the synovial joints, react with IgM antibody to produce immune complexes, complement activation, and tissue destruction. How IgG molecules become antigenic is still unknown, but they may be altered by aggregating with viruses or other antigens. Techniques for detecting RF include the sheep cell agglutination test and the latex fixation test. Although the presence of this autoantibody is diagnostically useful, it may not be etiologically related to RA.

Purpose

■ To confirm RA, especially when clinical diagnosis is doubtful

Patient preparation

■ Explain to the patient that this test helps confirm RA.
■ Inform the patient that he need not restrict food or fluids.
■ Tell the patient that the test requires a blood sample. Explain who will perform the venipuncture and when.
■ Explain to the patient that he may experience discomfort from the needle puncture and the tourniquet.

Procedure and posttest care

- Perform a venipuncture, and collect the sample in a 7-ml clot-activator tube.
- Because a patient with RA may be immunologically compromised, keep the venipuncture site clean and dry for 24 hours.
- Check regularly for signs of infection.
- Apply direct pressure to the venipuncture site until bleeding stops.
- If a hematoma develops at the venipuncture site, apply warm soaks.

Reference values

Normal RF titer is less than 1:20; normal rheumatoid screening test is nonreactive.

Abnormal findings

Non-RA and RA populations aren't clearly separated with regard to the presence of RF: 25% of patients with RA have a nonreactive titer; 8% of non-RA patients are reactive at greater than 39 IU/ml, and only 3% of non-RA patients are reactive at greater than 80 IU/ml.

Patients with various non-RA diseases characterized by chronic inflammation may test positive for RF. These diseases include systemic lupus erythematosus, polymyositis, tuberculosis, infectious mononucleosis, syphilis, viral hepatic disease, and influenza.

Interfering factors

- Inadequately activated complement (possible false-positive)
- Serum with high lipid or cryoglobulin levels (possible false-positive, requiring repetition of the test after restricting fat intake)
- Serum with high IgG levels (possible false-negative due to competition with IgG on the surface of latex particles or sheep red blood cells used as substrate)

COLD AGGLUTININS

Cold agglutinins are antibodies, usually of the immunoglobulin (Ig) M type, that cause red blood cells (RBCs) to aggregate at low temperatures. They may occur in small amounts in healthy people. Transient elevations of these antibodies develop during certain infectious diseases, notably primary atypical pneumonia. This test reliably detects such pneumonia within 1 to 2 weeks after onset.

Patients with high cold agglutinin titers, such as those with primary atypical pneumonia, may develop acute transient hemolytic anemia after repeated exposure to cold; patients with persistently high titers may develop chronic hemolytic anemia.

Purpose

- To help confirm primary atypical pneumonia
- To provide additional diagnostic evidence for cold agglutinin disease associated with many viral infections and lymphoreticular cancer
- To detect cold agglutinins in patients with suspected cold agglutinin disease

Patient preparation

- Explain to the patient that this test detects antibodies in the blood that attack RBCs after exposure to low temperatures.
- Inform the patient that the test will be repeated to monitor his response to therapy, if appropriate.
- Inform the patient that he need not restrict food or fluids.
- Tell the patient that the test requires a blood sample. Explain who will perform the venipuncture and when.

- Explain to the patient that he may experience discomfort from the needle puncture and the tourniquet.
- If the patient is receiving antimicrobial drugs, note this on the laboratory request because the use of such drugs may interfere with the development of cold agglutinins.

Procedure and posttest care

- Perform a venipuncture, and collect the sample in a 7-ml tube without additives that has been p rewarmed to 98.6° F (37° C).
- If cold agglutinin disease is suspected, keep the patient warm. If the patient is exposed to low temperatures, agglutination may occur within peripheral vessels, possibly leading to frostbite, anemia, Raynaud's phenomenon and, rarely, focal gangrene.
- Watch for signs of vascular abnormalities, such as mottled skin, purpura, jaundice, pallor, pain in or swelling of extremities, and cramping of fingers and toes. Hemoglobinuria may result from severe intravascular hemolysis on exposure to severe cold.
- Apply direct pressure to the venipuncture site until bleeding stops.
- If a hematoma develops at the venipuncture site, apply warm soaks.

Precautions

- Handle the sample gently to prevent hemolysis, and send it to the laboratory immediately.
- Don't refrigerate the sample; cold agglutinins will coat the RBCs, leaving none in the serum for testing.

Reference values

Cold agglutinin screening results are reported as negative or positive. A positive result, indicating the presence of cold agglutinin, is titered. A normal titer is less than 1:64.

Abnormal findings

High titers may occur as primary phenomena or secondary to infections or lymphoreticular cancer. They may be present in infectious mononucleosis, cytomegalovirus infection, hemolytic anemia, multiple myeloma, scleroderma, malaria, cirrhosis of the liver, congenital syphilis, peripheral vascular disease, pulmonary embolism, trypanosomiasis, tonsillitis, staphylococcemia, scarlatina, influenza and, occasionally, pregnancy. Chronically elevated titers are most commonly associated with pneumonia and lymphoreticular cancer; an acute transient elevation typically accompanies many viral infections.

Extremely high titers (> 1:2,000) can occur with idiopathic cold agglutinin disease that precedes lymphoma development. Patients with titers this high are susceptible to intravascular agglutination, which causes significant clinical problems.

Interfering factors

- Hemolysis due to rough handling of the sample (possible false-low titer)
- Refrigeration of the sample before serum is separated from RBCs (possible false-low titer)
- Antimicrobial drugs

CRYOGLOBULINS

Cryoglobulins are abnormal serum proteins that precipitate at low laboratory temperatures (39.2° F [4° C]) and redissolve after being warmed. Their presence in the blood (cryoglobulinemia) is usually associated with immunologic disease, but can also occur without known immunopathology. If patients with cryoglobulinemia are subjected to cold, they may experience Raynaud-like symptoms (pain, cyanosis, and coldness of fingers and toes), which generally result from precipitation of cryoglobulins in cooler parts of the body. In some patients, for example, cryoglobulins may precipitate at temperatures as high as 86° F (30° C); such temperatures are possible in some peripheral blood vessels.

The cryoglobulin test involves refrigerating a serum sample at 33.8° F (1° C) for 24 hours and observing for formation of a heat-reversible precipitate. Such a precipitate requires further study by immunoelectrophoresis or double diffusion to identify cryoglobulin components.

Purpose

- To detect cryoglobulinemia in patients with Raynaud-like vascular symptoms

Patient preparation

- Explain to the patient that this test detects antibodies in blood that may cause sensitivity to low temperatures.
- Instruct the patient to fast for 4 to 6 hours before the test.
- Tell the patient that the test requires a blood sample. Explain who will perform the venipuncture and when.
- Explain to the patient that he may experience discomfort from the needle puncture and the tourniquet.

Procedure and posttest care

- Perform a venipuncture, and collect the sample in a prewarmed 10-ml tube without additives.
- Instruct the patient that he may resume his usual diet.
- Tell the patient to avoid cold temperatures or contact with cold objects, if the test is positive for cryoglobulins, as ordered.
- Apply direct pressure to the venipuncture site until bleeding stops.
- If a hematoma develops at the venipuncture site, apply warm soaks.
- Observe for signs of intravascular coagulation, such as decreased color and temperature in distal extremities, and increased pain.

Precautions

- Warm the syringe and collection tube to 98.6° F (37° C) before venipuncture and keep the tube at that temperature to prevent loss of cryoglobulins.
- Send the sample to the laboratory immediately.

Normal findings

Normally, serum is negative for cryoglobulins. Positive results are reported as a percentage based on the amount of sample cryoprecipitation.

Abnormal findings

The presence of cryoglobulins in the blood confirms cryoglobulinemia. This finding doesn't always indicate the presence of clinical disease.

Interfering factors

- Failure to adhere to dietary restrictions
- Failure to keep the sample at 98.6° F (37° C) before centrifugation (possible loss of cryoglobulins)
- Reading the sample before the 72-hour precipitation period ends (possible incorrect analysis of results because some cryoglobulins take several days to precipitate)

ACETYLCHOLINE RECEPTOR ANTIBODIES

The acetylcholine receptor (AChR) antibodies test is the most useful immunologic test for confirming acquired (autoimmune) myasthenia gravis (MG), a disorder of neuromuscular transmission. In MG, antibodies block and destroy AChR sites, causing muscle weakness that can be either generalized or localized to the ocular muscles.

Two test methods — a binding assay and a blocking assay — are now available to determine the relative concentration of AChR antibodies in serum. The blocking assay is relatively new, and its clinical significance isn't fully known. However, it's specific for the autoimmune form of MG and useful for research. Determination of AChR antibodies by either method also helps monitor immunosuppressive therapy for MG, although antibody levels don't usually parallel the severity of disease.

Purpose

- To confirm diagnosis of MG
- To monitor the effectiveness of immunosuppressive therapy for MG

Patient preparation

- Explain to the patient that this test helps confirm MG.
- Tell the patient that the test assesses the effectiveness of treatment, if appropriate.
- Inform the patient that he need not restrict food or fluids.
- Tell the patient that the test requires a blood sample. Explain who will perform the venipuncture and when.
- Explain to the patient that he may experience discomfort from the needle puncture and the tourniquet.
- Check the patient's history for immunosuppressive drugs that may affect test results, and note such use on the laboratory request.

Procedure and posttest care

- Perform a venipuncture, and collect the sample in a 7-ml tube without additives.
- Because a patient with an autoimmune disease has a compromised immune system, check the venipuncture site for infection, and promptly report changes.
- Keep a clean, dry bandage over the site for at least 24 hours.
- Apply direct pressure to the venipuncture site until bleeding stops.
- If a hematoma develops at the venipuncture site, apply warm soaks.

Precautions

- Keep the sample at room temperature, and send it to the laboratory immediately.

Normal findings

Normal serum is negative for AChR-binding antibodies and AChR-blocking antibodies.

Abnormal findings

Positive AChR antibodies in symptomatic adults confirm the diagnosis of MG. Patients who have only ocular symptoms have lower antibody titers than those who have generalized symptoms.

Interfering factors

- Failure to maintain the sample at room temperature and send the sample to the laboratory immediately
- Thymectomy, thoracic duct drainage, immunosuppressive therapy, and plasmapheresis (possible decrease)
- Amyotrophic lateral sclerosis (possible false-positive)

ANTI-INSULIN ANTIBODIES

Some patients with diabetes form antibodies to the insulin they take. These antibodies bind with some of the insulin, making less insulin available for glucose metabolism and necessitating increased insulin dosages. This phenomenon is known as insulin resistance.

Performed on the blood of a patient with diabetes who takes insulin, the anti-insulin antibody test detects insulin antibodies. Insulin antibodies are immunoglobulins, called anti-insulin Ab. The most common type of anti-insulin Ab is immunoglobulin (Ig) G , but anti-insulin Ab is also found in the other four classes of immunoglobulins — IgA, IgD, IgE, and IgM. IgM may cause insulin resistance, and IgE has been associated with allergic reactions.

Purpose

- To determine insulin allergy
- To confirm insulin resistance
- To determine if hypoglycemia is caused by insulin overuse

Patient preparation

- Tell the patient that this test is used to determine the most appropriate treatment for his diabetes and to determine if he has insulin resistance or an allergy to insulin.
- Tell the patient that the test requires a blood sample. Explain who will perform the venipuncture and when.
- Explain to the patient that he may experience discomfort from the needle puncture and the tourniquet.
- Tell the patient that he need not restrict food or fluids.
- Ask the patient if he has had a radioactive test recently; if so, note this on the laboratory request.

Procedure and posttest care

- Perform a venipuncture, and collect the sample in a 7-ml tube without additives.
- Apply direct pressure to the venipuncture site until bleeding stops.
- If a hematoma develops at the venipuncture site, apply warm soaks.

Precautions

- Handle the sample gently to prevent hemolysis.

Normal findings

There should be less than 3% binding of the patient's serum with labeled beef, human, and pork insulin.

Abnormal findings

Elevated levels may occur in insulin allergy or resistance and in factitious hypoglycemia.

Interfering factors

- Radioactive test performed within 1 week before the test

ANTI-DOUBLE-STRANDED DNA ANTIBODIES

About two-thirds of patients with active systemic lupus erythematosus (SLE) have measurable levels of autoantibodies to double-stranded (native) deoxyribonucleic acid (known as anti-ds-DNA). These antibodies are rarely detected in patients with other connective tissue diseases.

The anti-ds-DNA antibody test measures and differentiates these antibody levels in a serum sample, using radioimmunoassay, agglutination, complement fixation, or immunoelectrophoresis. If anti-ds-DNA antibodies are present, they combine with native DNA and form complexes that are too large to pass through a membrane filter. The test counts these oversized complexes.

Purpose

- To confirm a diagnosis of SLE

■ To monitor the SLE patient's response to therapy and determine his prognosis

Patient preparation

■ Explain to the patient that this test helps diagnose and determine the appropriate therapy for SLE.
■ Inform the patient that he need not restrict food or fluids.
■ Tell the patient that the test requires a blood sample. Explain who will perform the venipuncture and when.
■ Explain to the patient that he may experience discomfort from the needle puncture and the tourniquet.
■ Ask the patient if he has had a recent radioactive test; if so, note this on the laboratory request.

Procedure and posttest care

■ Perform a venipuncture, and collect the sample in a 7-ml tube without additives. (Some laboratories may specify a tube with either EDTA or sodium fluoride and potassium oxalate added).
■ Apply direct pressure to the venipuncture site until bleeding stops.
■ If a hematoma develops at the venipuncture site, apply warm soaks.

Precautions

■ Handle the sample gently to prevent hemolysis.

Reference values

An anti-ds-DNA antibody level less than 25 IU/ml (SI, < 25 kIU/L) is considered negative for SLE.

Abnormal findings

Elevated anti-ds-DNA antibody levels may indicate SLE. Values of 25 to 30 IU/ml (SI, 25 to 30 kIU/L) are considered borderline positive. Values of 31 to 200 IU/ml (SI, 31 to 200 kIU/L) are positive, and those greater than 200 IU/ml (SI, > 200 kIU/L) are strongly positive.

Depressed anti-ds-DNA antibody levels may follow immunosuppressive therapy, demonstrating effective treatment of SLE.

Interfering factors

■ A radioactive scan performed within 1 week before collection of a sample
■ Hemolysis due to rough handling of the sample

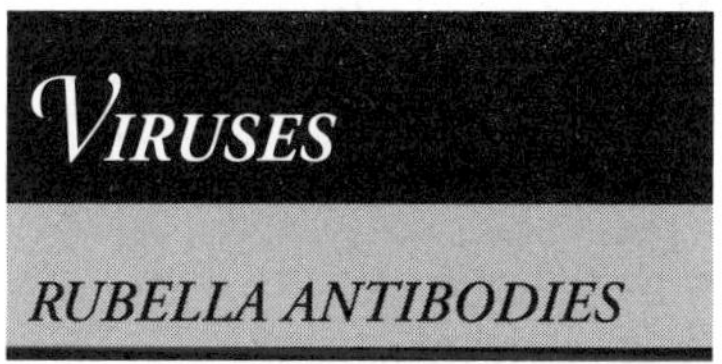

VIRUSES

RUBELLA ANTIBODIES

Although rubella (German measles) is generally a mild viral infection in children and young adults, it can produce severe infection in the fetus, resulting in spontaneous abortion, stillbirth, or congenital rubella syndrome. Because rubella infection normally induces immunoglobulin (Ig) G and IgM antibody production, measuring rubella antibodies can determine present infection as well as immunity resulting from past infection. The hemagglutination inhibition test is the most commonly used serologic test for rubella antibodies.

Purpose

■ To diagnose rubella infection, especially congenital infection
■ To determine susceptibility to rubella in children and in women of childbearing age

Patient preparation

■ Explain to the patient that this test diagnoses or evaluates susceptibility to rubella.

- Inform the patient that she need not restrict food or fluids before the test.
- Tell her that this test requires a blood sample and that if a current infection is suspected, a second blood sample will be needed in 2 to 3 weeks to identify a rise in the titer.
- Explain who will perform the venipuncture and when.
- Explain to the patient that she may experience slight discomfort from the needle puncture and the tourniquet.

Procedure and posttest care

- Perform a venipuncture, and collect the sample in a 7-ml clot-activator tube.
- Apply direct pressure to the venipuncture site until bleeding stops.
- If a hematoma develops at the venipuncture site, apply warm soaks.
- Instruct the patient to return for an additional blood test, when appropriate.
- If a woman of childbearing age is found to be susceptible to rubella, explain that vaccination can prevent rubella and that she must wait at least 3 months after the vaccination to become pregnant or risk permanent damage or death to the fetus.
- If the pregnant patient is found to be susceptible to rubella, instruct her to return for follow-up rubella antibody tests to detect possible subsequent infection.
- If the test confirms rubella in a pregnant patient, provide emotional support. As needed, refer her for appropriate counseling.

Precautions

- Handle the specimen gently to prevent hemolysis.

Reference values

Titer of 1:8 or less indicates little or no immunity against rubella; titer more than 1:10 indicates adequate protection against rubella.

IgM results are reported as positive or negative. The presence of rubella specific IgM class antibody indicates congenital or recent infection.

Abnormal findings

Hemagglutination inhibition antibodies normally appear 2 to 4 days after the onset of the rash, peak in 3 to 4 weeks, and then slowly decline but remain detectable for life. A fourfold or greater rise from the acute to the convalescent titer indicates a recent rubella infection.

The presence of rubella-specific IgM antibodies indicates recent infection in an adult and congenital rubella in an infant.

Interfering factors

- Hemolysis due to rough handling of the sample

HEPATITIS B SURFACE ANTIGEN

Hepatitis B surface antigen (HBsAg), also called hepatitis-associated antigen or Australia antigen, appears in the sera of patients with hepatitis B virus. It can be detected by radioimmunoassay or, less commonly, reverse passive hemagglutination during the extended incubation period and usually during the first 3 weeks of acute infection or if the patient is a carrier.

Because transmission of hepatitis is one of the gravest complications associated with blood transfusion, all donors must be screened for hepatitis B before their blood is stored. This screening, required by the Food and Drug Administration's Bureau of Biologics, has helped reduce the incidence of hepatitis. This test doesn't screen for hepatitis A virus (infectious hepatitis).

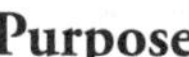

Purpose

- To screen blood donors for hepatitis B
- To screen people at high risk for contracting hepatitis B such as hemodialysis nurses
- To aid differential diagnosis of viral hepatitis

Patient preparation

- Explain to the patient that this test helps identify a type of viral hepatitis.
- Inform the patient that he need not restrict food or fluids.
- Tell the patient that the test requires a blood sample. Explain who will perform the venipuncture and when.
- Explain to the patient that he may experience discomfort from the needle puncture and the tourniquet.
- Check the patient's history for administration of hepatitis B vaccine.
- If the patient is giving blood, explain the donation procedure to him.

Procedure and posttest care

- Perform a venipuncture, and collect the sample in a 10-ml clot-activator tube.
- Report confirmed viral hepatitis to public health authorities. This is a reportable disease in most states.

Precautions

- Wash your hands carefully after the procedure.
- Remember to wear gloves when drawing blood and dispose of the needle properly.

Normal findings

Normal serum is negative for HBsAg.

Abnormal findings

The presence of HBsAg in a patient with hepatitis confirms hepatitis B. In chronic carriers and in people with chronic active hepatitis, HBsAg may be present in the serum several months after the onset of acute infection. It may also occur in more than 5% of patients with certain diseases other than hepatitis, such as hemophilia, Hodgkin's disease, and leukemia. If HbsAg is found in donor blood, that blood must be discarded because it carries a risk of transmitting hepatitis. Blood samples that test positive should be retested because inaccurate results do occur.

Interfering factors

- Hepatitis B vaccine (possible positive)

HETEROPHIL ANTIBODIES

Heterophil antibody tests detect and identify two immunoglobulin (Ig) M antibodies in human serum that react against foreign red blood cells (RBCs): Epstein-Barr virus (EBV) antibodies and Forssman antibodies.

In the Paul-Bunnell test — also called the presumptive test — EBV antibodies, found in the sera of patients with infectious mononucleosis, agglutinate with sheep RBCs in a test tube. Forssman antibodies, present in the sera of some normal persons as well as in the sera of patients with conditions, such as serum sickness, also agglutinate with sheep RBCs, thus rendering test results inconclusive for infectious mononucleosis.

If the Paul-Bunnell test establishes a presumptive titer, the Davidsohn differential absorption test can then distinguish between EBV antibodies and Forssman antibodies. (See *Monospot test for infectious mononucleosis,* page 300.)

Monospot test for infectious mononucleosis

Several screening tests can detect the heterophil infectious mononucleosis (IM) antibody. One of these tests — the monospot — converts the Paul-Bunnell and the Davidsohn differential absorption tests into one rapid slide test without titration. Monospot relies on agglutination of horse red blood cells (RBCs) by heterophil antibodies.

DISTINGUISHING ANTIBODIES

Because horse RBCs contain Forssman and IM antigens, differential absorption of the patient's serum is necesary to distinguish between them. This is done by mixing the serum sample with guinea pig kidney antigen (containing only Forssman antigen) on one end of a slide and with beef RBC stroma (containing only IM antigen) on the other end of the slide. Each absorbs only the heterophil antibody specific to it. After addition of horse RBCs to each spot, agglutination on the beef cell end of the slide indicates the presence of the IM heterophil antibody and confirms IM.

Monospot rivals the classic heterophil agglutination test for sensitivity. False-positives may occur in the presence of lymphoma, hepatitis A and B, leukemia, and pancreatic cancer.

Purpose

■ To aid differential diagnosis of infectious mononucleosis

Patient preparation

■ Explain to the patient that this test helps detect infectious mononucleosis.
■ Tell the patient that the test requires a blood sample. Explain who will perform the venipuncture and when.
■ Explain to the patient that he may experience discomfort from the needle puncture and the tourniquet.

Procedure and posttest care

■ Perform a venipuncture, and collect the sample in a 7-ml clot-activator tube.
■ Apply direct pressure to the venipuncture site until bleeding stops.
■ If a hematoma develops at the venipuncture site, apply warm soaks.
■ If the titer is positive and infectious mononucleosis is confirmed, instruct the patient in the treatment plan.
■ If the titer is positive but infectious mononucleosis isn't confirmed, or if the titer is negative but symptoms persist, explain that additional testing will be necessary in a few days or weeks to confirm the diagnosis and plan effective treatment.

Precautions

■ Handle the sample gently to prevent hemolysis.

Reference values

Normally, the titer is less than 1:56, but it may be higher in elderly people. Some laboratories refer to a normal titer as "negative" or as having "no reaction."

Abnormal findings

Although heterophil antibodies are present in the sera of about 80% of patients with infectious mononucleosis 1 month after onset, a positive finding—a titer higher than 1:56—doesn't confirm this disorder; a high titer can also result from systemic lupus erythematosus, syphilis, cryoglobulinemia, or the presence of antibodies to nonsyphilitic treponemata (yaws, pinta, bejel). A gradual increase in titer during week 3 or 4 followed by a gradual decrease during weeks 4 to 8 proves most conclusive for infectious mononucleosis. A negative titer doesn't always rule out this disorder; occasionally, the titer becomes reactive 2 weeks later. Therefore, if symptoms persist, the test should be repeated in 2 weeks.

Confirmation of infectious mononucleosis depends on heterophil agglutination and hematologic tests that show absolute lymphocytosis, with 10% or more atypical lymphocytes.

Interfering factors

- Hemolysis due to rough handling of the sample
- Narcotic use, lymphomas, hepatitis, leukemia, and phenytoin therapy (false-positive)

EPSTEIN-BARR VIRUS ANTIBODIES

Epstein-Barr virus (EBV), a member of the herpesvirus group, is the causative agent of heterophil-positive infectious mononucleosis, Burkitt's lymphoma, and nasopharyngeal carcinoma. Although the virus doesn't replicate in standard cell cultures, most EBV infections can be recognized by testing the patient's serum for heterophil antibodies (monospot test), which usually appear within the first 3 weeks of illness and then decline rapidly within a few weeks.

In about 10% of adults and a larger percentage of children, the monospot test is negative, despite primary infection with EBV. Further, EBV has been associated with lymphoproliferative processes in immunosuppressed patients. These disorders occur with reactivated, rather than primary, EBV infections and therefore are also monospot-negative.

Alternatively, EBV-specific antibodies, which develop to several antigens of the virus during active infection, can be measured with a high level of sensitivity and specificity by indirect immunofluorescence.

Purpose

- To provide a laboratory diagnosis of heterophil- (or monospot-) negative cases of infectious mononucleosis
- To determine the antibody status to EBV of immunosuppressed patients with lymphoproliferative processes

Patient preparation

- Explain to the patient the purpose of the test.
- Tell the patient that the test requires a blood sample. Explain who will perform the venipuncture and when.
- Explain to the patient that he may experience slight discomfort from the needle puncture and the tourniquet.

Procedure and posttest care

- Perform a venipuncture, and collect 5 ml of sterile blood in a clot-activator tube.
- Allow the blood to clot for at least 1 hour at room temperature.
- Apply direct pressure to the venipuncture site until bleeding stops.
- If a hematoma develops at the venipuncture site, apply warm soaks.

Precautions

- Handle the sample gently to prevent hemolysis.
- Transfer the serum to a sterile tube or vial and send it to the laboratory immediately.
- If transfer must be delayed, store the serum at 39.2° F (4° C) for 1 to 2 days or at –4° F (–20° C) for longer periods to prevent contamination.

Reference values

Sera from patients who have never been infected with EBV have no detectable antibodies to the virus as measured by either the monospot test or the indirect immunofluorescence test. The monospot test is positive only during the acute phase of infection with EBV; the indirect immunofluorescence test detects and discriminates between acute and past infection with the virus.

Abnormal findings

EBV infection can be ruled out if no antibodies to EBV antigens are detected in the indirect immunofluorescence test. A positive monospot test or an indirect immunofluorescence test that is either immunoglobulin M (IgM)-positive or Epstein-Barr nuclear antigen (EBNA)-negative indicates acute EBV infection.

A monospot-negative result doesn't necessarily rule out acute or past infection with EBV. Conversely, IgG class antibody to viral capsid antigen and EBNA antigens (IgM-negative) indicates remote (more than 2 months) infection with EBV. Recognize that most cases of monospot-negative infectious mononucleosis are caused by cytomegalovirus infections.

Interfering factors

- Hemolysis due to rough handling of the sample

RESPIRATORY SYNCYTIAL VIRUS ANTIBODIES

Respiratory syncytial virus (RSV), a member of the paramyxovirus group, is the major viral cause of severe lower respiratory tract disease in infants, but may cause infections in people of any age. RSV infections are most common and produce the most severe disease during the first 6 months of life. Initial infection involves viral replication in epithelial cells of the upper respiratory tract, but in younger children especially, the infection spreads to the bronchi, the bronchioles, and even the parenchyma of the lungs.

In this test, immunoglobulin (Ig) G and IgM class antibodies are quantified using indirect immunofluorescence.

Purpose

- To diagnose infections caused by RSV

Patient preparation

- Explain to the patient (or, to the patient's parents) the purpose of the test.
- Tell the patient or parents that the test requires a blood sample. Explain who will perform the venipuncture and when.
- Tell the patient he may experience discomfort from the needle puncture and the tourniquet.

Procedure and posttest care

- Perform a venipuncture, and collect 5 ml of sterile blood in a clot-activator tube.
- Allow the blood to clot for at least 1 hour at room temperature.
- Apply direct pressure to the venipuncture site until bleeding stops.
- If a hematoma develops at the venipuncture site, apply warm soaks.

Precautions

- Handle the sample gently to prevent hemolysis.
- Transfer the serum to a sterile tube or vial, and send it to the laboratory promptly.
- If transfer must be delayed, store the serum at 39.2° F (4° C) for 1 to 2 days

or at –4° F (–20° C) for longer periods to avoid contamination.

Reference values

Sera from patients who have never been infected with RSV have no detectable antibodies to the virus (less than 1:5).

Abnormal findings

The qualitative presence of IgM or a fourfold or greater increase in IgG antibodies indicates active RSV infection. Note that, in infants, serologic diagnosis of RSV infections is difficult because of the presence of maternal IgG antibodies. Thus, the presence of IgM antibodies is most significant.

Interfering factors

- Hemolysis due to rough handling of the sample

HERPES SIMPLEX ANTIBODIES

Herpes simplex virus (HSV), a member of the herpesvirus group, causes various clinically severe manifestations, including genital lesions, keratitis or conjunctivitis, generalized dermal lesions, and pneumonia. Severe involvement is associated with intrauterine or neonatal infections and encephalitis; such infections are most severe in immunosuppressed patients. Of the two closely related antigenic types, Type 1 usually causes infections above the waistline; Type 2 infections predominantly involve the external genitalia. Primary contact with this virus occurs in early childhood as acute stomatitis or, more commonly, as an inapparent infection.

Sensitive assays, such as indirect immunofluorescence and enzyme immunoassay, are used to demonstrate immunoglobulin (Ig) M class antibodies to HSV or to detect a fourfold or greater increase in IgG class antibodies between acute- and convalescent-phase sera.

Purpose

- To confirm infections caused by HSV
- To detect recent or past HSV infection

Patient preparation

- Explain to the patient the purpose of the test.
- Tell the patient that the test requires a blood sample. Explain who will perform the venipuncture and when.
- Explain to the patient that he may experience discomfort from the needle puncture and the tourniquet.

Procedure and posttest care

- Perform a venipuncture, and collect 5 ml of sterile blood in a tube designated by the laboratory.
- Allow the blood to clot for at least 1 hour at room temperature.
- Apply direct pressure to the venipuncture site until bleeding stops.
- If a hematoma develops at the venipuncture site, apply warm soaks.
- If the patient's immune system is compromised, check the venipuncture site for changes and report them promptly.

Precautions

- Handle the sample gently to prevent hemolysis.
- Transfer the serum to a sterile tube or vial, and send it to the laboratory promptly.
- If transfer must be delayed, store the serum at 39.2° F (4° C) for 1 to 2 days or at –4° F (–20° C) for longer periods to avoid contamination.

- Because the patient may have a compromised immune system, keep the venipuncture site clean and dry.

Reference values

Sera from patients who have never been infected with HSV have no detectable antibodies (less than 1:5).

Abnormal findings

HSV infection can be ruled out in patients whose serum shows no detectable antibodies to the virus. The presence of IgM or a fourfold or greater increase in IgG antibodies indicates active HSV infection.

Interfering factors

- Hemolysis due to rough handling of the sample

CYTOMEGALOVIRUS ANTIBODY SCREEN

After primary infection, cytomegalovirus (CMV) remains latent in white blood cells (WBCs). The presence of CMV antibodies indicates past infection with this virus. In an immunocompromised patient, CMV can be reactivated to cause active infection. Administration of blood or tissue from a seropositive donor may cause active CMV infection in CMV-seronegative organ transplant recipients or neonates, especially those born prematurely.

Antibodies to CMV can be detected by several methods, including passive hemagglutination, latex agglutination, enzyme immunoassay, and indirect immunofluorescence. The complement fixation test is only 60% sensitive compared with other assays and shouldn't be used to screen for CMV antibodies. Screening tests for CMV antibodies are qualitative; they detect the presence of antibody at a single low dilution. In quantitative methods, several dilutions of the serum sample are tested to indicate acute infection with CMV.

Purpose

- To detect CMV infection in donors and recipients of organs and blood and in immunocompromised patients
- To screen for CMV infection in infants who require blood transfusions or tissue transplants

Patient preparation

- Explain the purpose of the test to the patient or the parents of an infant, as appropriate.
- Tell the patient that the test requires a blood sample. Explain who will perform the venipuncture and when.
- Explain to the patient that he may experience slight discomfort from the needle puncture and the tourniquet.

Procedure and posttest care

- Perform a venipuncture, and collect the sample in a 5-ml tube as designated by the laboratory.
- Allow the blood to clot for at least 1 hour at room temperature.
- Apply direct pressure to the venipuncture site until bleeding stops.
- If a hematoma develops at the venipuncture site, apply warm soaks.

Precautions

- Handle the sample gently to prevent hemolysis.
- Transfer the serum to a sterile tube or vial, and send it to the laboratory.
- If transfer must be delayed, store the serum at 39.2° F (4° C) for 1 to 2 days or at –4° F (–20° C) for longer periods to avoid contamination.
- Because the patient may have a compromised immune system, keep the venipuncture site clean and dry.

Reference values

Patients who have never been infected with CMV have no detectable antibodies to the virus. Immunoglobulin (Ig) G and IgM are normally negative.

Abnormal findings

A serum sample collected early during the acute phase or late in the convalescent stage may not contain detectable IgG or IgM antibodies to CMV. Therefore, a negative result doesn't preclude recent infection. More than a single sample is needed to ensure accurate results.

A serum sample that tests positive for antibodies at this single dilution indicates that the patient has been infected with CMV and that his WBCs contain latent virus capable of being reactivated in an immunocompromised host. Immunosuppressed patients who lack antibodies to CMV should receive blood products or organ transplants from donors who are also seronegative. Patients with CMV antibodies don't require seronegative blood products.

Interfering factors

- Hemolysis due to rough handling of the sample

HUMAN IMMUNODEFICIENCY VIRUS ANTIBODIES

The human immunodeficiency virus (HIV) antibodies test detects antibodies to HIV in serum. HIV is the virus that causes acquired immunodeficiency syndrome (AIDS). Transmission occurs by direct exposure of a person's blood to body fluids containing the virus. The virus may be transmitted from one person to another through exchange of contaminated blood and blood products, during sexual intercourse with an infected partner, when I.V. drugs are shared, and from an infected mother to her child during pregnancy or breast-feeding.

Initial identification of HIV is usually achieved through enzyme-linked immunosorbent assay. Positive findings are confirmed by Western blot test and immunofluorescence. There are also other tests available, which may be performed to detect antibodies. (See *Testing for HIV,* page 306.)

Purpose

- To screen for HIV in high-risk patients
- To screen donated blood for HIV

Patient preparation

- Explain to the patient that this test detects HIV infection.
- Provide adequate counseling about the reasons for performing the test, which is usually requested by the patient's physician.
- If the patient has questions about his condition, be sure to provide full and accurate information.
- Tell the patient that the test requires a blood sample. Explain who will perform the venipuncture and when.
- Explain to the patient that he may experience slight discomfort from the needle puncture and the tourniquet.

Procedure and posttest care

- Perform a venipuncture, and collect the sample in a 10-ml barrier tube. Barrier tubes help prevent contamination when pouring the serum in the laboratory.
- Apply direct pressure to the venipuncture site until bleeding stops.
- If a hematoma develops at the venipuncture site, apply warm soaks.
- Keep test results confidential.

Testing for HIV

Newer tests are available to help identify human immunodeficiency virus (HIV)-infected antibodies quicker and more conveniently, including a test to identify genetic changes that may alter the patient's course of treatment.

ORAQUICK RAPID HIV-1 ANTIBODY TEST
For the large number of people a year who don't check back for test results, rapid HIV testing may be done by the patient in any outpatient setting. The OraQuick rapid HIV-1 antibody test, approved by the Food and Drug Administration (FDA), allows results to be obtained in less than 20 minutes using 1 drop of blood. A color indicator similar to a home pregnancy test is used. If it's positive, a confirmatory test must be done to validate the results.

NUCLEIC ACID TEST (NAT)
The FDA has also approved a nucleic acid test to screen plasma donation for HIV and hepatitis C. This test has been shown to dramatically reduce the waiting time involved until blood and products may be used.

GENE-BASED TESTS
Spikes of HIV virus in the bloodstream commonly mean that the individual being treated for HIV is growing resistant to the drug treatment being used. The government has approved the first gene-based test to help determine if an HIV infected person's virus is mutating, making the therapy fail. This test can help physician's select more appropriate treatment.

- When the patient receives the results, give him another opportunity to ask questions.
- Encourage the patient with positive screening tests to seek medical follow-up care, even if he's asymptomatic.
- Tell the patient to report early signs of AIDS, such as fever, weight loss, axillary or inguinal lymphadenopathy, rash, and persistent cough or diarrhea. Women should also report gynecologic symptoms.
- Tell the patient to assume that he can transmit HIV to others until conclusively proved otherwise. To prevent possible contagion, advise him about safer sex practices.
- Instruct the patient not to share razors, toothbrushes, or utensils (which may be contaminated with blood) and to clean such items with household bleach diluted 1:10 in water.
- Advise the patient against donating blood, tissues, or an organ.
- Warn the patient to inform his physician and dentist about his condition so that they can take proper precautions.

Precautions

- Observe standard precautions when drawing a blood sample.
- Use gloves, properly dispose of needles, and use blood-fluid precaution labels on tubes, as necessary.
- Because the patient may have a compromised immune system, keep the venipuncture site clean and dry.

Normal findings

Test results are normally negative.

Abnormal findings

The test detects previous exposure to the virus. However, it doesn't identify patients who have been exposed to the virus but haven't yet made antibodies. Most patients with AIDS have antibodies to HIV. A positive test for the HIV antibody can't determine whether a patient harbors actively replicating virus or when the patient will manifest signs and symptoms of AIDS.

Many apparently healthy people have been exposed to HIV and have circulating antibodies. The test results for such people aren't false-positives. Furthermore, patients in the later stages of AIDS may exhibit no detectable antibody in their sera because they can no longer mount an antibody response.

Interfering factors

None known

PARVOVIRUS B-19 ANTIBODIES

Parvovirus B-19, a small, single-stranded deoxyribonucleic acid virus belonging to the family Parvoviridae, destroys red blood cell (RBC) precursors and interferes with normal RBC production. It's also associated with erythema infectiosum (a self-limiting, low-grade fever and rash in young children) and aplastic crisis (in patients with chronic hemolytic anemia and immunodeficient patients with bone marrow failure). Immunoglobulin (Ig) G and IgM antibodies can be detected by enzyme-linked immunosorbent assay and immunofluorescence.

Purpose

- To detect parvovirus B-19 antibody, especially in prospective organ donors
- To diagnose erythema infectiosum, parvovirus B-19 aplastic crisis, and related parvovirus B-19 diseases

Patient preparation

- Explain to the patient the test purpose and procedure. To a potential organ donor, explain that the test is part of a panel of tests performed before organ donation to protect the organ recipient from potential infection.
- Tell the patient that the test requires a blood sample. Explain who will perform the venipuncture and when.
- Explain to the patient that he may experience discomfort from the needle puncture and the tourniquet.

Procedure and posttest care

- Perform a venipuncture, collect the blood sample in a 5-ml clot-activator tube, and store it on ice.
- Apply direct pressure to the venipuncture site until bleeding stops.
- If a hematoma develops at the venipuncture site, apply warm soaks.

Precautions

- Handle the sample gently to prevent hemolysis.

Normal findings

Normally, results are negative for IgM- and IgG-specific antibodies to parvovirus B-19.

Abnormal findings

About 50% of all adults lack immunity to parvovirus B-19, with as many as 20% of susceptible adults becoming infected after exposure. Positive results have been associated with joint arthralgia, hydrops fetalis, fetal loss, transient aplastic anemia, chronic anemia in immunocompromised patients, and bone marrow failure.

Abnormal findings for the parvovirus B 19 should be confirmed using the Western blot test.

Interfering factors

- Failure to send the sample on ice
- Hemolysis due to rough handling of the sample

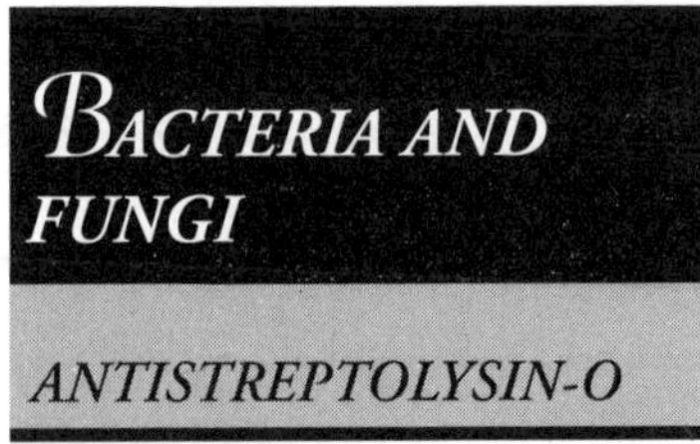

The antistreptolysin-O test measures the relative serum concentrations of the antibody to streptolysin O (known as ASO). A serum sample is diluted with a commercial preparation of streptolysin O and incubated. After the addition of human red blood cells, the tube is reincubated and examined visually. Failure of hemolysis to develop indicates recent streptococcal infection.

Purpose

- To confirm recent or ongoing streptococcal infection
- To help diagnose rheumatic fever and poststreptococcal glomerulonephritis in the presence of clinical symptoms
- To distinguish between rheumatic fever and rheumatoid arthritis when joint pains are present

Patient preparation

- Explain to the patient that this test detects an immunologic response to certain bacteria (streptococci).
- Inform the patient that he need not restrict food or fluids.
- Tell the patient that the test requires a blood sample. Explain who will perform the venipuncture and when.
- Explain to the patient that he may experience discomfort from the needle puncture and the tourniquet.
- If the test is to be repeated at regular intervals to identify active and inactive states of rheumatic fever or to confirm acute glomerulonephritis, tell the patient that measuring changes in antibody levels helps determine the effectiveness of therapy.
- Check the patient's history for drugs that may suppress the streptococcal antibody responses. If such drugs must be continued, note this on the laboratory request.

Procedure and posttest care

- Perform a venipuncture, and collect the sample in a 7-ml tube without additives.
- Apply direct pressure to the venipuncture site until bleeding stops.
- If a hematoma develops at the venipuncture site, apply warm soaks.

Precautions

- Handle the sample gently to prevent hemolysis.

Reference values

Even healthy people have some detectable ASO titers from previous minor streptococcal infections. Normal ASO titers range as follows:

- School-age children: 170 Todd units/ml
- Preschoolers and adults: 85 Todd units/ml.

Abnormal findings

High ASO titers usually occur only after prolonged or recurrent infections. Generally, a titer higher than 166 Todd units is considered a definite elevation. A low titer is good evidence for the absence of active rheumatic fever. A higher titer doesn't necessarily mean that rheumatic fever or glomerulonephritis is present; however, it does indicate the presence of a streptococcal infection.

Serial titers, determined at 10- to 14-day intervals, provide more reliable information than a single titer. An increase in titer 2 to 5 weeks after the acute infection, which peaks 4 to 6 weeks after the initial increase, confirms poststreptococcal disease.

Interfering factors

- Streptococcal skin infections, seldom producing abnormal ASO titers even with poststreptococcal disease (probable false-negative)
- Antibiotic or corticosteroid therapy (possible suppression of the streptococcal antibody response)
- Hemolysis due to rough handling of the sample

FEBRILE AGGLUTINATION

Sometimes bacterial infections (such as tularemia, brucellosis, and the disorders caused by *Salmonella*) and rickettsial infections (such as Rocky Mountain spotted fever and typhus) cause puzzling fevers, called fevers of undetermined origin (FUO). In these infections and others in which microorganisms are difficult to isolate from blood or excreta, febrile agglutination tests can provide important diagnostic information.

The Weil-Felix test for rickettsial disease, Widal's test for *Salmonella,* and tests for brucellosis and tularemia are essentially the same. In these tests, a serum sample is mixed with a few drops of prepared antigens in normal saline solution on a slide and the reaction is observed.

The Weil-Felix test establishes rickettsial antibody titers. It uses three forms of *Proteus* antigens (OX-19, OX-2, and OX-K) that cross-react with the various strains of rickettsiae. Antibodies to certain rickettsial strains react with more than one *Proteus* antigen, whereas antibodies to other strains fail to react with any *Proteus* antigens.

Widal's test establishes the titers for flagellar (H) and somatic (O) antigens, which may indicate *Salmonella* gastroenteritis and extraintestinal focal infections caused by *S. enteritidis* or enteric (typhoid) fever, caused by *S. typhosa.* A third antigen, the Vi or envelope antigen, may indicate typhoid carrier status, which often tests negative for H and O antigens. Widal's test isn't recommended for diagnosing *Salmonella* gastroenteritis.

Slide agglutination and tube dilution tests, using killed suspensions of the disease organisms as antigens, establish titers for the gram-negative coccobacilli *Brucella* and *Francisella tularensis*, which cause brucellosis and tularemia, respectively.

Purpose

- To support clinical findings in diagnosis of disorders caused by *Salmonella, Rickettsia, F. tularensis,* and *Brucella* organisms
- To identify the cause of FUO

Patient preparation

- Explain to the patient that this test detects and quantifies microorganisms that may cause fever and other symptoms.
- Inform the patient that he need not restrict food or fluids.
- Tell the patient that the test requires a blood sample. Explain who will perform the venipuncture and when.
- Explain to the patient that he may experience discomfort from the needle puncture and the tourniquet.

- Explain to the patient that this test requires a series of blood samples to detect a pattern of titers characteristic of the suspected disorder if appropriate. Reassure him that a positive titer only suggests a disorder.
- Note on the laboratory request when antimicrobial therapy began, if appropriate.

Procedure and posttest care

- Perform a venipuncture, and collect the sample in a 7-ml clot-activator tube.
- Apply direct pressure to the venipuncture site until bleeding stops.
- If a hematoma develops at the venipuncture site, apply warm soaks.
- In FUO and suspected infection, contact the facility's infection-control department. Isolation may be necessary.

Precautions

- Use standard hospital isolation procedures when collecting and handling samples.
- Send samples to the laboratory immediately.

Reference values

Results are reported as negative or positive, and positive results are titered. Normal dilutions are:

- *Salmonella* antibody: < 1:80
- Brucellosis antibody: < 1:80
- Tularemia antibody: < 1:40
- Rickettsial antibody: < 1:40.

Abnormal findings

Observed rise and fall of titers is crucial for detecting active infection. If this isn't possible, certain titer levels can suggest the disorder. For all febrile agglutinins, a fourfold increase in titers is strong evidence of infection.

The Weil-Felix test is positive for rickettsiae with antibodies to *Proteus* 6 to 12 days after infection; titers peak in 1 month and usually drop to negative in 5 to 6 months. This test can't be used to diagnose rickettsialpox or Q fever because the antibodies of these diseases don't cross-react with *Proteus* antigens; the test shows positive titers in *Proteus* infections and, in such cases, is nonspecific for rickettsiae.

In *Salmonella* infection, H and O agglutinins usually appear in serum after 1 week, and titers rise for 3 to 6 weeks. O agglutinins usually fall to insignificant levels in 6 to 12 months. Agglutinin titers may remain elevated for years.

In brucellosis, titers usually rise after 2 to 3 weeks and reach their highest levels between 4 and 8 weeks. The absence of *Brucella* agglutinins doesn't rule out brucellosis. In tularemia, titers usually become positive during the second week of infection, exceed 1:320 by the third week, peak within 4 to 7 weeks, and usually decline gradually 1 year after recovery.

Interfering factors

- Failure to send the sample to the laboratory immediately
- Vaccination or continuous exposure to bacterial or rickettsial infection, resulting in immunity (high titers)
- Antibody cross-reaction with bacteria causing other infectious diseases such as tularemia antibodies cross-reacting with *Brucella* antigens
- Immunodeficiency (negative titers even during symptomatic infection due to inability to form antibodies)
- Antibiotics (low titers early in the course of infection)
- Elevated immunoglobulin levels due to hepatic disease or excessive drug use (high *Salmonella* titers)
- Skin tests with *Brucella* antigen (possible high *Brucella* titers)
- *Proteus* infections (possible positive Weil-Felix titers for rickettsial disease)

FUNGAL SEROLOGY

Most fungal organisms enter the body as spores inhaled into the lungs or infiltrated through wounds in the skin or mucosa. If the body's defenses can't destroy the organisms initially, the fungi multiply to form lesions; blood and lymph vessels may then spread the mycoses throughout the body. Most healthy people easily overcome initial mycotic infection, but elderly people and others with a deficient immune system are more susceptible to acute or chronic mycotic infection and to disorders secondary to such infection. Mycosis may be deep-seated or superficial: Deep-seated mycosis occurs primarily in the lungs; superficial mycosis, in the skin or mucosal linings.

Although cultures are usually performed to diagnose mycoses by identifying the causative organism, serologic tests occasionally provide the sole evidence for mycosis. Such serologic tests use immunodiffusion, complement fixation, precipitin, latex agglutination, or agglutination methods to demonstrate the presence of specific mycotic antibodies. (See *Serum test methods for fungal infections,* pages 312 and 313.)

Purpose

- To rapidly detect the presence of antifungal antibodies, aiding in the diagnosis of mycoses
- To monitor effectiveness of therapy for mycoses

Patient preparation

- Explain to the patient that this test aids diagnosis of certain fungal infections. If appropriate, tell him that this test monitors his response to antimycotic therapy and that it may be necessary to repeat the test.
- Tell the patient that the test requires a blood sample. Explain who will perform the venipuncture and when.
- Explain to the patient that he may experience discomfort from the needle puncture and the tourniquet.

Procedure and posttest care

- Perform a venipuncture, and collect the sample in a 10-ml sterile clot-activator tube.
- Apply direct pressure to the venipuncture site until bleeding stops.
- If a hematoma develops at the venipuncture site, apply warm soaks.

Precautions

- Send the sample to the laboratory immediately.
- If transport to the laboratory is delayed, store the sample at 39.2° F (4° C).

Normal findings

Depending on the test method, a negative finding, or normal titer, usually indicates the absence of mycosis.

Abnormal findings

The chart on pages 312 and 313 explains the significance of findings for specific organisms.

Interfering factors

- Failure to observe dietary restrictions
- Failure to send a sterile sample to the laboratory immediately or to properly store the sample in case of delay in transportation
- Cross-reaction of antibodies with other antigens, such as blastomycosis and histoplasmosis antigens (possible false-positive or high titers)
- Recent skin testing with fungal antigens (possible high titers)
- Mycosis-caused immunosuppression (low titers or false-negative)

Serum test methods for fungal infections

DISEASE AND NORMAL VALUES	CLINICAL SIGNIFICANCE OF ABNORMAL RESULTS
Blastomycosis	
Complement fixation: titers < 1:8	Titers ranging from 1:8 to 1:16 suggest infection; titers > 1:32 denote active disease. A rising titer in serial samples taken every 3 to 4 weeks indicates disease progression; a falling titer indicates regression. This test has limited diagnostic value because of a high percentage of false-negatives.
Immunodiffusion: negative	A more sensitive test for blastomycosis; detects 80% of infected people.
Coccidioidomycosis	
Complement fixation: titers < 1:2	Most sensitive test for this fungus. Titers ranging from 1:2 to 1:4 suggest active infection; titers > 1:16 usually denote active disease. Test may remain active in mild infections.
Immunodiffusion: negative	Most useful for screening, followed by complement fixation test for confirmation.
Precipitin titers < 1:16	Good screening test, titers > 1:16 usually indicate infection. About 80% of infected people show positive titers by 2 weeks; most revert to negative by 6 months. Early primary disease is shown by positive precipitin and negative complement fixation test. A positive complement fixation and negative precipitin test indicate chronic disease.
Histoplasmosis	
Complement fixation (histoplasmin): titers < 1:8	Titers ranging from 1:8 to 1:16 suggest infection; titers > 1:32 indicate active disease. Antibodies generally appear 10 to 21 days after initial infection. Test is positive in 10% to 15% of cases.
Complement fixation: titers < 1:18	Titers ranging from 1:8 to 1:16 suggest infection; titers > 1:32 indicate active disease. More sensitive than histoplasmin complement fixation test; gives positive results in 75% to 80% of cases. (Histoplasmin and yeast antigens are positive in 10% of cases.) A rising titer in serial samples taken every 2 to 3 weeks indicates progressive infection; a decreasing titer indicates regression.
Immunodiffusion (histoplasmin): negative	Appearance of both H and M bands indicates active infection. If the M band appears first and lasts longer than the H band, the infection may be regressing. The M band alone may indicate early infection, chronic disease, or a recent skin test.

Serum test methods for fungal infections *(continued)*

DISEASE AND NORMAL VALUES	CLINICAL SIGNIFICANCE OF ABNORMAL RESULTS
Aspergillosis	
Complement fixation: titers < 1:8	Titers > 1:8 suggest infection; 70% to 90% of patients with known pulmonary aspergillosis or aspergillus allergy present antibodies. This test can't detect invasive aspergillosis because patients with this disease don't have antibodies; biopsy is required.
Immunodiffusion: negative	One or more precipitin bands suggests infection. The number of bands is related to complement fixation titers; the more precipitin bands, the higher the titer.
Sporotrichosis	
Agglutination: titers < 1:40	Titers of > 1:80 usually indicate active infection. The test usually is negative in cutaneous infections and positive in extracutaneous infections.
Cryptococcosis	
Latex agglutination for cryptococcal antigen: negative	About 90% of patients with cryptococcal meningitis exhibit positive latex agglutination in cerebrospinal fluid (CSF). (Serum is less frequently positive than CSF.) Culturing is definitive because false-positives do occur. (Presence of rheumatoid factor may cause a positive reaction.) Serum antigen tests are positive in 33% of patients with pulmonary cryptococcosis; biopsy is usually required.

CANDIDA ANTIBODIES

Commonly present in the body, *Candida albicans* is a saprophytic yeast that can become pathogenic when the environment favors proliferation or the host's defenses have been significantly weakened.

Candidiasis is usually limited to the skin and mucous membranes but may cause life-threatening systemic infection. Susceptibility to candidiasis is associated with antibacterial, antimetabolic, and corticosteroid therapy as well as with immunologic defects, pregnancy, obesity, diabetes, and debilitating diseases. Oral candidiasis is common and benign in children; in adults, it may be an early indication of acquired immunodeficiency syndrome.

Diagnosis of candidiasis is usually made by culture or histologic study. When such diagnosis can't be made, identifying *Candida* antibodies may be helpful in diagnosing systemic candidiasis. Be cautioned that serologic testing to detect antibodies in candidiasis isn't reliable, and investigators continue to disagree about its usefulness.

Purpose

■ To aid diagnosis of candidiasis when culture or histologic study can't confirm the diagnosis

Patient preparation

■ Explain the purpose of the test to the patient, as appropriate.
■ Inform the patient that he need not restrict food or fluids.
■ Tell the patient that the test requires a blood sample. Explain who will perform the venipuncture and when.
■ Explain to the patient that he may experience discomfort from the needle puncture and the tourniquet.

Procedure and posttest care

■ Perform a venipuncture, and collect the sample in a 5-ml sterile collection tube without additives.
■ Apply direct pressure to the venipuncture site until bleeding stops.
■ If a hematoma develops at the venipuncture site, apply warm soaks.

Precautions

■ Handle the sample gently to prevent hemolysis.
■ Send the sample to the laboratory promptly.
■ Note recent antimicrobial therapy on the laboratory request form.
■ Because the patient's immune system may be compromised, keep the veniuncture site clean and dry.

Normal findings

A normal test result is negative for *Candida* antibodies.

Abnormal findings

A positive test for *C. albicans* antibodies is common in patients with disseminated candidiasis. However, this test yields a significant percentage of false-positive results.

Interfering factors

■ Hemolysis due to rough handling of the sample

BACTERIAL MENINGITIS ANTIGEN

The bacterial meningitis antigen test can detect specific antigens of *Streptococcus pneumoniae, Neisseria meningitidis,* and *Haemophilus influenzae* type B, the principal etiologic agents in meningitis. It can be performed on samples of serum, cerebrospinal fluid (CSF), urine, pleural fluid, and joint fluid, but CSF and urine are preferred.

Purpose

■ To identify the etiologic agent in meningitis
■ To aid diagnosis of bacterial meningitis
■ To aid diagnosis of meningitis when the Gram stain smear and culture are negative

Patient preparation

■ Explain the purpose of the test to the patient, as appropriate.
■ Inform the patient that this test requires a specimen of urine or CSF.
■ If a CSF specimen is required, describe how it will be obtained.
■ Tell who will perform the procedure and when.
■ Explain to the patient that he may experience discomfort from the needle puncture.
■ Advise the patient that a headache is the most common complication of lumbar puncture, but that his cooperation during the test minimizes such an effect.

■ Make sure the patient or a family member has signed an informed consent form.

Procedure and posttest care

■ Collect a 10-ml urine specimen or a 1-ml CSF specimen in a sterile container. (For detailed instructions on collecting a CSF specimen, see "Cerebrospinal fluid analysis" in chapter 7.)

Precautions

■ Maintain specimen sterility during collection.
■ Wear gloves when obtaining or handling the specimen.
■ Make sure the cap is tightly fastened on the specimen container.
■ Place the specimen on a refrigerated coolant and send it to the laboratory promptly.

Normal findings

Normally, results are negative for bacterial antigens.

Abnormal findings

Positive results identify the specific bacterial antigen: *S. pneumoniae, N. meningitidis, H. influenzae* type B, or group B streptococci.

Interfering factors

■ Previous antimicrobial therapy
■ Failure to maintain sterility during specimen collection

LYME DISEASE SEROLOGY

Lyme disease is a multisystem disorder characterized by dermatologic, neurologic, cardiac, and rheumatic manifestations in various stages. Epidemiologic and serologic studies implicate a common tickborne spirochete, *Borrelia burgdorferi*, as the causative agent. Serologic tests for Lyme disease, both indirect immunofluorescent and enzyme-linked immunosorbent assays, measure antibody response to this spirochete and indicate current infection or past exposure. Serologic tests can identify 50% of patients with early-stage Lyme disease and all patients with later complications of carditis, neuritis, and arthritis or patients in remission.

Purpose

■ To confirm a diagnosis of Lyme disease

Patient preparation

■ Explain to the patient that this test helps determine whether his symptoms are caused by Lyme disease.
■ Instruct the patient to fast for 12 hours before the sample is drawn, but to drink fluids as usual.
■ Tell the patient that the test requires a blood sample. Explain who will perform the venipuncture and when.
■ Explain to the patient that he may experience slight discomfort from the needle puncture and the tourniquet.

Procedure and posttest care

■ Perform a venipuncture, and collect the sample in a 7-ml clot-activator tube.
■ Apply direct pressure to the venipuncture site until bleeding stops.
■ If a hematoma develops at the venipuncture site, apply warm soaks.

Precautions

■ Handle the specimen carefully to prevent hemolysis.
■ Send the specimen to the laboratory immediately.

Reference values

Normal serum values are nonreactive.

Abnormal findings

A positive Lyme serology can help confirm diagnosis, but isn't definitive. Other treponemal diseases and high rheumatoid factor titers can cause false-positive results. More than 15% of patients with Lyme disease fail to develop antibodies.

Interfering factors

- High serum lipid levels (possible inaccurate results, requiring repetition of the test after a period of restricted fat intake)
- Samples contaminated with other bacteria (possible false-positive)
- Hemolysis due to rough handling of the sample

HELICOBACTER PYLORI *ANTIBODIES*

Helicobacter pylori is a spiral, gram-negative bacterium associated with chronic gastritis and idiopathic chronic duodenal ulceration. Although a gastric specimen can be obtained by endoscopy and cultured for *H. pylori,* the *H. pylori* antibody blood test is a more useful noninvasive screening procedure and may be performed using the enzyme-linked immunosorbent assay.

Purpose

- To help diagnose *H. pylori* infection in patients with GI symptoms

Patient preparation

- Inform the patient that this test is used to diagnose the infection that may cause ulcers.
- Inform the patient that he need not restrict food or fluids.
- Tell the patient that the test requires a blood sample. Explain who will perform the venipuncture and when.
- Explain to the patient that he may experience slight discomfort from the needle puncture and the tourniquet.

Procedure and posttest care

- Perform a venipuncture, and collect the sample in a 7-ml clot-activator tube.
- Send the sample to the laboratory immediately.
- Apply direct pressure to the venipuncture site until bleeding stops.
- If a hematoma develops at the venipuncture site, apply warm soaks.

Precautions

- This test should be performed only on patients with GI symptoms because of the large number of healthy people who have *H. pylori* antibodies.

Normal findings

Normally, no antibodies to *H. pylori* are revealed. Test results are reported as negative or positive.

Abnormal findings

A positive *H. pylori* test result indicates that the patient has antibodies to the bacterium. The serologic results should be interpreted in light of the clinical findings.

Interfering factors

- None significant

Miscellaneous Tests

Venereal Disease Research Laboratory Test

The Venereal Disease Research Laboratory (VDRL) test is widely used to screen for primary and secondary syphilis. Usually, a serum sample is used in the VDRL test, but this test may also be performed on a cerebrospinal fluid (CSF) specimen obtained by lumbar puncture to test for tertiary syphilis. The VDRL test of CSF is less sensitive than the fluorescent treponemal antibody absorption test.

Purpose

- To screen for primary and secondary syphilis
- To confirm primary or secondary syphilis in the presence of syphilitic lesions
- To monitor response to treatment

Patient preparation

- Explain to the patient that this test detects syphilis.
- Inform the patient that the disease usually goes undetected in the general population because infected people remain untreated.
- Tell the patient that he need not restrict food, fluids, or medications, but should abstain from alcohol for 24 hours before the test.
- Tell the patient that the test requires a blood sample. Explain who will perform the venipuncture and when.
- Explain to the patient that he may experience discomfort from the needle puncture and the tourniquet; collecting the sample takes less than 3 minutes.

Procedure and posttest care

- Perform a venipuncture, and collect the sample in a 7-ml clot-activator tube.
- Apply direct pressure to the venipuncture site until bleeding stops.
- If a hematoma develops at the venipuncture site, apply warm soaks.
- If the test is nonreactive or borderline, but syphilis hasn't been ruled out, instruct the patient to return for follow-up testing. Explain that borderline test results don't necessarily mean that he's free from the disease.
- If the test is reactive, explain the importance of proper treatment. Provide the patient with further information about sexually transmitted diseases and how they're spread, and stress the need for antibiotic therapy. Report the results to state public health authorities, and prepare the patient for mandatory inquiries.
- If the test is reactive, but the patient shows no clinical signs of syphilis, explain that many uninfected people show false-positive reactions. Stress the need for further specific tests to rule out syphilis.

Precautions

- Handle the specimen carefully to prevent hemolysis.

Normal findings

Normal serum shows no flocculation and is reported as a nonreactive test.

Abnormal findings

Definite flocculation is reported as a reactive test; slight flocculation is reported as a weakly reactive test. A reactive VDRL test occurs in about 50% of patients with primary syphilis and in nearly all patients with secondary syphilis. If syphilitic lesions exist, a reactive VDRL test is diagnostic. If no lesions are evident, a reactive VDRL test necessitates repeated testing. Biological false-positive reactions can be caused by conditions unrelated to syphilis; for example, infectious mononucleosis, malaria, leprosy, hepatitis, systemic lupus erythematosus, rheumatoid arthritis, and nonsyphilitic treponemal diseases, such as pinta and yaws.

A nonreactive test doesn't rule out syphilis because *Treponema pallidum* causes no detectable immunologic changes in the serum for 14 to 21 days after infection. Darkfield microscopy of exudate from suspicious lesions can provide early diagnosis by identifying the causative spirochetes.

A reactive VDRL test using a CSF specimen indicates neurosyphilis, which can follow the primary and secondary stages in patients who remain untreated.

Interfering factors

- Ingestion of alcohol within 24 hours of the test (possible transient nonreactive results)
- Immunosuppression (possible nonreactive results)
- Hemolysis due to rough handling of the sample

FLUORESCENT TREPONEMAL ANTIBODY ABSORPTION TEST

The fluorescent treponemal antibody absorption (FTA-ABS or simply FTA) test uses indirect immunofluorescence to detect antibodies to the spirochete *Treponema pallidum* in serum. This spirochete causes syphilis.

Although the FTA-ABS test is generally performed on a serum sample to detect primary or secondary syphilis, a cerebrospinal fluid (CSF) specimen is required to detect tertiary syphilis. Because antibody levels remain constant for long periods, the FTA-ABS test isn't recommended for monitoring response to therapy. (See *Two tests for* Treponema pallidum.)

Purpose

- To confirm primary and secondary syphilis
- To screen for suspected false-positive results of Venereal Disease Research Laboratories tests

Patient preparation

- Explain to the patient that this test can confirm or rule out syphilis.
- Inform the patient that he need not restrict food or fluids.
- Tell the patient that the test requires a blood sample. Explain who will perform the venipuncture and when.
- Explain to the patient that he may experience discomfort from the needle puncture and the tourniquet.

Procedure and posttest care

- Perform a venipuncture, and collect the sample in a 7-ml clot-activator tube.
- Apply direct pressure to the venipuncture site until bleeding stops.
- If a hematoma develops at the venipuncture site, apply warm soaks.
- If the test is reactive, explain the nature of syphilis, and stress the importance of proper treatment and the need to find and treat the patient's sexual contacts.
- Provide the patient with additional information about syphilis and how it's spread; emphasize the need for antibiotic therapy, if appropriate. Report positive results to state public health authorities, and prepare the patient for mandatory inquiries.
- If the test is nonreactive or findings are borderline, but syphilis hasn't been ruled out, instruct the patient to return

Two tests for *Treponema pallidum*

The microhemagglutination assay for the *Treponema pallidum* antibody increases the specificity of syphilis testing by eliminating methodologic interference. In this assay, tanned sheep red blood cells are coated with *T. pallidum* antigen and combined with absorbed test serum. Hemagglutination occurs in the presence of specific anti-*T. pallidum* antibodies in the serum.

In the enzyme-linked immunosorbent assay, tubes coated with *T. pallidum* are washed and then treated with enzyme-labeled antihuman globulin. After the substrate for the enzymes is added to the tubes, the enzymatic activity is measured by quantitating the reaction product formed.

for follow-up testing; explain that inconclusive results don't necessarily indicate that he's free from the disease.

Precautions

- Handle the sample gently to prevent hemolysis.

Normal findings

Normally, results of the FTA-ABS test are nonreactive.

Abnormal findings

The presence of treponemal antibodies in the serum — a reactive test result — doesn't indicate the stage or severity of infection. (The presence of these antibodies in CSF is strong evidence of tertiary neurosyphilis.) Elevated antibody levels appear in most patients with primary syphilis and in almost all patients with secondary syphilis. Higher antibody levels persist for several years, with or without treatment.

The absence of treponemal antibodies — a nonreactive test result — doesn't necessarily rule out syphilis. *T. pallidum* causes no detectable immunologic changes in the blood for 14 to 21 days after initial infection. Organisms may be detected earlier by examining suspicious lesions with a darkfield microscope. Low antibody levels and other nonspecific factors produce borderline findings. In such cases, repeated testing and a thorough review of the patient's history may be productive.

Although the FTA-ABS test is specific, some patients with nonsyphilitic conditions, such as systemic lupus erythematosus, genital herpes, and increased or abnormal globulins, or those who are pregnant may show minimally reactive levels. In addition, the FTA-ABS test doesn't always distinguish between *T. pallidum* and certain other treponemas, such as those that cause pinta, yaws, and bejel.

Interfering factors

- Hemolysis due to rough handling of the sample

CARCINOEMBRYONIC ANTIGEN

Carcinoembryonic antigen (CEA) is a protein normally found in embryonic entodermal epithelium and fetal GI tissue. Production of CEA stops before birth, but it may begin again later if a neoplasm develops. Because CEA levels are also raised by biliary obstruction, alcoholic hepatitis, chronic heavy smoking, and other conditions, this test can't be used as a general indicator of cancer. The measurement of enzyme CEA levels by immunoassay is useful for staging and monitoring treatment of certain cancers.

Purpose

- To monitor the effectiveness of cancer therapy
- To assist in preoperative staging of colorectal cancers, assess adequacy of surgical resection, and test for recurrence of colorectal cancers

Patient preparation

- Explain to the patient that this test detects and measures a special protein that isn't normally present in adults.
- Inform the patient that the test will be repeated to monitor the effectiveness of therapy, if appropriate.
- Inform the patient that he need not restrict food, fluids, or medications.
- Tell the patient that the test requires a blood sample. Explain who will perform the venipuncture and when.
- Explain to the patient that he may experience discomfort from the needle puncture and the tourniquet.

Procedure and posttest care

- Perform a venipuncture, and collect the sample in a 7-ml tube without additives.
- Apply direct pressure to the venipuncture site until bleeding stops.
- If a hematoma develops at the venipuncture site, apply warm soaks.

Precautions

- Handle the sample gently to prevent hemolysis.
- Send the sample to the laboratory immediately.

Reference values

Normal serum CEA values are less than 5 ng/ml (SI, < 5 mg/L).

Abnormal findings

Persistent elevation of CEA levels suggests residual or recurrent tumor. If levels exceed normal before surgical resection, chemotherapy, or radiation therapy, their return to normal within 6 weeks suggests successful treatment.

High CEA levels are characteristic in various malignant conditions, particularly entodermally derived neoplasms of the GI organs and lungs, and in certain nonmalignant conditions, such as benign hepatic disease, hepatic cirrhosis, alcoholic pancreatitis, and inflammatory bowel disease.

Elevated CEA concentrations may occur in nonendodermal carcinomas, such as breast and ovarian cancers.

Interfering factors

- Chronic cigarette smoking (possible increase)
- Hemolysis due to rough handling of the sample

ALPHA-FETOPROTEIN

Alpha-fetoprotein (AFP) is a glycoprotein produced by fetal tissue and tumors that differentiate from midline embryonic structures. During fetal development, AFP levels in serum and amniotic fluid rise. AFP crosses the placenta and appears in maternal serum.

High maternal serum AFP levels may suggest fetal neural tube defects, such as spina bifida and anencephaly, but positive confirmation requires amniocentesis and ultrasonography. Other congenital anomalies, such as Down syndrome and other chromosomal disorders, may be associated with low maternal serum AFP concentrations.

Elevated AFP levels in patients who aren't pregnant may occur in cancers, such as hepatocellular carcinoma, or certain nonmalignant conditions such as ataxia-telangiectasia. In these conditions, AFP assays are more useful for monitoring response to therapy than for diagnosis. AFP levels are best determined by enzyme immunoassay on amniotic fluid or serum.

Purpose

- To monitor the effectiveness of therapy in malignant conditions, such as hepatomas and germ cell tumors, and certain nonmalignant conditions such as ataxia-telangiectasia
- To screen for the need for amniocentesis or high-resolution ultrasonography in a pregnant woman

Patient preparation

- Explain that this test helps in monitoring fetal development, screens for a need for further testing, helps detect possible congenital defects in the fetus, and monitors her response to therapy by measuring a specific blood protein, as appropriate.
- Inform the patient that she need not restrict food, fluids, or medications.
- Tell the patient that the test requires a blood sample. Explain who will perform the venipuncture and when.
- Explain to the patient that she may experience slight discomfort from the needle puncture and the tourniquet.

Procedure and posttest care

- Perform a venipuncture, and collect the sample in a 7-ml clot-activator tube.
- Record the patient's age, race, weight, and gestational period on the laboratory request.
- Apply direct pressure to the venipuncture site until bleeding stops.
- If a hematoma develops at the venipuncture site, apply warm soaks.

Precautions

- Handle the sample gently to prevent hemolysis.

Reference values

When testing by immunoassay, AFP values are less than 15 ng/ml (SI, < 15 mg/L) in men and nonpregnant women. Values in maternal serum are less than 2.5 multiples of median for fetal gestational age.

Abnormal findings

Elevated maternal serum AFP levels may suggest neural tube defects or other tube anomalies. Maternal AFP levels rise sharply in the maternal blood of about 90% of women carrying a fetus with anencephaly and in 50% of those carrying a fetus with spina bifida. Definitive diagnosis requires ultrasonography and amniocentesis. High AFP levels may indicate intrauterine death. Sometimes high levels indicate other anomalies, such as duodenal atresia, omphalocele, tetralogy of Fallot, and Turner's syndrome.

Elevated serum AFP levels occur in 70% of nonpregnant patients with hepatocellular carcinoma. Elevated levels are also related to germ cell tumor of gonadal, retroperitoneal, or mediastinal origin. Serum AFP levels rise in ataxia-telangiectasia and sometimes in cancer of the pancreas, stomach, or biliary system and in nonseminiferous testicular tumors. Transient modest elevations can occur in nonneoplastic hepatocellular disease, such as alcoholic cirrhosis and acute or chronic hepatitis. Elevation of AFP levels after remission suggests tumor recurrence.

In hepatocellular carcinoma, a gradual decrease in serum AFP levels indicates a favorable response to therapy. In germ cell tumors, serum AFP levels and serum human chorionic gonadotropin levels should be measured concurrently.

Interfering factors

- Hemolysis due to rough handling of the sample
- Multiple pregnancies (possible false-positive)

TORCH TEST

The TORCH test helps detect exposure to pathogens involved in congenital and neonatal infections. TORCH is an acronym for toxoplasmosis, rubella, cytomegalovirus, and herpes simplex antibodies. These pathogens are commonly associated with congenital and neonatal infections that aren't clinically apparent and may cause severe central nervous system impairment. This test detects specific immunoglobulin M-associated antibodies in infant blood.

Purpose

- To aid diagnosis of acute, congenital, and intrapartum infections

Patient preparation

- Explain to the infant's parents the purpose of the test and mention that the test requires a blood sample.
- Tell the parent's who will perform the venipuncture and when.
- Explain that the infant may experience discomfort from the needle puncture and the tourniquet.

Procedure and posttest care

- Obtain a 3-ml sample of venous or cord blood.
- Apply direct pressure to the venipuncture site until bleeding stops.
- If a hematoma develops at the venipuncture site, apply warm soaks.

Precautions

- Handle the sample gently to prevent hemolysis.
- Send the sample to the laboratory immediately.
- Don't freeze the sample.

Normal findings

Normal test results are negative for TORCH agents.

Abnormal findings

Toxoplasmosis is diagnosed by sequential examination that shows rising antibody titers, changing titers, and serologic conversion from negative to positive; a titer of 1:256 suggests recent *Toxoplasma* infection.

In infants less than 6 months old, rubella infection is associated with a marked and persistent rise in complement-fixing antibody titer over time. Persistence of rubella antibody in an infant after age 6 months strongly suggests congenital infection. Congenital rubella is associated with cardiac anomalies, neurosensory deafness, growth retardation, and encephalitic symptoms.

Detection of herpes antibodies in cerebrospinal fluid with signs of herpetic encephalitis and persistent herpes simplex virus type 2 antibody levels confirms herpes simplex infection in a neonate without obvious herpetic lesions.

Interfering factors

- Hemolysis due to rough handling of the sample

TUBERCULIN SKIN TESTS

Tuberculin skin tests are used to screen for previous infection by the tubercle bacillus. They're routinely performed in children, young adults, and patients with radiographic findings that suggest this infection. In the old tuberculin (OT) and purified protein derivative (PPD) tests, intradermal injection of the tuberculin antigen causes a delayed hypersensitivity reaction in patients with active or dormant tuberculosis.

The Mantoux test uses a single-needle intradermal injection of PPD, permitting precise measurement of the dose. Multipuncture tests, such as the tine test, MonoVacc tests, and Aplitest, use intradermal injections with tines impregnated with OT or PPD. Because they require less skill and are more rapidly administered, multipuncture tests are generally used for screening. A positive multipuncture test usually requires a Mantoux test for confirmation.

Purpose

- To distinguish tuberculosis (TB) from blastomycosis, coccidioidomycosis, and histoplasmosis
- To identify people who need diagnostic investigation for TB because of possible exposure

Patient preparation

- Explain to the patient that this test helps detect TB.
- Tell the patient that the test requires an intradermal injection, which may cause him discomfort.
- Check the patient's history for active TB, the results of previous skin tests, and hypersensitivities.
- If the patient has had TB, don't perform a skin test.
- If he's had a positive reaction to previous skin tests, consult the physician or follow facility policy.
- If he's had an allergic reaction to acacia, don't perform an OT test because this product contains acacia.
- If you're performing a tuberculin test on an outpatient, instruct the patient to return at the specified time so that test results can be read.
- Inform the patient that a positive reaction to a skin test appears as a red, hard, raised area at the injection site. Although the area may itch, instruct him not to scratch it.
- Stress that a positive reaction doesn't always indicate active TB.

Procedure and posttest care

- Ask the patient to sit and support his extended arm on a flat surface.
- Clean the volar surface of the upper forearm with alcohol, and allow the area to dry completely.

Mantoux test

- Perform an intradermal injection.

Multipuncture test

- Remove the protective cap on the injection device to expose the four tines.
- Hold the patient's forearm in one hand, stretching the skin of the forearm tightly. Then, with your other hand, firmly depress the device into the patient's skin, without twisting it.
- Hold the device in place for at least 1 second before removing it.
- If you've applied sufficient pressure, you'll see four puncture sites and a circular depression made by the device on the patient's skin.

Both tests

- Record where the test was given, the date and time, and when the results are to be read. Tuberculin skin tests are generally read 48 to 72 hours after injection; the MonoVacc test can be read 48 to 96 hours after the test.
- If ulceration or necrosis develops at the injection site, apply cold soaks or a topical steroid.

Precautions

- Tuberculin skin tests are contraindicated in patients with current reactions to smallpox vaccinations, a rash, a skin disorder, or active TB.

- Don't perform a skin test in areas with excessive hair, acne, or insufficient subcutaneous tissue, such as over a tendon or bone.
- If the patient is known to be hypersensitive to skin tests, use a first-strength dose in the Mantoux test to avoid necrosis at the puncture site.
- Have epinephrine available to treat a possible anaphylactic or acute hypersensitivity reaction.

Normal findings

In tuberculin skin tests, normal findings show negative or minimal reactions. In the Mantoux test, no induration may appear or the patient may develop induration less than 5 mm in diameter.

In the tine and Aplitest tests, no vesiculation or induration may appear or the patient may develop induration less than 2 mm in diameter. In the MonoVacc tests, no induration appears.

Abnormal findings

A positive tuberculin reaction indicates previous infection by tubercle bacilli. It doesn't distinguish between an active and a dormant infection or provide a definitive diagnosis. If a positive reaction occurs, sputum smear and culture and chest radiography are necessary for further information.

In the Mantoux test, induration 5 to 9 mm in diameter indicates a borderline reaction; larger induration, a positive reaction. Because patients infected with atypical mycobacteria other than tubercle bacilli may have borderline reactions, repeat testing is necessary.

In the tine or Aplitest tests, vesiculation indicates a positive reaction; induration 2 mm in diameter without vesiculation requires confirmation by the Mantoux test. Any induration in the MonoVacc test indicates a positive reaction; however, it requires confirmation by the Mantoux test.

Interfering factors

- Subcutaneous injection, usually indicated by erythema greater than 10 mm in diameter without induration
- Corticosteroids, other immunosuppressants, and live vaccine viruses, such as measles, mumps, rubella, and polio, within 4 to 6 weeks before the test (possible suppression of skin reaction)
- In elderly people and patients with viral infection, malnutrition, febrile illness, uremia, immunosuppressive disorders, or miliary TB (possible suppression of skin reaction)
- Less than 10-week period since infection (possible suppression of skin reaction)
- Improper dilution, dosage, or storage of the tuberculin

TUMOR MARKER TESTS (CA-125; CA 19-9; CA-50; AND CA 15-3 [27,29])

Tumor markers are substances produced and secreted by tumor cells to help determine tumor activity. They can be found in the serum of cancer patients. Specific tests are ordered depending on the type of cancer the patient has. The CA 15-3 antigen (breast-cystic fluid protein or BCFP) may be used in conjunction with CEA and is helpful particularly in breast cancer patients (CA 27, metastatic breast cancer, breast-cystic fluid protein 29, BCFP). CA 19-9 carbohydrate antigen may be ordered in patients with pancreas, hepatobiliary, or lung cancers. The CA-125 glycoprotein antigen and serum carbohydrate antigen is commonly associated with types of ovarian cancers. The CA-

50 may be ordered in patients with GI or pancreatic cancer.

A combination of markers may be used due to low sensitivity and specificity of the markers. Few tumor markers meet Food and Drug Administration approval due to their controversy of their role in cancer diagnosis and treatment.

Purpose

- To assist tumor staging and identify possible metastasis
- To monitor and detect disease recurrence
- To assess therapeutic response to therapy

Patient preparation

- Explain the purpose of the particular test ordered and that it may be helpful in the patient's disorder, as appropriate.
- Specific directions from the laboratory or cancer center should be followed for the particular test ordered. Fasting may be involved and factors may be identified that may interfere with test results. Note interfering factors on the appropriate laboratory requests.
- Tell the patient that the test requires a blood sample. Explain who will perform the venipuncture and when.
- Explain to the patient that he may experience discomfort from the needle puncture and the tourniquet.

Procedure and posttest care

- Obtain a 10-ml venous sample as ordered in the tube specified by the laboratory or cancer center, and transport the sample as directed.
- Apply direct pressure to the venipuncture site until bleeding stops.
- If a hematoma develops at the venipuncture site, apply warm soaks.

Precautions

- Consult the laboratory or cancer center as to specific patient preparation required (fasting, identifying interfering factors).
- Transport the specimen as directed.
- Handle the sample gently to prevent hemolysis.

Reference values

Normal values for these tumor markers are:

- CA 15-3 (27,29): < 30 U/ml
- CA 19-9: < 70 U/ml
- CA-125: < 34 U/ml
- CA-50: < 17 U/ml.

Abnormal findings

CA 15-3 (27,29) is greatly increased in metastatic breast cancer; it's also increased in pancreas, lung, colorectal, ovarian, and liver cancers. It decreases with therapy; an increase after therapy suggests progressive disease.

CA 19-9 is increased in pancreas, hepatobiliary, and lung cancers. It may be mildly increased in gastric and colorectal cancers.

CA-125 is increased in epithelial ovary, fallopian tube, endometrial, endocervix, pancreas, and liver cancers. It's less increased in colon, breast, lung, and GI cancers.

CA-50 is increased in GI and pancreatic cancers.

Interfering factors

- CA 15-3 (27,29) increased in benign breast or ovarian disease
- CA 19-9 increased in pancreatitis, cholecystitis, cirrhosis, gallstones, and cystic fibrosis (minimal elevations)
- CA-125 increased in pregnancy, endometriosis, pelvic inflammatory disease, menstruation, acute and chronic hepatitis, ascites, peritonitis, pancreatitis, GI disease, Meig's syndrome, pleural effusion, and pulmonary disease

6

Urine tests

URINALYSIS

ROUTINE URINALYSIS

A routine urinalysis tests for urinary and systemic disorders. This test evaluates physical characteristics (color, odor, turbidity, and opacity) of urine; determines specific gravity and pH; detects and measures protein, glucose, and ketone bodies; and examines sediment for blood cells, casts, and crystals.

Diagnostic laboratory methods include visual examination, reagent strip screening, refractometry for specific gravity, and microscopic inspection of centrifuged sediment.

Purpose

- To screen patient's urine for renal or urinary tract disease
- To help detect metabolic or systemic disease unrelated to renal disorders
- To detect substances (drugs)

Patient preparation

- Explain to the patient that this test aids in the diagnosis of renal or urinary tract disease and helps evaluate overall body function.
- Inform the patient that food or fluids need not be restricted before the test.
- Notify the laboratory and physician of medications the patient is taking that may affect laboratory results; they may need to be restricted.

Procedure and posttest care

- Collect a random urine specimen of at least 15 ml.
- Obtain a first-voided morning specimen if possible.
- Instruct the patient to resume his usual diet and medication schedule as ordered.

Precautions

- Strain the specimen to catch stones or stone fragments if the patient is being evaluated for renal colic.
- Carefully pour the urine through an unfolded 4″ × 4″ gauze pad or a fine-mesh sieve placed over the specimen container.
- Send the specimen to the laboratory immediately.
- Refrigerate the specimen if analysis will be delayed longer than 1 hour.

Normal findings

See *Normal findings in routine urinalysis.*

Abnormal findings

Nonpathologic variations in normal values may result from diet, nonpathologic conditions, specimen collection time, and other factors.

Urine pH, which is greatly affected by diet and medications, influences the appearance of urine and the composition of crystals. An alkaline pH (above 7.0) — characteristic of a vegetarian diet — causes turbidity and the formation of phosphate, carbonate, and amorphous crystals. An acid pH (below 7.0) — typical of a high-protein diet — produces turbidity and the formation of oxalate, cystine, leucine, tyrosine, amorphous urate, and uric acid crystals.

Protein, normally absent from the urine, may be present in a benign condition known as orthostatic (postural) proteinuria. Most common in patients ages 10 to 20, this condition is intermittent, appears after prolonged standing, and disappears after recumbency. Transient benign proteinuria can also occur with fever, exposure to cold, emotional stress, or strenuous exercise. Systemic diseases that may cause proteinuria include lymphoma, hepatitis, diabetes mellitus, toxemia, hyperten-

Normal findings in routine urinalysis

ELEMENT	FINDINGS
Macroscopic	
Color	◆ Straw to dark yellow
Odor	◆ Slightly aromatic
Appearance	◆ Clear
Specific gravity	◆ 1.005 to 1.035
pH	◆ 4.5 to 8
Protein	◆ None
Glucose	◆ None
Ketone bodies	◆ None
Bilirubin	◆ None
Urobilinogen	◆ Normal
Hemoglobin	◆ None
Erythrocytes (RBCs)	◆ None
Nitrites (bacteria)	◆ None
Leukocytes (WBCs)	◆ None
Microscopic	
RBCs	◆ 0 to 2/high-power field
WBCs	◆ 0 to 5/high-power field
Epithelial cells	◆ 0 to 5/high-power field
Casts	◆ None, except 1 to 2 hyaline casts/low-power field
Crystals	◆ Present
Bacteria	◆ None
Yeast cells	◆ None
Parasites	◆ None

sion, lupus erythematosus, and febrile illnesses.

Sugars, usually absent from the urine, may appear under normal conditions. The most common sugar in urine is glucose. Transient nonpathologic glycosuria may result from emotional stress or pregnancy and may follow ingestion of a high-carbohydrate meal.

Centrifuged urine sediment contains cells, casts, crystals, bacteria, yeast, and parasites. Red blood cells (RBCs) commonly don't appear in urine without pathologic significance; however, strenuous exercise can cause hematuria.

The following abnormal findings generally suggest pathologic conditions:

■ *Color:* Color change can result from diet, drugs, and many diseases.

■ *Odor:* In diabetes mellitus, starvation, and dehydration, a fruity odor accompanies formation of ketone bodies. In urinary tract infections, a fetid odor commonly is associated with *Escherichia coli.* Maple syrup urine disease and phenylketonuria also cause distinctive odors. Other abnormal odors include those similar to a brewery, sweaty feet, cabbage, fish and sulfur.

■ *Turbidity:* Turbid urine may contain red or white cells, bacteria, fat, or chyle and may reflect renal infection.

■ *Specific gravity:* Low specific gravity (< 1.005) is characteristic of diabetes insipidus, nephrogenic diabetes insipidus, acute tubular necrosis, and pyelonephritis. Fixed specific gravity, in which values remain 1.010 regardless of fluid intake, occurs in chronic glomerulonephritis with severe renal damage. High specific gravity (> 1.035) occurs in nephrotic syndrome, dehydration, acute glomerulonephritis, heart failure, liver failure, and shock.

■ *pH:* Alkaline urine pH may result from Fanconi's syndrome, urinary tract infection, and metabolic or respiratory alkalosis. Acid urine pH is associated with renal tuberculosis, pyrexia, phenylketonuria, alkaptonuria, and acidosis.

■ *Protein:* Proteinuria suggests renal failure or disease (including nephrosis, glomerulosclerosis, glomerulonephritis, nephrolithiasis, nephrotic syndrome, and polycystic kidney disease) or, possibly, multiple myeloma.

■ *Sugars:* Glycosuria usually indicates diabetes mellitus but may result from pheochromocytoma, Cushing's syndrome, impaired tubular reabsorption, advanced renal disease, and increased intracranial pressure. I.V. solutions containing glucose and total parenteral nutrition containing from 10% to 50% glucose can cause glucose to spill over the renal threshold, leading to glycosuria. Fructosuria, galactosuria, and pentosuria generally suggest rare hereditary metabolic disorders (except for lactosuria during pregnancy and breastfeeding). However, an alimentary form of pentosuria and fructosuria may follow excessive ingestion of pentose or fructose. When the liver fails to metabolize these sugars, they spill into the urine because the renal tubules don't reabsorb them.

■ *Ketone bodies:* Ketonuria occurs in diabetes mellitus when cellular energy needs exceed available cellular glucose. In the absence of glucose, cells metabolize fat for energy. Ketone bodies — the end products of incomplete fat metabolism — accumulate in plasma and are excreted in the urine. Ketonuria may also occur in starvation states, low or no carbohydrate diets and following diarrhea or vomiting.

■ *Bilirubin:* Bilirubin in urine may occur in liver disease resulting from obstructive jaundice or hepatotoxic drugs or toxins or from fibrosis of the biliary canaliculi (which may occur in cirrhosis).

■ *Urobilinogen:* Intestinal bacteria in the duodenum change bilirubin into urobilinogen. The liver reprocesses the remainder into bile. Increased urobilinogen in the urine may indicate liver damage, hemolytic disease, or severe infection. Decreased levels may occur with biliary obstruction, inflammatory disease, antimicrobial therapy, severe diarrhea, or renal insufficiency.

■ *Cells:* Hematuria indicates bleeding within the genitourinary tract and may result from infection, obstruction, inflammation, trauma, tumors, glomerulonephritis, renal hypertension, lupus nephritis, renal tuberculosis, renal vein thrombosis, renal calculi, hydronephrosis, pyelonephritis, scurvy, malaria, parasitic infection of the bladder, subacute bacterial endocarditis, polyarteritis nodosa, and hemorrhagic disorders. Strenuous exercise or exposure to toxic chemicals may also cause hematuria. An excess of white blood cells (WBCs) in urine usually implies urinary tract inflammation, especially cystitis or pyelonephritis. WBC and WBC casts in urine suggest renal infection or noninfective inflammatory disease. Numerous epithelial cells suggest renal tubular degeneration, such as heavy metal poisoning, eclampsia and kidney transplant rejection.

■ *Casts (plugs of gelled proteinaceous material [high-molecular-weight mucoprotein]):* Casts form in the renal tubules and collecting ducts by agglutination of protein cells or cellular debris and are flushed loose by urine flow. Excessive numbers of casts indicate renal disease. Hyaline casts are associated with renal parenchymal disease, inflammation, trauma to the glomerular capillary membrane, and some physiologic states (such as after exercise); epithelial casts, with renal tubular damage, nephrosis, eclampsia, amyloidosis, and heavy metal poisoning; coarse and fine granular casts, with acute or chronic renal failure, pyelonephritis, and chronic lead intoxication; fatty and waxy casts, with nephrotic syndrome, chronic renal disease, and diabetes mellitus; RBC casts, with renal parenchymal disease (especially glomerulonephritis), renal infarction, subacute bacterial endocarditis, vascular disorders, sickle cell anemia, scurvy, blood dyscrasias, malignant hypertension, collagen disease, and acute inflammation; and white blood cell casts, with acute pyelonephritis and glomerulonephritis, nephrotic syndrome, pyogenic infection, and lupus nephritis.

■ *Crystals:* Some crystals normally appear in urine, but numerous calcium oxalate crystals suggest hypercalcemia or ethylene glycol ingestion. Cystine crystals (cystinuria) reflect an inborn error of metabolism.

■ *Other components:* Bacteria, yeast cells, and parasites in urine sediment reflect genitourinary tract infection or contamination of external genitalia. Yeast cells, which may be mistaken for RBCs, are identifiable by their ovoid shape, lack of color, variable size and, frequently, signs of budding. The most common parasite in sediment is *Trichomonas vaginalis,* which causes vaginitis, urethritis, and prostatovesiculitis.

Interfering factors

■ Strenuous exercise before routine urinalysis may cause transient myoglobulinuria

■ Insufficient urinary volume, less than 2 ml (possible limitation of the range of procedures)

■ Failure to send specimen to the laboratory immediately after the collection is completed (false-low urobilinogen)

■ Foods, such as beets, berries, and rhubarb (false change in color)

■ Certain drugs may influence the results

■ Highly dilute urine such as in diabetes insipidus

URINARY CALCULI

Urinary calculi (urolithiasis or, more commonly, urinary stones) are insoluble substances most commonly formed of the mineral salts—calcium oxalate, calcium phosphate, magnesium ammonium phosphate, urate, or cystine. They may appear anywhere in the urinary tract and range in size from microscopic to several centimeters.

Formation of calculi can result from reduced urinary volume, increased excretion of mineral salts, urinary stasis, pH changes, and decreased protective substances. Calculi commonly form in the kidney, pass into the ureter, and are excreted in the urine. Because not all calculi pass spontaneously, they may require surgical extraction or pulverization using extracorporeal shock-wave lithotripsy. Calculi don't always cause symptoms, but when they do, hematuria is most common. If calculi obstruct the ureter, they may cause severe flank pain, dysuria, and urinary retention, frequency, and urgency.

Purpose

- To detect and analyze calculi in the urine

Patient preparation

- Explain to the patient that this test detects urinary calculi and that laboratory analysis will reveal their composition.
- Tell the patient that his urine will be collected and strained.
- Advise the patient that no prior restriction of food or fluids is required.
- Inform the patient that medication to control pain will be administered.

Equipment

Strainer (an unfolded 4″ × 4″ dressing or a fine-mesh sieve), specimen container

Procedure and posttest care

- Have the patient void into the strainer.
- Inspect the strainer carefully because calculi may be minute, looking like gravel or sand.
- Document the appearance of the calculi and the number if possible.
- Place the calculi in a properly labeled container.
- Send the container to the laboratory immediately for prompt analysis.
- Observe for severe flank pain, dysuria, and urinary retention, frequency, or urgency. Hematuria should subside.

Precautions

- Keep the strainer and urinal or bedpan within the patient's reach if he has received analgesics because he may be drowsy and unable to get out of bed to void.

Normal findings

Normally, calculi aren't present in urine.

Abnormal findings

More than one-half of all calculi in urine are of mixed composition, containing two or more mineral salts; calcium oxalate is the most common component. Determination of the composition of calculi helps identify various metabolic disorders, guiding proper treatment and prevention measures.

Interfering factors

- Improper collection technique

PHENOLSULFONPHTHALEIN EXCRETION

The phenolsulfonphthalein (PSP) excretion test evaluates kidney function. This test is indicated in patients with abnormal results in the urine concentration test, one of the earliest signs of renal dysfunction.

Purpose

- To determine renal plasma flow
- To evaluate tubular function

Patient preparation

- Explain to the patient that this test evaluates kidney function.
- Inform him that he need not restrict food before the test. Encourage the patient to drink fluids before and during the test to maintain adequate urine flow.
- Tell the patient the test requires an I.V. injection and collection of urine specimens 15 minutes, 30 minutes, 1 hour and, if ordered, 2 hours after the I.V. injection.

■ Inform the patient who will administer the I.V. injection and when.
■ Explain to the patient that he may experience discomfort from the needle puncture and the tourniquet, and that the dye temporarily turns the urine red.
■ If the patient can't void and requires catheterization, tell him that he may have the urge to void when the catheter is in place.
■ Notify the laboratory and physician of medications the patient is taking that may affect test results; they may need to be restricted. If they must be continued, however, note this on the laboratory request.

Equipment

PSP dye (6 mg in 1 ml of solution), equipment for indwelling urinary catheterization, four urine specimen containers

Procedure and posttest care

■ Instruct the patient to empty his bladder, and discard the urine.
■ The physician will administer 1 ml of PSP, which equals 6 mg of dye, I.V.
■ Collect a urine specimen at 15 minutes, 30 minutes, 1 hour and, if ordered, 2 hours after the injection.
■ Encourage fluid intake because 40 ml of urine is required for each specimen.
■ If the patient is catheterized, be sure to clamp the catheter between collections.
■ Record the PSP dosage on the laboratory request.
■ Properly label each specimen, and include the collection time.
■ Elevate the arm and apply warm soaks if phlebitis develops at the I.V. site.
■ If the patient is catheterized, make sure he voids within 8 hours after the catheter is removed.
■ Instruct the patient to resume his usual medication schedule as ordered.

Precautions

■ Use this test cautiously in a patient with cardiac dysfunction or renal insufficiency because the increased fluid intake necessary for proper hydration may precipitate heart failure.
■ Keep epinephrine, histamine-1 (H_1) receptor antagonists (diphenhydramine), and a glucocorticoid (Solu-Medrol) available because allergic reactions to PSP occasionally occur.
■ Don't use the urine in the drainage bag if the patient already has a catheter in place.
■ Empty the bag, and clamp the catheter for 1 hour before the test.
■ Send the specimen to the laboratory immediately after each collection.
■ Refrigerate the specimen if more than 10 minutes will elapse before transport.

Normal findings

Normally, 25% of the PSP dose is excreted in 15 minutes, 50% to 60% in 30 minutes, 60% to 70% in 1 hour, and 70% to 80% in 2 hours. Normal excretion for children (excluding infants) is 5% to 10% higher than for adults.

Abnormal findings

The 15-minute value is the most sensitive indicator of both tubular function and renal plasma flow because depressed excretion at this interval, with normal excretion later, suggests relatively mild or early-stage bilateral renal disease. However, a depressed 2-hour value may reveal moderate-to-severe renal impairment. Depressed PSP excretion is also characteristic in renal vascular disease, urinary tract obstruction, heart failure, and gout.

Elevated PSP excretion is characteristic in hypoalbuminemia, hepatic disease, and multiple myeloma.

Interfering factors

- Failure to collect an adequate specimen at required times
- Radiographic contrast agents, aspirin, chlorothiazide, salicylates, sulfonamides, penicillin, cascara sagrada, ethanol, indomethacin, nitrofurantoin, phenylbutazone, probenecid, and vitamins (possible increase or decrease)
- Beets, carrots, and rhubarb (possible increase or decrease)
- Incorrect PSP dosage (possible increase or decrease)
- High serum protein levels (decrease)
- Severe hypoalbuminemia, excessive albuminuria, or severe liver disease (possible effect on excretion)

CONCENTRATION AND DILUTION

The kidneys normally concentrate or dilute urine according to fluid intake. When such intake is excessive, the kidneys excrete more water in the urine; when intake is limited, they excrete less. The concentration and dilution test evaluates renal capacity to concentrate urine in response to fluid deprivation or to dilute it in response to fluid overload. This test may also be referred to as the water loading or water deprivation test.

Purpose

- To evaluate renal tubular function
- To detect renal impairment
- To diagnose disorders such as diabetes insipidus

Patient preparation

- Explain to the patient that this test evaluates kidney function.
- Tell him the test requires multiple urine specimens. Explain how many specimens will be collected and at what intervals.
- Instruct him to discard urine voided for a specific time, as per laboratory protocol, such as all urine collected during the night.
- Withhold diuretics as needed.

Concentration test

- Provide a high-protein meal and only 200 ml of fluid the night before the test.
- Instruct him to restrict food and fluids for at least 14 hours before the test. (Some concentration tests require that water be withheld for 24 hours but permit relatively normal food intake.)
- Limit salt intake at the evening meal to prevent excessive thirst.
- Emphasize to the patient that his cooperation is necessary to obtain accurate results.

Dilution test

- Generally, this test directly follows the concentration test and necessitates no additional patient preparation. If it's performed alone, simply withhold breakfast.

Procedure and posttest care

Concentration test

- Collect urine specimens at 6 a.m., 8 a.m., and 10 a.m.

Dilution test

- Instruct the patient to void and discard the first urine sample.
- Give the patient 1,500 ml of water to drink within a 30-minute period.
- Collect urine specimens every half hour or every hour for 4 hours thereafter.

Both tests

- Provide a balanced meal or a snack after collecting the final specimen.

■ Make sure the patient voids within 8 hours after the catheter is removed.

Precautions

■ May be contraindicated in patients with advanced renal disease or cardiac dysfunction because fluid overload can precipitate water intoxication, sodium diuresis, or heart failure.
■ Send each specimen to the laboratory immediately after collection.
■ Provide the patient with a clean bedpan, urinal, or toilet specimen pan if he's unable to urinate into the specimen containers.
■ Rinse the collection device after each use.
■ If the patient is catheterized, empty the drainage bag before the test. Obtain the specimens from the catheter, and clamp the catheter between collections.

Reference values

Normal specific gravity ranges from 1.005 to 1.035; osmolality normally ranges from 300 to 900 mOsm/kg.

Concentration test: Specific gravity ranges from 1.025 to 1.032 and osmolality rises above 800 mOsm/kg of water (SI, > 800 mmol/kg) in patients with normal renal function.

Dilution test: Normally, specific gravity falls below 1.003 and osmolality below 100 mOsm/kg for at least one specimen; 80% or more of the ingested water is eliminated in 4 hours. In elderly persons, depressed values can be associated with normal renal function.

Abnormal findings

Decreased renal capacity to concentrate urine in response to fluid deprivation, or to dilute urine in response to fluid overload, may indicate tubular epithelial damage, decreased renal blood flow, loss of functional nephrons, or pituitary or cardiac dysfunction.

Interfering factors

■ Failure to observe pretest restrictions
■ Use of radiographic contrast agents within 7 days of test (possible increase in osmolality)
■ Diuretics and nephrotoxic drugs (possible increase or decrease in specific gravity and osmolality)
■ Glycosuria

TUBULAR REABSORPTION OF PHOSPHATE

The test for tubular reabsorption of phosphate is an indirect measure of parathyroid hormone (PTH) levels. PTH helps maintain optimum blood levels of ionized calcium and controls renal excretion of calcium and phosphate. This test measures urine and serum phosphate and creatinine levels. These values are then used to calculate the tubular reabsorption of phosphate.

Purpose

■ To evaluate parathyroid function
■ To aid diagnosis of primary hyperparathyroidism
■ To aid differential diagnosis of hypercalcemia

Patient preparation

■ Explain to the patient that this test evaluates the function of the parathyroid glands.
■ Advise the patient that the test requires a blood sample and urine collection over a 24-hour period.
■ Tell the patient who will perform the venipuncture and when.
■ Advise the patient that he may experience transient discomfort from the needle puncture and the pressure of the tourniquet.

■ Instruct the patient to maintain a normal phosphate diet for 3 days before the test because low phosphate intake (< 500 mg/day) may elevate tubular reabsorption values and a high-phosphate diet (3,000 mg/day) may lower them. Common nutritional sources of phosphorus include legumes, nuts, milk, egg yolks, meat, poultry, fish, cereals, and cheese. These foods should be eaten in moderate amounts.
■ Instruct the patient to fast after midnight the night before the test.
■ Notify the laboratory and physician of medications the patient is taking that may affect test results; they may need to be restricted. If they must be continued, however, note this on the laboratory request.

Procedure and posttest care

■ Perform a venipuncture, and collect the blood sample in a 10-ml clot-activator tube.
■ Instruct the patient to empty his bladder, and discard the urine; record this as time zero.
■ Collect the patient's urine over a 24-hour period with the first sample discarded and the last sample retained; occasionally, a 4-hour collection or a random collection is ordered instead.
■ Allow the patient to eat, and encourage fluid intake to maintain adequate urine flow after the venipuncture.
■ Apply direct pressure to the venipuncture site until bleeding stops. Apply warm soaks if a hematoma develops at the venipuncture site.
■ Instruct the patient to resume his usual diet and medication schedule as ordered.

Precautions

■ Handle the blood collection tube gently to prevent hemolysis.
■ Keep the urine specimen container refrigerated or on ice during the collection period.
■ Tell the patient to avoid contaminating the specimen with toilet paper or stool.
■ Label the specimen and send it to the laboratory as soon as the collection period has ended.

Normal findings

Renal tubules normally reabsorb 80% or more of phosphate.

Abnormal findings

Reabsorption of less than 74% of phosphate strongly suggests primary hyperparathyroidism. Hypercalcemia is the most common manifestation of primary hyperparathyroidism. However, a patient with hypercalcemia may still require additional testing to confirm primary hyperparathyroidism as the cause.

Interfering factors

■ Uremia, renal tubular disease, osteomalacia, myeloma, and sarcoidosis (possible increase)
■ Furosemide and gentamicin (possible increase)
■ Renal calculi in patients not having parathyroid tumor, amphotericin B, thiazide diuretics (possible decrease)
■ Contamination of the specimen with toilet tissue or stool
■ Hemolysis caused by rough handling of the blood sample
■ Failure to keep the specimen on ice or to send it to the laboratory immediately after the collection is completed
■ Failure to follow dietary restrictions

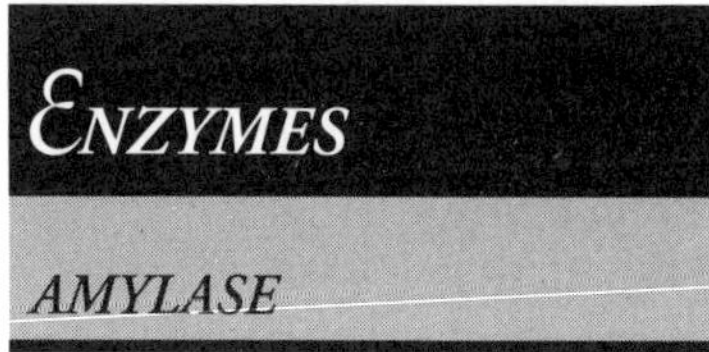

Amylase is a starch-splitting enzyme produced primarily in the pancreas and salivary glands, which is usually secreted into the alimentary tract and absorbed into the blood; small amounts of amylase are also absorbed into the blood directly from these organs. Following glomerular filtration, amylase is excreted in the urine.

In the presence of adequate renal function, serum and urine levels usually rise in tandem. However, within 2 to 3 days of the onset of acute pancreatitis, serum amylase levels fall to normal, but elevated urine amylase persists for 7 to 10 days. One method for determining urine amylase levels is the dye-coupled starch method.

Purpose

- To diagnose acute pancreatitis when serum amylase levels are normal or borderline
- To aid diagnosis of chronic pancreatitis and salivary gland disorders

Patient preparation

- Explain to the patient that this test evaluates the function of the pancreas and the salivary glands.
- Inform the patient that he need not restrict food or fluids.
- Tell the patient the test requires urine collection for 2, 6, 8, or 24 hours, and teach him how to collect a timed specimen.
- Notify the laboratory and physician of medications the patient is taking that may affect test results; they may need to be restricted.

Procedure and posttest care

- Collect the patient's urine over a 2-, 6-, 8-, or 24-hour period.

Precautions

- Cover and refrigerate the specimen during the collection period.
- If the patient is catheterized, keep the collection bag on ice.
- Instruct the patient not to contaminate the specimen with toilet tissue or stool.
- Send the specimen to the laboratory as soon as the test is complete.

Normal findings

Urine amylase is reported in various units of measure; therefore, values differ from laboratory to laboratory. The Mayo Clinic reports normal urinary excretion of 1 to 17 U/hour (SI, 0.017 to 0.29 µkat/h).

Abnormal findings

Elevated amylase levels occur in acute pancreatitis; obstruction of the pancreatic duct, intestines, or salivary duct; carcinoma of the head of the pancreas; mumps; acute injury of the spleen; renal disease, with impaired absorption; perforated peptic or duodenal ulcers; and gallbladder disease.

Depressed levels occur in pancreatitis, cachexia, alcoholism, cancer of the liver, cirrhosis, hepatitis, and hepatic abscess.

Interfering factors

- Salivary amylase in the urine due to coughing or talking over the sample (possible increase)
- Failure to collect all urine during the test period, to properly store the specimen, or to send the specimen to the laboratory immediately after the collection is completed
- High levels of bacterial contamination of the specimen or blood in the urine

- Morphine, meperidine, codeine, pentazocine, bethanechol, thiazide diuretics, indomethacin, or alcohol within 24 hours of the test (possible increase)
- Fluorides (possible decrease)

ARYLSULFATASE A

Arylsulfatase A (ARSA), a lysosomal enzyme found in every cell except the mature erythrocyte, is principally active in the liver, pancreas, and kidneys, where exogenous substances are detoxified into ester sulfates.

Urine ARSA levels rise in transitional bladder cancer, colorectal cancer, and leukemia. However, research hasn't resolved whether elevated ARSA levels provoke malignant growths or are simply an enzymatic response to them. This test measures urine ARSA levels by colorimetric or kinetic techniques.

Purpose

- To aid diagnosis of bladder, colon, or rectal cancer; myeloid (granulocytic) leukemia; and metachromatic leukodystrophy (an inherited lipid storage disease)

Patient preparation

- Tell the patient that this test measures an enzyme that's present throughout the body.
- Advise the patient that he need not restrict food or fluids before the test.
- Tell the patient the test requires urine collection over a 24-hour period, and teach him how to collect a timed specimen.

Procedure and posttest care

- Collect the patient's urine over a 24-hour period, discarding the first sample and retaining the last sample in the appropriate container.

Precautions

- If a female patient is menstruating, the test may have to be rescheduled.
- Tell the patient not to contaminate the urine specimen with toilet tissue or stool.
- Keep the collection container refrigerated or on ice during the collection period.
- Send the specimen to the laboratory as soon as the collection period has ended.
- If the patient has an indwelling urinary catheter in place, keep the collection bag on ice for the duration of the test.
- Begin the test period with a new, unused continuous urinary drainage apparatus.

Reference values

Normally, random values are 16 to 42 μ/g creatinine; 24-hour urine values are 0.37 to 3.60 μ/day creatinine; 1-hour test values are 2 to 19 μ/1 hour (SI, 2 to 19 μ/hour); 2-hour test values are 4 to 37 μ/2 hours (SI, 4 to 37 μ/hour); 24-hour test values are 170 to 2000 μ/24 hours (SI, 2.89 to 34.0 μkat/L).

Abnormal findings

Elevated ARSA levels may result from cancer of the bladder, colon, or rectum; or from myeloid leukemia.

Depressed ARSA levels can result from metachromatic leukodystrophy. In patients with this condition, urine studies show metachromatic granules in the urinary sediment.

Interfering factors

- Failure to collect all urine during the test period, to properly store the specimen, or to send the specimen to the

laboratory immediately after the collection is completed
- Contamination of the specimen with toilet tissue, stool, or menstrual blood
- Surgery within 1 week before the test (possible increase)

LYSOZYME

Lysozyme (or muramidase), a low-molecular-weight enzyme, is present in mucus, saliva, tears, skin secretions, and various internal body cells and fluids. This enzyme splits, or lyses, the cell walls of gram-positive bacteria and, with complement and other blood factors, acts to destroy them. Lysozyme seems to be synthesized in granulocytes and monocytes, and it first appears in serum after the destruction of such cells. When the serum lysozyme level exceeds three times the normal level, the enzyme appears in the urine. However, because renal tissue also contains lysozyme, renal injury alone can cause measurable excretion of this enzyme.

This test measures urine lysozyme levels with a turbidimeter. Serum lysozyme determinations, using the same method, confirm the results of urine testing.

Purpose

- To aid diagnosis of acute monocytic or granulocytic leukemia and to monitor the progression of these diseases
- To evaluate proximal tubular function and to diagnose renal impairment
- To detect rejection or infarction of kidney transplantation

Patient preparation

- Explain to the patient that this test evaluates renal function and the immune system.
- Advise the patient that he need not restrict food or fluids before the test.
- Tell the patient the test requires collection of urine over a 24-hour period, and teach him how to collect the specimen correctly.

Procedure and posttest care

- Collect the patient's urine over a 24-hour period, discarding the first specimen and retaining the last specimen in the appropriate container.

Precautions

- If a female patient is menstruating, the test may have to be rescheduled for a later date.
- Tell the patient to avoid contaminating the urine specimen with toilet tissue or stool.
- Cover and refrigerate the specimen throughout the collection period.
- Keep the collection bag on ice if the patient has an indwelling urinary catheter in place.
- Send the specimen to the laboratory as soon as the test is complete.

Reference values

Normally, urine lysozyme values are 0 to 3 mg/24 hours.

Abnormal findings

Elevated urine lysozyme levels are characteristic of impaired renal proximal tubular reabsorption, acute pyelonephritis, nephrotic syndrome, tuberculosis of the kidney, severe extrarenal infection, rejection or infarction of kidney transplantation (levels normally increase during the first few days after transplantation), and polycythemia vera.

Urine levels rise markedly after acute onset or relapse of monocytic or myelomonocytic leukemia and rise moderately after acute onset or relapse of granulocytic (myeloid) leukemia.

Urine lysozyme levels remain normal or decrease in lymphocytic leukemia and remain normal in myeloblastic and myelocytic leukemias.

Interfering factors

- Failure to collect all urine
- Bacteriuria (decrease)
- Blood or saliva in the specimen (increase)

CYCLIC ADENOSINE MONOPHOSPHATE

Formed from adenosine triphosphate by the action of the enzyme adenylate cyclase, the nucleotide cyclic adenosine monophosphate (cAMP) influences the protein synthesis rate within cells. Measurement of the urinary excretion of cAMP after an I.V. infusion of a standard dose of parathyroid hormone (PTH) can show renal tubular resistance in a patient with hypoparathyroid symptoms and high levels of PTH. Such findings suggest type I pseudohypoparathyroidism, a rare inherited disorder. (Urinary cAMP levels respond normally with type II pseudohypoparathyroidism because the defect is beyond the level of cAMP generation.)

Purpose

- To aid differential diagnosis of hypoparathyroidism and pseudohypoparathyroidism

Patient preparation

- Explain to the patient that this test evaluates parathyroid function.
- Tell the patient the test requires a 15-minute I.V. infusion of PTH and a 3- to 4-hour urine specimen collection.

CLINICAL ALERT *Perform a skin test to detect an allergy to PTH; keep epinephrine or an H1-receptor antagonist, such as diphenhydramine or glucocorticoids (Solu-Medrol), readily available in case of an adverse reaction.*

- Just before the procedure is performed, instruct the patient not to touch the I.V. line or exert pressure on the arm receiving the infusion.
- Tell the patient he may experience discomfort from the needle puncture. Ask him to notify you if he feels severe burning or if the site becomes inflamed or swollen.

Equipment

PTH (300 units, in refrigerated ampules), vial of sterile water (saline solution causes precipitate to form), urine collection container with hydrochloric acid added as a preservative

Procedure and posttest care

- Instruct the patient to empty his bladder.
- If the patient has an indwelling urinary catheter in place, replace the collection apparatus with an unused one.
- Send this specimen to the laboratory, if ordered; otherwise, discard it.
- Prepare the PTH for infusion as directed, using sterile water for dilution.
- Start the infusion with dextrose 5% in water, and infuse the PTH over 15 minutes. Record the start of the infusion as time zero.
- Collect a urine specimen 3 to 4 hours after infusion.
- Discontinue the I.V. infusion as ordered.
- Observe the patient for symptoms of hypercalcemia, including lethargy, anorexia, nausea, vomiting, vertigo, and abdominal cramps.
- Apply warm soaks if a hematoma or irritation develops at the venipuncture site.

Precautions

■ The cAMP test is contraindicated in patients with a positive PTH test as well as in patients with high calcium levels because PTH further raises calcium levels. It should be performed cautiously in patients receiving a cardiac glycoside and in those with sarcoidosis or renal or cardiac disease.
■ Tell the patient to avoid contaminating the urine specimen with toilet tissue or stool.
■ Send the specimen to the laboratory immediately after the collection is completed; if transport is delayed, refrigerate the specimen.
■ Keep the collection bag on ice if the patient has a catheter in place.

Reference values

Levels of cAMP are normally 0.3 to 3.6 mg/day (SI, 100 to 723 μmol/day) or 0.29 to 2.1 mg/g creatinine (SI, 100 to 723 μmol/mol creatinine).

Abnormal findings

Failure to respond to PTH, indicated by normal urinary excretion of cAMP, suggests type I pseudohypoparathyroidism.

Interfering factors

■ Contamination or improper storage of the specimen or failure to acidify the urine with hydrochloric acid

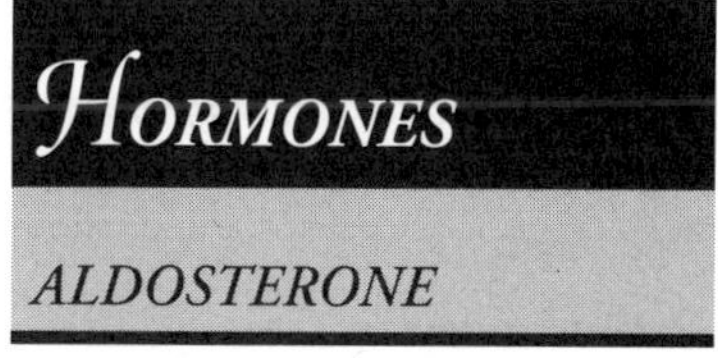

The aldosterone test measures urine levels of aldosterone, the principal mineralocorticoid secreted by the adrenal cortex. Aldosterone promotes retention of sodium and excretion of potassium by the renal tubules, thereby helping to regulate blood pressure and fluid and electrolyte balance. In turn, aldosterone secretion is controlled by the renin-angiotensin system. This feedback mechanism is vital to maintaining fluid and electrolyte balance.

Urine aldosterone levels, measured through radioimmunoassay, are usually evaluated after measurement of serum electrolyte and renin levels.

Purpose

■ To aid diagnosis of primary and secondary aldosteronism

Patient preparation

■ Explain to the patient that this test evaluates hormonal balance.
■ Instruct the patient to maintain a normal sodium diet (3 g/day) before the test and to avoid sodium-rich foods, such as bacon, barbecue sauce, corned beef, bouillon cubes or powder, pickles, snack foods (potato chips), and olives.
■ Advise the patient to avoid strenuous physical exercise and stressful situations during the collection period.
■ Tell the patient the test requires collection of urine during a 24-hour period, and teach him the proper collection technique.
■ Notify the laboratory and physician of medications the patient is taking that may affect test results; they may need to be restricted.

Procedure and posttest care

■ Collect the patient's urine over a 24-hour period, discarding the first specimen and retaining the last. Use a bottle containing a preservative, such as boric acid, to keep the specimen at a pH of 4.0 to 4.5.
■ Instruct the patient to resume his usual activities, diet, and medication schedule as ordered.

Precautions

- Refrigerate the specimen or place it on ice during the collection period.
- Send the specimen to the laboratory as soon as the collection is completed.

Reference values

Normally, urine aldosterone levels range from 3 to 19 μg/24 hours (SI, 8 to 51 nmol/day).

Abnormal findings

Elevated urine aldosterone levels suggest primary or secondary aldosteronism. The primary form usually arises from an aldosterone-secreting adenoma of the adrenal cortex but may also result from adrenocortical hyperplasia. Secondary aldosteronism, the more common form, results from external stimulation of the adrenal cortex such as that produced when the renin-angiotensin system is activated by hypertensive and edematous disorders.

Disorders that may result in secondary aldosteronism are malignant hypertension, heart failure, cirrhosis of the liver, nephrotic syndrome, and idiopathic cyclic edema.

Low urine aldosterone levels may result from Addison's disease, salt-losing syndrome, and toxemia of pregnancy. These levels normally rise during pregnancy but rapidly decline following parturition.

Interfering factors

- Failure to maintain normal dietary sodium intake as well as excess intake of licorice or glucose can influence the test results.
- Failure to avoid strenuous physical exercise and emotional stress before the test (possible increase due to stimulation of adrenocortical secretions)
- Radioactive scan performed within 1 week before the test
- Failure to collect all urine during the collection period, to properly store the specimen, or to send it to the laboratory immediately after the collection is completed
- Antihypertensive drugs (possible decrease due to sodium and water retention)
- Diuretics and most steroids (possible increase due to sodium excretion)
- Some corticosteroids, such as fludrocortisone, which mimic mineralocorticoid activity (possible decrease)

FREE CORTISOL

Used as a screen for adrenocortical hyperfunction, the free cortisol test measures urine levels of the portion of cortisol not bound to the corticosteroid-binding globulin transcortin. It's one of the best diagnostic tools for detecting Cushing's syndrome.

Unlike a single measurement of plasma cortisol, radioimmunoassay determinations of free cortisol levels in a 24-hour urine specimen reflect overall secretion levels instead of diurnal variations. Concurrent measurements of plasma cortisol and corticotropin, with urine 17-hydroxycorticosteroids and the dexamethasone suppression test, may be used to confirm the diagnosis.

Purpose

- To aid diagnosis of Cushing's syndrome
- To evaluate adrenal cortical function

Patient preparation

- Explain to the patient that this test helps evaluate adrenal gland function.
- Inform the patient that he need not restrict food or fluids before the test but should avoid stressful situations and ex-

cessive physical exercise during the collection period.

■ Tell the patient the test requires collection of urine over a 24-hour period.

■ Teach the patient the proper collection technique for a 24-hour urine specimen.

■ Notify the laboratory and physician of medications the patient is taking that may affect test results; they may need to be restricted.

Procedure and posttest care

■ Collect the patient's urine over a 24-hour period, discarding the first specimen and retaining the last specimen. Use a bottle containing a preservative to keep the specimen at a pH of 4.0 to 4.5.

■ Instruct the patient to resume his usual activities and medication schedule as ordered.

Precautions

■ Refrigerate the specimen or place it on ice during the collection period.

Reference values

Normal free cortisol values are less than 50 μg/24 hours (SI, < 138 mmol/24 hours)

Abnormal findings

Elevated free cortisol levels may indicate Cushing's syndrome resulting from adrenal hyperplasia, adrenal or pituitary tumor, or ectopic corticotropin production. Hepatic disease and obesity, which can raise plasma cortisol levels, generally don't appreciably raise urine levels of free cortisol. Low levels have little diagnostic significance and don't necessarily indicate adrenocortical hypofunction.

Interfering factors

■ Failure to collect all urine during the test period or to properly store the specimen

■ Pregnancy (possible increase)

■ Reserpine, phenothiazines, morphine, amphetamines, oral contraceptives, danazol, aldactone, and prolonged steroid therapy (possible increase)

■ Dexamethasone, ethacrynic acid, thiazides, and ketoconazole (decrease)

CATECHOLAMINES

The test for catecholamines uses spectrophotofluorometry to measure urine levels of the major catecholamines — epinephrine, norepinephrine, and dopamine. Epinephrine is secreted by the adrenal medulla; dopamine, by the central nervous system; and norepinephrine, by both. Catecholamines help regulate metabolism and prepare the body for the fight-or-flight response to stress. Certain tumors can also secrete catecholamines.

The specimen of choice for this test is a 24-hour urine specimen because catecholamine secretion fluctuates diurnally and in response to pain, heat, cold, emotional stress, physical exercise, hypoglycemia, injury, hemorrhage, asphyxia, and drugs. However, a random specimen may be useful for evaluating catecholamine levels after a hypertensive episode.

For a complete diagnostic workup of catecholamine secretion, urine levels of catecholamine metabolites are also measured. These metabolites — metanephrine, normetanephrine, homovanillic acid (HVA), and vanillylmandelic acid (VMA) — normally appear in the urine in greater quantities than the catecholamines.

Purpose

■ To aid diagnosis of pheochromocytoma in a patient with unexplained hypertension

■ To aid diagnosis of neuroblastoma, ganglioneuroma, and dysautonomia

Patient preparation

■ Explain to the patient that this test evaluates adrenal function.
■ Inform the patient that he should avoid chocolate, coffee and bananas for 7 hours before the test and should avoid stressful situations and excessive physical activity during the collection period.
■ Tell the patient that the test requires either a specimen collected over 24 hours or a random specimen, and explain the collection procedure.
■ Notify the laboratory and physician of medications the patient is taking that may affect test results; they may need to be restricted.

Procedure and posttest care

■ Collect the patient's urine over a 24-hour period. Use a bottle containing a preservative to keep the specimen acidified to a pH of 3.0 or less. (If a random specimen is ordered, collect it immediately after a hypertensive episode.)
■ Instruct the patient to resume his usual activities, diet, and medication schedule as ordered.

Precautions

■ Refrigerate a 24-hour specimen or place it on ice during the collection period.
■ Send the specimen to the laboratory as soon as the collection is complete.

Reference values

Values for catecholamine fractionalization range as follows.
Epinephrine: 0 to 20 μg/24 hours (SI, 0 to 109 nmol/24 hours)
Norepinephrine: 15 to 80 μg/24 hours (SI, 89 to 473 nmol/24 hours)
Dopamine: 65 to 400 μg/24 hours (SI, 425 to 2610 nmol/24 hours)

Abnormal findings

In a patient with undiagnosed hypertension, elevated urine catecholamine levels following a hypertensive episode usually indicate a pheochromocytoma. If tests indicate a pheochromocytoma, the patient may also be tested for multiple endocrine neoplasia. With the exception of HVA — a metabolite of dopamine — catecholamine metabolites may also be elevated. Abnormally high HVA levels rule out a pheochromocytoma because this tumor mainly secretes epinephrine, whose primary metabolite is VMA, not HVA.

Elevated catecholamine levels, without marked hypertension, may be due to a neuroblastoma or a ganglioneuroma, although HVA levels reflect these conditions more accurately. Elevated levels are also seen in severe systemic situations (burns, peritonitis, shock, and septicemia), cor pulmonale, manic depressive disorders, or depressive neurosis. Myasthenia gravis and progressive muscular dystrophy commonly cause urine catecholamine levels to rise above normal, but this test is rarely performed to diagnose these disorders. Consistently low-normal catecholamine levels may indicate dysautonomia marked by orthostatic hypotension.

Interfering factors

■ Failure to comply with drug restrictions, to collect all urine during the collection period, or to properly store the specimen
■ Excessive physical exercise or emotional stress (increase)
■ Caffeine, insulin, nitroglycerin, aminophylline, sympathomimetics, methyldopa, tricyclic antidepressants, chloral hydrate, quinidine, quinine, tetracycline, B-complex vitamins, isoproterenol, levodopa, and monoamine oxidase inhibitors (possible increase)

■ Clonidine, guanethidine, reserpine, and iodine-containing contrast media (possible decrease)
■ Phenothiazines, erythromycin, and methenamine compounds (possible increase or decrease)

TOTAL URINE ESTROGENS

The total urine estrogens test is a quantitative analysis of total urine levels of estradiol, estrone, and estriol — the major estrogens present in significant amounts in urine. A common method for measuring total urine estrogen levels involves purification by gel filtration, followed by spectrophotofluorometry. Supplementary tests that may provide further information about ovarian function include cytologic examination of vaginal smears, measurement of urine levels of pregnanediol and follicle-stimulating hormone, and evaluation of response to an injection of progesterone.

Purpose

■ To evaluate ovarian activity and to help determine the cause of amenorrhea and female hyperestrogenism
■ To aid diagnosis of tumors of ovarian, adrenocortical, or testicular origin
■ To assess fetoplacental status

Patient preparation

■ Explain to the female patient that this test helps evaluate ovarian function; to the pregnant patient that this test helps evaluate fetal development and placental function; and to the male patient that this test helps evaluate testicular function.
■ Inform the patient that the test requires collection of urine over a 24-hour period.
■ Advise the patient that no pretest restrictions of food or fluids are necessary.
■ If the 24-hour specimen is to be collected at home, teach the patient the proper collection technique.
■ Notify the laboratory and physician of medications the patient is taking that may affect test results; they may need to be restricted.

Procedure and posttest care

■ Collect the patient's urine over a 24-hour period, discarding the first specimen and retaining the last. Use a bottle containing a preservative to keep the specimen at a pH of 3.0 to 5.0.
■ If the patient is pregnant, note the approximate week of gestation on the laboratory request.
■ If the patient is a nonpregnant female, note the stage of her menstrual cycle.
■ Instruct the patient to resume her usual medication schedule as ordered.

Precautions

■ Refrigerate the specimen or keep it on ice during the collection period.

Normal findings

In nonpregnant females, total urine estrogen levels rise and fall during the menstrual cycle, peaking shortly before midcycle, decreasing immediately after ovulation, increasing through the life of the corpus luteum, and decreasing greatly as the corpus luteum degenerates and menstruation begins.

Total estrogen levels range as follows.

Nonpregnant females
■ 4 to 60 µg/24 hours

Pregnant females
■ First trimester: 0 to 800 µg/24 hours
■ Second trimester: 800 to 5,000 µg/24 hours

- Third trimester: 5,000 to 50,000 μg/24 hours

In postmenopausal females, values are less than 10 μg/24 hours. In males, total estrogen levels range from 4 to 25 μg/24 hours.

Abnormal findings

Decreased total urine estrogen levels may reflect ovarian agenesis, primary ovarian insufficiency (due to Stein-Leventhal syndrome, for example), or secondary ovarian insufficiency (due to pituitary or adrenal hypofunction or metabolic disturbances).

Elevated total estrogen levels in non-pregnant females may indicate tumors of ovarian or adrenocortical origin, adrenocortical hyperplasia, or a metabolic or hepatic disorder. In males, elevated total estrogen levels are associated with testicular tumors.

Elevated total urine estrogen levels are normal during pregnancy; serial determinations should show a rising titer.

Interfering factors

- Steroid hormones, methenamine mandelate, phenazopyridine hydrochloride, phenothiazines, tetracyclines, phenolphthalein, ampicillin, meprobamate, senna, cascara sagrada, and hydrochlorothiazide (possible increase or decrease)

PLACENTAL ESTRIOL

The placental estriol test, also referred to as maternal urine estriol, monitors fetal viability by measuring urine levels of placental estriol, the predominant estrogen excreted in urine during pregnancy. A steady rise in estriol reflects a properly functioning placenta and, in most cases, a healthy, growing fetus. Normally, estriol is secreted in much smaller amounts by the ovaries in non-pregnant females, by the testes in males, and by the adrenal cortex in both sexes.

The usual clinical indication for this test is high-risk pregnancy. Serial testing is necessary to plot the expected rise in estriol levels or to show the absence of such a rise. The specimen of choice for this test is a 24-hour urine specimen because estriol levels fluctuate diurnally. Radioimmunoassay is the usual test method. Generally, serum estriol levels are considered more reliable than urine levels.

Purpose

- To assess fetoplacental status, especially in high-risk pregnancy.

Patient preparation

- Explain to the patient that this test helps determine if the placenta is functioning properly, which is essential to the health of the fetus.
- Tell the patient that she need not restrict food or fluids.
- Advise the patient that this test requires urine collection over a 24-hour period, and instruct her how to collect the specimen. Emphasize that proper collection technique is necessary for the results to be valid.
- Notify the laboratory and physician of medications the patient is taking that may affect test results; they may need to be restricted.

Procedure and posttest care

- Collect the patient's urine over a 24-hour period, discarding the first specimen and retaining the last. Use a bottle containing a preservative to keep the specimen at a pH of 3.0 to 5.0. The test may also be done serially, requiring collection twice a week.

Urine estriol levels

Because urine estriol levels rise as normal gestation proceeds (as shown below) any significant changes in serial urine determinations suggest abnormal conditions that may require prompt medical interventions.

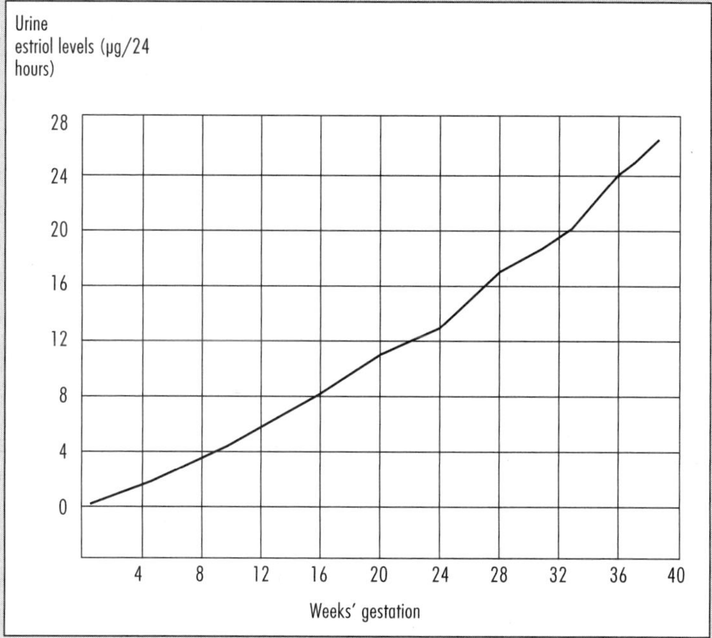

Urine estriol levels (µg/24 hours)

28
24
20
16
12
8
4
0

4 8 12 16 20 24 28 32 36 40

Weeks' gestation

■ Send the specimen to the laboratory. If the patient is pregnant, note the week of gestation on the laboratory request.

■ Instruct the patient to resume her usual medication schedule as ordered.

Precautions

■ Refrigerate the specimen or keep it on ice during the collection period.

■ Some physicians may use an average of 3 previous values as a control because levels vary daily and false-positive and false-negative results are possible.

Normal findings

Normal urine estriol values vary considerably, but serial measures of urine estriol levels, when plotted on a graph, should share a steadily rising curve. (See *Urine estriol levels.*)

Abnormal findings

A 40% drop from baseline values that occurs on 2 consecutive days strongly suggests placental insufficiency and impending fetal distress. A 20% drop over 2 weeks or failure of consecutive estriol levels to rise in a normal curve similarly indicates inadequate placental function and undesirable fetal status. These developments may necessitate cesarean section, depending on the patient's condition and other apparent signs of fetal distress.

A chronically low urine estriol curve may result from fetal adrenal insufficiency, congenital anomalies (such as anencephaly), Rh isoimmunization, or placental sulfatase deficiency.

A high-risk pregnancy in which the maternal glomerular filtration rate decreases may cause a low-normal estriol curve. Such a pregnancy may occur in a patient with hypertension or diabetes mellitus, for example. The pregnancy may continue, as long as no complications develop and estriol levels continue to rise. However, falling estriol levels or a sudden drop from baseline values indicates severe fetal distress.

High urine estriol levels may occur in multiple pregnancy.

Interfering factors

- Failure to collect all urine during the 24-hour period and properly store the specimen during the collection period
- Failure to refrigerate the specimen or keep it on ice.
- Failure to maintain prescribed pH level of the specimen.
- Steroid hormones, methenamine mandelate, phenothiazines, phenazopyridine, tetracyclines, phenolphthalein, ampicillin, meprobamate, senna, cascara sagrada, and hydrochlorothiazide
- Maternal hemoglobinopathy, anemia, malnutrition, hepatic or intestinal diseases (decrease)

HUMAN CHORIONIC GONADOTROPIN

Qualitative analysis of urine levels of human chorionic gonadotropin (hCG) allows for the detection of pregnancy as early as 14 days after ovulation. Production of hCG, a glycoprotein, which prevents degeneration of the corpus luteum at the end of the normal menstrual cycle, begins after conception. During the first trimester, hCG levels rise steadily and rapidly, peaking around the 10th week of gestation, subsequently tapering off to less than 10% of peak levels.

The most common method of evaluating hCG in urine is hemagglutination inhibition. This laboratory procedure can provide both qualitative and quantitative information. The qualitative urine test is easier and less expensive than the serum hCG test (beta-subunit assay); therefore, it's used more frequently to detect pregnancy.

Purpose

- To detect and confirm pregnancy
- To aid diagnosis of hydatidiform mole or hCG-secreting tumors, threatened abortion, or dead fetus

Patient preparation

- If appropriate, explain to the patient that this test determines whether she's pregnant or the status of her pregnancy. Alternatively, explain how the test functions as a screen for some types of cancer.
- Tell the patient she need not restrict food, but should restrict fluids for 8 hours before the test.
- Inform the patient that the test requires a first-voided morning specimen or urine collection over a 24-hour peri-

od, depending on whether the test is qualitative or quantitative.

- Notify the laboratory and physician of medications the patient is taking that may affect test results; they may need to be restricted.

Procedure and posttest care

- For verification of pregnancy (qualitative analysis), collect a first-voided morning specimen. If this isn't possible, collect a random specimen.
- For quantitative analysis of hCG, collect the patient's urine over a 24-hour period in the appropriate container, discarding the first specimen and retaining the last.
- Specify the date of the patient's last menstrual period on the laboratory request.
- Instruct the patient to resume her usual fluid and medication schedule as ordered.

Precautions

- Refrigerate the 24-hour specimen or keep it on ice during the collection period.
- The test should be performed at least 5 days after a missed period to avoid a false-negative result.

Normal findings

In a qualitative immunoassay analysis, results are reported as negative (nonpregnant) or positive (pregnant) for hCG. In quantitative analysis, urine hCG levels in the first trimester of a normal pregnancy may be as high as 500,000 IU/24 hours; in the second trimester, they range from 10,000 to 25,000 IU/24 hours; and in the third trimester, from 5,000 to 15,000 IU/24 hours.

Measurable hCG levels don't normally appear in the urine of men or nonpregnant women.

Abnormal findings

During pregnancy, elevated urine hCG levels may indicate multiple pregnancy or erythroblastosis fetalis; depressed urine hCG levels may indicate threatened abortion or ectopic pregnancy.

Measurable levels of hCG in males and nonpregnant females may indicate choriocarcinoma, ovarian or testicular tumors, melanoma, multiple myeloma, or gastric, hepatic, pancreatic, or breast cancer.

Interfering factors

- Gross proteinuria (> 1 g/24 hours), hematuria, or an elevated erythrocyte sedimentation rate (possible false-positive, depending on the laboratory method)
- Early pregnancy, ectopic pregnancy, or threatened abortion (possible false-negative)
- Phenothiazine (possible false-negative or false-positive)

METABOLITES

PREGNANETRIOL

Using spectrophotometry, the pregnanetriol test determines urine levels of pregnanetriol, the metabolite of the cortisol precursor 17-hydroxyprogesterone. Pregnanetriol is normally excreted in the urine in minute amounts. However, when cortisol biosynthesis is impaired at the point of 17-hydroxyprogesterone conversion, urinary excretion of pregnanetriol rises significantly.

Elevated urine pregnanetriol levels suggest adrenogenital syndrome. Urine 17-ketosteroids and urine 17-ketogenic steroids may be measured concurrently to assess androgen levels. Elevated androgen levels are characteristic of adrenogenital syndrome (congenital adrenal hyperplasia).

Purpose

- To aid diagnosis of adrenogenital syndrome
- To monitor cortisol replacement
- To detect anterior pituitary hypofunction or adrenocortical hyperfunction.

Patient preparation

- Explain to the patient (or to the parents if the patient is a child) that this test evaluates hormonal secretion.
- Inform the patient that he need not restrict food or fluids before the test.
- Tell the patient the test requires collection of urine over a 24-hour period, and teach him the proper collection technique.
- Notify the laboratory and physician of medications the patient is taking that may affect test results; they may need to be restricted.

Procedure and posttest care

- Collect the patient's urine over a 24-hour period, discarding the first specimen and retaining the last. Use a bottle containing a preservative to keep the specimen at a pH of 4.0 to 4.5.
- Instruct the patient to resume his usual medication schedule as ordered.

Precautions

- Refrigerate the specimen or keep it on ice during the collection period.
- Send the specimen to the laboratory as soon as the collection is complete.

Reference values

The normal value of pregnanetriol excretion for males age 16 and over are 0.4 to 2.5 mg/24 hours (SI, 1.2 to 7.5 µmol/day). For females age 16 and over, 0.1 to 1.8 mg/24 hours (SI, 0.3 to 5.3 µmol/day).

Abnormal findings

Elevated urine pregnanetriol levels suggest adrenogenital syndrome: excessive adrenal androgen secretion and resulting virilization. Females with this condition fail to develop normal secondary sex characteristics and show marked masculinization of external genitalia at birth. Males usually appear normal at birth but later develop signs of somatic and sexual precocity.

In monitoring treatment with cortisol replacement, elevated urine pregnanetriol levels indicate insufficient dosage of cortisol. When cortisol replacement adequately inhibits hypersecretion of corticotropin and subsequent overproduction of 17-hydroxyprogesterone, pregnanetriol levels fall within the normal range.

Interfering factors

- Corticotropin (increase)
- Oral contraceptives, progesterone (decrease)
- Failure to store the specimen properly during the collection period or to send the sample to the laboratory immediately after the collection is completed

17-HYDROXYCORTICOSTEROIDS

The 17-hydroxycorticosteroids (17-OHCS) test measures urine levels of 17-OHCS — metabolites of the hormones that regulate glyconeogenesis. More than 80% of all urinary 17-OHCS are metabolites of cortisol, the primary adrenocortical steroid. Test findings thus reflect cortisol secretion and, indirectly, adrenocortical function.

Urine 17-OHCS levels are most accurately determined from a 24-hour specimen because cortisol secretion varies diurnally and in response to stress and many other factors. Column chromatography and spectrophotofluorometry with the Porter-Silber reagent are used to measure 17-OHCS levels.

Levels of plasma cortisol, urine free cortisol, and urine 17-ketosteroids may be measured and corticotropin stimulation and suppression testing performed to confirm results of this test. Of these, urine free cortisol is a more sensitive and specific test for hypercortisolism.

Purpose

- To assess adrenocortical function

Patient preparation

- Explain to the patient that this test evaluates how his adrenal glands are functioning.
- Inform the patient that he should restrict food or fluids that will alter test results (coffee, tea) and avoid excessive physical exercise and stressful situations during the collection period.
- Tell the patient the test requires collection of urine over a 24-hour period, and instruct him in the proper collection technique.
- Notify the laboratory and physician of medications the patient is taking that may affect test results; they may need to be restricted.

Procedure and posttest care

- Collect the patient's urine over a 24-hour period, discarding the first specimen and retaining the last. Use a bottle containing a preservative to prevent deterioration of the specimen. Label the specimen appropriately, including the patient's gender on the request forms.
- Instruct the patient to resume his usual activities, diet, and medication schedule as ordered.

Precautions

- Refrigerate the specimen or place it on ice during the collection period.

Reference values

Normally, urine 17-OHCS values range from 4.5 to 12 mg/24 hours in males (SI, 12.4 to 33.1 μmol/day), and from 2.5 to 10 mg/24 hours in females (SI, 6.9 to 27.6 μmol/day). In children ages 8 to 12, levels range from less than 4.5 mg/24 hours (SI, < 12.4 μmol/day); in children younger than age 8, levels are normally less than 1.5 mg/24 hours (SI, < 4.14 μmol/day).

Abnormal findings

Elevated urine 17-OHCS levels may indicate Cushing's syndrome, adrenal carcinoma or adenoma, or pituitary tumor. Increased levels may also occur in patients with virilism, hyperthyroidism, and severe hypertension. Extreme stress induced by such conditions as acute pancreatitis and eclampsia also causes urine 17-OHCS levels to rise above normal.

Low urine 17-OHCS levels may indicate Addison's disease, hypopituitarism, or myxedema.

Interfering factors

- Failure to observe restrictions, to collect all urine during the test period, or to properly store the specimen
- Meprobamate, phenothiazines, spironolactone, ascorbic acid, chloral hydrate, glutethimide, chlordiazepoxide, penicillin G, hydroxyzine, quinidine, quinine, iodides, and methenamine (possible increase)
- Hydralazine, phenytoin, thiazide diuretics, estrogens, oral contraceptives, phenothiazines, nalidixic acid, and reserpine (possible decrease)

Normal values for the 17-ketosteroid fractionation test

Through gas-liquid chromatography, this fractionation test shows which specific steroids in the 17-ketosteroid (17-KS) group are elevated or suppressed and thus aids differential diagnosis of conditions suggested by abnormal 17-KS levels. Note that 17-KS levels are measured in milligrams per 24 hours.

STEROID	ADULT MALE	ADULT FEMALE	MALE AGES 10 TO 15	FEMALE AGES 10 TO 15
Androsterone	0.9 to 6.1	0 to 3.1	0.2 to 2	0.5 to 2.5
Dehydroepiandrosterone	0 to 3.1	0 to 1.5	< 0.4	< 0.4
Etiocholanolone	0.9 to 5.2	0.1 to 3.5	0.1 to 1.6	0.7 to 3.1
11-Hydroxyandrosterone	0.2 to 1.6	0 to 1.1	0.1 to 1.1	0.2 to 1
11-Hydroxyetiocholanolone	0.1 to 0.9	0.1 to 0.8	< 0.3	0.1 to 0.5
11-Ketoandrosterone	0 to 0.5	0 to 0.3	< 0.1	< 0.1
11-Ketoetiocholanolone	0 to 1.6	0 to 1	< 0.3	0.1 to 0.5
Pregnanetriol	0.2 to 2	0 to 1.4	0.2 to 0.6	0.1 to 0.6

17-KETOSTEROIDS

The 17-ketosteroids (17-KS) is a fractionation test that uses the spectrophotofluorometric technique to measure urine levels of 17-KS. Steroids and steroid metabolites characterized by a ketone group on carbon 17 in the steroid nucleus, 17-KS originate primarily in the adrenal glands, but also in the testes and ovaries.

Although not all 17-KS are androgens, they cause androgenic effects. For example, excessive secretion of 17-KS may result in hirsutism and may increase clitoral or phallic size; in utero, elevated 17-KS levels may cause a female fetus to develop a male urogenital tract. Because 17-KS don't include all the androgens (testosterone, for example, the most potent androgen, isn't a 17-KS), these levels provide only a rough estimate of androgenic activity. To provide additional information about androgen secretion, plasma testosterone levels may be measured concurrently.

Purpose

- To aid diagnosis of adrenal and gonadal dysfunction

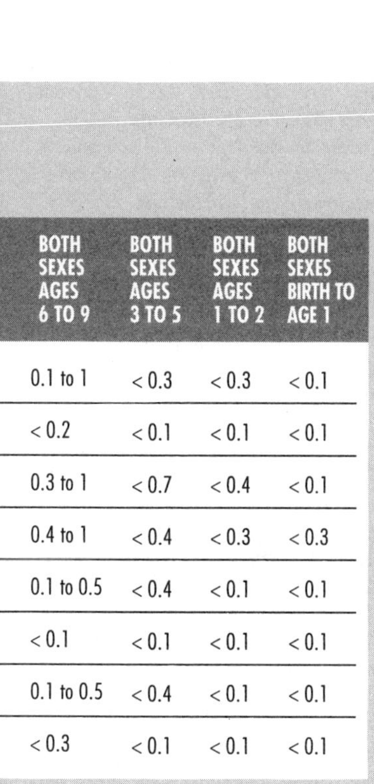

BOTH SEXES AGES 6 TO 9	BOTH SEXES AGES 3 TO 5	BOTH SEXES AGES 1 TO 2	BOTH SEXES BIRTH TO AGE 1
0.1 to 1	< 0.3	< 0.3	< 0.1
< 0.2	< 0.1	< 0.1	< 0.1
0.3 to 1	< 0.7	< 0.4	< 0.1
0.4 to 1	< 0.4	< 0.3	< 0.3
0.1 to 0.5	< 0.4	< 0.1	< 0.1
< 0.1	< 0.1	< 0.1	< 0.1
0.1 to 0.5	< 0.4	< 0.1	< 0.1
< 0.3	< 0.1	< 0.1	< 0.1

■ To aid diagnosis of adrenogenital syndrome (congenital adrenal hyperplasia)
■ To monitor cortisol therapy in the treatment of adrenogenital syndrome

Patient preparation

■ Explain to the patient that this test evaluates hormonal balance.
■ Inform the patient that he need not restrict food or fluids before the test but should avoid excessive physical exercise and stressful situations during the collection period.
■ Tell the patient the test requires urine collection over a 24-hour period, and instruct him in the proper collection technique.
■ Notify the laboratory and physician of medications the patient is taking that may affect test results; they may need to be restricted.

Procedure and posttest care

■ Collect the patient's urine over a 24-hour period, discarding the first sample and retaining the last. Use a bottle containing a preservative to keep the specimen at a pH of 4.0 to 4.5. Appropriately label the specimen and laboratory requisition requests with the patient's gender.
■ Instruct the patient to resume his usual activities and medication schedule as ordered.

Precautions

■ Refrigerate the specimen or place it on ice during the collection period.
■ Send the specimen to the laboratory immediately after the collection is completed.

Reference values

Normally, urine 17-KS values range from 10 to 25 mg/24 hours (SI, 35 to 87 μmol/day) in men and from 4 to 6 mg/24 hours (SI, 4 to 21 μmol/day) in women. Children between ages 10 and 14 excrete 1 to 6 mg/24 hours (SI, 2 to 21 μmol/day); children younger than age 10 excrete less than 3 mg/24 hours (SI, < 10 μmol/day).

For more information about specific steroids in the 17-KS group, the 17-KS fractionation test may be performed. (See *Normal values for the 17-ketosteroid fractionation test.*)

Abnormal findings

Elevated urine 17-KS levels may result from adrenal hyperplasia, carcinoma or adenoma, or adrenogenital syndrome. In women, elevated levels may also indicate ovarian dysfunction, such as polycystic ovary disease (Stein-Leventhal syndrome), lutein cell tumor of the ovary, or androgenic arrhenoblastoma. In men, elevated 17-KS levels may indicate interstitial cell tumor of the testis. Characteristically, 17-KS levels also rise during pregnancy, severe stress, chronic illness, or debilitating disease.

Depressed urine 17-KS levels may result from Addison's disease, panhypopituitarism, eunuchoidism, or castration and may occur in cretinism, myxedema, and nephrosis. When this test is used to monitor cortisol therapy for adrenogenital syndrome, 17-KS levels typically return to normal with adequate cortisol administration.

Interfering factors

- Failure to observe restrictions, to collect all urine during the collection period, to properly store the specimen, or to send it to the laboratory immediately after the collection is completed
- Presence of menstrual blood in the specimen
- Meprobamate, phenothiazines, corticotropin, antibiotics, dexamethasone, spironolactone, and oleandomycin (possible increase)
- Estrogens, penicillin, ethacrynic acid, and phenytoin (possible decrease)
- Nalidixic acid and quinine (possible increase or decrease)

17-KETOGENIC STEROIDS

Using spectrophotofluorometry, the 17-ketogenic steroids (17-KGS) test determines urine levels of 17-KGS, which consist of the 17-hydroxycorticosteroids—cortisol and its metabolites, for example—and other adrenocortical steroids, such as pregnanetriol, that can be oxidized in the laboratory to 17-ketosteroids. Because 17-KGS represent such a large group of steroids, this test provides an excellent overall assessment of adrenocortical function. For accurate diagnosis of a specific disease, 17-KGS levels must be compared with results of other tests, including plasma corticotropin, plasma cortisol, corticotropin stimulation, single-dose metyrapone, and dexamethasone suppression.

Purpose

- To evaluate adrenocortical and testicular function.
- To aid diagnosis of Cushing's syndrome and Addison's disease

Patient preparation

- Explain to the patient that this test evaluates adrenal function.
- Inform the patient that he need not restrict food or fluids before the test but should avoid excessive physical exercise and stressful situations during the collection period.
- Tell the patient the test requires urine collection over a 24-hour period, and teach him how to collect the specimen correctly.
- Notify the laboratory and physician of medications the patient is taking that may affect test results; they may need to be restricted.

Procedure and posttest care

- Collect the patient's urine over a 24-hour period, discarding the first specimen and retaining the last. Use a bottle containing a preservative to keep the specimen at a pH of 4.0 to 4.5. Appropriately label the specimen and laboratory requisition requests with the patient's gender.

■ Instruct the patient to resume his usual activities and medication schedule as ordered.

Precautions

■ Refrigerate the specimen or keep it on ice during the collection period.
■ Send the specimen to the laboratory as soon as the collection is complete.

Reference values

Normally, urine 17-KGS levels range from 4 to 14 mg/24 hours (SI, 13 to 49 μmol/day) in men and from 2 to 12 mg/24 hours (SI, 7 to 42 μmol/day) in women. Children ages 11 to 14 excrete 2 to 9 mg/24 hours (SI, 7 to 31 μmol/day); younger children and infants excrete 0.1 to 4 mg/24 hours (SI, 0.3 to 14 μmol/day).

Abnormal findings

Elevated urine 17-KGS levels indicate hyperadrenalism, which may occur in Cushing's syndrome, adrenogenital syndrome (congenital adrenal hyperplasia), and adrenal carcinoma or adenoma. Levels also rise with severe physical stress (burns, infections, or surgery, for example) or emotional stress.

Low levels may reflect hypoadrenalism, which may occur in Addison's disease and may also be associated with panhypopituitarism, cretinism, and general wasting.

Interfering factors

■ Failure to observe restrictions, to collect all urine during the collection period, to properly store the specimen, or to send it to the laboratory immediately after the collection is completed
■ Corticotropin, meprobamate, phenothiazines, spironolactone, penicillin, oleandomycin, and hydralazine (possible increase)
■ Estrogens, quinine, reserpine, thiazide diuretics, and long-term corticosteroid therapy (possible decrease)
■ Nalidixic acid and dexamethasone, carbamazepine, cephalothin, tiaprofenic acid (possible increase or decrease)

VANILLYLMANDELIC ACID

Using spectrophotofluorometry, the vanillylmandelic acid (VMA) test determines urine levels of VMA, a phenolic acid. VMA is the catecholamine metabolite that's normally most prevalent in the urine and is the product of hepatic conversion of epinephrine and norepinephrine; urine VMA levels reflect endogenous production of these major catecholamines. Like the test for urine total catecholamines, this test helps to detect catecholamine-secreting tumors — especially pheochromocytoma — and helps evaluate the function of the adrenal medulla, the primary site of catecholamine production.

The VMA test ideally should be performed on a 24-hour urine specimen (not a random specimen) to overcome the effects of diurnal variations in catecholamine secretion. Other catecholamine metabolites — metanephrine, normetanephrine, and homovanillic acid (HVA) — may be measured at the same time. If evaluating hypertension, specimen collection may be of greatest value during the hypertensive episode.

Purpose

■ To help detect pheochromocytoma, neuroblastoma, and ganglioneuroma
■ To evaluate the function of the adrenal medulla

Patient preparation

■ Explain to the patient that this test evaluates hormonal secretion.

■ Instruct the patient to restrict foods and beverages containing phenolic acid, such as coffee, tea, bananas, citrus fruits, chocolate, and vanilla, and carbonated beverages for 3 days before the test.

■ Advise the patient to avoid stressful situations and excessive physical activity during the urine collection period.

■ Tell the patient the test requires collection of urine over a 24-hour period, and teach him the proper collection technique.

■ Notify the laboratory and physician of medications the patient is taking that may affect test results; they may need to be restricted.

Procedure and posttest care

■ Collect the patient's urine over a 24-hour period, discarding the first specimen and retaining the last. Use a bottle containing a preservative to keep the specimen at a pH of 3.0.

■ Instruct the patient to resume his usual activities, diet, and medication schedule as ordered.

Precautions

■ Refrigerate the specimen or keep it on ice during the collection period.

■ Send the specimen to the laboratory immediately after the collection is completed.

Reference values

Normally, VMA levels in adults are 1.4 to 6.5 mg/24 hours (SI, 7 to 33 μmol/day).

Abnormal findings

Elevated urine VMA levels may result from a catecholamine-secreting tumor. Further testing, such as measurement of urine HVA levels to rule out pheochromocytoma, is necessary for precise diagnosis. If pheochromocytoma is confirmed, the patient may be tested for multiple endocrine neoplasia, an inherited condition commonly associated with pheochromocytoma. (Family members of a patient with confirmed pheochromocytoma should also be carefully evaluated for multiple endocrine neoplasia.)

Interfering factors

■ Excessive exercise or emotional stress (increase)

■ Failure to observe restrictions, to properly store the specimen during the collection period, or to send the sample to the laboratory immediately after the collection is completed

■ Epinephrine, norepinephrine, lithium carbonate, methocarbamol (increase); chlorpromazine, guanethidine, reserpine, monoamine oxidase inhibitors, clonidine (lower); levodopa, and salicylates (raise or lower)

HOMOVANILLIC ACID

The homovanillic acid (HVA) test is a quantitative analysis of urine levels of HVA, which is a metabolite of dopamine, one of the three major catecholamines. Synthesized primarily in the brain, dopamine is a precursor to epinephrine and norepinephrine, the other principal catecholamines. The liver breaks down most dopamine into HVA for eventual excretion; a minimal amount of dopamine appears in the urine.

Using two-dimensional chromatography, urine HVA levels are usually measured simultaneously with the major catecholamines and other catecholamine metabolites — metanephrine, normetanephrine, and vanillylmandelic acid.

Purpose

- To aid diagnosis of neuroblastoma and ganglioneuroma
- To rule out pheochromocytoma

Patient preparation

- Explain to the patient that this test assesses hormone secretion.
- Inform the patient that he need not restrict food or fluids before the test but should avoid stressful situations and excessive physical exercise during the collection period.
- Tell the patient the test requires collection of urine over a 24-hour period, and teach him the proper collection technique.
- Notify the laboratory and physician of medications the patient is taking that may affect test results; they may need to be restricted.

Procedure and posttest care

- Collect the patient's urine over a 24-hour period, discarding the first specimen and retaining the last. Use a bottle containing a preservative to keep the specimen at a pH of 2.0 to 4.0.
- Instruct the patient to resume his usual activities and medication schedule as ordered.

Precautions

- Refrigerate the specimen or keep it on ice during the collection period.
- Send the specimen to the laboratory immediately after the collection is completed.

Reference values

The normal urine HVA value for adults is less than 10 mg/24 hours (SI, < 55 µmol/day).

Abnormal findings

Elevated urine HVA levels suggest neuroblastoma, a malignant soft-tissue tumor that develops in infants and young children; or ganglioneuroma, a tumor of the sympathetic nervous system that develops in older children and adolescents and rarely metastasizes. HVA levels don't usually rise in patients with pheochromocytoma because this tumor secretes mainly epinephrine, which metabolizes primarily into vanillylmandelic acid. Thus, an abnormally high urine HVA level generally rules out pheochromocytoma.

Interfering factors

- Failure to observe restrictions, to collect all urine during the test period, to store the specimen properly, or to send the sample to the laboratory immediately after the collection is completed
- Excessive physical exercise or emotional stress during the collection period (possible increase)
- Monoamine oxidase inhibitors (decrease due to inhibition of dopamine metabolism)
- Aspirin, methocarbamol, and levodopa (possible increase or decrease)

5-HYDROXYINDOLEACETIC ACID

The quantitative analysis of urine levels of 5-hydroxyindoleacetic acid (5-HIAA) is used mainly to screen for carcinoid tumors (argentaffinomas). Such tumors, found generally in the intestine or appendix, secrete an excessive amount of serotonin, which is reflected by high 5-HIAA levels. This test measures 5-HIAA levels by the colorimetric technique and is most accurate when performed with a 24-hour urine specimen, which can detect small or intermittently secreting carcinoid tumors.

Purpose

- To aid diagnosis of carcinoid tumors (argentaffinomas)

Patient preparation

- Explain to the patient what serotonin is and why this test is important.
- Instruct the patient not to eat foods containing serotonin, such as bananas, plums, pineapples, avocados, eggplants, tomatoes, or walnuts, for 4 days before the test.
- Tell the patient the test requires collection of urine over a 24-hour period, and teach him the proper collection technique.
- Notify the laboratory and physician of medications the patient is taking that may affect test results; they may need to be restricted.

Procedure and posttest care

- Collect the patient's urine over a 24-hour period, discarding the first specimen and retaining the last. Use a bottle containing a preservative to keep the specimen at a pH of 2.0 to 4.0.
- Instruct the patient to resume his usual diet and medication schedule as ordered.

Precautions

- Refrigerate the specimen or keep it on ice during the collection period.
- Send the specimen to the laboratory as soon as the collection is complete.

Reference values

Normally, urine 5-HIAA values are qualitatively reported as negative; quantitative results are 2 to 7 mg/24 hours (SI, 10.4 to 36.6 µmol/day).

Abnormal findings

Marked elevation of urine 5-HIAA levels, possibly as high as 200 to 600 mg/24 hours (SI, 1040 to 3120 µmol/day), indicates a carcinoid tumor. However, because these tumors vary in their capacity to store and secrete serotonin, some patients with carcinoid syndrome (metastatic carcinoid tumors) may not show elevated levels. Repeated testing is often necessary.

Interfering factors

- Failure to observe pretest restrictions, to collect all urine during the test period, to properly store the specimen, or to send the sample to the laboratory immediately after the collection is completed
- Severe GI disturbance or diarrhea
- Melphalan, reserpine, methamphetamine, and fluorouracil (increase)
- Ethanol, tricyclic antidepressants, monoamine oxidase inhibitors, methyldopa, and isoniazid (decrease in most cases)
- Methenamine compounds, phenothiazines, salicylates, guaifenesin, methamphetamine, methocarbamol, and acetaminophen (possible increase or decrease)

PREGNANEDIOL

Using gas chromatography or radioimmunoassay, this test measures urine levels of pregnanediol, the chief metabolite of progesterone. Although biologically inert, pregnanediol has diagnostic significance because it reflects about 10% of the endogenous production of its parent hormone.

Progesterone is produced in nonpregnant females by the corpus luteum during the latter half of each menstrual cycle, preparing the uterus for implantation of a fertilized ovum. If implantation doesn't occur, progesterone secretion drops sharply; if implantation does occur, the corpus luteum secretes more progesterone to further prepare the uterus for pregnancy and to begin development of the placenta. Toward the end of the first trimester, the placenta becomes the primary source of progesterone secretion, producing the progressively larger amounts needed to maintain pregnancy.

Normally, urine levels of pregnanediol reflect variations in progesterone secretion during the menstrual cycle and during pregnancy. Direct measurement of plasma progesterone levels by radioimmunoassay may also be done.

Purpose

- To evaluate placental function in pregnant females
- To evaluate ovarian function in nonpregnant females
- To aid in the diagnosis of menstrual disorder

Patient preparation

- Explain to the patient that this test evaluates placental or ovarian function.
- Inform the patient that she need not restrict food or fluids.
- Tell the patient the test requires collection of urine over a 24-hour period, and teach her the proper collection technique.
- Advise the pregnant patient that this test may be repeated several times to obtain serial measurements.
- Notify the laboratory and physician of medications the patient is taking that may affect test results; they may need to be restricted.

Procedure and posttest care

- Collect the patient's urine over a 24-hour period, discarding the first specimen and retaining the last.
- Instruct the patient to resume her usual medication schedule as ordered.

Precautions

- Refrigerate the specimen or keep it on ice during the collection period.
- If the patient is pregnant, note the approximate week of gestation on the laboratory request.
- For premenopausal women who aren't pregnant, note the stage of the menstrual cycle on the laboratory request.

Normal findings

In nonpregnant females, urine pregnanediol values normally range from 0.5 to 1.5 mg/24 hours during the follicular phase of the menstrual cycle. In pregnant females, the values are:

- first trimester: 10 to 30 mg/24 hours
- second trimester: 35 to 70 mg/24 hours
- third trimester: 70 to 100 mg/24 hours.

Normal postmenopausal values range from 0.2 to 1 mg/24 hours. In males, urine pregnanediol levels are 0 to 1 mg/24 hours.

Abnormal findings

During pregnancy, a marked decrease in urine pregnanediol levels based on a single 24-hour urine specimen or a steady decrease in pregnanediol levels in serial measurements may indicate placental insufficiency and requires immediate investigation. A precipitous drop in pregnanediol values may suggest fetal distress — for example, threatened abortion or preeclampsia — or fetal death. However, pregnanediol measurements aren't reliable indicators of fetal viability because levels can remain normal even after fetal death, as long as maternal circulation to the placenta remains adequate.

In nonpregnant females, abnormally low urine pregnanediol levels may occur with anovulation, amenorrhea, or other menstrual abnormalities. Low to normal pregnanediol levels may be associated with hydatidiform mole. Elevations may indicate luteinized granulosa or theca cell tumors, diffuse thecal luteinization, or metastatic ovarian cancer.

Adrenal hyperplasia or biliary tract obstruction may elevate urine pregnanediol values in males or females. Some forms of primary hepatic disease produce abnormally low levels in both sexes.

Interfering factors

- Failure to properly store the specimen during the collection period
- Methenamine mandelate, methenamine hippurate, progestogens, combination oral contraceptives, and drugs containing corticotropin (possible increase or decrease)

PROTEINS AND PROTEIN METABOLITES

PROTEINS

A protein test is a quantitative test for proteinuria. Normally, the glomerular membrane allows only proteins of low molecular weight to enter the filtrate. The renal tubules then reabsorb most of these proteins, normally excreting a small amount that's undetectable by a screening test. A damaged glomerular capillary membrane and impaired tubular reabsorption allow excretion of proteins in the urine.

A qualitative screening often precedes this test. A positive result requires quantitative analysis of a 24-hour urine specimen by acid precipitation tests. Electrophoresis can detect Bence Jones proteins, hemoglobins, myoglobins, or albumin.

Purpose

- To aid diagnosis of pathologic states characterized by proteinuria, primarily renal disease

Patient preparation

- Explain to the patient that this test detects proteins in the urine.
- Inform the patient that he need not restrict food or fluids.
- Tell the patient that the test usually requires urine collection over a 24-hour period; random collection can be done.
- Notify the laboratory and physician of medications the patient is taking that may affect test results; they may need to be restricted.

Procedure and posttest care

- Collect the patient's urine over a 24-hour period, discarding the first specimen and retaining the last. A special specimen container can be obtained from the laboratory.
- Instruct the patient to resume his usual medication schedule as ordered.

Precautions

- Tell the patient not to contaminate the urine with toilet tissue or stool.
- Refrigerate the specimen or place it on ice during the collection period.

Nomal findings

At rest, normal urine protein values range from 50 to 80 mg/24 hours (SI, 50 to 80 mg/day).

Abnormal findings

Proteinuria is a chief characteristic of renal disease. When proteinuria is present in a single specimen, a 24-hour urine collection is required to identify specific renal abnormalities.

Proteinuria can result from glomerular leakage of plasma proteins (a major cause of protein excretion), from overflow of filtered proteins of low molecular weight (when these are present in excessive concentrations), from impaired tubular reabsorption of filtered proteins, and from the presence of renal proteins derived from the breakdown of kidney tissue.

Persistent proteinuria indicates renal disease resulting from increased glomerular permeability. *Minimal proteinuria* (< 0.5 g/24 hours), however, is commonly associated with renal diseases in which glomerular involvement isn't a major factor, as in chronic pyelonephritis.

Moderate proteinuria (0.5 to 4 g/24 hours) occurs in several types of renal disease — acute or chronic glomerulonephritis, amyloidosis, toxic nephropathies — or in diseases in which renal failure often develops as a late complication (diabetes or heart failure, for example). *Heavy proteinuria* (> 4 g/24 hours) is commonly associated with nephrotic syndrome.

When accompanied by an elevated white blood cell (WBC) count, proteinuria indicates urinary tract infection. When accompanied by hematuria, proteinuria indicates local or diffuse urinary tract disorders. Other pathologic states (infections and lesions of the central nervous system, for example) can also result in detectable amounts of proteins in the urine.

Many drugs (such as amphotericin B, gold preparations, aminoglycosides, polymyxins, and trimethadione) inflict renal damage, causing true proteinuria. This makes the routine evaluation of urine proteins essential during such treatment. In all forms of proteinuria, fractionation results obtained by electrophoresis provide more precise information than the screening test. For example, excessive hemoglobin in the urine indicates intravascular hemolysis; elevated myoglobin suggests muscle damage; albumin, increased glomerular permeability; and Bence Jones protein, multiple myeloma.

Not all forms of proteinuria have pathologic significance. *Benign proteinuria* can result from changes in body position. *Functional proteinuria* is associated with exercise as well as emotional or physiologic stress and is usually transient.

Interfering factors

- Contamination of the specimen with toilet tissue or stool
- Tolbutamide, para-aminosalicylic acid, acetazolamide, sodium bicarbonate, penicillin, sulfonamides, cephalosporins, and iodine-containing contrast media (possible false-positive or false-negative)
- Very dilute urine (such as from forcing fluids) may depress protein values and cause false-negative results.

BENCE JONES PROTEINS

Bence Jones proteins are abnormal light-chain immunoglobulins of low molecular weight that are derived from the clone of a single plasma cell. This globulin appears in the urine of 50% to 80% of patients with multiple myeloma and in most patients with Waldenström's macroglobulinemia.

Screening tests, such as thermal coagulation and Bradshaw's test, can detect Bence Jones proteins, but urine immunoelectrophoresis is usually the method of choice for quantitative studies. Serum immunoelectrophoresis, which is sometimes used, is less sensitive than other tests. Nevertheless, both urine and serum studies are frequently used when multiple myeloma is suspected.

Purpose

- To confirm the presence of multiple myeloma in patients with characteristic clinical signs, such as bone pain (especially in the back and the thorax) and persistent anemia and fatigue

Patient preparation

- Tell the patient that this test can detect an abnormal protein in the urine.
- Tell the patient the test requires an early-morning urine specimen; teach him how to collect a mid-stream clean-catch specimen.

Procedure and posttest care

- Collect an early-morning urine specimen of at least 50 ml.

Precautions

- Instruct the patient not to contaminate the urine specimen with toilet tissue or stool.
- Send the specimen to the laboratory immediately after collection, or refrigerate it if transport is delayed. A refrigerated specimen must be analyzed within 24 hours, or it should be discarded.

Normal findings

Normal urine should contain no Bence Jones proteins.

Abnormal findings

The presence of Bence Jones proteins in urine suggests multiple myeloma or Waldenström's macroglobulinemia. Very low levels, in the absence of other symptoms, may result from benign monoclonal gammopathy. However, clinical evidence figures prominently in the diagnosis of multiple myeloma.

Interfering factors

- Connective tissue disease, renal insufficiency, and certain cancers (possible false-positive)
- Contamination of the specimen with menstrual blood, prostatic secretions, or semen (possible false-positive)
- Contamination of the specimen with toilet tissue or stool
- Failure to properly store the specimen during the collection period or to send the sample to the laboratory immediately after the collection is completed (possible false positive from deterioration of protein)

AMINO ACID SCREENING

Amino acid screening tests screen for aminoaciduria — elevated urine amino acid levels — a condition that may result from inborn errors of metabolism due to the absence of specific enzymatic activities. Abnormal metabolism causes an excess of one or more amino acids to appear in plasma and, as the renal threshold is exceeded, in urine. (See *Chromatographic identification of amino acid disorders,* pages 364 and 365.)

Aminoacidurias may be classified as either primary (overflow) aminoacidopathies or as secondary (renal) aminoacidopathies. The latter type is associated with conditions marked by defective tubular reabsorption from congenital disorders. A more specific defect, such as cystinuria, may cause one or more amino acids to appear in urine.

To screen newborns, children, and adults for congenital aminoacidurias, plasma or urine specimens may be used. The plasma test is the better indicator of overflow aminoacidurias; urine testing is used to confirm or monitor certain amino acid disorders and to screen for renal aminoacidurias.

Various laboratory techniques are available to screen for aminoacidurias, but chromatography is the preferred method. Positive findings on chromatography can be elaborated by fractionation, showing specific amino acid levels. Testing for specific amino acid levels is also necessary for infants or young children with acidosis, severe vomiting and diarrhea, and abnormal urine odor. Such testing is especially important in newborns because early diagnosis and prompt treatment of aminoacidurias may prevent mental retardation.

Purpose

- To screen for renal aminoacidurias
- To follow up on plasma test findings when results of these tests suggest overflow aminoacidurias

Patient preparation

- Explain to the patient (or the parents if the patient is an infant or a child) that this test helps detect amino acid disorders. Advise him that additional tests may be necessary.
- Inform the patient that he need not restrict food or fluids before the test.
- Tell the patient the test requires a urine specimen.
- Notify the laboratory and physician of medications the patient is taking that may affect test results; they may need to be restricted. If such drugs must be continued, however, note this on the laboratory request. (If the patient is a breast-fed infant, record any drugs the mother is receiving.)

Procedure and posttest care

- If the patient is an infant, clean and dry the genital area, attach the collection device, and observe for voiding. Transfer urine — at least 20 ml — to a specimen container. Remove the collection device carefully to prevent skin irritation, and be sure to remove all adhesive residues.
- If the patient is an adult or a child, collect a fresh random specimen.

Precautions

- For an infant, apply the adhesive flanges of the collection device securely to the skin to prevent leakage.
- Send the specimen to the laboratory immediately after collection.

Normal findings

Reported values are age-dependent and are indicated as normal or abnormal.

Abnormal findings

If thin-layer chromatography shows gross changes or abnormal patterns, blood and 24-hour urine quantitative column chromatography are performed to identify specific amino acid abnormalities and to differentiate overflow and renal aminoacidurias.

Interfering factors

- Failure to send the urine specimen to the laboratory immediately after collection
- In neonates, failure to ingest dietary protein during the 48 hours preceding the test

(Text continues on page 366.)

Chromatographic identification of amino acid disorders

In chromatography — the preferred method for screening aminoacidurias — amino acids migrate into multicolored bands. The sequence of amino acids and their corresponding band numbers, as listed below, reflect these standard migratory patterns. When congenital enzyme deficiencies and subsequent metabolic disorders increase plasma and urine amino acid levels, these bands intensify.

		METABOLIC AMINO ACID DISORDERS					
		Phenylketonuria		Maple syrup urine disease		Cystinuria	
Chromatographic band number	Amino acids	Plasma	Urine	Plasma	Urine	Plasma	Urine
1	Leucine, isoleucine			+	+		
2	Phenylalanine	+	+				
3	Valine, methionine			+	+		
4	Tryptophan, beta-amino isobutyric acid						
5	Tyrosine						
6	Proline			+			
7	Alanine, ethanolamine						
8	Threonine, glutamic acid						
9	Homocitrulline, glycine, serine, hydroxyproline, aspartic acid, glutamine, citrulline			+			
10	Homocystine, asparagine						
11	Argininosuccinic acid, histidine, arginine, lysine, ornithine, cystathionine, cystine, cysteine, hydroxylysine						+

KEY: + = increased amino acids in plasma or urine

Homocystinuria		Hartnup disease		Argininosuccinicaciduria		Histidinemia		Hyperprolinemia type A		Citrullinuria	
Plasma	Urine	Plasma	Urine	Plasma	Urine	Plasma	Urine	Plasma	Urine	Plasma	Urine
			+								
			+								
+			+							+	
			+								
			+								
								+	+		
			+				+				+
							+				+
			+		+				+	+	+
	+										
			+		+	+	+				+

HYDROXYPROLINE

Total urine levels of hydroxyproline, an amino acid found mainly in collagen (a component of skin and bone), are a good index of bone matrix turnover because levels increase when collagen breaks down during bone resorption. Bone matrix turnover and hydroxyproline levels normally rise in children during periods of rapid skeletal growth. However, they also rise in disorders that increase bone resorption, such as Paget's disease, metastatic bone tumors, and certain endocrine disorders.

Hydroxyproline levels are most often determined colorimetrically on a timed urine sample; they may also be determined by ion-exchange or gas-liquid chromatography. A collagen-restricted diet is essential for this test because hydroxyproline levels reflect collagen intake. Free hydroxyproline, a small component of total hydroxyproline and a sensitive indicator of dietary collagen intake, may be measured to validate results.

Purpose

- To monitor treatment for disorders characterized by bone resorption, including Paget's disease, metastatic bone tumors, certain endocrine disorders (hyperthyroidism), rheumatoid arthritis, and osteoporosis.
- To aid diagnosis of disorders characterized by bone resorption

Patient preparation

- Explain to the patient that this test helps monitor treatment or detect an amino acid disorder related to bone formation.
- Inform the patient that he must follow a collagen-free diet and avoid eating ice cream, candy, meat, fish, poultry, jelly, and any foods containing gelatin for 24 hours before the test and during the test period itself.
- Tell the patient the test requires urine collection over a 2-hour or 24-hour period, and teach him the correct collection technique.
- Note the patient's age and sex on the laboratory request.
- Notify the laboratory and physician of medications the patient is taking that may affect test results; they may need to be restricted.

Procedure and posttest care

- Collect the patient's urine over a 2-hour or 24-hour period. In a 24-hour collection, discard the first sample and retain the last. Use a container that has a preservative to prevent degradation of hydroxyproline.
- Instruct the patient to resume his usual diet and medication schedule as ordered.

Precautions

- Refrigerate the specimen or keep it on ice during the collection period.
- Send the specimen to the laboratory immediately after the collection is completed.

Normal findings

Normal values typically range from 1 to 9 mg/24 hours (SI, 1.0 to 3.4 IU/day).

Abnormal findings

Hydroxyproline levels should decrease slowly during therapy for bone resorption disorders. Elevated levels may indicate bone disease, metastatic bone tumors, or endocrine disorders that stimulate hormonal secretion.

Interfering factors

- Failure to observe restrictions, to collect all urine during the collection period, to properly store the specimen, or to send the specimen to the laboratory immediately after the collection is completed

- Ascorbic acid, vitamin D, aspirin, glucocorticoids, antineoplastic agents, calcium gluconate, corticosteroids, estradiol, propranolol. calcitonin, and mithramycin (used to treat Paget's disease) (possible decrease)
- Psoriasis and burns (possible increase due to collagen turnover)
- Growth hormone, parathyroid hormone, phenobarbital, sulfonylureas (increase)

CREATININE

The creatinine test measures urine levels of creatinine, the chief metabolite of creatine. Produced in amounts proportional to total body muscle mass, creatinine is removed from the plasma primarily by glomerular filtration and is excreted in the urine. Because the body doesn't recycle it, creatinine has a relatively high, constant clearance rate, making it an efficient indicator of renal function. However, the creatinine clearance test, which measures both urine and plasma creatinine clearance, is a more precise index than this test. A standard method for determining urine creatinine levels is based on Jaffé's reaction, in which creatinine treated with an alkaline picrate solution yields a bright orange-red complex.

Purpose

- To help assess glomerular filtration
- To check the accuracy of 24-hour urine collection, based on the relatively constant levels of creatinine excretion

Patient preparation

- Explain to the patient that this test helps evaluate kidney function.
- Inform the patient that he need not restrict fluids but that he shouldn't eat an excessive amount of meat before the test.
- Advise the patient that he should avoid strenuous physical exercise during the collection period.
- Tell the patient the test usually requires urine collection over a 24-hour period, and teach him the proper collection technique.
- Notify the laboratory and physician of medications the patient is taking that may affect test results; they may need to be restricted.

Procedure and posttest care

- Collect the patient's urine over a 24-hour period, discarding the first specimen and retaining the last. Use a specimen bottle that contains a preservative to prevent the degradation of creatinine.
- Instruct the patient to resume his usual activities, diet, and medication schedule as ordered.

Precautions

- Refrigerate the specimen or keep it on ice during the collection period.
- Send the specimen to the laboratory immediately after the collection is completed.

Reference values

Normally, urine creatinine levels range from 14 to 26 mg/kg body weight/24 hours (SI, 124 to 230 μmol/kg body weight/day) in males; and from 11 to 20 mg/kg body weight/24 hours (SI, 97 to 177 μmol/kg body weight/day) in females.

Abnormal findings

Decreased urine creatinine levels may result from impaired renal perfusion (associated with shock, for example) or from renal disease due to urinary tract obstruction. Chronic bilateral pyelonephritis, acute or chronic glomerulonephritis, and polycystic kidney disease may also depress creatinine levels. Increased levels generally have little diagnostic significance.

Interfering factors

- Failure to observe restrictions, to collect all urine during the test period, to properly store the specimen, or to send the specimen to the laboratory immediately after the collection is completed
- Corticosteroids, gentamycin, tetracyclines, diuretics, and amphotericin B (possible decrease)

CREATININE CLEARANCE

An anhydride of creatine, creatinine is formed and excreted in constant amounts by an irreversible reaction and functions solely as the main end product of creatine. Creatinine production is proportional to total muscle mass and is relatively unaffected by urine volume or normal physical activity or diet.

An excellent diagnostic indicator of renal function, the creatinine clearance test determines how efficiently the kidneys are clearing creatinine from the blood. The rate of clearance is expressed in terms of the volume of blood (in milliliters) that can be cleared of creatinine in 1 minute. Creatinine levels become abnormal when more than 50% of the nephrons have been damaged.

Purpose

- To assess renal function (primarily glomerular filtration)
- To monitor progression of renal insufficiency

Patient preparation

- Explain to the patient that this test assesses kidney function.
- Inform the patient that he may need to avoid meat, poultry, fish, tea, or coffee for 6 hours before the test.
- Advise the patient that he should avoid strenuous physical exercise during the collection period.
- Tell the patient the test requires a timed urine specimen and at least one blood sample.
- Tell the patient how the urine specimen will be collected. Also inform him who will perform the venipuncture and when and that he may feel some discomfort from the needle puncture.
- Explain that more than one venipuncture may be necessary.
- Notify the laboratory and physician of medications the patient is taking that may affect test results; they may need to be restricted.

Procedure and posttest care

- Collect a timed urine specimen at 2, 6, 12, or 24 hours in a bottle containing a preservative to prevent degradation of creatinine.
- Perform a venipuncture anytime during the collection period, and collect the sample in a 7-ml tube without additives.
- Apply direct pressure to the venipuncture site until bleeding stops. Apply warm soaks to ease discomfort if a hematoma develops at the venipuncture site.
- Instruct the patient to resume his usual activities, diet, and medication schedule as ordered.

Precautions

- Refrigerate the urine specimen or keep it on ice during the collection period.
- Send the specimen to the laboratory as soon as the collection is completed.

Reference values

Normal creatinine clearance varies with age; in males, it ranges from 94 to

140 mL/min/1.73m^2 (SI, 0.91 to 1.35 mL/s/m^2); in females, 72 to 110 mL/min/1.73m^2 (SI, 0.69 to 1.06 mL/s/m^2)

Abnormal findings

Low creatinine clearance may result from reduced renal blood flow (associated with shock or renal artery obstruction), acute tubular necrosis, acute or chronic glomerulonephritis, advanced bilateral chronic pyelonephritis, advanced bilateral renal lesions (which may occur in polycystic kidney disease, renal tuberculosis, and cancer), nephrosclerosis, heart failure, or severe dehydration.

High creatinine clearance can suggest poor hydration.

Interfering factors

- Failure to observe restrictions, to collect all urine during the test period, to properly store the specimen, or to send the sample to the laboratory immediately after the collection is completed
- Amphotericin B, thiazide diuretics, furosemide, and aminoglycosides (possible decrease)
- High-protein diet, strenuous exercise (increase)

URIC ACID

A quantitative analysis of urine uric acid levels may supplement serum uric acid testing when seeking to identify disorders that alter production or excretion of uric acid (such as leukemia, gout, and renal dysfunction).

The most specific laboratory method for detecting uric acid is spectrophotometric absorption after treatment of the specimen with the enzyme uricase.

Purpose

- To detect enzyme deficiencies and metabolic disturbances that affect uric acid production, such as gout
- To help measure the efficiency of renal clearance and to determine the risk of stone formation

Patient preparation

- Explain to the patient that this test measures the body's production and excretion of a waste product known as uric acid.
- A diet low or high in purines may be ordered before or during the urine collection.
- Tell the patient the test requires urine collection over a 24-hour period, and teach him the proper collection technique.
- Notify the laboratory and physician of medications the patient is taking that may affect test results; they may need to be restricted.

Procedure and posttest care

- Collect the patient's urine over a 24-hour period, discarding the first specimen and retaining the last.
- Instruct the patient to resume his usual diet and medication schedule as ordered.

Precautions

- Send the specimen to the laboratory immediately after the collection is completed.

Reference values

Normal urine uric acid values vary with diet but generally are 250 to 750 mg/ 24 hours (SI, 1.48 to 4.43 mmol/day).

Abnormal findings

Elevated urine uric acid levels may result from chronic myeloid leukemia, polycythemia vera, multiple myeloma, early remission in pernicious anemia, lymphosarcoma and lymphatic leukemia during radiotherapy, or tubular reabsorption defects, such as Fanconi's syndrome and hepatolenticular degeneration (Wilson's disease).

Low urine uric acid levels occur in gout (when associated with normal uric acid production but inadequate excretion) and in severe renal damage, such as that resulting from chronic glomerulonephritis, diabetic glomerulosclerosis, and collagen disorders.

Interfering factors

- Failure to send the sample to the laboratory immediately after the collection is completed
- Diuretics, such as benzthiazide, furosemide, and ethacrynic acid (decrease); pyrazinamide, salicylates, phenylbutazone, probenecid, and allopurinol (increase)
- High-purine diet (increase)
- Low-purine diet (decrease)

PIGMENTS

HEMOGLOBIN

An abnormal finding, free hemoglobin (Hb) in the urine may occur in hemolytic anemias, infection, strenuous exercise, or severe intravascular hemolysis from a transfusion reaction. Contained in red blood cells (RBCs), Hb consists of an iron-protoporphyrin complex (heme) and a polypeptide (globin). Usually, RBC destruction occurs within the reticuloendothelial system. However, when RBC destruction occurs within the circulation, free Hb enters the plasma and binds with haptoglobin. If the plasma level of Hb exceeds that of haptoglobin, the excess of unbound Hb is excreted in the urine (hemoglobinuria).

Heme proteins act like enzymes that catalyze oxidation of organic substances. This reaction produces a blue coloration; the intensity of color varies with the amount of Hb present. Microscopic examination is required to identify intact RBCs in urine (hematuria), which can occur in the presence of unbound Hb.

Purpose

- To aid diagnosis of hemolytic anemias, infection, or severe intravascular hemolysis from a transfusion reaction

Patient preparation

- Explain to the patient that this test detects excessive RBC destruction.
- Inform the patient that he need not restrict food or fluid.
- Tell the patient the test requires a random urine specimen, and teach him the proper collection technique.
- If the female patient is menstruating, reschedule the test as results may be altered.
- Notify the laboratory and physician of medications the patient is taking that may affect test results; they may need to be restricted.

Procedure and posttest care

- Collect a random urine specimen. (See *Bedside testing for urine blood pigments.*)
- Instruct the patient to resume his usual medication schedule as ordered

Precautions

- A female patient who is menstruating should reschedule her test because contamination of the specimen with menstrual blood alters results.
- Send the specimen to the laboratory immediately after collection.

Bedside testing for urine blood pigments

To test a patient's urine for blood pigments at bedside, use one of the methods that follow.

DIPSTICK, MULTISTIX, OR CHEMSTRIP

- ◆ Collect a urine specimen.
- ◆ Dip the stick into the specimen and withdraw it.
- ◆ After 30 seconds, compare the stick to the color chart. Blue indicates a positive reaction; the intensity of color indicates pigment concentration.

OCCULT TABLET

- ◆ Collect a urine specimen.
- ◆ Put one drop of urine on the filter paper. Place the tablet on the urine, and then put two drops of water on the tablet.
- ◆ After 2 minutes, inspect the filter paper around the tablet. Blue indicates a positive reaction; the intensity of color indicates pigment concentration.

OCCULT SOLUTION

- ◆ Collect a urine specimen.
- ◆ After placing one drop of urine on the filter paper, close the package and turn it over. Open the opposite ends, and place two drops of solution on the filter paper.
- ◆ After 30 seconds, inspect the filter paper. Blue indicates a positive reaction; the intensity of color indicates pigment concentration.

DISTINGUISHING HEMOGLOBIN

Because these methods detect only blood pigments, immunochemical studies are necessary to differentiate hemoglobin from other blood pigments such as myoglobin.

Normal findings

Normally, Hb isn't present in the urine.

Abnormal findings

Hemoglobinuria may result from severe intravascular hemolysis due to a blood transfusion reaction, burns, or a crushing injury. It may result from acquired hemolytic anemias caused by chemical or drug intoxication or malaria; congenital hemolytic anemias, such as hemoglobinopathies or enzyme defects; or paroxysmal nocturnal hemoglobinuria (another type of hemolytic anemia). Less commonly, it may signal cystitis, ureteral calculi, or urethritis.

Hemoglobinuria and hematuria occur in renal epithelial damage (which may result from acute glomerulonephritis or pyelonephritis), renal tumor, and tuberculosis.

Interfering factors

- Failure to send the specimen to the laboratory immediately after collection
- Nephrotoxic drugs, anticoagulants (positive results)
- Large doses of vitamin C or drugs that contain vitamin C as a preservative (false negative)
- Lysis of RBCs in stale or alkaline urine and contamination of the specimen by menstrual blood
- Bacterial peroxidases in highly infected specimens (false-positive)

MYOGLOBIN

The myoglobin test detects the presence of myoglobin — a red pigment found in the cytoplasm of cardiac and skeletal muscle cells — in the urine.

When muscle cells are extensively damaged, as by disease or severe crushing trauma, myoglobin is released into the blood, quickly cleared by renal glomerular filtration, and eliminated in the urine (myoglobinuria). For example, myoglobin appears in the urine within 24 hours after a myocardial infarction (MI).

Urine myoglobin must be differentiated from urine hemoglobin because of their marked structural similarities. The most commonly used test method is the differential precipitation test. Hemoglobin — bound to haptoglobin — precipitates when urine is mixed with ammonium sulfate. Myoglobin, however, remains soluble and can be measured.

Purpose

- To aid diagnosis of muscular disease of rhabdomyolysis
- To detect extensive infarction of muscle tissue
- To assess the extent of muscular damage from crushing trauma

Patient preparation

- Explain to the patient that this test detects a red pigment found in muscle cells and helps evaluate muscle injury or disease.
- Inform the patient that he need not restrict food or fluids before the test.
- Tell the patient that this test requires a random urine specimen, and teach him the proper collection technique.

Procedure and posttest care

- Collect a random urine specimen.

Precautions

- Send the specimen to the laboratory immediately after collection.

Normal findings

Normally, myoglobin doesn't appear in urine.

Abnormal findings

Myoglobinuria occurs in acute or chronic muscular disease, alcoholic polymyopathy, familial myoglobinuria, extensive MI, and in severe trauma to the skeletal muscles (which may result from a crushing injury, extreme hyperthermia, or severe burns). It also occurs in strenuous or prolonged exercise, but disappears after rest.

Interfering factors

- Extremely dilute urine reduces sensitivity
- Contamination with iodine during surgery (positive results)
- Recent ingestion of large amounts of vitamin C (inhibits reaction if testing is performed with chemstrip or other regent strips)
- Failure to send the specimen to the laboratory immediately after collection

PORPHYRINS

The test for porphyrins is a quantitative analysis of urine porphyrins (most notably, uroporphyrins and coproporphyrins) and their precursors (porphyrinogens, such as porphobilinogen [PBG]). Tests for prophyrins may include PBG and urine δ-aminolevulinic acid. Porphyrins are red-orange fluorescent compounds, consisting of four pyrrole rings that are produced during heme biosynthesis. They're present in all protoplasm, figure in energy storage and utilization, and are normally excreted in urine in small amounts. Elevated urine levels of porphyrins or porphyrinogens, therefore, reflect impaired heme biosynthesis. Such impairment may result from inherited enzyme deficiencies (congenital porphyrias) or from defects due to such disorders as hemolytic anemias and hepatic disease (acquired porphyrias).

Determination of the specific porphyrins and porphyrinogens found in a urine specimen can help identify the impaired metabolic step in hemebiosynthesis. Occasionally, a preliminary qualitative screening is performed on a random specimen. However, a positive finding on the screening test must be confirmed by the quantitative analysis of a 24-hour specimen. For correct diagnosis of a specific porphyria, urine porphyrin levels should be correlated with plasma and fecal porphyrin levels.

Purpose

- To aid diagnosis of congenital or acquired porphyrias

Patient preparation

- Explain to the patient that this test detects abnormal hemoglobin formation.
- Inform the patient that he need not restrict food or fluids before the test.
- Tell the patient the test requires urine collection over a 24-hour period, and teach him the proper collection technique.
- Notify the laboratory and physician of medications the patient is taking that may affect test results; they may need to be restricted.

Procedure and posttest care

- Collect the patient's urine over a 24-hour period, discarding the first specimen and retaining the last. Use a light-resistant specimen bottle containing a preservative to prevent degradation of the light-sensitive porphyrins and their precursors.
- Instruct the patient to resume his usual medication schedule as ordered.

Precautions

- Be aware that pregnancy or menstruation may affect the accuracy of test results.
- Refrigerate the specimen or keep it on ice during the collection period.
- Send it to the laboratory as soon as the collection is completed.
- Protect the specimen from light exposure if a light-resistant container is not available.
- Put the collection bag in a dark plastic bag if an indwelling urinary catheter is in place.

Normal findings

Normal urine porphyrin and precursor values fall in the following ranges:

- uroporphyrins: 27 to 52 µg/24 hours (SI, 32 to 63 nmol/day)
- coproporphyrins: 34 to 230 µg/24 hours (SI, 52 to 351 nmol/day).

Abnormal findings

Increased urine levels of porphyrins and porphyrin precursors are characteristic of porphyria. (See *Urine porphyrin levels in porphyria,* page 374.) Infectious hepatitis, Hodgkin's disease, central nervous system disorders, cirrhosis, and heavy metal, benzene, or carbon tetrachloride toxicity may also increase porphyrin levels.

Interfering factors

- Failure to properly store the specimen during the collection period, to protect it from exposure to light, or to send the specimen to the laboratory immediately after the collection is completed
- Barbiturates, chloral hydrate, chloropropamide, sulfonamides, meprobamate, chlordiazepoxide (induce porphyria or porphyrinuria); discontinue 12 days before the test if possible (possible increase or decrease)
- Oral contraceptives, griseofulvin (increase)

Urine porphyrin levels in porphyria

In porphyria, defective heme biosynthesis increases urinary porphyrins and their corresponding precursors.

PORPHYRIA	PORPHYRINS		PORPHYRIN PRECURSORS	
	Uroporphyrins	Coproporphyrins	δ-aminolevulinic acid	Porphobilinogen
Erythropoietic porphyria	Highly increased	Increased	Normal	Normal
Erythropoietic protoporphyria	Normal	Normal	Normal	Normal
Acute intermittent porphyria	Variable	Variable	Highly increased	Highly increased
Variegate porphyria	Normal or slightly increased; may be highly increased during acute attack	Normal or slightly increased; may be highly increased during acute attack	Highly increased during acute attack	Normal or slightly increased; highly increased during acute attack
Coproporphyria	Not applicable	May be highly increased during acute attack	Increased during acute attack	Increased during acute attack
Porphyria cutanea tarda	Highly increased	Increased	Variable	Variable

- Pregnancy or menstruation (possible increase or decrease)
- Rifampin (elevated urine urobilinogen)

δ-AMINOLEVULINIC ACID

Using the colorimetric technique, the quantitative analysis of urine δ-aminolevulinic acid (ALA) levels helps diagnose porphyrias, hepatic disease, and lead poisoning. In an emergency, a simple qualitative screening test may be performed.

ALA, the basic precursor of the porphyrins, normally converts to porphobilinogen during heme synthesis. Impaired conversion, which occurs in porphyrias and lead poisoning, causes urine ALA levels to rise before other chemical or hematologic changes occur.

Purpose

- To screen for lead poisoning
- To aid diagnosis of porphyrias and certain hepatic disorders, such as hepatitis and hepatic carcinoma

Patient preparation

- Explain to the patient that this test detects abnormal hemoglobin formation.
- If lead poisoning is suspected, tell the patient (or parents, because the patient is usually a child) that the test helps detect the presence of excessive lead in the body.
- Inform the patient or his parents that he need not restrict food or fluids.
- Tell the patient that the test requires urine collection over a 24-hour period, and teach him or his parents the proper collection technique.
- Notify the laboratory and physician of medications the patient is taking that may affect test results; they may need to be restricted.

Procedure and posttest care

- Collect the patient's urine over a 24-hour period, discarding the first specimen and retaining the last. Use a light-resistant bottle containing a preservative (usually glacial acetic acid) to prevent degradation of ALA.
- Instruct the patient to resume his usual medication schedule as ordered.

Precautions

- Refrigerate the specimen or keep it on ice during the collection period.
- Send the specimen to the laboratory as soon as the collection is complete.
- Protect the specimen from direct sunlight.
- Insert the drainage bag in a dark plastic bag if the patient has an indwelling urinary catheter in place.
- Blood levels for lead aren't sensitive indicators of lead poisoning in children.

Reference values

Normally, urine ALA values range from 1.3 to 7.0 mg/24 hours (SI, 10 to 53 μmol/day).

Abnormal findings

Elevated urine ALA levels may occur in lead poisoning, hereditary tyrosinemia, acute porphyria, hepatic carcinoma, or hepatitis.

Interfering factors

- Failure to collect all urine during the test period, to properly store the specimen and protect it from light, or to send the specimen to the laboratory immediately after the collection is completed
- Barbiturates and griseofulvin (increase due to accumulation of porphyrins in the liver)
- Vitamin E in pharmacologic doses (possible decrease)

BILIRUBIN

The bilirubin screening test, based on a color reaction with a specific reagent, detects water-soluble direct (conjugated) bilirubin in the urine. Detectable amounts of bilirubin in the urine may indicate liver disease caused by infections, biliary disease, or hepatotoxicity.

When combined with urobilinogen measurements, the bilirubin test helps identify disorders that can cause jaundice. The analysis can be performed at the bedside, using a bilirubin reagent strip, or in the laboratory.

Purpose

- To help identify the cause of jaundice
- To compare urine and serum bilirubin levels and other liver enzyme tests.

Comparative values of bilirubin and urobilinogen

CAUSES OF JAUNDICE	SERUM		URINE		STOOL
	Indirect bilirubin	Direct bilirubin	Bilirubin	Urobilinogen	Urobilinogen
Unconjugated hyperbilirubinemia					
Hemolytic disorders: hemolytic anemia, erythroblastosis fetalis	↑	N	O	N↑	↑
Gilbert's disease: constitutional hepatic dysfunction	↑↑	N	O	N↓	N↓
Crigler-Najjar syndrome: congenital hyperbilirubinemia	↑↑↑	N	O	N↓	N↓
Conjugated hyperbilirubinemia					
Extrahepatic obstruction: calculi, tumor, scar tissue in common bile duct or hepatic excretory duct	N	↑	+	↓O	↓O
Hepatocellular disorders: viral, toxic, or alcoholic hepatitis; cirrhosis; parenchymal injury	↑	↑	+	↓N↑	N↑
Hepatocanalicular disorders or intrahepatic obstruction: drug-induced cholestasis; some familial defects, such as Dubin-Johnson and Rotor's syndromes; viral hepatitis; and primary biliary cirrhosis	↑	↑	+	↓N↑	N↑

KEY:

↑	Increased	0	Absent
N↑	May be increased	+	Present
↑↑	Moderately increased	N↓	Normal or reduced
↑↑↑	Markedly increased	↓0	Decreased or absent
N	Normal	↓N↑	Variable

Patient preparation

■ Explain to the patient that this test helps determine the cause of jaundice.
■ Inform the patient that he need not restrict food or fluids before the test.
■ Tell the patient the test requires a random urine specimen.
■ Advise the patient that the specimen will be tested at bedside or in the laboratory.
■ Notify the laboratory and physician of medications the patient is taking that may affect test results; they may need to be restricted.

Procedure and posttest care

■ Collect a random urine specimen in the container provided.
Bedside analysis using the dipstrip procedure
■ Dip the reagent strip into the specimen and remove it immediately.
■ Compare the strip color with the color standards after 20 seconds.
■ Record the test results on the patient's chart.
Bedside analysis using the ictotest procedure
■ Place five drops of urine on the asbestos-cellulose test mat. If bilirubin is present, it will be absorbed into the mat.
■ Put a reagent tablet on the wet area of the mat, and place two drops of water on the tablet. If bilirubin is present, a blue to purple coloration will develop on the mat. Pink or red indicates absence of bilirubin.
■ Instruct the patient to resume his usual medication schedule as ordered.

Precautions

■ Use only a freshly voided specimen. Bilirubin disintegrates after 30 minutes of exposure to room temperature or light.
■ If the specimen is to be analyzed in the laboratory, send it there at once.
■ If the specimen is tested at the bedside, make sure 20 seconds elapse before interpreting the color change on the dipstrip.
■ Make sure lighting is adequate to make this color determination.

Normal findings

Normally, bilirubin isn't found in urine in a routine screening test.

Abnormal findings

High concentrations of direct bilirubin in urine may be evident from the specimen's appearance (dark, with a yellow foam). To diagnose jaundice, however, the presence or absence of direct bilirubin in urine must be correlated with serum test results and with urine and fecal urobilinogen levels. (See *Comparative values of bilirubin and urobilinogen.*)

Interfering factors

■ Failure to test the specimen promptly or to send it to the laboratory immediately after collection
■ Phenazopyridine, phenothiazine derivatives (chlorpromazine and acetophenazine maleate) (false-positive)
■ Large amounts of ascorbic acid and nitrite (false-negative if using dipstick testing, such as chemstrip or N-multistix)
■ Exposure of specimen to room temperature or light (decrease due to bilirubin degradation)

UROBILINOGEN

The urobilinogen test detects impaired liver function by measuring urine levels of urobilinogen, the colorless, water-soluble product that results from the reduction of bilirubin by intestinal bacteria. Absent or altered urobilinogen levels can indicate hepatic damage or dysfunction. Increased urine urobilinogen levels may indicate hemolysis of red blood cells.

Quantitative analysis of urine urobilinogen involves the addition of a reagent to a 2-hour urine specimen. The resulting color reaction is read promptly by spectrophotometry.

Purpose

- To aid diagnosis of extrahepatic obstruction, such as blockage of the common bile duct
- To aid differential diagnosis of hepatic and hematologic disorders

Patient preparation

- Explain to the patient that this test helps assess liver and biliary tract function.
- Inform the patient that he need not restrict fluids or food, except for bananas, which he should avoid for 48 hours before the test.
- Tell the patient that the test requires a 2-hour urine specimen, and teach him how to collect it.
- Notify the laboratory and physician of medications the patient is taking that may affect test results; they may need to be restricted.

Procedure and posttest care

- Most laboratories request a random urine specimen; others prefer a 2-hour specimen, usually during the afternoon (ideally, between 1 p.m. and 3 p.m.), when urobilinogen levels peak.
- Instruct the patient to resume his usual diet and medication schedule as ordered.

Precautions

- Send the specimen to the laboratory immediately after collection. This test must be performed within 30 minutes of collection because urobilinogen quickly oxidizes into an orange compound called urobilin.

Reference values

Normally, urine urobilinogen values are 0.1 to 0.8 EU/2 hours (SI, 0.1 to 0.8 EU/2 hours) or 0.5 to 4.0 EU/24 hours (SI, 0.5 to 4.0 EU/day).

Abnormal findings

Absence of urine urobilinogen may result from complete obstructive jaundice or treatment with broad-spectrum antibiotics, which destroy the intestinal bacterial flora. Low urine urobilinogen levels may result from congenital enzymatic jaundice (hyperbilirubinemia syndromes) or from treatment with drugs that acidify urine, such as ammonium chloride or ascorbic acid.

Elevated levels may indicate hemolytic jaundice, hepatitis, or cirrhosis.

Interfering factors

- Failure to observe pretest restrictions or to send the specimen to the laboratory immediately after collection
- Para-aminosalicylic acid, phenazopyridine, procaine, phenothiazines, and sulfonamides (possible decrease)
- Acetazolamide, sodium bicarbonate (increase)
- Bananas eaten up to 48 hours before the test (increase)

SUGARS, KETONES, AND MUCOPOLY-SACCHARIDES

GLUCOSE OXIDASE

The glucose oxidase test — which involves the use of commercial, plastic-coated reagent strips (Clinistix, Diastix) or Tes-Tape — is a specific, qualitative test for glycosuria. The test is used primarily to monitor urine glucose in patients with diabetes. Patients can perform this test at home because of its simplicity and convenience.

Purpose

- To detect glycosuria and determine the renal threshold for glucose.
- To monitor urine glucose levels during insulin therapy

Patient preparation

- Explain to the patient that this test determines urine glucose concentration.
- If the patient is a newly diagnosed with diabetes, teach him how to perform a reagent strip test.
- If he's receiving levodopa, ascorbic acid, phenazopyridine, salicylates, peroxides, or hypochlorites, use Clinitest tablets instead.

Equipment

Specimen container, glucose test strips, reference color blocks

Procedure and posttest care

- Have the patient void; then give him a drink of water.
- Collect a second-voided specimen after 30 to 45 minutes.

Clinistix test

- Dip the test area of the reagent strip in the specimen for 2 seconds.
- Remove excess urine by tapping the strip against a clean surface or the side of the container, and begin timing.
- Hold the strip in the air, and "read" the color *exactly 10 seconds* after taking the strip out of the urine by comparing it with the reference color blocks on the label of the container.
- Record the results.
- Ignore color changes that develop after 10 seconds.

Diastix test

- Dip the reagent strip in the specimen for 2 seconds.
- Remove excess urine by tapping the strip against the container, and begin timing.
- Hold the strip in the air, and compare the color to the color chart *exactly 30 seconds* after taking the strip out of the urine.
- Record the results.
- Ignore color changes that develop after 30 seconds.

Tes-Tape

- Withdraw about 1″ (2.5 cm) of the reagent tape from the dispenser; dip ¼″ (0.6 cm) in the specimen for 2 seconds.
- Remove excess urine by tapping the strip against the side of the container, and begin timing.
- Hold the tape in the air, and compare the color of the darkest part of the tape to the color chart *exactly 60 seconds* after taking the strip out of the urine.
- If the tape indicates 0.5% or higher, wait an additional 60 seconds to make the final color comparison.
- Record the results.

Precautions

- Instruct the patient not to contaminate the urine specimen with toilet tissue or stool.

■ Keep the test strip container tightly closed to prevent deterioration of strips by exposure to light or moisture.
■ Store it in a cool place (under 86° F [30° C]) to avoid heat degradation.
■ Don't use discolored or darkened Clinistix or Diastix or dark yellow or yellow-brown Tes-Tape.

Normal findings

Normally, no glucose is present in urine.

Abnormal findings

Glycosuria occurs in diabetes mellitus, adrenal and thyroid disorders, hepatic and central nervous system diseases, conditions involving low renal threshold (such as Fanconi's syndrome), toxic renal tubular disease, heavy metal poisoning, glomerulonephritis, and nephrosis; in pregnant women; and in those receiving total parenteral nutrition. It also occurs with the administration of large amounts of glucose and of certain drugs, such as asparaginase, corticosteroids, carbamazepine, ammonium chloride, thiazide diuretics, dextrothyroxine, large doses of nicotinic acid, lithium carbonate, and prolonged use of phenothiazines.

Interfering factors

■ Dilute, stale urine or contamination of the specimen due to toilet tissue, stool, or bacteria
■ Use of reagent strips after the expiration date, failure to keep the reagent strip container tightly closed, or failure to record the reagent strip method used
■ Presence of reducing substances, such as levodopa, ascorbic acid, phenazopyridine, methyldopa, and salicylates (possible false-negative)
■ Tetracyclines (false-negative)

KETONES

In the ketone test, a routine, semiquantitative screening test, a commercially prepared product is used to measure the urine level of ketone bodies. Ketone bodies are the by-products of fat metabolism; they include acetoacetic acid, acetone, and beta-hydroxybutyric acid. Excessive amounts may appear in patients with carbohydrate dehydration, which may occur in starvation or diabetic ketoacidosis (DKA).

Commercially available tests include the Acetest tablet, Chemstrip K, Ketostix, or Keto-Diastix. Each product measures a specific ketone body. For example, Acetest measures acetone and Ketostix measures acetoacetic acid.

Purpose

■ To screen for ketonuria
■ To identify DKA and carbohydrate deprivation
■ To distinguish between a diabetic and a nondiabetic coma
■ To monitor control of diabetes mellitus, ketogenic weight reduction, and treatment of DKA

Patient preparation

■ Explain to the patient that this test evaluates fat metabolism.
■ If the patient is newly diagnosed with diabetes, tell him how to perform the test.
■ If the patient is taking levodopa or phenazopyridine or has recently received sulfobromophthalein, Acetest tablets must be used because reagent strips may produce inaccurate results.

Procedure and posttest care

■ Instruct the patient to void; then give him a drink of water.

- Collect a second-voided midstream specimen about 30 minutes later.

Acetest

- Lay the tablet on a piece of white paper, and place one drop of urine on the tablet.
- Compare the tablet color (white, lavender, or purple) with the color chart after 30 seconds.

Ketostix

- Dip the reagent stick into the specimen, and remove it immediately.
- Compare the stick color (buff or purple) with the color chart after 15 seconds.
- Record the results as negative, small, moderate, or large amounts of ketones.

Keto-Diastix

- Dip the reagent strip into the specimen, and remove it immediately.
- Tap the edge of the strip against the container or a clean, dry surface to remove excess urine.
- Hold the strip horizontally to prevent mixing the chemicals from the two areas.
- Interpret each area of the strip separately. Compare the color of the ketone section (buff or purple) with the appropriate color chart after exactly 15 seconds; compare the color of the glucose section after 30 seconds.
- Ignore color changes that occur after the specified waiting periods.
- Record the results as negative or positive for small, moderate, or large amounts of ketones.

Precautions

- Test the specimen within 60 minutes after it's obtained, or you must refrigerate it.
- Allow refrigerated specimens to return to room temperature before testing.
- Don't use tablets or strips that have become discolored or darkened.

Normal findings

Normally, no ketones are present in urine.

Abnormal findings

Ketonuria may occur in uncontrolled diabetes mellitus or starvation. It also occurs as a metabolic complication of total parenteral nutrition.

Interfering factors

- Failure to keep the reagent container tightly closed to prevent absorption of light or moisture or bacterial contamination of the specimen (false-negative)
- Failure to test the specimen within 1 hour or to refrigerate it
- Levodopa, phenazopyridine, and sulfobromophthalein (false-positive results when Ketostix or Keto-Diastix is used instead of Acetest)

ACID MUCOPOLYSACCHARIDES

The acid mucopolysaccharides test is a quantitative test that helps detect mucopolysaccharidosis, a rare disorder that may affect the skeleton, joints, liver, spleen, eye, ear, skin, teeth, and the cardiovascular, respiratory, and central nervous systems. This test measures the urine level of acid mucopolysaccharides, a group of polysaccharides or carbohydrates.

Purpose

- To diagnose mucopolysaccharidosis in infants with a family history of the disease

Patient preparation

- Explain to the parents of the infant that this test helps determine the efficiency of carbohydrate metabolism.

■ Inform them that they need not restrict the child's food or fluids.
■ Tell the parents that the test requires urine collection for 24 hours, and instruct them on the proper way to collect the specimen at home.
■ If the child is receiving therapy with heparin and must continue it, note this on the laboratory request.

Equipment
Pediatric urine collectors, 24-hour collection container, 20 ml toluene (usually obtained from the laboratory)

Procedure and posttest care
■ Collect the patient's urine over a 24-hour period, discarding the first specimen and retaining the last.
■ Add 20 ml toluene (as a preservative) to the collection container at the start of the collection.
■ Indicate the patient's age on the laboratory request.
■ Send the specimen to the laboratory immediately after the 24-hour collection period.
■ Make sure all adhesive from the urine collector is removed from the infant's perineum.
■ Wash the area gently with soap and water, and watch for irritation.

Precautions
■ Refrigerate the specimen or place it on ice during the collection period.

Normal findings
The acid mucopolysaccharide value is expressed as milligrams of glucuronic acid divided by the amount of creatinine in the same specimen (which reflects glomerular filtration rate) to overcome irregularities in the 24-hour urine collection.

Normal acid mucopolysaccharide values for adults are less than 13.3 μg glucuronic acid/mg/creatinine/24 hours. For children, values vary with age.

Abnormal findings
Elevated acid mucopolysaccharide levels reliably indicate mucopolysaccharidosis. Supplementary quantitative analysis and detailed blood studies can identify the defective enzyme.

Interfering factors
■ Failure to collect all urine during the test period, to properly store the specimen, or to send the specimen to the laboratory immediately after the collection is completed
■ Heparin (increase)

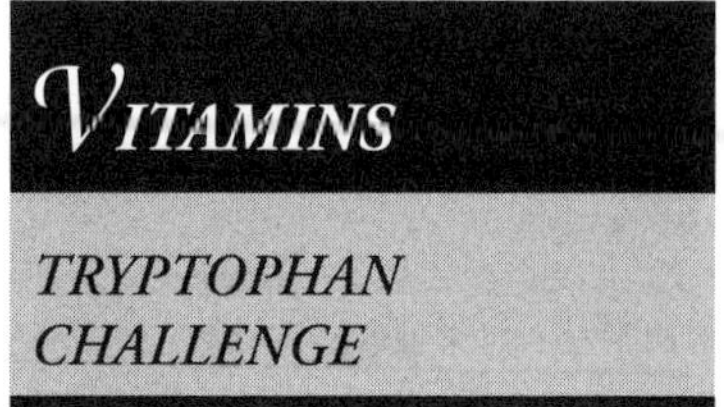

VITAMINS

TRYPTOPHAN CHALLENGE

Measurement of urine xanthurenic acid after a challenge dose of tryptophan confirms deficiency of vitamin B_6 long before symptoms appear.

Although vitamin B_6 isn't directly involved in energy metabolism, it's essential for reactions that occur in protein metabolism and for amino acid synthesis. Vitamin B_6 deficiency can cause hypochromic microcytic anemia without iron deficiency and central nervous system disturbances. When normal magnesium levels accompany a vitamin B_6 deficiency, urinary citrate and oxalate solubility may decrease, causing formation of urinary calculi.

Purpose
■ To detect vitamin B_6 deficiency

Patient preparation

- Explain to the patient that this test determines the body's stores of vitamin B_6.
- Tell the patient he'll receive an oral dose of medication.
- Explain that this test requires urine collection over a 24-hour period.
- Notify the laboratory and physician of medications the patient is taking that may affect test results; they may need to be restricted.

Procedure and posttest care

- Administer L-tryptophan by mouth (usually, 50 mg/kg for children and up to 2 g/kg for adults).
- Have the patient void and discard the urine. Immediately begin collection of a 24-hour urine specimen.
- Inform the patient with vitamin B_6 deficiency that yeast, wheat, corn, liver, and kidneys are good sources of pyridoxine.
- Instruct the patient to resume his usual medication schedule as ordered.

Precautions

- Make sure the specimen bottle contains a crystal of thymol, a preservative.
- Tell the patient not to contaminate the urine specimen with toilet tissue or stool.
- Refrigerate the specimen, or place it on ice during the collection period.

Normal findings

Normal excretion of xanthurenic acid after a tryptophan challenge dose is less than 50 mg/24 hours.

Abnormal findings

Urine levels of xanthurenic acid exceeding 100 mg/24 hours indicate vitamin B_6 deficiency. This rare disorder may result from malnutrition, malignancy, pregnancy, familial xanthurenic aciduria, or use of oral contraceptives, hydralazine, D-penicillamine, or isoniazid.

Interfering factors

- Contamination of the specimen with toilet tissue or stool
- Failure to properly handle the specimen
- Oral contraceptives, hydralazine, D-penicillamine, and isoniazid (decrease)

VITAMIN C

Through colorimetric measurement of urinary levels, the vitamin C test determines body stores of vitamin C (ascorbic acid). This water-soluble vitamin, which is easily absorbed by the intestine, acts as a reversible reducing agent in metabolic processes, aids collagen formation, and helps maintain connective and osteoid tissues.

This analysis is particularly useful in diagnosing scurvy, an extreme deficiency of vitamin C characterized by the degeneration of connective and osteoid tissues, dentin, and endothelial membranes. Although now uncommon in North America, scurvy may occur in alcoholics, people on low-residue or low-citrus diets, and infants who have been weaned to cow's milk that doesn't contain a vitamin C supplement.

Purpose

- To aid diagnosis of scurvy, scurvy-like conditions, and metabolic disorders, such as malnutrition, that interfere with oxidative processes

Patient preparation

- Explain to the patient that this test detects vitamin C deficiency.
- Inform the patient that he should maintain a normal diet.

■ Tell the patient the test requires urine collection over a 24-hour period.
■ If the specimen is to be collected at home, instruct the patient on proper collection technique.

Procedure and posttest care

■ Collect the patient's urine over a 24-hour period, discarding the first specimen and retaining the last.
■ Advise the patient with vitamin C deficiency that citrus fruits, tomatoes, potatoes, cabbage, and strawberries are good dietary sources of vitamin C.

Precautions

■ Tell the patient not to contaminate the specimen with toilet tissue or stool.
■ Refrigerate the specimen, or place it on ice during the collection period.

Reference values

Normal urine vitamin C excretion is 30 mg/24 hours.

Abnormal findings

Depressed urine vitamin C levels are common in patients with infection, cancer, burns, or other stress-producing conditions. Decreased vitamin C levels may also indicate malnutrition, malabsorption, renal deficiencies, or prolonged I.V. therapy without vitamin C replacement. Severe vitamin C deficiency causes scurvy.

Interfering factors

■ Improper specimen collection or storage or exposure to light
■ Contamination of the specimen with toilet tissue or stool

MINERALS

SODIUM AND CHLORIDE

The sodium and chloride test determines urine levels of sodium, the major extracellular cation, and of chloride, the major extracellular anion. Less significant than serum levels and, consequently, performed less frequently, the measurement of urine sodium and chloride concentrations is used to evaluate renal conservation of these two electrolytes and to confirm serum sodium and chloride values.

In the body, sodium and chloride help maintain osmotic pressure and water and acid-base balance. Normal ranges of sodium and chloride in the urine vary greatly with dietary salt intake and perspiration.

Purpose

■ To help evaluate fluid and electrolyte imbalance
■ To monitor the effects of a low-salt diet
■ To help evaluate renal and adrenal disorders

Patient preparation

■ Explain to the patient that this test helps determine the balance of salt and water in the body.
■ Advise the patient that no special restrictions are necessary.
■ Tell the patient the test requires urine collection over a 24-hour period.
■ If the specimen is to be collected at home, instruct the patient on proper collection technique.
■ Notify the laboratory and physician of medications the patient is taking that

may affect test results; they may need to be restricted.

Procedure and posttest care

- Collect the patient's urine over a 24-hour period, discarding the first specimen and retaining the last.
- Instruct the patient to resume his usual medication schedule as ordered.

Precautions

- Tell the patient not to contaminate the specimen with toilet tissue or stool.
- Tell the patient not to use a metallic bedpan for specimen collection.

Reference values

Normal urine sodium excretion in an adult ranges from 40 to 220 mEq/L/24 hours (SI, 40 to 220 mmol/day); in a child, 41 to 115 mEq/L/24 hours (SI, 41 to 115 mmol/day). Normal urine chloride excretion in an adult ranges from 110 to 250 nmol/24 hours (SI, 110 to 250 mmol/day); in a child, from 15 to 40 nmol/24 hours (SI, 15 to 40 mmol/day); in infants, 2 to 10 mmol/24 hours (SI, 2 to 10 mmol/day).

Abnormal findings

Most commonly, urine sodium and urine chloride levels are parallel, rising and falling in tandem. Abnormal levels of both minerals may indicate the need for more specific testing.

Elevated urine sodium levels may reflect increased salt intake, adrenal failure, salicylate toxicity, diabetic acidosis, salt-losing nephritis, and water-deficient dehydration.

Decreased urine sodium levels suggest decreased salt intake, primary aldosteronism, acute renal failure, and heart failure.

Elevated urine chloride levels may result from water-deficient dehydration, salicylate toxicity, diabetic ketoacidosis, adrenocortical insufficiency (Addison's disease), or salt-losing renal disease. Decreased levels may result from excessive diaphoresis, heart failure, hypochloremic metabolic alkalosis, or prolonged vomiting or gastric suctioning.

To evaluate fluid-electrolyte imbalance, results must be correlated with findings of serum electrolyte studies.

Interfering factors

- Failure to collect all urine during the test period.
- Sodium bicarbonate and thiazide diuretics (increase sodium)
- Steroids (decrease sodium)
- Ammonium chloride and potassium chloride (increase in chloride)

POTASSIUM

The potassium test is a quantitative test that measures urine levels of potassium, a major intracellular cation that helps regulate acid-base balance and neuromuscular function. Potassium imbalance may cause such signs and symptoms as muscle weakness, nausea, diarrhea, confusion, hypotension, and electrocardiogram changes; severe imbalance may lead to cardiac arrest.

Most commonly, a serum potassium test is performed to detect hyperkalemia (abnormally high levels) or hypokalemia (abnormally low levels). A urine potassium test may be performed to evaluate hypokalemia when a history and physical examination fail to uncover the cause. If results suggest a renal disorder, additional renal function tests may be ordered.

Purpose

- To determine whether hypokalemia is caused by renal or extrarenal disorders

Patient preparation

- Explain to the patient that this test evaluates his kidney function.
- Advise the patient that no special dietary restrictions are necessary.
- Tell the patient that the test requires urine collection over a 24-hour period.
- If the specimen is to be collected at home, teach the patient the correct collection technique.
- Notify the laboratory and physician of medications the patient is taking that may affect test results; they may need to be restricted.

Procedure and posttest care

- Collect the patient's urine over a 24-hour period, discarding the first specimen and retaining the last.
- Administer potassium supplements and monitor serum levels as appropriate.
- Provide dietary supplements and nutritional counseling as necessary.
- Replace fluid volume loss with I.V. or oral fluids as necessary.
- Instruct the patient to resume his usual medication schedule as ordered.
- Don't use a metallic bedpan for collection.

Precautions

- Tell the patient not to contaminate the specimen with toilet tissue or stool.
- Refrigerate the specimen, or place it on ice during the collection period.
- Send the specimen to the laboratory immediately after the collection is completed, or refrigerate it.

Reference values

Normal potassium excretion in adults is 25 to 125 mmol/24 hours (SI, 25 to 125 mmol/day) and varies with diet. In children, normal excretion is 22 to 57 mmol/24 hours (SI, 22 to 57 mmol/day).

Abnormal findings

In a patient with hypokalemia, potassium concentration less than 10 mmol/24 hours (SI, 10 mmol/day) suggests normal renal function, indicating that potassium loss is most likely the result of a GI disorder such as malabsorption syndrome.

In a patient with hypokalemia lasting more than 3 days, urine potassium concentration above 10 mmol/24 hours (SI, 10 mmol/day) indicates renal loss of potassium. These losses may result from such disorders as aldosteronism, renal tubular acidosis, or chronic renal failure. However, extrarenal disorders, such as dehydration, starvation, Cushing's disease, or salicylate intoxication, may also elevate urine potassium levels.

Interfering factors

- Excess dietary potassium (increase)
- Contamination of the specimen with toilet tissue or stool
- Failure to collect all urine and send the specimen to the laboratory immediately after collection or to refrigerate it
- Potassium-wasting medications, such as ammonium chloride, thiazide diuretics, and acetazolamide (increase)
- Excess vomiting or stomach suctioning

CALCIUM AND PHOSPHATES

The calcium and phosphates test measures the urine levels of calcium and phosphates, elements essential for the formation and resorption of bone. Urine calcium and phosphate levels generally parallel serum levels.

Normally absorbed in the upper intestine and excreted in stool and urine, calcium and phosphates help maintain tissue and fluid pH, electrolyte balance in cells and extracellular fluids, and permeability of cell membranes. Calcium promotes enzymatic processes, aids blood coagulation, and lowers neuromuscular irritability; phosphates aid carbohydrate metabolism.

Purpose

- To evaluate calcium and phosphate metabolism and excretion
- To monitor treatment of calcium or phosphate deficiency

Patient preparation

- Explain to the patient that this test measures the amount of calcium and phosphates in the urine.
- Encourage the patient to be as active as possible before the test.
- Tell the patient the test requires urine collection over a 24-hour period.
- If the patient is to collect the specimen, teach him the proper technique.
- Provide a diet that contains about 130 mg of calcium/24 hours for 3 days before the test or provide a copy of the diet for the patient to follow at home.
- Notify the laboratory and physician of medications the patient is taking that may affect test results; they may need to be restricted.

Procedure and posttest care

- Collect the patient's urine over a 24-hour period, discarding the first specimen and retaining the last.
- Observe a patient with low urine calcium levels for tetany.

Precautions

- Tell the patient not to contaminate the specimen with toilet tissue or stool.

Reference values

Normal values depend on dietary intake. For a normal diet, urine calcium levels for a 24-hour period range from 100 to 300 mg/24 hours (SI, 2.50 to 7.50 mmol/day). Normal excretion of phosphate is less than 1,000 mg/24 hours.

Abnormal findings

A variety of disorders may affect calcium and phosphorus levels. (See *Disorders that affect urine calcium and urine phosphorus levels,* page 388.)

Interfering factors

- Failure to collect all urine during the test period
- Parathyroid hormones (increases excretion of phosphates and decreases urinary excretion of calcium)
- Thiazide diuretics (decreases excretion of calcium)
- Prolonged inactivity and ingestion of corticosteroids, sodium phosphate, calcitonin (increases excretion of calcium)
- Vitamin D (increases phosphate absorption and excretion)

MAGNESIUM

Measurement of urine magnesium is especially useful because magnesium deficiency is detectable in urine before it changes serum magnesium levels. This test may be used to rule out magnesium deficiency as the cause of neurologic symptoms and to help evaluate glomerular function in suspected renal disease.

Magnesium is a cation found primarily in the bones and in intracellular fluid; a small amount is present in extracellular fluid. This element activates many enzyme systems, helps transport sodium and potassium across cell membranes, affects nucleic acid and protein metabolism, and influences intracellular calcium levels through its effect on secretion of parathyroid hormone.

Disorders that affect urine calcium and urine phosphorus levels

DISORDER	URINE CALCIUM LEVEL	URINE PHOSPHATE LEVEL
Hyperparathyroidism	Elevated	Elevated
Vitamin D intoxication	Elevated	Suppressed
Metastatic carcinoma	Elevated	Normal
Sarcoidosis	Elevated	Suppressed
Renal tubular acidosis	Elevated	Elevated
Multiple myeloma	Elevated or normal	Elevated or normal
Paget's disease	Normal	Normal
Milk-alkali syndrome	Suppressed or normal	Suppressed or normal
Hypoparathyroidism	Suppressed	Suppressed
Acute nephrosis	Suppressed	Suppressed or normal
Chronic nephrosis	Suppressed	Suppressed
Acute nephritis	Suppressed	Suppressed
Renal insufficiency	Suppressed	Suppressed
Osteomalacia	Suppressed	Suppressed
Steatorrhea	Suppressed	Suppressed

Purpose

- To rule out magnesium deficiency in patients with symptoms of central nervous system irritation
- To detect excessive urinary excretion of magnesium
- To help evaluate glomerular function in renal disease

Patient preparation

- Explain to the patient that this test determines urine magnesium levels.
- Tell the patient that this test requires urine collection over a 24-hour period.
- Notify the laboratory and physician of medications the patient is taking that may affect test results; they may need to be restricted.

Procedure and posttest care

- Collect the patient's urine over a 24-hour period, discarding the first specimen and retaining the last.

Precautions

- Tell the patient to be careful not to contaminate the urine specimen with toilet tissue or stool.
- Tell the patient not to use a metallic bedpan for collection.

Reference values

Normal urinary excretion of magnesium is 6 to 10 mEq/24 hours (SI, 3.0 to 5.0 mmol/day).

Abnormal findings

Low urine magnesium levels may result from malabsorption, acute or chronic diarrhea, diabetic ketoacidosis, dehydration, pancreatitis, advanced renal failure, and primary aldosteronism. They may also result from decreased dietary intake of magnesium.

Elevated urine magnesium levels may result from early chronic renal disease, adrenocortical insufficiency (Addison's disease), chronic alcoholism, or chronic ingestion of magnesium-containing antacids.

Interfering factors

- Failure to collect all urine during the test period
- Spirolactone (decrease)
- Increased calcium intake (decrease)
- Magnesium-containing antacids, ethacrynic acid, thiazide diuretics, and aldosterone (possible increase)

COPPER

The copper test measures the urine level of copper, an essential trace element and a component of several metalloenzymes and proteins necessary for hemoglobin synthesis and oxidation reduction. Most copper in plasma is bound to and transported by an alpha$_2$-globulin (plasma protein) called ceruloplasmin. When copper is unbound, the ions can inhibit many enzyme reactions, resulting in copper toxicity. Urine normally contains only a small amount of free copper.

Determination of urine copper levels is frequently used to detect Wilson's disease, a rare, inborn metabolic error that is most common among people of eastern European Jewish, southern Italian, or Sicilian ancestry.

Purpose

- To help detect Wilson's disease, chronic active hepatitis, or environmental exposure.
- To screen infants with family histories of Wilson's disease

Patient preparation

- Explain to the patient that this test determines the amount of copper in urine.
- Inform the patient that no special restrictions are necessary.
- Tell the patient the test requires urine collection over a 24-hour period. If the specimen is to be collected at home, describe the proper collection technique.
- Notify the laboratory and physician of medications the patient is taking that may affect test results; they may need to be restricted.

Procedure and posttest care

- Collect the patient's urine over a 24-hour period, discarding first specimen and retaining the last, using no preservatives.
- Refrigerate the specimen during the collection period.
- Instruct the patient to resume his usual medication schedule as ordered.

Precautions

■ Tell the patient not to contaminate the urine specimen with toilet tissue or stool.

Reference values

Normal urinary excretion of copper is 3 to 35 μg/24 hours (SI, 0.05 to 0.55 μmol/day).

Abnormal findings

Elevated urine copper levels usually indicate Wilson's disease (a liver biopsy helps establish this diagnosis). Wilson's disease is marked by decreased ceruloplasmin, increased urinary excretion of copper, and accumulation of copper in the interstitial tissues of the liver and brain. Early detection and treatment (low-copper diet and D-penicillamine) are vital to prevent irreversible changes, such as nerve tissue degeneration and cirrhosis of the liver.

Elevated copper levels may also occur in nephrotic syndromes, chronic active hepatitis, biliary cirrhosis, and rheumatoid arthritis.

Interfering factors

■ D-penicillamine (increase)

■ Failure to collect all urine during the test period and to refrigerate specimen

HEMOSIDERIN

The test for hemosiderin measures the urine level of hemosiderin — a colloidal iron oxide and one of the two forms of iron that are stored and deposited in body tissue.

When iron storage mechanisms fail to manage iron overload, excess iron may escape to cells unaccustomed to high iron concentrations and may produce toxic effects. Toxicity may affect the liver, myocardium, bone marrow, pancreas, kidneys, and skin. Subsequent tissue damage is referred to as hemochromatosis. Hemochromatosis may occur in a rare hereditary form (primary hemochromatosis) and in exogenous forms.

Purpose

■ To aid diagnosis of hemochromatosis, hemolytic anemia associated with intravascular hemolysis.

Patient preparation

■ Explain to the patient that this test helps determine if the body is accumulating excessive amounts of iron.

■ Inform the patient that no restrictions are necessary and that the test requires a urine specimen.

Procedure and posttest care

■ Collect a random urine specimen of approximately 30 ml, preferably the first void of the morning.

■ Instruct the patient to resume his usual medication schedule as ordered.

Precautions

■ Seal the container securely, and send the specimen to the laboratory immediately after collection.

Normal findings

Normally, hemosiderin is not found in urine.

Abnormal findings

The presence of hemosiderin, appearing as yellow-brown granules in urinary sediment, indicates hemochromatosis; liver or bone marrow biopsy is necessary for confirmation of primary hemochromatosis. Hemosiderin may also suggest pernicious anemia, chronic hemolytic anemia, multiple blood transfusions, and paroxysmal nocturnal hemoglobinuria, the result of excessive iron injections or dietary intake of iron.

Interfering factors

- Failure to send the specimen to the laboratory immediately after collection

OXALATE

Oxalate, a salt of oxalic acid, is an end product of metabolism and is excreted almost exclusively in the urine. Measuring urine levels of oxalate detects hyperoxaluria, a disorder in which oxalate accumulates in the soft and connective tissue, especially in the kidneys and bladder, causing chronic inflammation and fibrosis. Calcium oxalate deposits are the most common cause of renal calculi, which may produce kidney damage.

Purpose

- To detect primary hyperoxaluria in infants
- To rule out hyperoxaluria in renal insufficiency

Patient preparation

- Explain to the patient (or to the parents if the patient is a child) that this test determines if the urine contains excess oxalate.
- Tell the patient or parents that the test requires urine collection over a 24-hour period.
- Tell the patient to avoid foods high in oxalate — such as tomatoes, strawberries, rhubarb, and spinach — for 1 week before the test.

Procedure and posttest care

- Collect the patient's urine over a 24-hour period, discarding first specimen and retaining the last. Use a light-protected container with 30 ml of 6 N hydrochloric acid.

Precautions

- Tell the patient not to urinate directly into the 24-hour specimen container, but to use an appropriate container.
- Advise him not to contaminate the urine specimen with toilet tissue or stool.
- Oxalate in acidified urine is stable for up to 7 days at room temperature or when refrigerated at 35.6° to 46.4° F (2° to 8° C)

Reference values

Urine oxalate levels of less than or equal to 40 mg/24 hours (SI, ≤ 456 μmol/day)

Abnormal findings

Elevated urine oxalate levels (hyperoxaluria) may result from excessive metabolic production of oxalate or increased oxalate intake. Levels as high as 400 mg/24 hours (≤ 4560 μmol/day) can occur.

Primary hyperoxaluria, a rare inborn metabolic disorder, causes excessive production and urinary excretion of oxalate. In this type of hyperoxaluria, urine oxalate levels become elevated before serum levels become elevated.

Secondary hyperoxaluria can result from pancreatic insufficiency, diabetes mellitus, cirrhosis, pyridoxine deficiency, Crohn's disease, ileal resection, or ingestion of antifreeze (ethylene glycol) or stain-remover, or it can occur as a reaction to a methoxyflurane anesthetic.

Interfering factors

- Tomatoes, strawberries, rhubarb, and spinach (possible false increase)
- Vitamin C (increases oxalate excretion which may be a risk for calcium oxalate nephrolithiasis in individuals consuming megadoses of this vitamin)
- Failure to collect all urine during the test period or properly store the specimen

Additional specimen tests

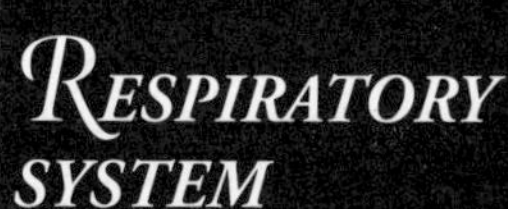

RESPIRATORY SYSTEM

OVA AND PARASITES IN SPUTUM

Parasitic infestation is rare in North America but may result from exposure to *Entamoeba histolytica, Ascaris lumbricoides, Echinococcus granulosus, Strongyloides stercoralis, Paragonimus westermani,* or *Necator americanus.* A sputum specimen is obtained by expectoration or tracheal suctioning to evaluate for parasites.

Purpose

- To identify pulmonary parasites

Patient preparation

- Explain to the patient that this test helps identify parasitic pulmonary infection.
- Tell him the test requires a sputum specimen or, if necessary, tracheal suctioning.
- Inform him that early morning collection is preferred because secretions accumulate overnight.
- Encourage the patient to help sputum production by drinking fluids the night before collection.
- Teach the patient how to expectorate by taking three deep breaths and forcing a deep cough.
- Tell him that he'll experience some discomfort from the catheter during tracheal suctioning.
- Notify the laboratory and physician of medications the patient is taking that may affect test results; they may need to be restricted.

Equipment

For expectoration: Sterile, disposable, impermeable container with screw cap or tight-fitting cap, nebulizer, intermittent positive-pressure breathing ventilator, and 10% sodium chloride, acetylcysteine, or sterile or distilled water aerosols, to induce cough

For tracheal suctioning: #16 or #18 French suction catheter, sterile gloves, sterile specimen container or sputum trap, sterile normal saline solution, and protective eyewear.

Procedure and posttest care

Expectoration

- Instruct the patient to breathe deeply a few times and then to "deep cough" and expectorate into the container.
- Use chest physiotherapy, or heated aerosol spray (nebulization), if cough is unproductive.
- Take proper precautions in sending the specimen to the laboratory.

Tracheal suctioning

- Administer oxygen before and after the procedure, if necessary.
- Attach a sputum trap to the suction catheter.
- Wearing a sterile glove, lubricate the tip of the catheter; then pass the catheter through the patient's nostril without suction. (The patient will cough when the catheter passes into the larynx.)
- Advance the catheter into the trachea.
- Apply suction for no longer than 15 seconds to obtain the specimen.
- Stop suction, and gently remove the catheter.
- Discard the catheter and glove in a proper receptacle.
- Detach the sputum trap from the suction apparatus, and cap the opening.
- Label all specimens carefully.
- Provide proper mouth care. After suctioning, offer water.

■ Monitor vital signs every hour until the patient is stable.

Precautions

■ Be sure to wear gloves and protective eyewear when performing procedures and handling specimens.

◆ CLINICAL ALERT *Don't perform tracheal suctioning on patients with esophageal varices.*

■ If the patient has asthma or chronic bronchitis, watch for aggravated bronchospasms with use of more than 10% concentration of sodium chloride or acetylcysteine in an aerosol.

◆ CLINICAL ALERT *Suction for only 5 to 10 seconds at a time during tracheal suctioning. Never suction for longer than 15 seconds. If the patient shows signs of hypoxia or cyanosis, remove the suctioning catheter immediately and administer oxygen.*

■ Send the specimen to the laboratory or place it in preservative immediately after collection.

Normal findings

Normally, no parasites or ova are present in sputum.

Abnormal findings

The parasite identified indicates the type of pulmonary infection as well as the presence and stage of intestinal infection.

■ *E. histolytica* trophozoites: pulmonary amebiasis

■ *A. lumbricoides* larvae and adults: pneumonitis

■ *E. granulosus* cysts of larval stage: hydatid disease

■ *P. westermani* ova: paragonimiasis

■ *S. stercoralis* larvae: strongyloidiasis

■ *N. americanus* larvae: hookworm disease

Interfering factors

■ Improper collection technique or failure to send the specimen to the laboratory immediately after collection

■ Recent therapy with antihelmintics or amebicides

PLEURAL FLUID ANALYSIS

The pleura, a two-layer membrane that covers the lungs and lines the thoracic cavity, maintains a small amount of lubricating fluid between its layers to minimize friction during respiration. Increased fluid in this space may result from diseases such as cancer or tuberculosis, or from blood or lymphatic disorders, and can cause respiratory difficulty.

In pleural fluid aspiration (thoracentesis), the thoracic wall is punctured to obtain a specimen of pleural fluid for analysis or to relieve pulmonary (and possibly cardiac) compression and resultant respiratory distress.

Purpose

■ To determine the cause and nature of pleural effusion

■ To permit better radiographic visualization of a lung with large effusions

Patient preparation

■ Explain to the patient that the test assesses the space around the lungs for fluid.

■ Inform him that he need not restrict food or fluids.

■ Tell him who will perform the test and where.

■ Explain that chest X-rays or an ultrasound study may precede the test to help locate the fluid.

■ Check the patient's history for hypersensitivity to local anesthetics.
■ Warn the patient that he may feel a stinging sensation on injection of the anesthetic and some pressure during withdrawal of the fluid.
■ Advise him not to cough, breathe deeply, or move during the test to minimize the risk of injury to the lung.

Equipment

Sterile collection bottles, sterile gloves, personal protective eyewear, adhesive tape, sterile thoracentesis tray (a prepackaged, disposable tray with the following: 70% alcohol or povidone-iodine solution for disinfection, drapes, local anesthetic [usually 1% lidocaine], 5-ml sterile syringe and 25 G needle for local anesthetic, 50-ml syringe for removing fluid, 17G thoracentesis aspiration needle, sterile specimen bottle or tube, three-way stopcock or sterile tubing to prevent air from entering the pleural cavity, small sterile dressing)

Procedure and posttest care

■ Record baseline vital signs.
■ If necessary, shave the area around the needle insertion site.
■ Position the patient to widen intercostal spaces and to allow easier access to the pleural cavity. He must be well-supported and comfortable, preferably seated at the edge of the bed with a chair or stool supporting his feet and his head and arms resting on a padded overbed table. If the patient can't sit up, he may be positioned on his unaffected side, with the arm on the affected side elevated above his head.
■ Remind him not to cough, breathe deeply, or move suddenly during the procedure.
■ After positioning, the physician disinfects the skin, drapes the area, injects a local anesthetic into the subcutaneous tissue, and inserts the thoracentesis needle above the rib to avoid lacerating intercostal vessels. When the needle reaches the pocket of fluid, the 50-ml syringe is attached and the stopcock and clamps are opened on the tubing to aspirate the fluid into the container.
■ During aspiration, observe the patient for signs of respiratory distress, such as weakness, dyspnea, pallor, cyanosis, changes in heart rate, tachypnea, diaphoresis, blood-tinged frothy mucus, and hypotension.
■ After the needle is withdrawn, apply slight pressure and a small adhesive bandage to the puncture site.
■ Label the specimen container, and record the date and time of the test and the amount, color, and character of the fluid (clear, frothy, purulent, bloody) on the laboratory request.
■ Note any signs of distress exhibited during the procedure.
■ Record the exact location from which the fluid was removed to aid diagnosis.
■ Reposition the patient comfortably on the affected side. Tell him to remain on this side for at least 1 hour to seal the puncture site. Elevate the head of the bed to facilitate breathing.
■ Monitor vital signs every 30 minutes for 2 hours, and then every 4 hours until they're stable.
■ Tell the patient to call a nurse immediately if he experiences difficulty breathing.

◆ **CLINICAL ALERT** *Watch for signs of pneumothorax, tension pneumothorax, fluid reaccumulation and, if a large amount of fluid was withdrawn, pulmonary edema or cardiac distress due to mediastinal shift. Usually, a posttest X-ray is ordered to detect these complications before clinical symptoms appear.*

■ Check the puncture site for any fluid leakage. A large amount of leakage is abnormal. Also check the site and surrounding area for subcutaneous emphysema.

Precautions

- Thoracentesis is contraindicated in patients who have a history of bleeding disorders or anticoagulant therapy.
- Use strict aseptic technique.
- Note the patient's temperature and whether he's receiving antimicrobial therapy on the laboratory request.
- Send the specimen to the laboratory immediately after collection.

Normal findings

Normally, the pleural cavity maintains negative pressure and contains < 20 ml of serous fluid.

Abnormal findings

Pleural effusion results from the abnormal formation or reabsorption of pleural fluid. Certain characteristics classify pleural fluid as either a transudate (a low-protein fluid leaked from normal blood vessels) or an exudate (a protein-rich fluid leaked from blood vessels with increased permeability).

Pleural fluid may contain blood (hemothorax), chyle (chylothorax), or pus (empyema) and necrotic tissue. Blood-tinged fluid may indicate a traumatic tap; if so, the fluid should clear as aspiration progresses.

Transudative effusion generally results from diminished colloidal pressure, increased negative pressure within the pleural cavity, ascites, systemic and pulmonary venous hypertension, heart failure, hepatic cirrhosis, and nephritis.

Exudative effusion results from disorders that increase pleural capillary permeability (possibly with changes in hydrostatic or colloid osmotic pressures), lymphatic drainage interference, infections, pulmonary infarctions, and neoplasms. Exudative effusion associated with depressed glucose levels, elevated lactate dehydrogenase (LD) isoenzymes, rheumatoid arthritis cells, and negative smears, cultures, and cytologic examination may indicate pleurisy associated with rheumatoid arthritis.

The most common pathogens that appear in culture studies of pleural fluid are *Mycobacterium tuberculosis, Staphylococcus aureus, Streptococcus pneumoniae* and other streptococci, *Haemophilus influenzae* and, in the case of a ruptured pulmonary abscess, anaerobes such as *Bacteroides.* Cultures are usually positive during the early stages of infection; however, antibiotic therapy may produce a negative culture despite a positive Gram stain and grossly purulent fluid. Empyema may result from complications of pneumonia, pulmonary abscess, perforation of the esophagus, or penetration from mediastinitis. A high percentage of neutrophils suggests septic inflammation; predominating lymphocytes suggest tuberculosis, or fungal or viral effusions.

Serosanguineous fluid may indicate pleural extension of a malignant tumor. Elevated LD in a nonpurulent, nonhemolyzed, nonbloody effusion may also suggest malignancy. Pleural fluid glucose levels that are 30 to 40 mg/dl lower than blood glucose levels may indicate a malignant tumor, a bacterial infection, nonseptic inflammation, or metastasis. Increased amylase levels occur in pleural effusions associated with pancreatitis.

Interfering factors

- Failure to use aseptic technique
- Failure to send the specimen to the laboratory immediately after collection
- Antimicrobial therapy before aspiration of fluid for culture (possible decrease in numbers of bacteria, making it difficult to isolate the infecting organism)

GASTROINTESTINAL SYSTEM

BASAL GASTRIC SECRETION

The basal gastric secretion test measures basal secretion during fasting by aspirating stomach contents through a nasogastric (NG) tube. It's indicated in patients with obscure epigastric pain, anorexia, and weight loss. Because external factors — such as the sight or odor of food — and psychological stress stimulate gastric secretion, accurate testing requires that the patient be relaxed and isolated from all sources of sensory stimulation. Although abnormal basal secretion can suggest various gastric and duodenal disorders, a complete evaluation of secretion requires the gastric acid stimulation test.

Purpose

- To determine gastric output while the patient is fasting

Patient preparation

- Explain to the patient that this test measures the stomach's secretion of acid.
- Instruct him to restrict food for 12 hours and fluids and smoking for 8 hours before the test.
- Tell him who will perform the test and that the procedure takes approximately 1¼ hours (or 2¼ hours, if followed by the gastric acid stimulation test).
- Inform the patient that the test requires insertion of a tube through the nose and into the stomach and that he may initially experience discomfort and may cough or gag.
- Notify the laboratory and physician of medications the patient is taking that may affect test results; they may need to be restricted. If these drugs must be continued, note this on the laboratory request.
- Check the patient's pulse rate and blood pressure just before the test. Then encourage him to relax.

Procedure and posttest care

- Insert the NG tube after seating the patient comfortably.
- Attach a 20-ml syringe to it, and aspirate the stomach contents.
- To ensure complete emptying of the stomach, ask the patient to assume three positions in sequence — supine and right and left lateral decubitus — while stomach contents are aspirated.
- Label the specimen container RESIDUAL CONTENTS.
- Connect the NG tube to the suction machine. Aspirate gastric contents by continuous low suction for 1 hour. Aspiration can also be performed manually with a syringe.
- Collect a specimen every 15 minutes, but discard the first two; this eliminates the specimens that could be affected by the stress of the intubation.
- Record the color and odor of each specimen, and note the presence of food, mucus, bile, or blood.
- Label these specimens BASAL CONTENTS, and number them 1 through 4.
- Next, secretion volume and acid concentration are measured.
- If the NG tube is to be left in place, clamp it or attach it to low intermittent suction as ordered.
- Watch for complications, such as nausea, vomiting, and abdominal distention or pain, following removal of the NG tube.
- If the patient complains of a sore throat, provide soothing lozenges as ordered.

■ Instruct the patient to resume his usual diet and medication schedule, as ordered, unless the gastric acid stimulation test will also be performed.

Precautions

■ The basal gastric secretion test is contraindicated in patients with conditions that prohibit NG intubation.
■ During insertion, make sure the NG tube enters the esophagus and not the trachea; remove it immediately if the patient develops cyanosis or paroxysmal coughing.
■ Monitor vital signs during intubation, and observe carefully for arrhythmias.
■ To prevent contamination of the specimens with saliva, instruct the patient to expectorate excess saliva.
■ Send the specimens to the laboratory immediately after the collection is completed.

Reference values

Normally, basal secretion ranges from 1 to 5 mEq/hour in males and from 0.2 to 3.3 mEq/hour in females.

Abnormal findings

Abnormal basal secretion findings are nonspecific and must be considered with the results of the gastric acid stimulation test. Elevated secretion may suggest duodenal or jejunal ulcer (after partial gastrectomy); markedly elevated secretion, Zollinger-Ellison syndrome. Depressed secretion may indicate gastric carcinoma or benign gastric ulcer. Absence of secretion may indicate pernicious anemia.

Interfering factors

■ Failure to observe pretest restrictions (increase)
■ Psychological stress (possible increase)
■ Cholinergics, reserpine, alcohol, adrenergic blockers, and adrenocorticosteroids (possible increase)
■ Antacids, anticholinergics, histamine-2 blockers, proton pump inhibitors (possible decrease)

GASTRIC ACID STIMULATION

The gastric acid stimulation test measures the secretion of gastric acid for 1 hour after subcutaneous injection of pentagastrin or a similar drug that stimulates gastric acid output. This test is indicated when the basal secretion test suggests abnormal gastric secretion and is commonly performed immediately afterward. Although this test detects abnormal gastric secretion, radiographic studies and endoscopy are necessary to determine the cause.

Purpose

■ To aid diagnosis of duodenal ulcer, Zollinger-Ellison syndrome, pernicious anemia, and gastric carcinoma

Patient preparation

■ Explain to the patient that this test determines if the stomach is secreting acid properly.
■ Instruct him to refrain from eating, drinking, and smoking after midnight before the test.
■ Tell him who will perform the test, where it will take place, and that it takes 1 hour.
■ Explain that the test requires passing a tube through the nose and into the stomach and a subcutaneous injection of pentagastrin.
■ Describe the possible adverse effects of the test, such as abdominal pain, nausea, vomiting, flushing, and transi-

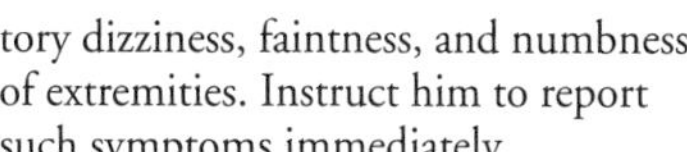

tory dizziness, faintness, and numbness of extremities. Instruct him to report such symptoms immediately.

- Check the patient's history for hypersensitivity to pentagastrin.
- Notify the laboratory and the physician of medications the patient is taking that may affect test results; they may need to be restricted. If these drugs must be continued, however, note this on the laboratory request.
- Record baseline vital signs before beginning the procedure.

Procedure and posttest care

- After basal gastric secretions have been collected, the NG tube remains in place.
- Pentagastrin is injected subcutaneously. After 15 minutes, collect a specimen every 15 minutes for 1 hour.
- Record the color and odor of each specimen, and note the presence of food, mucus, bile, or blood.
- Label the specimens STIMULATED CONTENTS, and number them 1 through 4.
- If the NG tube is kept in place, it should be clamped or attached to low intermittent suction, as ordered.
- Watch for nausea, vomiting, and abdominal distention and pain after the NG tube is removed.
- If the patient complains of a sore throat, provide soothing lozenges, as ordered.
- Instruct the patient to resume his usual diet and medication schedule as ordered.

Precautions

- The gastric acid stimulation test is contraindicated in patients with hypersensitivity to pentagastrin or with conditions that prohibit NG intubation.
- Observe for adverse effects of pentagastrin.
- To prevent contamination of the specimens with saliva, instruct the patient to expectorate excess saliva.
- Send the specimens to the laboratory immediately after the collection is completed.

Reference values

Following stimulation, gastric acid secretion ranges from 18 to 28 mEq/hour for males and from 11 to 21 mEq/hour for females.

Abnormal findings

Elevated gastric secretion may indicate duodenal ulcer; markedly elevated secretion suggests Zollinger-Ellison syndrome. Depressed secretion may indicate gastric carcinoma; achlorhydria may indicate pernicious anemia.

Interfering factors

- Failure to observe pretest restrictions
- Cholinergics, adrenergic blockers, and reserpine (increase)
- Antacids, anticholinergics, histamine-2 blockers, and proton pump inhibitors (decrease)

PERITONEAL FLUID ANALYSIS

Peritoneal fluid analysis assesses a specimen of peritoneal fluid obtained by paracentesis. This procedure requires inserting a trocar and cannula through the abdominal wall while the patient receives a local anesthetic. If the fluid specimen is removed for therapeutic purposes, the trocar may be connected to a drainage system. However, if only a small amount of fluid is removed for diagnostic purposes, an 18G needle may be used in place of the trocar and cannula. In a four-quadrant tap, fluid is aspirated from each quadrant of the abdomen to verify abdominal trauma and confirm the need for surgery.

Purpose

■ To determine the cause of ascites
■ To detect abdominal trauma

Patient preparation

■ Explain to the patient that this procedure helps determine the cause of ascites or detects abdominal trauma.
■ Inform him that he need not restrict food or fluids before the test.
■ Tell him that the test requires a peritoneal fluid specimen, that he'll receive a local anesthetic to minimize discomfort, and that the procedure takes about 45 minutes to perform.
■ Provide psychological support to decrease the patient's anxiety, and assure him that complications are rare.
■ If the patient has severe ascites, inform him that the procedure will relieve his discomfort and allow him to breathe more easily.
■ Make sure the patient or responsible family member has signed a consent form.
■ Record baseline vital signs, weight, and abdominal girth.
■ Tell him a blood sample may be taken for analysis.
■ Tell the patient to void just before the test. This helps to prevent accidental bladder injury during needle insertion.
■ X-rays may be performed prior to peritoneal analysis to ensure reliability.

Procedure and posttest care

■ Have the patient sit on a bed or in a chair with his feet flat on the floor and his back well supported. If he can't tolerate being out of bed, place him in high Fowler's position and make him as comfortable as possible.
■ Except for the puncture site, keep him covered to prevent chilling.
■ Provide a plastic sheet or absorbent pad to collect spillage and to protect the patient and bed linens.
■ The puncture site is shaved, the skin prepared, and the area draped.
■ The local anesthetic is injected.
■ The examiner inserts the needle or trocar and cannula 1″ to 2″ (2.5 to 5 cm) below the umbilicus. (However, it may also be inserted through the flank, the iliac fossa, the border of the rectus, or at each quadrant of the abdomen.)
■ If a trocar and cannula are used, a small incision is made to facilitate insertion. When the needle pierces the peritoneum, it "gives" with an audible sound. The trocar is removed and a sample of fluid is aspirated with a 50-ml luer-lock syringe.
■ If additional fluid is to be drained, assist in attaching one end of an I.V. tube to the cannula and the other end to a collection bag. The fluid is then aspirated (no more than 1500 ml). If aspirating is difficult, reposition as ordered.
■ After aspiration, the trocar needle is removed and a pressure dressing is applied. Occasionally, the wound may be sutured first.
■ Label the specimens in the order they were drawn. If the patient has received antibiotic therapy, note this on the laboratory request.
■ Carefully and properly dispose of needles and contaminated articles according to the Center for Disease Control and Prevention guidelines; incinerate disposable items and return reusable ones to the central supply area.
■ Apply a gauze dressing to the puncture site. Make sure it's thick enough to absorb all drainage. Check the dressing frequently (for example, whenever you check vital signs) and reinforce or apply a pressure dressing, if needed.
■ Monitor vital signs until stable. If the patient's recovery is poor, check vital signs every 15 minutes. Weigh the pa-

tient and measure abdominal girth; compare these with baseline values.

- Allow the patient to rest and, if possible, withhold treatment or procedures that may cause undue stress, such as linen changes.
- Monitor urine output for at least 24 hours, and watch for hematuria, which may indicate bladder trauma.
- If a large amount of fluid was aspirated, watch for signs of vascular collapse (color change, elevated pulse and respiratory rates, decreased blood pressure and central venous pressure, mental changes, and dizziness). Administer fluids orally if the patient is alert and can accept them.

◆ **CLINICAL ALERT** *Watch for signs of hemorrhage or shock and for increasing pain or abdominal tenderness. These may indicate a perforated intestine or, depending on the site of the tap, puncture of the inferior epigastric artery, hematoma of the anterior cecal wall, or rupture of the iliac vein or bladder.*

◆ **CLINICAL ALERT** *Observe the patient with severe hepatic disease for signs of hepatic coma, which may result from loss of sodium and potassium accompanying hypovolemia. Watch for mental changes, drowsiness, and stupor. Such a patient is also prone to uremia, infection, hemorrhage, and protein depletion.*

- As ordered, administer I.V. infusions and albumin. Check the laboratory report for electrolytes (especially sodium) and serum protein levels.

Precautions

- Peritoneal fluid analysis should be performed cautiously in pregnant patients and in patients with bleeding tendencies or unstable vital signs.
- Check vital signs every 15 minutes during the procedure. Watch for deviations from baseline findings. Observe for dizziness, pallor, perspiration, and increased anxiety.
- If rapid fluid aspiration induces hypovolemia and shock, reduce the vertical distance between the trocar and the collection bag to slow the drainage rate. If necessary, stop the drainage by turning off the stopcock or clamping the tubing.
- Avoid contamination of the specimens, which alters their bacterial content. Send them to the laboratory immediately after collection.

Reference values

For normal peritoneal fluid values, see *Normal findings in peritoneal fluid analysis,* page 402.

Abnormal findings

Milk-colored peritoneal fluid may result from chyle or lymph fluid escaping from a thoracic duct that is damaged or blocked by a malignant tumor, lymphoma, tuberculosis, parasitic infestation, adhesion, or hepatic cirrhosis; a pseudochylous condition may result from the presence of leukocytes or tumor cells. Differential diagnosis of true chylous ascites depends on the presence of elevated triglyceride levels ($\geq$ 400 mg/dl [SI $\geq$ 4.36 mmol/L]) and microscopic fat globules.

Cloudy or turbid fluid may indicate peritonitis due to primary bacterial infection, ruptured bowel (after trauma), pancreatitis, strangulated or infarcted intestine, or appendicitis. Bloody fluid may result from a benign or malignant tumor, hemorrhagic pancreatitis, or a traumatic tap; however, if the fluid fails to clear on continued aspiration, a traumatic tap isn't the cause. Bile-stained green fluid may indicate a ruptured

Normal findings in peritoneal fluid analysis

ELEMENT	NORMAL VALUE OR FINDING
Gross appearance	Sterile, odorless, clear to pale yellow color; scant amount (< 50 ml)
Red blood cells	None
White blood cells	< 300 /µl (SI, < 300 × 10^9/L)
Protein	0.3 to 4.1 g/dl (SI, 3 to 41 g/L)
Glucose	70 to 100 mg/dl (SI, 3.5 to 5 mmol/L)
Amylase	138 to 404 U/L (SI, 138 to 404 U/L)
Ammonia	< 50 µg/dl (SI, < 29 µmol/L)
Alkaline phosphatase	Males over age 18: 90 to 239 U/L (SI, 90 to 239 U/L) Females < 45: 76 to 196 U/L (SI, 76 to 196 U/L) Females > 45: 87 to 250 U/L (SI, 87 to 250 U/L)
Cytology	No malignant cells present
Bacteria	None
Fungi	None

gallbladder, acute pancreatitis, or a perforated intestine or duodenal ulcer.

A red blood cell count > 100/µl (SI, 100/L) indicates neoplasm or tuberculosis; a count > 100,000/µl (SI, 100,000/L) indicates intra-abdominal trauma. An elevated white blood cell count with more than 25% neutrophils occurs in 90% of patients with spontaneous bacterial peritonitis and in 50% of those with cirrhosis. A high percentage of lymphocytes suggest tuberculous peritonitis or chylous ascites. Numerous mesothelial cells indicate tuberculous peritonitis.

Protein levels rise above 3 g/dl in malignancy (SI, 3 g/L) and above 4 g/dl (SI, 4 g/L) in tuberculosis. Peritoneal fluid glucose levels fall in patients with tuberculous peritonitis and peritoneal carcinomatosis.

Amylase levels rise with pancreatic trauma, pancreatic pseudocyst, or acute pancreatitis and may also rise in intestinal necrosis or strangulation.

Peritoneal alkaline phosphatase levels rise to more than twice the normal serum levels in patients with ruptured or strangulated small intestines. Peritoneal ammonia levels also exceed twice the normal serum levels in ruptured or strangulated large and small intestines, and in ruptured ulcer or appendix.

A protein ascitic fluid to serum ratio of 0.5 or greater may suggest a malignancy, tuberculous, or pancreatic ascites. The presence of this finding indicates a nonhepatic cause; its absence suggests uncomplicated hepatic disease. An albumin gradient between ascitic fluid and serum greater than 1 g/dl (SI > 1g/L) indicates chronic hepatic disease; a lesser value suggests malignancy.

Cytologic examination of peritoneal fluid accurately detects malignant cells. Microbiological examination can reveal coliforms, anaerobes, and enterococci, which can enter the peritoneum from a ruptured organ or from infections accompanying appendicitis, pancreatitis, tuberculosis, or ovarian disease. Gram-positive cocci often indicate primary peritonitis; gram-negative organisms, secondary peritonitis. The presence of fungi may indicate histoplasmosis, candidiasis, or coccidioidomycosis.

Interfering factors

- Unsterile collection technique or failure to send the specimen to the laboratory immediately after collection
- Contamination of the specimen with blood, bile, urine, or stool due to injury to underlying structures during paracentesis

DUODENAL PARASITES

The test for duodenal parasites evaluates duodenal contents for the presence of parasites in a specimen obtained by duodenal intubation and aspiration or by the string test (Entero test). Such parasites include trophozoites of *Giardia lamblia* and *Giardia duodenalis,* the ova and larvae of *Strongyloides stercoralis,* and the ova of *Entamoeba histolytica, Necator americanus,* or *Ancylostoma duodenale* in various stages of cleavage. This test can also detect ova of the liver flukes *Clonorchis sinensis* and *Fasciola hepatica* in the biliary tract. However, liver fluke infestations are rare in North America.

Examination of duodenal contents for ova and parasites is performed only in a symptomatic patient with negative stool examinations.

Purpose

- To detect parasitic infestation when stool examinations are negative

Patient preparation

- Explain to the patient that this test detects parasitic infestation of the GI tract.
- Instruct him to restrict food and fluids for 12 hours before the test.
- Tell him who will perform the test and when.
- If the test will be done with a nasoenteric tube, warn him that he may gag during the tube's passage, but assure him that following the examiner's instructions about positioning, breathing, and swallowing will minimize discomfort.
- Instruct the patient to empty his bladder just before the procedure.

Equipment

Gloves, double-lumen tube with olive tip (or weighted gelatin capsule with string attached, for string test), water-soluble jelly, 30-ml sterile syringe, emesis basin, sterile specimen container, ½″ adhesive tape

Procedure and posttest care

Nasoenteric tube

- After inserting the tube, place the patient in a left lateral decubitus position, with his feet elevated, to allow peristalsis to move the tube into the duodenum.

■ The pH of a small amount of aspirated fluid determines tube position: If the tube is in the stomach, the pH is lower than 7.0; if it's in the duodenum, the pH is higher than 7.0.
■ Fluoroscopy can also determine correct positioning. When position is confirmed, residual duodenal contents are aspirated.
■ Transfer the entire specimen to a sterile container, and label the container appropriately.
Entero test capsule with string
■ Tape the free end of the string to the patient's cheek.
■ Instruct him to swallow the capsule (on the other end of the string) with water.
■ As ordered, leave the string in place for 4 hours; then pull it out gently and place it in a sterile container.
■ Label the container appropriately.
■ Dispose of the equipment properly.
■ Provide oral hygiene and offer the patient water.
■ Observe carefully for signs of perforation, such as dysphagia or fever.
■ Tell the patient he can resume his normal diet.

Precautions

■ Use gloves when performing the procedure and handling specimens.
■ Duodenal intubation is contraindicated for pregnant women and for patients with acute cholecystitis; acute pancreatitis; esophageal varices, stenosis, diverticula, or malignant neoplasms; recent severe gastric hemorrhage; aortic aneurysm; or heart failure.
■ When possible, obtain the specimen before the start of drug therapy.
■ Send the specimen to the laboratory immediately.
■ As ordered, withdraw the tube slowly (about 6″ to 8″ [15 to 20 cm] every 10 minutes) to the esophagus; then clamp the tube and remove it quickly. *Never* force the tube.

Normal findings

Normally, no ova or parasites appear in duodenal contents.

Abnormal findings

Finding *G. lamblia* or *G. duodenalis* indicates giardiasis, possibly causing malabsorption syndrome; *S. stercoralis* suggests strongyloidiasis; *A. duodenale* and *N. americanus* imply hookworm disease; and *C. sinensis* and *F. hepatica* signify histopathologic changes in the bile ducts.

Interfering factors

■ Failure to observe pretest restrictions (possible dilution of the specimen)
■ Previous drug therapy or delay in transporting the specimen to the laboratory

FECAL OCCULT BLOOD

Fecal occult blood is detected by microscopic analysis or by chemical tests for hemoglobin, such as the guaiac test. Normally, stool contains small amounts of blood (2 to 2.5 ml/day); therefore, tests for occult blood detect quantities larger than this. Testing is indicated when clinical symptoms and preliminary blood studies suggest GI bleeding. Additional tests are required to pinpoint the origin of the bleeding. (See *Common sites and causes of GI blood loss.*)

Purpose

■ To detect GI bleeding
■ To aid early diagnosis of colorectal cancer

Common sites and causes of GI blood loss

Illustrated below are potential areas that can cause blood loss, resulting in positive fecal occult blood testing. Further clinical assessment and testing is necessary to determine the area involved.

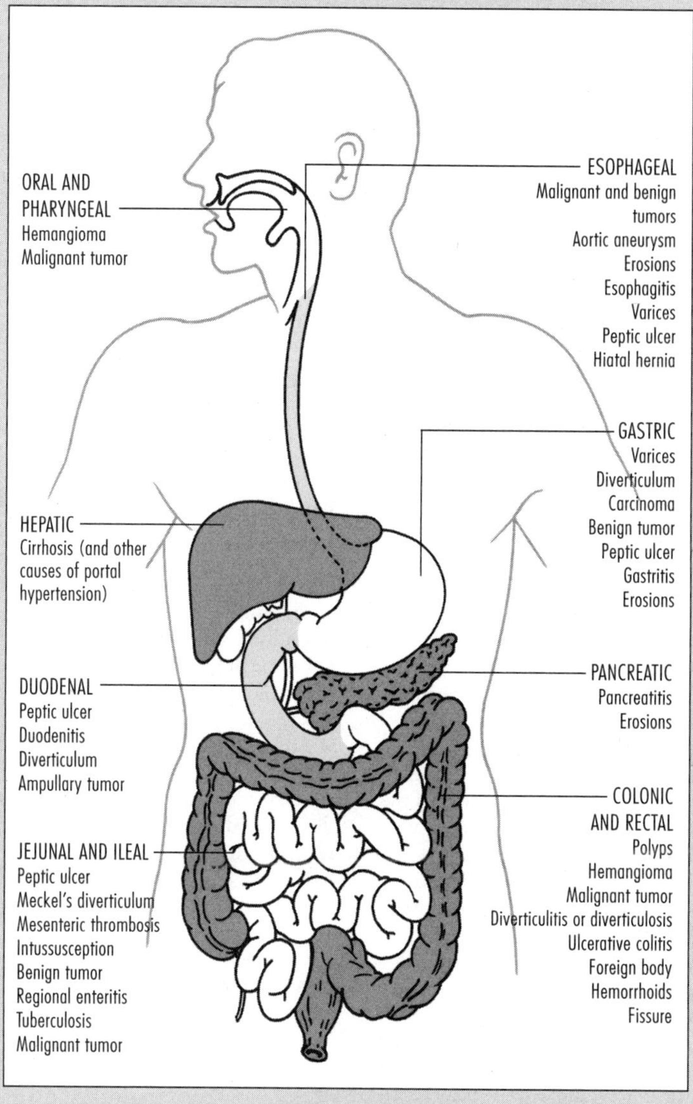

Patient preparation

■ Explain to the patient that this test helps detect abnormal GI bleeding.

■ Instruct him to maintain a high-fiber diet and to refrain from eating red meats, turnips, and horseradish for 48 to 72 hours before the test as well as throughout the collection period.

■ Tell him the test requires collection of three stool specimens. Occasionally, only a random specimen is collected.

■ Notify the laboratory and physician of medications the patient is taking that may affect test results; they may need to be restricted. If these drugs must be continued, note this on the laboratory request.

Procedure and posttest care

■ Collect three stool specimens or a random specimen, as ordered. Obtain specimens from two different areas of each stool. Testing may take place in the laboratory or in a utility room on the nursing unit, depending on the facility's policy. Two of the most commonly used screening tests are Hematest and Hemoccult. Hematest uses orthotoluidine to detect hemoglobin, and Hemoccult uses guaiac.

Hemtest reagent tablet test

■ Use a wooden applicator to smear a bit of the stool specimen on the filter paper supplied with the kit. Alternatively, after performing a digital rectal examination, wipe the finger you used for the examination on a square of the filter paper. Place the filter paper with the stool smear on a glass plate.

■ Remove a reagent tablet from the bottle, and immediately replace the cap tightly. Place the tablet in the center of the stool smear on the filter paper. Add one drop of water to the tablet, and allow it to soak in for 5 to 10 seconds. Add a second drop, letting it run from the tablet onto the specimen and filter paper. If necessary, tap the plate gently to dislodge any water from the top of the tablet.

■ After 2 minutes, the filter paper will turn blue if the test is positive. Don't read the color that appears on the tablet itself or develops on the filter paper after the 2-minute period. Note the results, and discard the filter paper. Remove and discard your gloves, and wash your hands thoroughly.

Hemoccult slide test

■ Open the flap on the slide pack, and use a wooden applicator to apply a thin smear of the stool specimen to the guaiac-impregnated filter paper exposed in box A. Alternatively, after performing a digital rectal examination, wipe the finger you used for the examination on a square of filter paper. Apply a second smear from another part of the specimen to the filter paper exposed in box B because some parts of the specimen may not contain blood.

■ Allow the specimen to dry for 3 to 5 minutes. Open the flap at the rear of the slide package, and place 2 drops of Hemoccult developing solution on the paper over each smear. A blue reaction will appear in 30 to 60 seconds if the test is positive. Record the results and discard the slide package. Remove and discard your gloves and wash your hands thoroughly.

Instant-View fecal occult blood test

■ Add a stool sample to the collection tube. Shake it to mix the sample with the extraction buffer; then dispense 4 drops into the sample well of the cassette. Results will appear on both the test region and the control region of the cassette in 5 to 10 minutes, indicating whether the level of hemoglobin is greater than 0.05 ug/ml of stool. Results will also indicate if the device is performing properly.

All tests

■ Tell the patient to resume his usual diet and medication schedule, as ordered.

Precautions

■ Instruct the patient to avoid contaminating the stool specimen with toilet tissue or urine.

■ Send the specimen to the laboratory or perform the test immediately.

Normal findings

Less than 2.5 ml of blood should be present in stool, resulting in a green reaction.

Abnormal findings

A positive test indicates GI bleeding, which may result from many disorders, such as varices, peptic ulcer, carcinoma, ulcerative colitis, dysentery, or hemorrhagic disease. This test is particularly important for early diagnosis of colorectal cancer. Further tests, such as barium swallow, analyses of gastric contents, and endoscopic procedures, are necessary to define the site and extent of the bleeding.

Interfering factors

■ Failure to observe pretest restrictions, to test the specimen immediately, or to send it to the laboratory immediately after collection

■ Iron preparations, bromides, rauwolfia derivatives, indomethacin, colchicine, phenylbutazone, and steroids (possible increase due to association with GI blood loss)

■ Ascorbic acid (false-normal, even with significant bleeding)

■ Ingestion of 2 to 5 ml of blood such as from bleeding gums

■ Active bleeding from hemorrhoids may produce false-positive results

FECAL LIPIDS

Lipids excreted in stool include monoglycerides, diglycerides, triglycerides, phospholipids, glycolipids, soaps (fatty acids and fatty acid salts), sterols, and cholesterol esters. When biliary and pancreatic secretions are adequate, emulsified dietary lipids are almost completely absorbed in the small intestine.

Excessive excretion of fecal lipids (steatorrhea) occurs in several malabsorption syndromes. Qualitative and quantitative tests are used to detect excessive excretion of lipids in patients exhibiting signs of malabsorption, such as weight loss, abdominal distention, and scaly skin.

The qualitative test involves staining a specimen of stool with Sudan III dye and then examining it microscopically for evidence of malabsorption, such as undigested muscle fibers and various fats. The quantitative test involves drying and weighing a 72-hour specimen and then using a solvent to extract the lipids, which are subsequently evaporated and weighed. Only the quantitative test confirms steatorrhea.

Purpose

■ To confirm steatorrhea

Patient preparation

■ Explain to the patient that this test evaluates fat digestion.

■ Instruct him to abstain from alcohol and to maintain a high-fat diet (100 g/day) for 3 days before the test and during the collection period.

■ Tell him the test requires a 72-hour stool collection.

■ Notify the laboratory and physician of medications the patient is taking that may affect test results; they may need to be restricted.

- Teach the patient how to collect a timed stool specimen, and provide him with the necessary equipment.
- Inform him that the laboratory requires 1 or 2 days to complete the analysis.

Procedure and posttest care

- Collect a 72-hour stool specimen.
- Instruct the patient to resume his usual diet and medication schedule as ordered.

Precautions

- Don't use a waxed collection container because the wax may become incorporated in the stool and interfere with accurate testing.
- Tell the patient to avoid contaminating the stool specimen with toilet tissue or urine.
- Refrigerate the collection container, and keep it tightly covered.

Normal findings

Fecal lipids normally comprise less than 20% of excreted solids, with excretion < 7 g/24 hours.

Abnormal findings

Both digestive and absorptive disorders cause steatorrhea. Digestive disorders may affect the production and release of pancreatic lipase or bile; absorptive disorders may affect the integrity of the intestine.

In pancreatic insufficiency, impaired lipid digestion may result from insufficient production of lipase. Pancreatic resection, cystic fibrosis, chronic pancreatitis, or ductal obstruction by stone or tumor may prevent the normal release or action of lipase.

In impaired hepatic function, faulty lipid digestion may result from inadequate production of bile salts. Biliary obstruction, which may accompany gallbladder disease, may prevent the normal release of bile salts into the duodenum.

Extensive small-bowel resection or bypass may also interrupt normal enterohepatic circulation of bile salts.

Diseases of the intestinal mucosa affect the normal absorption of lipids; regional ileitis and atrophy due to malnutrition cause gross structural changes in the intestinal wall; and celiac disease and tropical sprue produce mucosal abnormalities.

Scleroderma, radiation enteritis, fistulas, intestinal tuberculosis, small intestine diverticula, and altered intestinal flora may also cause steatorrhea.

Whipple's disease and lymphomas cause lymphatic obstruction that may inhibit fat absorption.

Interfering factors

- Failure to observe pretest restrictions or the use of a waxed collection container
- Contaminated or incomplete stool specimen (total weight < 300 g)
- Azathioprine, bisacodyl, cholestyramine, kanamycin, neomycin, colchicine, aluminum hydroxide, calcium carbonate, alcohol, potassium chloride, and mineral oil (possible increase or decrease due to inhibited absorption or altered chemical digestion)

FECAL UROBILINOGEN

Urobilinogen, the end product of bilirubin metabolism, is a brown pigment formed by bacterial enzymes in the small intestine. It's excreted in stool or reabsorbed into portal blood, where it's returned to the liver and excreted in bile; a small amount is excreted in urine. Proper bilirubin metabolism depends on normal hepatobiliary system functioning and normal erythrocyte life span.

Although measuring fecal urobilinogen is a useful indicator of hepatobiliary and hemolytic disorders, the test is rarely performed because it's easier to measure serum bilirubin and urine urobilinogen.

Purpose

- To aid diagnosis of hepatobiliary and hemolytic disorders

Patient preparation

- Explain to the patient that this test evaluates liver and bile duct function or detects red blood cell disorders.
- Inform him that he need not restrict food or fluids before the test.
- Tell him the test requires collection of a random stool specimen.
- Notify the laboratory and physician of medications the patient is taking that may affect test results; they may need to be restricted.

Procedure and posttest care

- Collect a random stool specimen.
- Tell the patient he may resume his usual medication schedule, as ordered.

Precautions

- Tell the patient not to contaminate the stool specimen with toilet tissue or urine.
- Use a light-resistant collection container because urobilinogen breaks down to urobilin when exposed to light.
- Send the specimen to the laboratory immediately after collection.
- Refrigerate the specimen if transport or testing is delayed more than 30 minutes; freeze the specimen if test is to be performed by an outside laboratory.

Reference values

Normally, fecal urobilinogen values range from 50 to 300 mg/24 hours (SI, 100 to 400 EU/100 g).

Abnormal findings

Absent or low levels of urobilinogen in the stool indicate obstructed bile flow, the result of intrahepatic disorders (such as hepatocellular jaundice due to cirrhosis or hepatitis) or extrahepatic disorders (such as choledocholithiasis or tumor of the head of the pancreas, ampulla of Vater, or bile duct). Low fecal urobilinogen levels are also characteristic of depressed erythropoiesis, as in aplastic anemia.

Interfering factors

- Contamination of the specimen or failure to use a light-resistant collection container
- Broad-spectrum antibiotics (possible decrease due to inhibition of bacterial growth in the colon)
- Sulfonamides, which react with the reagent used by the laboratory in this test, and large doses of salicylates (possible increase)

OVA AND PARASITES IN STOOL

Examination of a stool specimen can detect several types of intestinal parasites. Some of these parasites live in nonpathogenic symbiosis; others cause intestinal disease. In North America, the most common parasites include the roundworms *Ascaris lumbricoides* and *Necator americanus* (also called hookworms); the tapeworms *Diphyllobothrium latum, Taenia saginata,* and *Taenia solium* (rare); the amoeba *Entamoeba histolytica;* and the flagellate *Giardia lamblia*. Cyclospora can also be detected in stool exam for ova and parasites.

Purpose

■ To confirm or rule out intestinal parasitic infection and disease

Patient preparation

■ Explain to the patient that this test detects intestinal parasitic infection.
■ As ordered, instruct him to avoid treatments with castor or mineral oil, bismuth, magnesium or antidiarrheal compounds, barium enemas, and antibiotics for 7 to 10 days before the test.
■ Tell him the test requires three stool specimens—one every other day or every third day. Up to six specimens may be required to confirm the presence of *E. histolytica.*
■ Record recent dietary and travel history if the patient has diarrhea. Check the patient's history for antiparasitic drugs, such as carbarsone, tetracycline, paromomycin, metronidazole, and diiodohydroxyquin, within 2 weeks of the test.

Equipment

Gloves, waterproof container with tight-fitting lid, bedpan (if necessary), tongue blade

Procedure and posttest care

■ Put on gloves and collect a stool specimen directly into the container. (See *Collection procedure for pinworms.*)
■ Collect the specimen into a clean, dry bedpan if the patient is bedridden; then, using a tongue blade, transfer it into a properly labeled container.
■ Note on the laboratory request the date and time of collection and the specimen's consistency.
■ Also record any recent or current antimicrobial therapy and any pertinent travel or dietary history.
■ Commercial stool collection and preservation kits for the detection of ova and parasites are currently available. A two-vial system is available for transport; one vial contains 8 to 10 ml of 10% formalin, the other contains 8 to 10 ml of polyvinyl alcohol. To each vial add 2 to 3 ml of feces. Thoroughly mix the specimen and fluid. Cap each vial tightly.
■ Tell the patient he may resume his usual medication schedule, as ordered.
■ Past therapy specimens should be examined 3 to 4 weeks after treatment to verify eradication.

Precautions

■ Don't contaminate the stool specimen with urine, which can destroy trophozoites.
■ Don't collect stool from a toilet bowl because water is toxic to trophozoites and may contain organisms that interfere with test results.
■ Send the specimen to the laboratory immediately after collection. If a liquid or soft stool specimen can't be examined within 30 minutes of passage, place some of it in a preservative; if a formed stool specimen can't be examined immediately, refrigerate it or place it in preservative.
■ If the entire stool can't be sent to the laboratory, include macroscopic worms or worm segments and bloody and mucoid portions of the specimen.
■ Use gloves when performing the procedure and handling the specimen, disposing of equipment, sealing the container, and transporting it. Dispose of the gloves after specimen collection.

Normal findings

No parasites or ova appear in stool.

Abnormal findings

The presence of *E. histolytica* confirms amebiasis; *G. lamblia,* giardiasis. How-

Collection procedure for pinworms

The ova of the pinworm *Enterobius vermicularis* seldom appear in stool because the female migrates from the anus during the night and deposits the eggs in the perianal area. To collect them, place a piece of cellophane tape, sticky side out, on the end of a tongue depressor, and press it firmly on the anal area. Then transfer the tape, sticky side down, to a slide (kits with tape and a slide or a sticky paddle are available). If tape is unavailable, use an anal swab technique. Because the female usually deposits her ova at night, collect the specimen early in the morning before the patient bathes or defecates.

ever, the extent of infection depends on the degree of tissue invasion. If amebiasis is suspected but stool examinations are negative, specimen collection after a saline cathartic using buffered sodium biphosphate or during a sigmoidoscopy may be necessary. If giardiasis or the presence of *Strongyloides stercoralis* is suspected but stool examinations are negative, examination of duodenal contents may be necessary.

Injury to the host is difficult to detect — even when helminth ova or larvae appear — therefore, the number of worms is usually correlated with the patient's clinical symptoms to distinguish between helminth infestation and helminth diseases. Eosinophilia may also indicate parasitic infection.

Helminths may migrate from the intestinal tract, producing pathologic changes in other parts of the body. For example, the roundworm *Ascaris* may perforate the bowel wall, causing peritonitis, or may migrate to the lungs, causing pneumonitis. Hookworms can cause hypochromic microcytic anemia secondary to bloodsucking and hemorrhage, especially in patients with iron-deficient diets. The tapeworm *D. latum* may cause megaloblastic anemia by removing vitamin B_{12}.

Interfering factors

- Castor or mineral oil, bismuth, magnesium or antidiarrheal compounds, and barium enema
- Failure to observe pretest restrictions
- Improper collection technique, collection of too few specimens, or contamination of the sample with urine (possible false-negative)
- Failure to transport the specimen to the laboratory promptly or to refrigerate or preserve it
- Exposure of specimen to excessive heat or cold
- Any radiographic contrast media given to the patient within 5 to 10 days prior to specimen collection

ROTAVIRUS ANTIGEN IN STOOL

Rotaviruses are the most common cause of infectious diarrhea in infants and young children. They're most prevalent in children ages 3 months to 2 years during the winter months. Clinical features include diarrhea, vomiting, fever, and abdominal pain. Symptoms of infection may range from mild in adults to severe in young children, especially hospitalized infants.

Detection of human rotaviruses typically requires sensitive, specific enzyme immunoassays that provide results within minutes or hours (depending on the assay) because human rotaviruses don't replicate efficiently in laboratory cell cultures.

Purpose

- To obtain a laboratory diagnosis of rotavirus gastroenteritis

Patient preparation

- Explain the purpose of the test to the patient or his parents if the patient is a child.
- Inform him that the test requires a stool specimen.
- Collect the specimens during the prodromal and acute stages of clinical infection to ensure detection of the viral antigens by enzyme immunoassay.

Procedure and posttest care

- Usually, a stool specimen (1 g in a screw-capped tube or vial) is used to detect rotaviruses. If a microbiological transport swab is used, it must be heavily stained with stool to be diagnostically productive for rotavirus.
- Monitor the patient's intake and output and provide him with fluids to avoid dehydration caused by vomiting and diarrhea.

Precautions

- Avoid using collection containers with preservatives, metal ions, detergents, and serum, which may interfere with the assay.
- Store stool specimens for up to 24 hours at 35.6° to 46.4° F (2° to 8° C). If a longer period of storage or shipment is necessary, freeze specimens at − 4° F (− 20° C) or colder. Repeated freezing and thawing will cause the specimen to deteriorate and yield misleading results.
- Don't store the specimen in a self-defrosting freezer.
- Use gloves when obtaining or handling all specimens.

Normal findings

The detection of rotavirus by enzyme immunoassay is laboratory evidence of current infection with the organism.

Abnormal findings

- Rotavirus is not normally detectable in the stool. It can infect all age groups, but is generally more severe in young children than in adults. Rotavirus infections are easily transmitted in group settings, such as nursing homes, preschools, and day-care centers. Transmission is presumed to occur from person to person by the fecal-oral route. In a hospital setting, nosocomial spread of this viral infection can cause significant harm.

Interfering factors

- Collection of specimen in containers with preservatives such as metal ions, detergents, or serum (decreased number of pathogens)

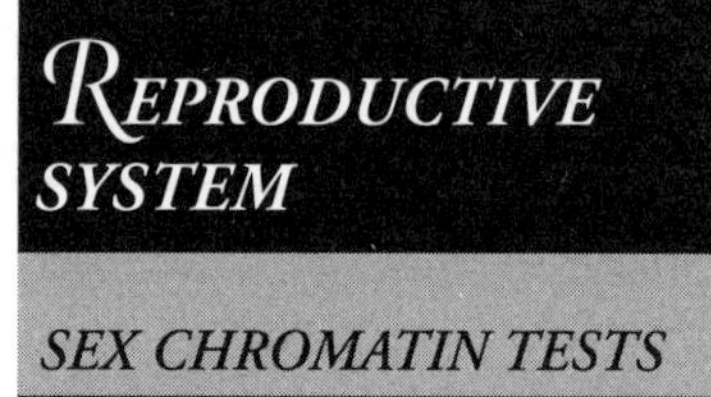

REPRODUCTIVE SYSTEM

SEX CHROMATIN TESTS

Although sex chromatin tests can screen for abnormalities in the number of sex chromosomes, the faster, simpler, and more accurate full karyotype (chromosome analysis) has all but replaced them. Sex chromatin tests are usually indicated for abnormal sexual development, ambiguous genitalia, amenorrhea, and suspected chromosomal abnormalities.

Purpose

■ To quickly screen for abnormal sexual development (both X and Y chromatin tests)
■ To aid assessment of an infant with ambiguous genitalia (X chromatin test only)
■ To determine the number of Y chromosomes in an individual (Y chromatin test only)

Patient preparation

■ Explain to the patient or his parents, if appropriate, why the test is being performed.
■ Tell him the test requires that the inside of his cheek be scraped to obtain a specimen and who will perform the test.
■ Assure the patient that the test takes only a few minutes but may require a follow-up chromosome analysis.
■ Inform him that the laboratory generally requires as long as 4 weeks to complete the analysis.

Equipment

Wooden or metal spatula, clean glass slide, cell fixative

Procedure and posttest care

■ Scrape the buccal mucosa firmly with a wooden or metal spatula at least twice to obtain a specimen of healthy cells (vaginal mucosa is occasionally used in young women).
■ Rub the spatula over the glass slide, making sure the cells are evenly distributed.
■ Spray the slide with cell fixative, and send it to the laboratory with a brief patient history and indications for the test.

Precautions

■ Make sure the buccal mucosa is scraped firmly to ensure a sufficient number of cells.
■ Check that the specimen isn't saliva, which contains no cells.

Normal findings

A normal female (XX) has only one X chromatin mass (the number of X chromatin masses discernible is one less than the number of X chromosomes in the cells examined). For various reasons, an X chromatin mass is ordinarily discernible in only 20% to 50% of the buccal mucosal cells of a normal woman.

A normal male (XY) has only one Y chromatin mass (the number of Y chromatin masses equals the number of Y chromosomes in the cells examined).

Abnormal findings

In most laboratories, if less than 20% of the cells in a buccal smear contain an X chromatin mass, some cells are presumed to contain only one X chromosome, necessitating full karyotyping. Persons with female phenotypes and positive Y chromatin masses run a high risk of developing malignancies in their intra-abdominal gonads. In such persons, removal of these gonads is indicated and should generally be performed before age 5.

The patient or his parents require genetic counseling after the cause of chromosomal abnormal sexual development has been identified. A medical team comprised of physicians, psychologists, psychiatrists, and educators must decide the child's sex if a child is phenotypically of one sex and genotypically of the other. This careful evaluation should be made early to prevent developmental problems related to incorrect gender identification. (See *Sex chromosome anomalies,* pages 414 and 415.)

(Text continues on page 416.)

Sex chromosomes anomalies

DISORDER AND CHROMOSOMAL ANEUPLOIDY	CAUSE AND INCIDENCE
Klinefelter's syndrome ◆ 47,XXY ◆ 48,XXXY ◆ 49,XXXXY ◆ 48,XX,YY ◆ 49,XXX,YY	◆ Nondisjunction or improper chromatid separation during anaphase I or II of oogenesis or spermatogenesis results in abnormal gamete ◆ 1 per 1,000 male births
Polysomy Y ◆ 47,XYY	◆ Nondisjunction during anaphase II of spermatogenesis causes both Y chromosomes to pass to the same pole and results in a YY sperm ◆ 1 per 1,000 male births
Turner's syndrome ◆ 45,XO ◆ Mosaics: XO/XX or XO/XXX ◆ Aberrations of X chromosomes, including deletion of short arm of one X chromosome, presence of a ring chromosome, or presence of an isochromosome on the long arm of an X chromosome	◆ Nondisjunction during anaphase I or II of spermatogenesis results in sperm without any sex chromosomes ◆ 1 per 3,500 female births (most common chromosome complement in first-trimester abortions)
Other X polysomes	◆ Nondisjunction at anaphase I or II of oogenesis
◆ 47,XXX	◆ 1 per 1,400 female births
◆ 48,XXXX	◆ Rare
◆ 49,XXXXX	◆ Rare

PHENOTYPIC FEATURES

- Syndrome usually inapparent until puberty
- Small penis and testes
- Sparse facial and abdominal hair; feminine distribution of pubic hair
- Somewhat enlarged breasts (gynecomastia)
- Sexual dysfunction
- Truncal obesity
- Sterility
- Possible mental retardation (greater incidence with increased X chromosomes)

- Above-average stature (commonly over 72″ [182.9 cm])
- Increased incidence of severe acne
- May display aggressive, psychopathic or criminal behavior
- Normal fertility
- Learning disabilities

- Short stature (usually under 57″ [144.8 cm])
- Webbed neck
- Low posterior hairline
- Broad chest with widely spaced nipples
- Underdeveloped breasts
- Juvenile external genitalia
- Primary amenorrhea common
- CHD (30% with coarctation of the aorta)
- Renal abnormalities
- Sterility from underdeveloped internal reproductive organs (ovaries are only strands of connective tissue)
- No mental retardation but possible problems with space perception and orientation

---

- Often, no obvious anatomical abnormalities
- Normal fertility

- Mental retardation
- Ocular hypertelorism
- Reduced fertility

- Severe mental retardation
- Ocular hypertelorism, with uncoordinated eye movement
- Abnormal development of sexual organs
- Various skeletal anomalies

Interfering factors

- Obtaining saliva instead of buccal cells (false specimen)
- Cell deterioration due to failure to apply cell fixative to the slide
- Presence of bacteria or wrinkles in the cell membrane, analysis of degenerative cells, or use of an outdated stain

CHROMOSOME ANALYSIS

Chromosome analysis studies the relationship between the microscopic appearance of chromosomes and an individual's phenotype — the expression of the genes in physical, biochemical, or physiologic traits.

Ideally, chromosomes are studied during metaphase, the middle phase of mitosis, when new cell poles appear. During metaphase, colchicine (a cell poison) is added to arrest cell division. Cells are harvested, stained, and then examined under a microscope. These cells are then photographed to record the karyotype — the systematic arrangement of chromosomes in groupings according to size and shape.

Only rapidly dividing cells, such as bone marrow or neoplastic cells, permit direct, immediate study. In other cells, mitosis is stimulated by the addition of phytohemagglutinin. Indications for the test determine the specimen required (blood, bone marrow, amniotic fluid, skin, or placental tissue) and the specific analytic procedure.

Purpose

- To identify chromosomal abnormalities, such as hypoploidy or hyperploidy, as the underlying cause of malformation, maldevelopment, or disease

Patient preparation

- Explain to the patient or his parents, if appropriate, the purpose of this test.
- Tell him who will perform the test and what kind of specimen will be required.
- Inform him when results will be available, according to the specimen required.

Procedure and posttest care

- Collect a blood sample (in a 5- to 10-ml heparinized tube), a tissue specimen, 1 ml of bone marrow, or at least 20 ml of amniotic fluid.
- Provide appropriate posttest care, depending on the procedure used to collect the specimen.
- Explain the test results and their implications to the patient or his parents if he's a child with a chromosomal abnormality.
- Recommend appropriate genetic or other counseling and follow-up care if necessary, such as an infant stimulation program for a patient with Down syndrome.

Precautions

- Keep all specimens sterile, especially those requiring a tissue culture.
- To facilitate interpretation of test results, send the specimen to the laboratory immediately after collection, with a brief patient history and the indication for the test.
- Refrigerate the specimen if transport is delayed, but *never* freeze it.
- Make sure the povidone-iodine solution is thoroughly removed with alcohol before a skin biopsy to prevent cell growth in tissue culture.

Normal findings

The normal cell contains 46 chromosomes: 22 pairs of nonsex chromosomes (autosomes) and 1 pair of sex chromosomes (Y for the male-determining chromosome, X for the female-determining chromosome). On a karyotype, chromosomes are arranged according to size and the location of their primary constrictions, or centromeres.

The centromere may be medial (metacentric), slightly to one end of the chromosome (submetacentric), or entirely to one end (acrocentric). The largest chromosomes are displayed first; the others are arranged in order of decreasing size, with the two sex chromosomes traditionally placed last. By convention, the centromere is always placed at the top in a karyotype. Thus, if the two pairs of chromosomal arms are of unequal length, the arm above the centromere will be shorter. The letter "p" designates the short arm; the letter "q," the long arm.

Special stains identify individual chromosomes and locate and enumerate particular portions of chromosomes. Trypsin, alkali, heat denaturation, and Giemsa stain are used for visible light microscopy; quinacrine stain, for ultraviolet microscopy. These techniques produce nonuniform staining of each chromosome in a repetitive, banded pattern. The mechanism of chromosome banding is unknown, but seems related to primary deoxyribonucleic acid sequence and protein composition of the chromosome.

Abnormal findings

Chromosomal abnormalities may be numerical or structural. Any numerical deviation from the norm of 46 chromosomes is called *aneuploidy.* Less than 46 chromosomes is called *hypoploidy;* more than 46, *hyperploidy.* Special designations exist for whole multiples of the haploid number 23: *diploidy* for the normal somatic number of 46, *triploidy* for 69, *tetraploidy* for 92, and so forth.

When the deviation occurs within a single pair of chromosomes, the suffix "–somy" is used, as in *trisomy* for the presence of three chromosomes instead of the usual pair or *monosomy* for the presence of only one chromosome.

Aneuploidy most commonly follows failure of the chromosomal pair to separate (nondisjunction) during anaphase, the mitotic stage that follows metaphase. It may also result from anaphase lag, in which one of the normally separated chromosomes fails to move to a pole and is left out of the daughter cells.

If nondisjunction or anaphase lag occurs during meiosis, the cells of the zygote will all be the same. Errors in mitotic division after zygote formation will produce more than one cell line (mosaicism).

Structural chromosomal abnormalities result from chromosome breakage. Intrachromosomal rearrangement occurs within a single chromosome in the following forms:

- *deletion:* loss of an end (terminal) or middle (interstitial) portion of a chromosome
- *inversion:* end-to-end reversal of a chromosome segment, which may be pericentric inversion (including the centromere) or paracentric inversion (occurring in only one arm of the chromosome)
- *ring chromosome formation:* breakage of both ends of a chromosome and reunion of the ends
- *isochromosome formation:* abnormal splitting of the centromere in a transverse rather than a longitudinal plane.

Interchromosomal rearrangements (of more than one chromosome, usually two) also occur. The most common rearrangement is translocation, or exchange, of genetic material between two chromosomes. Translocations may

Chromosome analysis findings

SPECIMEN AND INDICATION	RESULT	IMPLICATION
Blood		
◆ To evaluate abnormal appearance or development, suggesting chromosomal irregularity	◆ Abnormal chromosome number (aneuploidy) or arrangement	◆ Identifies specific chromosomal abnormality
◆ To evaluate couples with history of miscarriages or to identify balanced translocation carriers having unbalanced offspring	◆ Normal chromosomes ◆ Parental balanced translocation carrier	◆ Miscarriage unrelated to parental chromosomal abnormality ◆ Increased risk of repeated abortion or unbalanced offspring indicates need for amniocentesis in future pregnancies
◆ To detect chromosomal rearrangements in rare genetic diseases predisposing patient to malignant neoplasms	◆ Chromosomal rearrangements, gaps, and breaks	◆ Occurs in Bloom's syndrome, Fanconi's syndrome, telangiectasia; patient predisposed to malignant neoplasms
Blood or bone marrow		
◆ To identify Philadelphia chromosome and confirm chronic myelogenous leukemia	◆ Translocation of chromosome 22q (long arm) to another chromosome (often chromosome 9) ◆ Aneuploidy (usually due to abnormalities in chromosomes 8 and 12) ◆ Trisomy 21	◆ Aids diagnosis of chronic myelogenous leukemia ◆ Occurs in acute myelogenous leukemia ◆ Occasionally occurs in chronic lymphocytic leukemia cells
Skin		
◆ To evaluate abnormal appearance or development, suggesting chromosomal irregularity	◆ All chromosomal abnormalities possible	◆ Same as chromosomal abnormality in blood; rarely, mosaic individual has normal blood but abnormal skin chromosomes

Chromosome analysis findings *(continued)*

SPECIMEN AND INDICATION	RESULT	IMPLICATION
Amniotic fluid		
◆ To evaluate developing fetus with possible chromosomal abnormality	◆ All chromosomal abnormalities possible	◆ Same as chromosomal abnormality in blood or fetus
Placental tissue		
◆ To evaluate products of conception after a miscarriage to determine if abnormality is fetal or placental in origin	◆ All chromosomal abnormalities possible	◆ More than 50% of aborted tissue is chromosomally abnormal
Tumor tissue		
◆ For research purposes only	◆ Many chromosomal abnormalities possible	◆ Although malignant tumors aren't associated with specific chromosomal aberrations, most are aneuploid, usually hyperploid.

be balanced, in which the cell neither loses nor gains genetic material; unbalanced, in which a piece of genetic material is gained or lost from each cell; reciprocal (in children), in which two chromosomes exchange material; or Robertsonian, in which two chromosomes join to form one combined chromosome, with little or no loss of material.

Implications of chromosome analysis results depend on the specimen and indications for the test. (See *Chromosome analysis findings.*)

Interfering factors

- Chemotherapy (possible abnormal results due to chromosome breaks)
- Contamination of tissue with bacteria, fungus, or a virus (possible inhibition of culture growth)
- Inclusion of maternal cells in a specimen obtained by amniocentesis, with subsequent culturing (possible false results)

AMNIOTIC FLUID ANALYSIS

Amniocentesis produces a 10- to 20-ml sample for laboratory analysis. This analysis may be used to detect certain birth defects, such as Down syndrome or spina bifida; to determine fetal ma-

Chorionic villi sampling

Chorionic villi sampling (CVS) is a prenatal test for quick detection of fetal chromosomal and biochemical disorders that's performed during the first trimester of pregnancy. Preliminary results may be available within hours; complete results, within a few days. In contrast, amniocentesis can't be performed before the 16th week of pregnancy, and the results aren't available for at least 2 weeks. Thus, CVS can detect fetal abnormalities as much as 10 weeks sooner than amniocentesis.

The chorionic villi are fingerlike projections that surround the embryonic membrane and eventually give rise to the placenta. Cells obtained from an appropriate sample are of fetal, rather than maternal, origin and thus can be analyzed for fetal abnormalities.

COLLECTION TIME

Samples are best obtained between the 8th and 10th weeks of pregnancy. Before 7 weeks, the villi cover the embryo and make selective sampling difficult. After 10 weeks, maternal cells begin to grow over the villi, and the amniotic sac begins to fill the uterine cavity, making the procedure difficult and potentially dangerous.

COLLECTION METHOD

To collect a chorionic villi sample, the patient is placed in the lithotomy position. The physician checks the placement of the patient's uterus bimanually, and then inserts a Graves speculum and swabs the cervix with an antiseptic solution. If necessary, he may use a tenaculum to straighten an acutely flexed uterus, permitting cannula insertion. Guided by ultrasound and possibly endoscopy, he directs the catheter through the cannula to the villi. Suction is applied to the catheter to remove about 30 mg of tissue from the villi. The sample is withdrawn, placed in a Petri dish, and examined with a dissecting microscope. Part of the specimen is then cultured for further testing.

INTERPRETATION

CVS can be used to detect about 200 diseases prenatally. For example, direct analysis of rapidly dividing fetal cells

turity; to detect hemolytic disease of the newborn; or, through karyotyping, to detect gender and chromosomal abnormalities. This test can be performed only when the amniotic fluid level reaches 150 ml, usually after the 16th week of pregnancy.

Amniocentesis is indicated if the mother is over age 35; has a family history of genetic, chromosomal, or neural tube defects; or has had a miscarriage. Although adverse effects are rare, potential complications include spontaneous abortion, trauma to the fetus or placenta, bleeding, premature labor, infection, and Rh sensitization from fetal bleeding into the maternal circulation. Because of the severity of possible complications, amniocentesis is contraindicated as a general screening test. Abnormal test results or failure of the tissue cultures to grow may necessitate repetition of the test.

Another method of detecting fetal chromosomal and biochemical disorders in early pregnancy is chorionic villi sampling. (See *Chorionic villi sampling.*)

can detect chromosome disorders, deoxyribonucleic acid analysis can detect hemoglobinopathies, and lysosomal enzyme assays can screen for lysosomal storage disorders such as Tay-Sachs disease.

The test appears to provide reliable results except when the sample contains too few cells or the cells fail to grow in culture. Patient risks for this procedure appear to be similar to those for amniocentesis: a small chance of spontaneous abortion, cramps, infection, and bleeding. However, recent research reports an incidence of limb malformations in neonates when CVS has been performed.

Unlike amniocentesis, CVS can't detect complications in cases of Rh sensitization, uncover neural tube defects, or determine pulmonary maturity. However, it may prove to be the best way to detect other serious fetal abnormalities early in pregnancy.

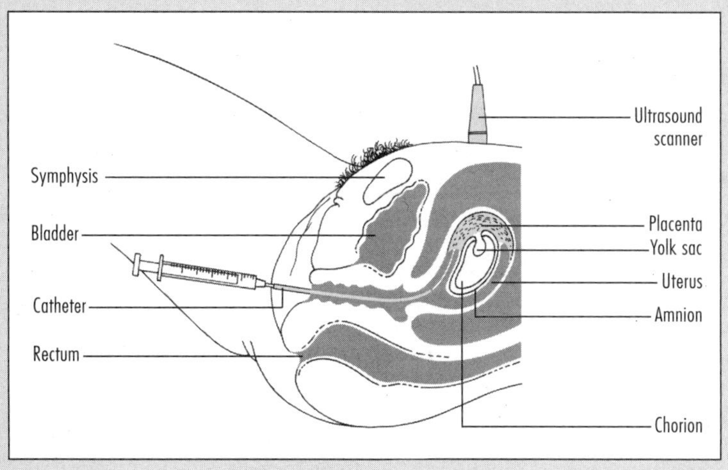

Purpose

- To detect fetal abnormalities, particularly chromosomal and neural tube defects
- To detect hemolytic disease of the neonate
- To diagnose metabolic disorders, amino acid disorders, and mucopolysaccharidosis
- To determine fetal age and maturity, especially pulmonary maturity (See *Shake test,* page 422.)
- To assess fetal health by detecting the presence of meconium or blood or measuring amniotic levels of estriol and fetal thyroid hormone
- To identify fetal gender when one or both parents are carriers of a sex-linked disorder

Patient preparation

- Describe the procedure to the patient, and explain that this test detects fetal abnormalities.
- Assess her understanding of the test, and answer any questions she may have.
- Inform her that she need not restrict food or fluids.

Shake test

Amniotic fluid from mature fetal lungs contains surfacants. In the shake test, also known as the foam stability test, bubbles should appear on the surface of a test tube of amniotic fluid that's shaken vigorously if adequate amounts of surfactants are present.

Using a chemically clean 13-mm × 100-mm glass tube with a Teflon-lined screw cap or a rubber stopper, combine 1 ml of amniotic fluid and 1 ml of 95% ethanol. In another tube, combine 0.5 ml of amniotic fluid, 0.5 ml of saline solution, and 1 ml of 95% ethanol. Shake both tubes vigorously for 15 seconds, and place them upright in a rack for 15 minutes.

If a complete ring of bubbles is still evident in both tubes after 15 minutes, as shown, the test is positive and the risk of respiratory distress is low. A positive result in the second tube indicates pulmonary maturity. Negative results indicate a risk of respiratory distress. Blood or meconium in the fluid invalidates the test.

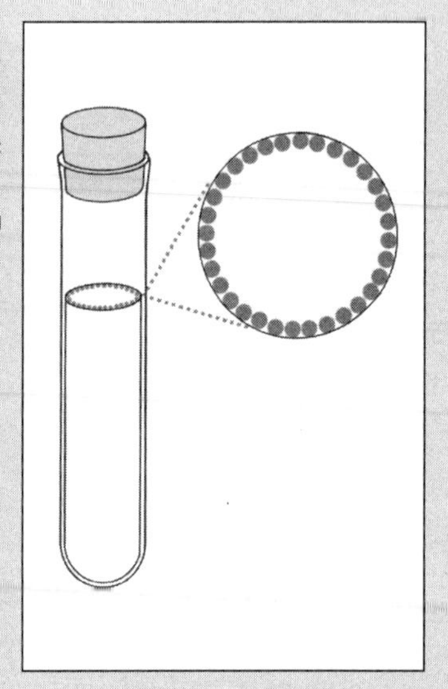

- Tell her the test requires a specimen of amniotic fluid and who will perform the test.
- Advise her that normal test results can't guarantee a normal fetus because some fetal disorders are undetectable.
- Make sure the patient has signed a consent form.
- Explain that she'll feel a stinging sensation when the local anesthetic is injected.
- Provide emotional support before and during the test.
- Ask her to void just before the test to minimize the risk of puncturing the bladder and aspirating urine instead of amniotic fluid.

Equipment

70% alcohol or povidone-iodine solution, sponge forceps, 2″ × 2″ gauze pads, local anesthetic (1% lidocaine), 25G sterile needle, 3-ml syringe, 20G sterile spinal needle with stylet, 10-ml syringe, amber or foil-covered sterile 10-ml test tube

Procedure and posttest care

- A pool of amniotic fluid is located after determining fetal and placental position, usually through palpation and ultrasonic visualization.
- The skin is prepared with antiseptic and alcohol; then 1 ml of 1% lidocaine is injected with a 25G needle, first intradermally and then subcutaneously.
- Then a 20G spinal needle, with a stylet, is inserted into the amniotic cavity and the stylet is withdrawn.
- A 10-ml syringe is attached to the needle; then the fluid is aspirated and

Apt test

Blood in the amniotic fluid can be of maternal or fetal origin. The Apt test, which is based on the premises that fetal hemoglobin is alkali-resistant and adult hemoglobin changes to alkaline hematin after the addition of alkali, can differentiate between the two. This test may be performed on all bloody amniotic fluid samples.

To perform this test, dilute 1 ml of amniotic fluid with water until it turns pink. Centrifuge for 10 minutes, then decant the supernatant. Add five parts supernatant to one part 0.25 N (1%) sodium hydroxide, and observe for 1 to 2 minutes. Fetal blood appears red; maternal blood, yellow-brown. To confirm the results, repeat the test with known maternal blood.

placed in an amber or foil-covered test tube.

- The needle is withdrawn, and an adhesive bandage is placed over the needle insertion site.
- Monitor fetal heart rate and maternal vital signs every 15 minutes for at least 30 minutes.
- Position the patient on her left side if she sweats profusely or feels faint or nauseated to counteract uterine pressure on the vena cava.
- Instruct the patient before she's discharged to immediately report abdominal pain or cramping, chills, fever, vaginal bleeding or leakage of serous vaginal fluid, or fetal hyperactivity or unusual fetal lethargy.

Precautions

- Instruct the patient to fold her hands behind her head to prevent her from accidentally touching the sterile field and causing contamination.
- Send the specimen to the laboratory immediately after collection.

Normal findings

Normal amniotic fluid is clear but may contain white flecks of vernix caseosa when the fetus is near term. For an analysis of the appearance and components of amniotic fluid, see *Findings in amniotic fluid analysis,* page 424.

Abnormal findings

Blood, which is found in about 10% of amniocenteses, results from a faulty tap and doesn't indicate an abnormality. However, it does inhibit cell growth and changes the level of other amniotic fluid constituents. "Port wine" fluid, on the other hand, may be a sign of abruptio placentae, and blood of fetal origin may indicate damage to the fetal, placental, or umbilical cord vessels by the amniocentesis needle. (See *Apt test.*)

Large amounts of *bilirubin,* a breakdown product of red blood cells, may indicate hemolytic disease of the newborn. Normally, the bilirubin level increases from the 14th to the 24th week of pregnancy, then declines as the fetus matures, essentially reaching zero at term. Testing for bilirubin usually isn't performed until the 26th week because that's the earliest time successful therapy for Rh sensitization can begin. Bilirubin level is determined by spectrophotometric measurement of the optic density of the amniotic fluid. The deviation of the scan at 450µ from a straight line drawn between 375µ and 525µ represents the bilirubin peak.

Meconium, a semisolid viscous material found in the fetal GI tract, consists of mucopolysaccharides, desquamated cells, vernix, hair, and cholesterol. Meconium passes into the amniotic flu-

Findings in amniotic fluid analysis

TEST	NORMAL FINDINGS	FETAL IMPLICATIONS OF ABNORMAL FINDINGS
Color	Clear, with white flecks of vernix caseosa in a mature fetus	Blood of maternal origin is usually harmless. "Port wine" fluid may indicate abruptio placentae. Fetal blood may indicate damage to the fetal, placental, or umbilical cord vessels.
Bilirubin	◆ Early: < 0.075 mg/dl (SI, < 1.3 Umol/L) ◆ Term: < 0.025 mg/dl (SI, < 0.41 Umol/L)	High levels indicate hemolytic disease of the newborn in isoimmunized pregnancy.
Meconium	Absent (except in breech presentation)	Presence indicates fetal hypotension or distress.
Creatinine	> 2 mg/dl (SI, 177 µmol/L)	Decreased levels may indicate Immature fetus (less than 37 weeks).
Lecithin-sphingomyelin ratio	> 2	< 2 indicates pulmonary immaturity
Phosphatidylglycerol	Present	Absence indicates pulmonary immaturity.
Glucose	< 45 mg/dl (SI, 2.3 mmol/L)	Excessive increases at term or near term indicates hypertrophy of fetal pancreas
Alpha-fetoprotein	Variable, depending on gestation age and laboratory technique	Inappropriate increases indicate neural tube defects, such as spina bifida or anencephaly, impending fetal death, congenital nephrosis, or contamination by fetal blood.
Bacteria	Absent	Presence indicates chorioamniotitis
Chromosome	Normal karyotype	Abnormal karyotype may indicate fetal sex and chromosome disorders.
Acetylcholinesterase	Absent	Presence may indicate neural tube defects, exomphalos, or other serious malformations.

id when hypoxia causes fetal distress and relaxation of the anal sphincter. Meconium is a normal finding in breech presentation. Meconium in the amniotic fluid produces a peak of 410 mμ on the spectrophotometric analysis. However, serial amniocentesis may show a clearing of meconium over a 2- to 3-week period. If meconium is present during labor, the newborn's nose and throat require thorough cleaning to prevent meconium aspiration.

Creatinine, a product of fetal urine, increases in the amniotic fluid as the fetal kidneys mature. Generally, the creatinine value exceeds 2 mg/dl in a mature fetus.

Alpha-fetoprotein (AFP) is a fetal alpha globulin produced first in the yolk sac and later in the parenchymal cells of the liver and GI tract. Fetal serum AFP levels are about 150 times higher than amniotic fluid levels; maternal serum AFP levels are far lower than amniotic fluid levels. High amniotic fluid levels indicate neural tube defects, but the AFP level may remain normal if the defect is small and closed. Elevated AFP levels may also occur in multiple pregnancy; in disorders such as omphalocele, congenital nephrosis, esophageal or duodenal atresia, cystic fibrosis, exomphalos, Turner's syndrome, and fetal bladder neck obstruction with hydronephrosis; and in impending fetal death.

The amount of *uric acid* in the amniotic fluid increases as the fetus matures, but these levels fluctuate widely and can't accurately predict maturity. Laboratory studies indicate that severe erythroblastosis fetalis, familial hyperuricemia, and Lesch-Nyhan syndrome tend to increase the level of uric acid.

Estrone, estradiol, estriol, and *estriol conjugates* appear in amniotic fluid in varying amounts. Levels of estriol, the most prevalent estrogen, increase substantially at term. Severe erythroblastosis fetalis decreases the estriol level.

The type II cells lining the fetal lung alveoli produce *lecithin* slowly in early pregnancy and then markedly increase production around the 35th week.

The *sphingomyelin* level parallels that of lecithin until the 35th week, when it gradually decreases. Measuring the ratio of lecithin to sphingomyelin (L/S) confirms fetal pulmonary maturity (L/S ratio > 2) or suggests a risk of respiratory distress (L/S ratio < 2). However, fetal respiratory distress may develop in the fetus of a patient with diabetes, even though the L/S ratio is greater than 2, a level that usually indicates pulmonary maturity.

Phosphatidylglycerol levels are present with pulmonary maturity; *phosphatidylinositol* levels decrease.

Measuring *glucose* levels in the fluid can aid in assessing glucose control in the patient with diabetes, but this isn't done routinely. A level greater than 45 mg/dl (SI, > 2.6 mmol/L) indicates poor maternal and fetal control. *Insulin* levels normally increase slightly from the 27th to the 40th week but increase sharply (up to 27 times normal) in a poorly controlled patient with diabetes.

Laboratory analysis can identify at least 25 different *enzymes* (usually in low concentrations) in amniotic fluid. The enzymes have few known clinical implications, although elevated acetylcholinesterase levels may occur with neural tube defects, exomphalos, and other serious malformations.

When the mother carries an *X-linked disorder,* determination of fetal sex is important. If chromosome karyotyping identifies a male fetus, there's a 50% chance he'll be affected; a female fetus won't be affected but has a 50% chance of being a carrier.

Interfering factors

- Use of plastic disposable syringes (possible toxicity to amniotic fluid cells)
- Failure to place the specimen in an appropriate amber or foil-covered tube (possible decrease in bilirubin)
- Blood or meconium in the fluid (effect on L-S ratio)
- Maternal blood in the fluid (possible decrease in creatinine)
- Any amount of fetal blood in the fluid specimen (possible doubling of AFP concentrations)
- Several disorders that aren't associated with pregnancy, including infectious mononucleosis, cirrhosis, hepatic cancer, teratoma, endodermal sinus tumor, gastric carcinoma, pancreatic carcinoma, and subacute hereditary tyrosinemia (possible increase in AFP levels)

PAPANICOLAOU TEST

The Papanicolaou (Pap) test is a widely known cytologic test for early detection of cervical cancer. A physician or specially trained nurse scrapes secretions from the patient's cervix and spreads them on a slide, which is sent to the laboratory for cytologic analysis. The test relies on the ready exfoliation of malignant cells from the cervix and shows cell maturity, metabolic activity, and morphology variations.

Although cervical scrapings are the most common test specimen, the test may involve cytologic evaluation of the vaginal pool, prostatic secretions, urine, gastric secretions, cavity fluids, bronchial aspirations, sputum, or solid tumor cells obtained by fine needle aspiration. If a Pap test is positive or suggests malignancy, cervical biopsy can confirm diagnosis.

Purpose

- To detect malignant cells
- To detect inflammatory tissue changes
- To assess response to chemotherapy and radiation therapy
- To detect viral, fungal and, occasionally, parasitic invasion

Patient preparation

- Explain to the patient that the test allows the study of cervical cells.
- Stress its importance as an aid for detection of cancer at a stage when the disease is often asymptomatic and still curable.
- The test shouldn't be scheduled during the menstrual period; the best time is midcycle.
- Instruct the patient to avoid having intercourse for 24 hours, not to douche for 48 hours, and not to insert vaginal medications for 1 week before the test because doing so can wash away cellular deposits and change the vaginal pH.
- Tell her the test requires that the cervix be scraped, who will perform the procedure and when, and that she may experience slight discomfort but no pain from the speculum (but may feel some pain when the cervix is scraped).
- Inform her that the procedure takes 5 to 10 minutes or slightly longer if the vagina, pelvic cavity, and rectum are examined bimanually.
- Obtain an accurate patient history, and ask the following questions: When did you last have a Pap test? Have you ever had an abnormal Pap test? When was your last menstrual period? Are your periods regular? How many days do they last? Is bleeding heavy or light? Have you taken or are you presently taking hormones or oral contraceptives? Do you use an intrauterine device? Do you have any vaginal discharge, pain, or itching? Which, if any, gynecologic disorders have occurred in your family?

Have you ever had gynecologic surgery, chemotherapy, or radiation therapy? If so, describe it fully. Note any pertinent patient history data on the laboratory request.

■ Provide emotional support if the patient is anxious; tell her that test results should be available in a few days.

■ Ask the patient to empty her bladder just before the test.

Equipment

Gloves; drape; vaginal speculum; collection device, such as a Pap stick (wooden spatula), endocervical brush; saline solution; glass microscopic slides; fixative (commercial spray or 95% ethyl alcohol solution in a jar) for slides

Procedure and posttest care

■ Instruct the patient to disrobe from the waist down and to drape herself.

■ Ask her to lie on the examining table and to place her heels in the stirrups. (She may be more comfortable if she keeps her shoes on.) Tell her to slide her buttocks to the edge of the table. Adjust the drape to minimize exposure.

■ To avoid startling the patient, tell her when the examination will begin.

■ The examiner puts on gloves and inserts an unlubricated speculum into the vagina. To make insertion easier, the speculum may be moistened with saline solution or warm water.

■ After the examiner locates the cervix, he collects secretions from the cervix and material from the endocervical canal. He places the endocervical brush inside the endocervix and rolls it firmly inside the canal. If using a Pap stick (wooden spatula), it's placed against the cervix with the longest protrusion in the cervical canal, then rotates the stick clockwise 360 degrees firmly against the cervix.

■ He then spreads the specimen on the slide according to laboratory recommendations and immediately immerses the slide in (or sprays it with) a fixative.

■ Alternatively, posterior vaginal pool secretions and pancervical material may be collected and smeared on a single slide, which must be fixed immediately according to laboratory instructions.

■ Label the specimen appropriately, including the date, the patient's name, age, the date of her last menstrual period, and the collection site and method.

■ A bimanual examination may follow removal of the speculum. Help the patient up and instruct her to dress when the examination is completed.

■ Supply the patient with a sanitary napkin if cervical bleeding occurs.

■ Tell the patient when to return for her next Pap test.

Precautions

■ Make sure the cervical specimen is aspirated and scraped from the cervix. A vaginal pool sample isn't recommended for cervical or endometrial cancer screening.

■ The specimen should be thick enough that it isn't transparent.

■ Scrapings taken directly from the lesion are preferred if vaginal or vulval lesions are present.

■ Use a small pipette, if necessary, in a patient whose uterus is involuting or atrophying from age, to aspirate cells from the squamocolumnar junction and the cervical canal.

■ Preserve the slides immediately after the specimen is collected.

Normal findings

Normally, no malignant cells or other abnormalities are present.

Abnormal findings

Malignant cells usually have relatively large nuclei and only small amounts of cytoplasm. They show abnormal nuclear chromatin patterns and marked

Testing for cervical cancer

To analyze cervical cells, the ThinPrep may be collected in the same manner as a Papanicolaou (Pap) test using a cytobrush and plastic spatula. The specimens are deposited in a bottle provided with a fixative and sent to the laboratory. A filter is then inserted into the bottle and excess mucus, blood, and inflammatory cells are filtered out by centrifuge. Remaining cells are then placed on a slide in a uniform, thin layer and read as a Pap test. This causes fewer slides to be classified as unreadable, significantly reducing the incidence of false negatives and the need for repeat tests.

When using the ThinPrep test, screening can also be easily done for the human papillomavirus (HPV), of which certain strains have been identified as the primary cause of cervical cancer. The Digene hc2 HPV deoxyribonucleic acid (DNA) test has been approved by the Food and Drug Administration to determine if those identified as high risk for developing cervical cancer have been exposed to HPV. The specimen is collected as a Pap smear, but is dispersed with ThinPrep solution. Separate aliquots are used for each test, from brushings of the endocervix. The brush is then inserted into the specialized tube and snapped off at the shaft, capping securely. The target solution in the tube disrupts the virus and releases target DNA, which combines with specific ribonucleic acid (RNA) probes creating RNA:DNA hybrids. The hybrids are captured, bound and able to be magnified and measured using a luminometer.

If the individual is found to be positive for HPV, it means she had been infected with the virus. Depending on the type of HPV found through DNA testing, those harboring high risk HPV strains have a high risk of developing cervical cancer. It is recommended that she undergo colposcopy in which the cervix is viewed under microscope and a biopsy taken from the tissue sample.

variation in size, shape, and staining properties and may have prominent nucleoli.

A Pap smear may be graded in different ways, so check your laboratory's reporting format. In the Bethesda system, the current standardized method, potentially premalignant squamous lesions fall into three categories: atypical squamous cells of undetermined significance, low-grade squamous intraepithelial lesions, and high-grade squamous intraepithelial lesions. The low-grade category includes mild dysplasia and the changes of the human papillomavirus. The high-grade category includes moderate to severe dysplasia and carcinoma in situ.

To confirm a suggestive or positive cytology report, the test may be repeated or followed by a biopsy. (See *Testing for cervical cancer*.)

Interfering factors

- Douching within 48 hours or having intercourse within 24 hours before the test (can wash away cellular deposits)
- Excessive use of lubricating jelly on the speculum (false-negative)
- Collection of the specimen during menstruation
- Exclusive use of a specimen collected from the vaginal fornix (possible false-negative)
- Delay in fixing the specimen (difficult cytologic interpretation due to dehydration of cells)
- Too thin or thick a specimen.

SEMEN ANALYSIS

Semen analysis is a simple, inexpensive, and reasonably definitive test that's used in a broad range of applications, including evaluation of a man's fertility. Fertility analysis usually includes measuring the volume of seminal fluid, performing sperm counts, and microscopic examination of spermatozoa. Sperm are counted in much the same way that white blood cells, red blood cells, and platelets are counted in a blood sample. Motility and morphology are studied microscopically after staining a drop of semen.

If analysis detects an abnormality, additional tests (for example, liver, thyroid, pituitary, or adrenal function tests) may be performed to identify the underlying cause and to screen for metabolic abnormalities (such as diabetes mellitus). Significant abnormalities — such as greatly decreased sperm count or motility, or marked increase in morphologically abnormal forms — may require testicular biopsy.

Purpose

- To evaluate male fertility in an infertile couple
- To substantiate the effectiveness of vasectomy
- To detect semen on the body or clothing of a suspected rape victim or elsewhere at the crime scene
- To identify blood group substances to exonerate or incriminate a criminal suspect
- To rule out paternity on grounds of complete sterility

Patient preparation

Evaluation of fertility

- Provide written instructions, and inform the patient that the most desirable specimen requires masturbation, ideally in a physician's office or a laboratory.
- Tell him to follow the instructions given to him regarding the period of sexual continence before the test because this may increase his sperm count. Some physicians specify a fixed number of days, usually between 2 and 5; others advise a period of continence equal to the usual interval between episodes of sexual intercourse.
- If the patient prefers to collect the specimen at home, emphasize the importance of delivering the specimen to the laboratory within 1 hour after collection. Warn him not to expose the specimen to extreme temperatures or to direct sunlight (which can also increase its temperature). Ideally, the specimen should remain at body temperature until liquefaction is complete (about 20 minutes). To deliver a semen specimen during cold weather, suggest that the patient keep the specimen container in a coat pocket on the way to the laboratory to protect the specimen from exposure to cold.
- Alternatives to collection by masturbation include coitus interruptus or the use of a condom. For collection by coitus interruptus, instruct the patient to withdraw immediately before ejaculation and to deposit the ejaculate in a suitable specimen container. For collection by condom, tell the patient to first wash the condom with soap and water, rinse it thoroughly, and allow it to dry completely. (Powders or lubricants applied to the condom may be spermicidal.) Special sheaths that don't contain spermacide are also available for semen collection. After collection, instruct him to tie the condom, place it in a glass jar, and promptly deliver it to the laboratory.
- Fertility may also be determined by collecting semen from the woman after coitus to assess the ability of the sper-

matozoa to penetrate the cervical mucus and remain active. For the postcoital cervical mucus test, instruct the patient to report for examination 1 to 2 days before ovulation as determined by basal temperature records. A urine luteinizing hormone-releasing hormone test may help predict ovulation in patients with irregular cycles. Instruct the couple to abstain from intercourse for 2 days and then to have sex 2 to 8 hours before the examination. Remind them to avoid using lubricants. Explain to the patient scheduled for this test that the procedure takes only a few minutes. Tell her that she'll be placed in the lithotomy position and that a speculum will be inserted into the vagina to collect the specimen. She may feel some pressure but no pain during this procedure.

Semen collection from rape victim

- Explain to the patient that the examiner will try to obtain a semen specimen from her vagina.
- Prepare her for insertion of the speculum as you would the patient scheduled for postcoital examination.
- Handle the victim's clothes as little as possible. If her clothes are moist, put them in a paper bag — not a plastic bag (which causes seminal stains and secretions to mold). Label the bag properly, and send it to the laboratory immediately.
- Provide emotional support by speaking to the patient calmly and reassuringly. Encourage her to express her fears and anxieties. Listen sympathetically.
- If she's scheduled for vaginal lavage, tell the rape victim to expect a cold sensation when saline solution is instilled to wash out the specimen.
- Help her relax during this procedure by instructing her to breathe deeply and slowly through her mouth.
- Instruct the victim to urinate just before the test, but warn her not to wipe the vulva afterward because this may remove semen.

Equipment

For semen collection by masturbation, coitus interruptus, or condom: clean plastic specimen container (for example, disposable urine or sputum container with lid)

For semen collection from rape victim: clean plastic specimen container, vaginal speculum, rubber gloves, cotton applicator sticks, glass microscopic slides with frosted ends, physiologic (0.85%) saline solution, Pap sticks, Coplin jars containing 95% ethanol, large syringe, rubber bulb or other device suitable for vaginal lavage

For a postcoital specimen collection: clean plastic specimen container, vaginal speculum, rubber gloves, cotton applicator sticks, glass microscopic slides with frosted ends, 1-ml tuberculin syringe without a cannula or needle

Procedure and posttest care

- Obtain a semen specimen for a fertility study by asking the patient to collect semen in a clean plastic specimen container.
- A specimen is obtained from the vagina of a rape victim by direct aspiration, saline lavage, or a direct smear of vaginal contents, using a Pap stick or, less desirably, a cotton applicator stick. Dried smears are usually collected from the suspected rape victim's skin by gently washing the skin with a small piece of gauze moistened with physiologic saline solution.
- Prepare direct smears on glass microscopic slides after labeling the frosted end. Immediately place smeared slides in Coplin jars containing 95% ethanol.
- Before postcoital examination, the examiner wipes any excess mucus from the external cervix and collects the specimen by direct aspiration of the cervical

canal, using a 1-ml tuberculin syringe without a cannula or needle.

- Inform a patient who is undergoing infertility studies that test results should be available in 24 hours.
- Refer the suspected rape victim to an appropriate specialist for counseling—a gynecologist, psychiatrist, clinical psychologist, nursing specialist, member of the clergy, or representative of a community support group, such as Women Organized Against Rape.

Precautions

- If the patient prefers to collect the specimen during coitus interruptus, tell him he must prevent any loss of semen during ejaculation.
- Deliver all specimens, regardless of the source or method of collection, to the laboratory within 1 hour.
- Protect semen specimens for fertility studies from extremes of temperature and direct sunlight during delivery to the laboratory.
- Never lubricate the vaginal speculum. Oil or grease hinders examination of spermatozoa by interfering with smear preparation and staining and by inhibiting sperm motility through toxic ingredients. Instead, moisten the speculum with water or physiologic saline solution.
- Use extreme caution in securing, labeling, and delivering all specimens to be used for medicolegal purposes. You may be asked to testify as to when, where, and from whom the specimen was obtained; the specimen's general appearance and identifying features; steps taken to ensure the specimen's integrity; and when, where, and to whom the specimen was delivered for analysis. If your hospital or clinic uses routing requests for such specimens, fill them out carefully, and place them in the permanent medicolegal file.

Normal findings

Normal semen volume ranges from 0.7 to 6.5 ml. Paradoxically, the semen volume of many men in infertile couples is increased. Abstinence for 1 week or more results in progressively increased semen volume. (With abstinence of up to 10 days, sperm counts increase, sperm motility progressively decreases, and sperm morphology stays the same.) Liquefied semen is generally highly viscid, translucent, and gray-white, with a musty or acrid odor. After liquefaction, specimens of normal viscosity can be poured in drops. Normally, semen is slightly alkaline, with a pH of 7.3 to 7.9

Other normal characteristics of semen: It coagulates immediately and liquefies within 20 minutes; the normal sperm count is 20 to 150 million/ml and can be greater; 40% of spermatozoa have normal morphology; and 20% or more of spermatozoa show progressive motility within 4 hours of collection.

The normal postcoital cervical mucus test shows 10 to 20 motile spermatozoa per microscopic high-power field and spinnbarkeit (a measurement of the tenacity of the mucus) of at least 4″ (10 cm). These findings indicate adequate spermatozoa and receptivity of the cervical mucus. Shaking or dead sperm may indicate antisperm antibodies.

Abnormal findings

Abnormal semen is *not* synonymous with infertility. Only one viable spermatozoon is needed to fertilize an ovum. Although a normal sperm count is 20 million/ml or more, many men with sperm counts below 1 million/ml have fathered normal children. Only men who can't deliver *any* viable spermatozoa in their ejaculate during sexual intercourse are absolutely sterile. Nevertheless, subnormal sperm counts, decreased sperm motility, and abnormal morphology are usually associated with decreased fertility.

Other tests may be necessary to evaluate the patient's general health, metabolic status, or the function of specific endocrine glands (pituitary, thyroid, adrenal, or gonadal).

Interfering factors

- Poor timing of test within the menstrual cycle (abnormal postcoital test results)
- Prior cervical conization or cryotherapy and some medications, such as clomiphene citrate (possible abnormal postcoital test results due to changes in cervical mucus)
- Delayed transport of the specimen, exposure to extreme temperatures or direct sunlight, or the presence of toxic chemicals in the container or the condom (possible decrease in number of viable sperm)
- An incomplete specimen — for example, from coitus interruptus or improper collection technique (decrease in specimen volume)

CONTRACTION STRESS TEST

The contraction stress test, also known as the oxytocin challenge test, measures the fetus's ability to withstand a decreased oxygen supply and the stress of contractions induced before actual labor begins. An infusion of oxytocin (Pitocin) is given to stimulate uterine contractions while the fetal heart rate (FHR) is assessed, to evaluate the placenta's ability to provide sufficient oxygen to the fetus.

Purpose

- To determine and evaluate the fetus's in utero risk of hypoxia or ability to withstand uterine contractions before labor begins
- To determine effects of maternal diabetes or hypertension on fetoplacental adequacy and fetal well-being
- To evaluate high-risk pregnancies
- To determine if vaginal delivery will place the fetus at risk
- To determine the need to terminate the pregnancy by labor induction and early birth when performed in conjunction with other diagnostic studies

Patient preparation

- Explain that the procedure takes about 2 hours and is performed within a controlled environment with specially trained nurses and a physician nearby.
- Inform the patient that food and fluid will be restricted for 4 to 8 hours before the study.
- Review breathing and relaxation techniques the patient may have learned in Lamaze or other childbirth classes, or teach these techniques before the test.
- Inform the patient that she will experience mild contractions and that the fetus and she will be evaluated at all times.
- Vital signs, FHR, assessment, and history will be performed before the test.

Equipment

External monitor for FHR, oxytocin in ordered dosages, I.V. tubing, I.V. access device, dextrose 50 in water, for infusion, ultrasound transducer, tocodynamometer

Procedure and posttest care

- Have the patient empty her bladder.

■ Assist her into a semi-Fowler, side-lying position, and drape her for privacy.
■ Take the patient's blood pressure before and every 10 minutes during the procedure.
■ Place the fetal monitor on her abdomen to monitor FHR and the tocodynamometer on the lower abdomen to monitor contractions. A baseline recording is made and then the FHR is monitored and recorded continuously for 20 minutes.
■ An I.V. line is inserted and I.V. oxytocin is administered via I.V. pump as ordered. The FHR and contractions are monitored and recorded to determine the FHR response to the contractions.
■ Encourage the patient to use deep-breathing and relaxation skills while the oxytocin is administered and she feels the contractions.
■ Continue to monitor the FHR for 30 minutes as uterine movements return to normal.
■ If premature labor begins, note the frequency, strength, and length of contractions, and prepare for labor or cesarean delivery.

Precautions

■ This test is contraindicated in multiple pregnancy, previous cesarean birth or surgical hysterotomy, previous premature labor, premature ruptured membranes, abruptio placentae, placenta previa, and fetus of less than 34 weeks' gestation.

Normal findings

A negative result occurs when the FHR is within normal range (120 to 160 beats/minute), indicating that the fetus can tolerate the stress of labor.

Abnormal findings

Late decelerations in FHR during 2 or more contractions or late decelerations that are inconsistent indicate risk of fetal asphyxia.

Interfering factors

■ Maternal hypotension (false-positive results due to diminished placental blood flow)
■ Full bladder

MISCELLANEOUS TESTS

CEREBROSPINAL FLUID ANALYSIS

For qualitative analysis, cerebrospinal fluid (CSF) is most commonly obtained by lumbar puncture (usually between the third and fourth lumbar vertebrae) and, rarely, by cisternal or ventricular puncture. A CSF specimen may also be obtained during other neurologic tests such as myelography.

Purpose

■ To measure CSF pressure as an aid in detecting obstruction of CSF circulation
■ To aid diagnosis of viral or bacterial meningitis, subarachnoid or intracranial hemorrhage, tumors, and brain abscesses
■ To aid diagnosis of neurosyphilis and chronic central nervous system infections
■ To check for Alzheimer's disease.

Patient preparation

■ Describe the procedure to the patient, and explain that this test analyzes the fluid around the spinal cord.
■ Inform him that he need not restrict food or fluids.

■ Tell him who will perform the procedure and where.
■ Advise the patient that a headache is the most common adverse effect of a lumbar puncture, but reassure him that his cooperation during the test helps minimize this effect.
■ Make sure the patient or his legal guardian has signed the appropriate consent form.
■ If the patient is unusually anxious, assess and report his vital signs.

Equipment

Lumbar puncture tray, sterile gloves, face mask, local anesthetic (usually 1% lidocaine), povidone-iodine solution, small adhesive bandage

Procedure and posttest care

■ Position the patient on his side at the edge of the bed, with his knees drawn up to his abdomen and his chin on his chest. Provide pillows to support the spine on a horizontal plane. This position allows full flexion of the spine and easy access to the lumbar subarachnoid space. Help him maintain this position by placing one arm around his knees and the other arm around his neck.
■ If the sitting position is preferred, have the patient sit up and bend his chest and head toward his knees. Help him maintain this position throughout the procedure.
■ After the skin is prepared for injection, the area is draped. Warn the patient that he'll probably experience a transient burning sensation when the local anesthetic is injected.
■ Tell him that when the spinal needle is inserted, he may feel some transient local pain as the needle transverses the dura mater.
■ Ask him to report any pain or sensations that differ from or continue after this expected discomfort because such sensations may indicate irritation or puncture of a nerve root, requiring repositioning of the needle.
■ Instruct the patient to remain still and breathe normally; movement and hyperventilation can alter pressure readings or cause injury.
■ The anesthetic is injected, and the spinal needle is inserted in the midline, between the spinous processes of the vertebrae (usually between the third and fourth lumbar vertebrae). At this point, initial (or opening) CSF pressure is measured and a specimen is obtained.
■ After the specimen is collected, label the containers in the order in which they were filled, and find out if any specific instructions are required for the laboratory.
■ Next, a final pressure reading is taken, and the needle is removed.
■ Clean the puncture site with a local antiseptic, such as povidone-iodine solution, and apply a small adhesive bandage.
■ Check whether the patient must lie flat or if the head of his bed may be slightly elevated. In most cases, you'll be instructed to keep the patient lying flat for 8 hours after lumbar puncture. Some physicians, however, allow a 30-degree elevation at the head of the bed. Remind the patient that although he must not raise his head, he can turn from side to side.
■ Encourage the patient to drink fluids. Provide a flexible straw.
■ Check the puncture site for redness, swelling, and drainage every hour for the first 4 hours, then every 4 hours for the first 24 hours.
■ If CSF pressure is elevated, assess neurologic status every 15 minutes for 4 hours. If the patient is stable, assess him every hour for 2 hours, and then every 4 hours or according to pretest schedule.

◆ **CLINICAL ALERT** *Watch for complications of lumbar puncture, such as reaction to the anesthetic, meningitis, bleeding* *into the spinal canal, and cerebellar tonsillar herniation and medullary compression. Signs of meningitis include fever, neck rigidity, and irritability; signs of herniation include decreased level of consciousness, changes in pupil size and equality, altered vital signs (including widened pulse pressure, decreased pulse rate, and irregular respirations), or respiratory failure.*

Precautions

- Infection at the puncture site contraindicates removal of CSF; in a patient with increased intracranial pressure, CSF should be removed with extreme caution because the rapid reduction in pressure that follows withdrawal of fluid can cause cerebellar tonsillar herniation and medullary compression.
- During the procedure, observe closely for adverse reactions, such as elevated pulse rate, pallor, or clammy skin. Report any significant changes immediately.
- Record the collection time on the test request form. Send the form and labeled specimens to the laboratory immediately after collection.

Normal findings

For a summary of normal and abnormal findings in CSF analysis, see *Findings in cerebrospinal fluid analysis.*

Normally, the CSF pressure is recorded and the appearance of the specimen is checked. Three tubes are collected routinely and are sent to the laboratory for analysis of protein, sugar, and cells as well as for serologic testing, such as the Venereal Disease Research Laboratory test for neurosyphilis. A separate specimen is also sent to the laboratory for culture and sensitivity testing. Electrolyte analysis and Gram stain may be ordered as supplementary

Findings in cerebrospinal fluid analysis

TEST	NORMAL	ABNORMAL	IMPLICATIONS
Pressure	50 to 180 mm H_2O	Increase	Increased intracranial pressure
		Decrease	Spinal subarachnoid obstruction above puncture site
Appearance	Clear, colorless	Cloudy	Infection
		Xanthochromic or bloody	Subarachnoid, intracerebral, or intraventricular hemorrhage; spinal cord obstruction; traumatic tap (usually noted only in initial specimen)
		Brown, orange, or yellow	Elevated protein levels, red blood cell (RBC) breakdown (blood present for at least 3 days)

(continued)

Findings in cerebrospinal fluid analysis *(continued)*

TEST	NORMAL	ABNORMAL	IMPLICATIONS
Protein	15 to 50 mg/dl (SI, 0.15 to 0.5 g/L)	Marked increase	Tumors, trauma, hemorrhage, diabetes mellitus, polyneuritis, blood in cerebrospinal fluid (CSF)
		Marked decrease	Rapid CSF production
Gamma globulin	3% to 12% of total protein	Increase	Demyelinating disease, neurosyphilis, Gullian-Barré syndrome
Glucose	50 to 80 mg/dl (SI, 2.8 to 4.4 mmol/L)	Increase	Systemic hyperglycemia
		Decrease	Systemic hypoglycemia, bacterial or fungal infection, meningitis, mumps, postsubarachnoid hemorrhage
Cell count	0 to 5 white blood cells	Increase	Active disease: meningitis, acute infection, onset of chronic illness, tumor, abscess, infarction, demyelinating disease
	No RBCs	RBCs	Hemorrhage or traumatic lumbar puncture
Venereal Disease Research Laboratories, test for syphilis, and other serologic tests	Nonreactive	Positive	Neurosyphilis
Chloride	118 to 130 mEq/L (SI, 118 to 130 mmol/L)	Decrease	Infected meninges
Gram stain	No organisms	Gram-positive or gram-negative organisms	Bacterial meningitis

Tests for Alzheimer's disease

Two tests are used for patients with symptoms of dementia. One test determines the level of tau protein in conjunction with beta amyloid in the cerebrospinal fluid and requires a lumbar puncture. Elevated levels of tau and reduced levels of beta amyloid are associated with Alzheimer's disease. The manufacturer claims that this test is 95% accurate in ruling out or confirming Alzheimer's disease in about 60% of symptomatic patients over age 60.

The second test determines apolipoprotein E (apoE) genotype, which is statistically significant in determining the probability of Alzheimer's. The presence of two copies of the apoE4 allele may increase the probability to over 90%.

Although these tests may prove helpful in diagnosing Alzheimer's disease, experts caution that further studies are necessary to confirm their reliability.

tests. CSF electrolyte levels are of special interest in patients with abnormal serum electrolyte levels or CSF infection and in those receiving hyperosmolar agents.

Interfering factors

- Patient position and activity (possible increase or decrease in CSF pressure)
- Crying, coughing, or straining (possible increase in CSF pressure)
- Delay between collection time and laboratory testing (possible invalidation of test results, especially cell counts)

SOLUBLE BETA AMYLOID PROTEIN PRECURSOR

The presence of the beta amyloid protein in the senile plaques of the brain is a hallmark of Alzheimer's disease, leading researchers to believe that this protein may be responsible for the disease's neurotoxic effects. Although amyloid is found in the cerebrospinal fluid (CSF) of healthy people, it's also found in smaller amounts in some patients with dementia, making it a useful diagnostic tool.

Purpose

- To assist in the diagnosis of Alzheimer's disease (See *Tests for Alzheimer's disease.*)

Patient preparation

- Explain to the patient that a specimen of CSF is collected by lumbar puncture, and a small portion is tested using the enzyme-linked immunosorbent assay (ELISA) test.
- Tell the patient who will perform the procedure and where.
- Inform him that he need not restrict food or fluids.
- Advise him that a headache is the most common adverse effect of lumbar puncture, but reassure him that his cooperation during the test helps minimize this effect.
- Make sure a signed consent form has been obtained.

Equipment

Lumbar puncture tray, sterile gloves, local anesthetic (1% lidocaine), povidone-iodine solution, small adhesive bandage

Procedure and posttest care

■ Position the patient on his side at the edge of the bed, with his knees drawn up to his abdomen and his chin on his chest. Provide pillows to support the spine on a horizontal plane. This position allows full flexion of the spine and easy access to the lumbar subarachnoid space. Help the patient maintain this position by placing one arm around his knees and the other arm around his neck.

■ If the sitting position is preferred, have the patient sit up and bend his chest and head toward his knees. Help him maintain this position throughout the procedure.

■ After the skin is prepared for injection, the area is draped. Warn the patient that he'll probably experience a transient burning sensation when the local anesthetic is injected.

■ Tell the patient that when the spinal needle is inserted, he may feel some transient local pain as the needle transverses the dura mater.

■ Ask him to report any pain or other sensations that differ from or continue after this expected discomfort because such sensations could indicate irritation or puncture of a nerve root, requiring repositioning of the needle.

■ Instruct the patient to remain still and breathe normally during the procedure; movement and hyperventilation can alter pressure readings or cause injury.

■ The anesthetic is injected, and the spinal needle is inserted in the midline, between the spinous processes of the vertebrae (usually between the third and fourth lumbar vertebrae). At this point, initial (or opening) CSF pressure is measured and a specimen is obtained.

■ After the specimen is collected, label the containers in the order in which they were filled, and determine if there are any specific instructions for the laboratory.

■ Next, a final pressure reading is taken, and the needle is removed.

■ Clean the puncture site with a local antiseptic such as povidone-iodine solution, and apply a small adhesive bandage.

■ Check whether the patient must lie flat or if the head of his bed may be slightly elevated. In most cases, you'll be instructed to keep the patient lying flat for 8 hours after lumbar puncture. Some physicians, however, allow a 30-degree elevation at the head of the bed. Remind the patient that although he should not raise his head, he can turn from side to side.

■ Encourage the patient to drink fluids. Provide a flexible straw.

■ Check the puncture site for redness, swelling, and drainage every hour for the first 4 hours, then every 4 hours the first 24 hours.

■ If CSF pressure is elevated, assess neurologic status every 15 minutes for 4 hours. If the patient is stable, assess him every hour for 2 hours, and then every 4 hours or according to pretest schedule.

Precautions

■ Infection at the puncture site contraindicates removal of CSF; in a patient with increased intracranial pressure, CSF should be removed with extreme caution because the rapid reduction in pressure that follows withdrawal of fluid can cause cerebellar tonsillar herniation and medullary compression.

■ During the procedure, observe the patient closely for adverse reactions, such as elevated pulse rate, pallor, or clammy skin. Report any significant changes immediately.

■ Record the collection time on the test request form. Send the form and labeled specimens to the laboratory immediately after collection.

Normal findings

Normal beta amyloid protein levels in CSF are greater than 450 units/L, based on age-matched controls using the ELISA test.

Abnormal findings

Soluble beta amyloid protein precursor is found in the CSF of healthy people. Low CSF levels suggest an alteration in the beta amyloid protein precursor processing and beta amyloid protein formation. Low soluble beta amyloid protein precursor levels correlate with clinically diagnosed and autopsy-confirmed Alzheimer's disease.

Interfering factors

- Patient positioning and activity (possible increase or decrease in CSF pressure)
- Crying, coughing, or straining (possible increase in CSF pressure)
- Delay in collection time and laboratory testing

SYNOVIAL FLUID ANALYSIS

In synovial fluid aspiration, or arthrocentesis, a sterile needle is inserted into a joint space — most commonly the knee — to obtain a fluid specimen for analysis. This procedure is indicated for patients with undiagnosed articular disease and symptomatic joint effusion, a condition marked by the excessive accumulation of synovial fluid. Although rare, complications associated with synovial fluid aspiration include joint infection and hemorrhage leading to hemarthrosis (accumulation of blood within the joint).

Purpose

- To aid differential diagnosis of arthritis, particularly septic or crystal-induced arthritis
- To identify the cause and nature of joint effusion
- To relieve the pain and distention resulting from accumulation of fluid within the joint
- To administer a drug locally (usually corticosteroids)

Patient preparation

- Describe the procedure to the patient, and answer any questions he may have.
- Explain that this test helps determine the cause of joint inflammation and swelling and also helps relieve the associated pain.
- Instruct him to fast for 6 to 12 hours before the test if glucose testing of synovial fluid is ordered; otherwise, inform him that he need not restrict food or fluids before the test.
- Tell him who will perform the test and where.
- Warn him that although he'll receive a local anesthetic, he may still feel transient pain when the needle penetrates the joint capsule.
- Make sure the patient or his legal guardian has signed a consent form.
- Check the patient's history for hypersensitivity to iodine compounds (such as povidone-iodine), procaine, lidocaine, or other local anesthetics.
- Administer a sedative, as ordered.

Equipment

Surgical detergent; skin antiseptic (usually tincture of povidone-iodine); alcohol pads; local anesthetic (procaine or lidocaine, 1% or 2%); sterile, disposable 1½" 25G needle; sterile, disposable

1½″ to 2½″ 20G needle; sterile 5-ml syringe for injecting anesthetic; sterile 20-ml syringe for aspiration, 3 ml syringe for administering sedative; sterile dressings; 2″ × 2″ sterile gauze pads; sterile drapes; elastic bandage; tubes for culture, cytologic, clot, and glucose analysis; anticoagulants (heparin, EDTA, and potassium oxalate); venipuncture equipment

For corticosteroid administration: corticosteroid suspension such as hydrocortisone, 2-ml and 5-ml syringes (or one 10-ml syringe if procaine and steroid are to be injected simultaneously)

Procedure and posttest care

- Position the patient, and explain that he'll need to maintain this position throughout the procedure.
- Clean the skin over the puncture site with surgical detergent and alcohol.
- Paint the site with tincture of povidone-iodine, and allow it to air-dry for 2 minutes.
- After the local anesthetic is administered, the aspirating needle is quickly inserted through the skin, subcutaneous tissue, and synovial membrane into the joint space.
- As much fluid as possible is aspirated into the syringe; at least 15 ml should be obtained, although a smaller amount is usually adequate for analysis.
- The joint (except for the area around the puncture site) may be wrapped with an elastic bandage to compress the free fluid into this portion of the sac, ensuring maximal collection of fluid.
- If a corticosteroid is being injected, prepare the dose as necessary. For instillation, the syringe is detached, leaving the needle in the joint, and the syringe containing the steroid is attached to the needle instead.
- After the steroid is injected and the needle withdrawn, wipe the puncture site with an alcohol pad.
- Apply pressure to the puncture site for about 2 minutes to prevent bleeding; then apply a sterile dressing.
- If synovial fluid glucose levels are being measured, perform a venipuncture to obtain a specimen for blood glucose analysis.
- Apply ice or cold packs to the affected joint for 24 to 36 hours after aspiration to decrease pain and swelling. Use pillows for support. If a large quantity of fluid was aspirated, apply an elastic bandage to stabilize the joint.
- If the patient's condition permits, tell him he may resume normal activity immediately after the procedure. However, warn him to avoid excessive use of the affected joint for a few days after the test even if pain and swelling subside.
- Watch for increased pain or fever; these symptoms may indicate joint infection.
- Be careful when handling the dressings and linens of patients with drainage from the joint space, especially if septic arthritis is confirmed or suspected.
- Tell the patient that he may resume his usual diet, as ordered.

Precautions

- Wear gloves when handling all specimens.
- Don't perform the test in areas of skin or wound infections.
- Use strict sterile technique throughout aspiration to prevent contamination of joint space or synovial fluid specimen.
- Add an anticoagulant to the specimen, according to the laboratory tests requested. Gently invert the tube several times to mix the specimen and anticoagulant adequately.
- *For cultures,* obtain 2 to 5 ml of synovial fluid and, if possible, inoculate the medium immediately. Otherwise, add

one or two drops of heparin to the specimen.

- *For cytologic analysis,* add 5 mg of EDTA or one or two drops of heparin to 2 to 5 ml of synovial fluid.
- *For glucose analysis,* add potassium oxalate, as specified by the laboratory, to 3 to 5 ml of fluid.
- *For crystal examination,* add heparin if specified by the laboratory.
- *For other studies,* such as general appearance and clot evaluation, obtain 2 to 5 ml of synovial fluid, but don't add an anticoagulant.
- Send the properly labeled specimens to the laboratory immediately after collection — gonococci are particularly labile. If a white blood cell (WBC) count is being obtained as well, clearly label the specimen "Synovial Fluid" and "Caution: Don't Use Acid Diluents."

Normal findings

Routine examination includes gross analysis for color, clarity, quantity, viscosity, pH, and the presence of a mucin clot as well as microscopic analysis for WBC count and differential. Special examination includes microbiological analysis for formed elements (including crystals) and bacteria, serologic analysis, and chemical analysis for such components as glucose, protein, and enzymes.

Abnormal findings

Examination of synovial fluid may reveal various joint diseases, including noninflammatory disease (traumatic arthritis and osteoarthritis), inflammatory disease (systemic lupus erythematosus, rheumatic fever, pseudogout, gout, and rheumatoid arthritis), and septic disease (tuberculous and septic arthritis).

Interfering factors

- Failure to adhere to dietary restrictions
- Specimen contamination
- Acid diluents added to the specimen for WBC count (alteration in cell count)
- Failure to adequately mix the specimen and the anticoagulant or to send the specimen to the laboratory immediately after collection

PERICARDIAL FLUID ANALYSIS

Analysis of the fluid inside the pericardial sac of the heart is usually done for patients with pericardial effusion (an accumulation of excess pericardial fluid), which may result from inflammation (as in pericarditis), rupture, or penetrating trauma.

Obtaining a specimen for analysis requires needle aspiration of pericardial fluid, a procedure called *pericardiocentesis.* This procedure must be performed cautiously because of the risk of potentially fatal complications, such as myocardial or coronary artery laceration, ventricular fibrillation or vasovagal arrest, pleural infection, or accidental puncture of the lung, liver, or stomach. If possible, echocardiography should determine the effusion site before pericardiocentesis is performed to minimize the risk of complications. (See *Aspirating pericardial fluid,* page 442.)

Purpose

- To assist in identifying the cause of pericardial effusion and to help determine appropriate therapy

Patient preparation

- Explain to the patient that this test detects excessive fluid around the heart, determines its cause, and helps determine appropriate therapy.

Aspirating pericardial fluid

In pericardiocentesis, a needle and syringe assembly is inserted through the chest wall into the pericardial sac, as illustrated below. Electrocardiographic (ECG) monitoring with a leadwire attached to the needle and electrodes placed on the limbs (right arm [RA], right leg [RL], left arm [LA], and left leg [LL]) helps to ensure proper needle placement and to avoid damage to the heart.

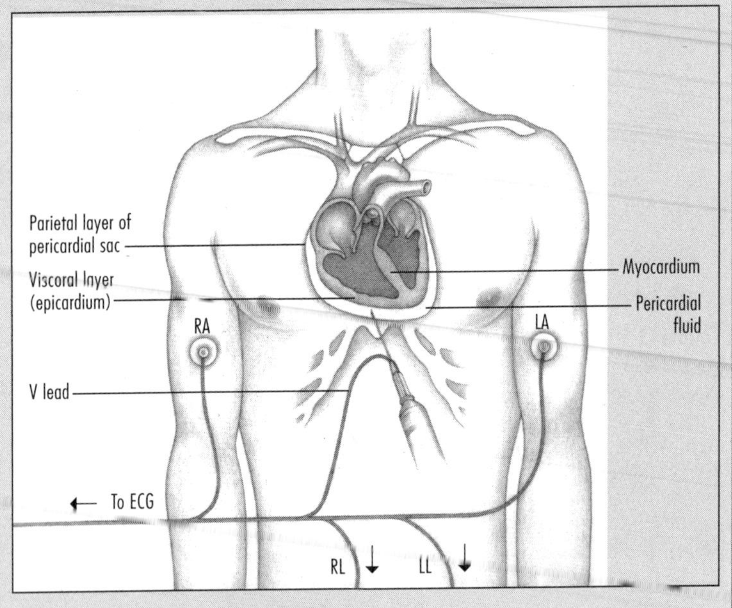

■ Inform him that he need not restrict food or fluids before the test.
■ Tell him who will perform the test and where.
■ Inform the patient that a local anesthetic will be injected before the aspiration needle is inserted.
■ Warn him that although fluid aspiration isn't painful, he may experience pressure upon insertion of the needle into the pericardial sac.
■ Advise him that he may be asked to briefly hold his breath to aid needle insertion and placement.
■ Tell the patient that an I.V. line will be started at a slow rate in case medications need to be administered.
■ Assure him that someone will remain with him during the test and that his pulse and blood pressure will be monitored after the procedure.
■ Check the patient's history for current antimicrobial usage, and record such usage on the test request form.
■ Make sure the patient or a responsible member of the family has signed a consent form.

■ Explain the test to the family if pericardiocentesis is performed to relieve cardiac tamponade and the patient is in shock.

Equipment

70% alcohol or povidone-iodine solution; local anesthetic (1% procaine or 1% lidocaine); sterile 25G needle for the anesthetic; sterile 14G, 16G, and 18G 4″ or 5″ cardiac needles; 50-ml syringe with luer-lock tip; 7-ml sterile test tubes (one clot-activator, one heparin, and one with EDTA); sterile specimen container for culture; vial of heparin 1:1,000; 4″ × 4″ gauze pads; bandage; three-way stopcock. All of these items may be included in a prepackaged pericardiocentesis tray.

Also needed: electrocardiograph (ECG) or bedside monitor, Kelly clamp, alligator clips, defibrillator, and emergency drugs.

Procedure and posttest care

■ Place the patient in the supine position with the thorax elevated 60 degrees.

■ When the patient is comfortable and well supported, instruct him to remain still during the procedure.

■ A local anesthetic is administered at the insertion site after the skin is prepared with alcohol or povidone-iodine solution from the left costal margin to the xiphoid process.

■ With the three-way stopcock open, a 50-ml syringe is aseptically attached to one end and the cardiac needle to the other end.

■ The ECG lead wire is attached to the hub of the needle with an alligator clip. The ECG is set to lead V and turned on (or the patient is connected to a bedside monitor).

■ The needle is inserted through the chest wall into the pericardial sac, maintaining gentle aspiration until fluid appears in the syringe.

■ The needle is angled 35 to 45 degrees toward the tip of the right scapula between the left costal margin and the xiphoid process. A Kelly clamp is attached at the skin surface after the needle is properly positioned so it won't advance further.

■ While the fluid is being aspirated, label and number the specimen tubes.

■ When the needle is withdrawn, apply pressure to the site *immediately* with sterile gauze pads for 3 to 5 minutes. Then apply a bandage.

■ Check blood pressure readings, pulse, respiration, and heart sounds every 15 minutes until stable, then every 1½ hour for 2 hours, every hour for 4 hours, and every 4 hours thereafter. Reassure the patient that such monitoring is routine.

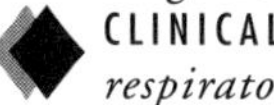

CLINICAL ALERT *Be alert for respiratory or cardiac distress. Watch especially for signs of cardiac tamponade: muffled and distant heart sounds, distended neck veins, paradoxical pulse, and shock. Cardiac tamponade may result from rapid reaccumulation of pericardial fluid or puncture of a coronary vessel causing bleeding into the pericardial sac.*

Precautions

■ Carefully observe the ECG tracing during insertion of the cardiac needle; an ST-segment elevation indicates that the needle has reached the epicardial surface and should be retracted slightly; an abnormally shaped QRS complex may indicate perforation of the myocardium. Premature ventricular contractions usually indicate that the needle has touched the ventricular wall.

■ Watch for grossly bloody aspirate — a sign of inadvertent puncture of a cardiac chamber.

■ Be sure to use specimen tubes with the proper additives. Although fibrin isn't a normal component of pericardial fluid, it does appear in fluid in some pericardial diseases and in carcinoma, and clotting is possible.

■ Clean the top of the culture and sensitivity tube with povidone-iodine solution to reduce the risk of extrinsic contamination.

■ If bacterial culture and sensitivity tests are scheduled, record any antimicrobial therapy the patient is receiving on the laboratory request.

■ If anaerobic organisms are suspected, consult the laboratory concerning the proper collection technique to avoid exposing the aspirate to air. The aspirate may be placed in an anaerobic collection tube or the syringe may be filled completely, displacing all air, and the collection tube capped tightly with a sterile rubber tip.

■ Send all specimens to the laboratory immediately after collection.

■ Have resuscitation equipment on hand.

Normal findings

Normally, 10 to 50 ml of sterile fluid is present in the pericardium. Pericardial fluid is clear and straw-colored, without evidence of pathogens, blood, or malignant cells. It normally contains fewer than 1,000/µl (SI, $< 1.0 \times 10^9$/L) white blood cells (WBCs). Its glucose concentration approximately equals the levels in whole blood.

Abnormal findings

Generally, pericardial effusions are classified as transudates or exudates. Transudates are protein-poor effusions that usually arise from mechanical factors altering fluid formation or resorption, such as increased hydrostatic pressure, decreased plasma oncotic pressure, or obstruction of the pericardial lymphatic drainage system by a tumor.

Most exudates result from inflammation and contain large amounts of protein. In these effusions, inflammation damages the capillary membrane, allowing protein molecules to leak into the pericardial fluid. Exudate effusions may occur in pericarditis, neoplasms, acute myocardial infarction, tuberculosis, rheumatoid disease, and systemic lupus erythematosus.

An elevated WBC count or neutrophil fraction may also accompany inflammatory conditions such as bacterial pericarditis; a high lymphocyte fraction may indicate fungal or tuberculous pericarditis. Turbid or milky effusions may result from the accumulation of lymph or pus in the pericardial sac, or from tuberculosis or rheumatoid disease.

Bloody pericardial fluid may indicate hemopericardium, hemorrhagic pericarditis, or a traumatic tap. Hemopericardium, the accumulation of blood in the pericardium, may result from myocardial rupture after infarction or aortic rupture secondary to a dissecting aortic aneurysm or thoracic trauma. In hemopericardium, the fluid has a hematocrit level similar to that of whole blood; in hemorrhagic pericarditis, it has a relatively low hematocrit and doesn't clot on standing.

Hemorrhagic effusions may indicate a malignant tumor, closed chest trauma, Dressler's syndrome, or postcardiotomy syndrome. A traumatic tap is easily distinguished from hemopericardium or hemorrhagic pericarditis because the fluid becomes progressively clearer.

Glucose concentrations below whole blood levels may reflect increased local metabolism due to malignancy, inflammation, or infection. Possible causes of bacterial pericarditis include *Staphylococcus aureus, Haemophilus influenzae,* and various gram-negative organisms;

possible causes of granulomatous pericarditis include *Mycobacterium tuberculosis* or various fungal agents; and possible causes of viral pericarditis include coxsackieviruses, echoviruses, and others.

Interfering factors

- Failure to use aseptic collection technique, allowing skin contaminants to be mistaken for the causative organism
- Failure to use proper additives in test tubes
- Antimicrobial therapy can prevent isolation of the causative organisms.

SWEAT TEST

The sweat test is a quantitative measurement of electrolyte concentrations (primarily sodium and chloride) in sweat, usually performed using pilocarpine iontophoresis (pilocarpine is a sweat inducer). Although this test is primarily used to confirm cystic fibrosis (CF) in children, it's also performed in adults to determine if they're homozygous or heterozygous for CF.

Purpose

- To confirm CF
- To exclude the diagnosis in siblings of those with CF

Patient preparation

- Explain the test to the child (if he's old enough to understand), using clear, simple terms.
- Inform the child and his parents that there are no restrictions on diet, medication, or activity before the test.
- Tell the child who will perform the test and where.
- Tell him he may feel a slight tickling sensation during the procedure but won't feel any pain.
- Encourage the parents to assist with preparations and to stay with their child during the test. Their presence will minimize the child's anxiety.

Equipment

Analyzer, two skin chloride electrodes (positive and negative), distilled water, two standardizing solutions (chloride concentrations), 2″ × 2″ sterile gauze pads (kept in airtight container), pilocarpine pads, forceps (for handling pads), straps (for securing electrodes), gram scale, normal saline solution

Procedure and posttest care

- Wash the area that will undergo iontophoresis with distilled water and dry it. (The flexor surface of the right forearm is commonly used or, when the patient's arm is too small to secure electrodes [as with an infant], the right thigh.)
- Place a gauze pad saturated with premeasured pilocarpine solution on the positive electrode; place the pad saturated with normal saline solution on the negative electrode.
- Apply both electrodes to the area to undergo iontophoresis, and secure them with straps. Lead wires to the analyzer are given a current of 4 milliamperes in 15 to 20 seconds. Iontophoresis will continue at 15- to 20-second intervals for 5 minutes.
- Try to distract the child with a book, television, toy, or another diversion if he becomes nervous or frightened during the test.
- Remove both electrodes after iontophoresis.
- Discard the pads, clean the skin with distilled water, and then dry it.
- Using forceps, place a dry gauze pad or filter paper (previously weighed on a gram scale) on the area that underwent iontophoresis.
- Cover the pad or filter paper with a slightly larger piece of plastic, and seal

the edges of the plastic with waterproof adhesive tape.

- Leave the gauze pad or filter paper in place for about 30 to 40 minutes. (The appearance of droplets on the plastic usually indicates induction of an adequate amount of sweat.)
- Remove the pad or filter paper with the forceps, place it immediately in the weighing bottle, and insert the stopper in the bottle. (The difference between the first and second weights indicates the weight of the sweat specimen collected.)
- Wash the area that underwent iontophoresis with soap and water, and dry it thoroughly. If the area looks red, reassure the patient that this is normal and will disappear within a few hours.
- Tell the patient or his parents that he may resume his usual activities.

Precautions

- Always perform iontophoresis on the right arm (or right thigh) rather than on the left.
- Never perform iontophoresis on the chest, especially in a child, because the current can induce cardiac arrest.
- Use battery-powered equipment to prevent electric shock if possible.
- Stop the test immediately if the patient complains of a burning sensation, which usually indicates that the positive electrode is exposed or positioned improperly. Adjust the electrode and continue the test.
- Make sure at least 100 mg of sweat is collected for analysis.
- Carefully seal the gauze pad or filter paper in the weighing bottle, and immediately send the bottle to the laboratory.

Reference values

Normal sodium values in sweat range from 10 to 30 mEq/L (SI, 10 to 30 nmol/L). Normal chloride values from 10 to 35 mEq/L (SI, 10 to 35 nmol/L).

Abnormal findings

Sodium concentrations of 50 to 60 mEq/L (SI, 50 to 60 mmol/L) strongly suggests CF. Concentrations above 60 mEq/L (SI, above 60 mmol/L) with typical clinical features confirm the diagnosis.

Only a few conditions other than CF result in elevated sweat electrolyte levels — most notably, untreated adrenal insufficiency, as well as type I glycogen storage disease, vasopressin-resistant diabetes insipidus, meconium ileus, and renal failure. In women, sweat electrolyte levels fluctuate cyclically; chloride concentrations usually peak 5 to 10 days before onset of menses, and most women retain fluid before menses. Men also show fluctuations up to 70 meq/L (SI, 70 mmol/L). However, CF is the only condition that raises sweat electrolyte levels above 80 mEq/L (SI, 80 mmol/L).

Interfering factors

- Dehydration or edema, especially in the area of collection
- Failure to obtain an adequate amount of sweat, a common problem in neonates
- Presence of pure salt depletion, common during hot weather (possible false normal)
- Failure to clean the skin thoroughly or to use sterile gauze pads (possible false high)
- Failure to seal the gauze pad or filter paper carefully (possible false-high electrolyte levels due to evaporation)

UROGENITAL SECRETIONS IN TRICHOMONADS

Microscopic examination of urine or vaginal, urethral, or prostatic secretions can detect urogenital infection by *Trichomonas vaginalis,* a parasitic, flagellate protozoan that's usually transmitted sexually. This test is more commonly performed on women than on men because women are more likely to exhibit symptoms of trichomoniasis; men may exhibit symptoms of urethritis or prostatitis.

Purpose

- To confirm trichomoniasis

Patient preparation

- Explain that this test can identify the cause of urogenital infection.
- If the patient is a woman, tell her the test requires a specimen of vaginal secretions or urethral discharge, and ask her not to douche before the test.
- If the patient is a man, tell him the test requires a specimen of urethral or prostatic secretions.
- Inform the patient who will perform the procedure and when.

Equipment

Gloves, cotton swab, test tube containing small amount of normal saline solution, vaginal speculum, specimen cup (if a urine specimen is being collected)

Procedure and posttest care

Vaginal secretions

- With the patient in the lithotomy position, an unlubricated vaginal speculum is inserted, and discharge is collected with a cotton swab. The swab is then placed in the tube containing normal saline solution, and the speculum is removed.
- Another method is to smear the specimen on a glass slide, allow it to air-dry, and then transport it to the laboratory.

Prostatic material

- After prostatic massage, collect secretions with a cotton swab, and place the swab in normal saline solution.

Urethral discharge

- Collect the discharge with a cotton swab, and place the swab in normal saline solution.

Urine

- Include the first portion of a voided random specimen (not midstream).

All procedures

- Label the specimen container appropriately, including the date and time of collection.
- Provide perineal care.

Precautions

- Remember to use gloves when performing procedures and handling specimens.
- If possible, obtain the urogenital specimen before treatment with a trichomonacide begins.
- Send the specimen to the laboratory immediately after collection because trichomonads can be identified only while they're still motile.

Normal findings

Trichomonads are normally absent from the urogenital tract.

Abnormal findings

Trichomonads confirm trichomoniasis. In approximately 25% of women and in most infected men, trichomonads may be present without associated pathology.

Interfering factors

- Improper collection technique
- Failure to send the specimen to the laboratory immediately after collection, causing trichomonads to lose motility
- Collection of the specimen after trichomonacide therapy begins (fewer trichomonads in the specimen)

8

Cultures

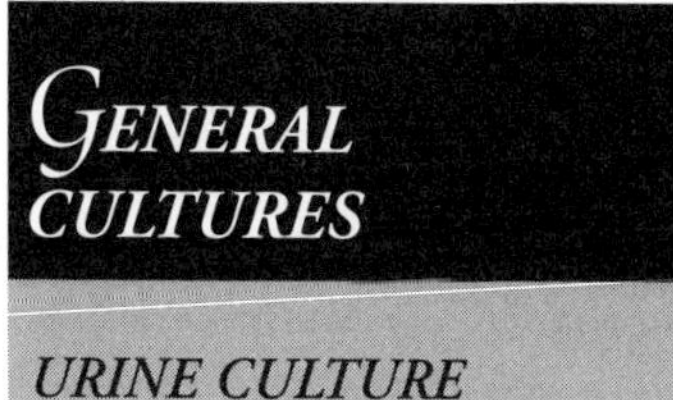

General Cultures

Urine Culture

Laboratory examination and culture of urine are used to evaluate urinary tract infections (UTIs), especially bladder infections. Urine in the kidneys and bladder is normally sterile, but a urine specimen may contain various organisms due to bacteria in the urethra and on external genitalia. Bacteriuria generally results from one prevalent bacteria type; the presence of more than two bacterial species in a specimen strongly suggests contamination during collection. A single negative culture doesn't always rule out infection; a quantitative examination of urine culture is needed.

Purpose

- To diagnose UTI
- To monitor microorganism colonization after urinary catheter insertion

Patient preparation

- Explain to the patient that this test is used to detect UTI.
- Inform the patient that the test requires a urine specimen and that no restriction of food or fluids is necessary.
- Instruct him how to collect a clean-voided midstream specimen; emphasize that external genitalia must be cleaned thoroughly.
- If appropriate, explain catheterization or suprapubic aspiration to the patient, and inform him that he may experience some discomfort during specimen collection.
- For the patient with suspected tuberculosis, specimen collection may be required on three consecutive mornings.
- Check the patient's history for current antimicrobial therapy.

Equipment

Gloves, sterile specimen cup, premoistened antiseptic towelettes (Commercial clean-catch urine kits are available. Many include instructions in several languages.)

Procedure and posttest care

- Collect a urine specimen as ordered.
- When obtaining a specimen from an indwelling catheter, clamp the tubing below the collection port to collect a specimen in the tubing. Then use an alcohol pad to clean the port. Next, using a sterile needle and syringe, aspirate a 4-ml specimen from the port, and transfer it into a sterile specimen cup.
- Seal the cup with a sterile lid, and send it to the laboratory immediately. If transport is delayed longer than 30 minutes, store the specimen at 39.2° F (4° C) or place it on ice, unless a urine transport tube containing preservative is used.
- Instruct the patient to wash his hands, then clean the urethral area with antiseptic towelettes. Tell the patient to begin urinating in the toilet, then stop and continue to urinate into the sterile cup, without touching the inside of the cup.
- Record on the laboratory request the suspected diagnosis, the collection time and method, current antimicrobial therapy, and fluid- or drug-induced diuresis.

Precautions

- Wear gloves when performing the procedure and handling specimens.
- Collect at least 3 ml of urine, but don't fill the specimen cup more than halfway.

Normal findings

Culture results of sterile urine are usually reported as "no growth," which usually indicates the absence of UTI.

Abnormal findings

Bacterial counts of 100,000/ml or more of a single microbe species indicate probable UTI. Counts under 100,000/ml may be significant, depending on the patient's age, sex, history, and other individual factors. Counts under 10,000/ml usually suggest that the organisms are contaminants, except in symptomatic patients, those with urologic disorders, and those whose urine specimens were collected by suprapubic aspiration. A special test for acid-fast bacteria isolates *Mycobacterium tuberculosis,* thus indicating tuberculosis of the urinary tract.

Isolation of more than two species of organisms or of vaginal or skin organisms usually suggests contamination and requires a repeat culture. Prolonged catheterization or urinary diversion may cause polymicrobial infection.

Interfering factors

- Failure to use proper collection technique
- Failure to preserve the specimen properly or to send it to the laboratory immediately
- Fluid- or drug-induced diuresis and antimicrobial therapy (possible decrease)

STOOL CULTURE

Normal bacterial flora in stool include several potentially pathogenic organisms. Bacteriologic examination is valuable for identifying pathogens that cause overt GI disease — such as typhoid and dysentery — and carrier states. A sensitivity test may follow isolation of the pathogen. Stool culture may also be used to detect certain viruses such as enterovirus, which can cause aseptic meningitis.

Purpose

- To identify pathogenic organisms caused by GI disease
- To identify carrier states

Patient preparation

- Explain to the patient that this test is used to determine the cause of GI distress or to determine if he's a carrier of infectious organisms.
- Advise him that food and fluids need not be restricted.
- Tell the patient that the test requires the collection of a stool specimen on 3 consecutive days.
- Check the patient's history for dietary patterns, recent antimicrobial therapy, and recent travel that might suggest endemic infections or infestations.

Equipment

Gloves, waterproof container with tight-fitting lid or sterile swab and commercial sterile collection and transport system, tongue blade, bedpan (if needed)

Procedure and posttest care

- Collect a stool specimen directly into the container. If the patient isn't ambulatory, collect the specimen in a clean, dry bedpan and, using a tongue blade, transfer the specimen to the container.
- If you must collect the specimen by rectal swab, insert the swab past the anal sphincter, rotate it gently, and withdraw it. Then place the swab in the appropriate container.

- Check with the laboratory for the proper collection procedure before obtaining a specimen for a virus test.
- Label the specimen with the patient's name, physician's name, facility number, and date and time of collection.
- Indicate the suspected cause of enteritis and current antimicrobial therapy on the laboratory request.

Precautions

- Wear gloves when performing the procedure and handling the specimen.
- If the patient uses a bedpan or a diaper, avoid contaminating the stool specimen with urine.
- The specimen must represent the first, middle, and last portion of the stool passed. Be sure to include mucoid and bloody portions.
- Put the specimen container in a leakproof bag.
- Send the specimen to the laboratory immediately. Trophozoites and cysts may be destroyed if exposed to heat, cold, or a delay in delivery to the laboratory.
- Specimens should be colleted before antimicrobial therapy is started.

Normal findings

A large percentage of normal fecal flora consists of anaerobes, including non-spore-forming bacilli, clostridia, and anaerobic streptococci. The remaining percentage consists of aerobes, including gram-negative bacilli (predominantly *Escherichia coli* and other Enterobacteriaceae, plus small amounts of *Pseudomonas*), gram-positive cocci (mostly enterococci), and a few yeasts.

Abnormal findings

The most common pathogenic organisms of the GI tract are *Shigella, Salmonella,* and *Campylobacter jejuni.* Less common pathogenic organisms include *Vibrio cholerae, V. parahaemolyticus, Clostridium botulinum, C. difficile, C. perfringens, Staphylococcus aureus,* enterotoxigenic *E. coli,* and *Yersinia enterocolitica.* Isolation of some pathogens indicates bacterial infection in patients with acute diarrhea and may require antimicrobial sensitivity tests. Normal fecal flora may include *C. difficile, E. coli,* and other organisms. Therefore, isolation of these organisms may require further tests to demonstrate invasiveness or toxin production.

Isolation of pathogens such as *C. botulinum* indicates food poisoning; the pathogens must also be isolated from the contaminated food. In a patient undergoing long-term antimicrobial therapy, isolation of large numbers of *S. aureus* or yeast may indicate infection. (Asymptomatic carrier states are also indicated by these enteric pathogens.) Isolation of enteroviruses may indicate aseptic meningitis.

If a stool culture shows no unusual growth, detection of viruses by immunoassay or electron microscopy may be used to diagnose nonbacterial gastroenteritis. Highly increased polymorphonuclear leukocytes in fecal material may indicate an invasive pathogen.

Interfering factors

- Failure to use proper collection technique
- Contamination of the specimen by urine (possible injury to or destruction of enteric pathogens)
- Antimicrobial therapy (possible decrease in bacterial growth)
- Failure to transport the specimen promptly or, if delivery is delayed, to use a transport medium such as buffered glycerol that stabilizes pH (possible loss of enteric pathogens or overgrowth of nonpathogenic organisms)

THROAT CULTURE

A throat culture is used primarily to isolate and identify pathogens. Culture results are considered in relation to the patient's clinical status, recent antimicrobial therapy, and amount of normal flora.

Purpose

- To isolate and identify group A beta-hemolytic streptococci
- To screen asymptomatic carriers of pathogens, especially *Neisseria meningitidis*

Patient preparation

- Explain to the patient that this test is used to identify microorganisms that may be causing his symptoms or to screen for asymptomatic carriers.
- Inform him that he need not restrict food or fluids before the test.
- Tell him that a specimen will be collected from his throat and who will collect the specimen and when.
- Describe the procedure, and warn him that he may gag during the swabbing.
- Check the patient's history for recent antimicrobial therapy. Determine immunization history if pertinent to preliminary diagnosis.

Equipment

Gloves, sterile swab and culture tube with transport medium or commercial collection and transport system

Procedure and posttest care

- Tell the patient to tilt his head back and close his eyes.
- With the throat well illuminated, check for inflamed areas, using a tongue blade.
- Swab the tonsillar areas from side to side; include inflamed or purulent sites.
- *Don't* touch the tongue, cheeks, or teeth with the swab.
- Immediately place the swab in the culture tube.
- If a commercial sterile collection and transport system is used, crush the ampule and force the swab into the medium to keep the swab moist.
- Note recent antimicrobial therapy on the laboratory request; label the specimen with the patient's name, the physician's name, the date and time of collection, and the origin of the specimen; indicate the suspected organism, especially *C. diphtheriae* (requires two swabs and special growth medium), *Bordetella pertussis* (requires a nasopharyngeal culture and a special growth medium), and *N. meningitidis* (requires enriched selective media).
- Nonculture antigen testing methods can be used to detect group A streptococcal antigen in as few as 5 minutes. Cultures are then performed on negative specimens.

Precautions

- Procure the throat specimen before beginning antimicrobial therapy.
- Wear gloves when performing the procedure and handling specimens.
- Send the specimen to the laboratory immediately. Unless a commercial sterile collection and transport system is used, keep the container upright during transport.

◆ **CLINICAL ALERT** *Laryngospasm may occur after the culture is obtained if the patient has epiglottiditis or diphtheria. Keep resuscitation equipment nearby.*

- Obtain the throat specimen before beginning microbial therapy.

Normal findings

Normal throat flora include nonhemolytic and alpha-hemolytic streptococci, *Neisseria* species, staphylococci, diphtheroids, some hemophilus, pneumococci, yeasts, enteric gram-negative rods, spirochetes, *Veillonella* species, and *Micrococcus* species.

Abnormal findings

Pathogens that may be cultured include group A beta-hemolytic streptococci *(S. Pyogenes),* which can cause scarlet fever and pharyngitis; *C. albicans,* which can cause thrush; *C. diphtheriae,* which can cause diphtheria; and *B. pertussis,* which can cause whooping cough. The laboratory report should indicate the prevalent organisms and the quantity of pathogens cultured.

Interfering factors

- Failure to report recent or current antimicrobial therapy on the laboratory request (possible false-negative)
- Failure to use the proper transport medium
- More than a 15-minute delay in sending the specimen to the laboratory

NASOPHARYNGEAL CULTURE

A nasopharyngeal culture is used to evaluate nasopharyngeal secretions for the presence of pathogenic organisms. It requires direct microscopic examination of a Gram-stained smear of the specimen. Preliminary identification of organisms may be used to guide clinical management and determine the need for additional testing. Cultured pathogens may then require susceptibility testing to determine appropriate antimicrobial therapy.

Purpose

- To identify pathogens causing upper respiratory tract symptoms
- To identify proliferation of normal nasopharyngeal flora, which may be pathogenic in debilitated and other immunocompromised patients
- To identify *B. pertussis* and *N. meningitidis,* especially in very young, elderly, or debilitated patients and asymptomatic carriers
- Infrequently, to isolate viruses, especially to identify carriers of influenza virus A and B

Patient preparation

- Explain to the patient that this test is used to isolate the cause of nasopharyngeal infection.
- Describe the procedure to the patient; tell him that secretions will be obtained from the back of the nose and the throat, using a cotton-tipped swab, and who will collect the specimen.
- Warn him that he may experience slight discomfort and gagging, but reassure him that obtaining the specimen takes less than 15 seconds.

Equipment

Gloves; penlight; sterile, flexible wire swab; small, sterile, open-ended glass tube or sterile nasal speculum; tongue blade; culture tube; transport medium (broth), sterile water or saline

Procedure and posttest care

- Put on gloves.
- Moisten the swab with sterile water or saline.
- Ask the patient to cough before you begin collecting the specimen.
- Position the patient with his head tilted back.
- Using a penlight and a tongue blade, inspect the nasopharyngeal area.
- Gently pass the swab through the nostril and into the nasopharynx, keep-

ing the swab near the septum and floor of the nose. Rotate the swab quickly and remove it.

- Alternatively, place the glass tube in the patient's nostril, and carefully pass the swab through the tube into the nasopharynx. Rotate the swab for 5 seconds; then place it in the culture tube with transport medium. Remove the glass tube.
- Label the specimen with the patient's name, the physician's name, the date and time of collection, the origin of the material, and the suspected organism.
- Ideally, specimens for *B. pertussis* should be inoculated to fresh culture medium at the patient's bedside because of the organism's susceptibility to environmental changes.
- If the purpose of specimen collection is to isolate a virus, follow the laboratory's recommended collection technique.

Precautions

- Wear gloves when performing the procedure and handling the specimen.
- *Don't* let the swab touch the sides of the patient's nostril or his tongue to prevent specimen contamination.

◆ CLINICAL ALERT *Laryngospasm may occur after the culture is obtained if the patient has epiglottitis or diphtheria. Keep resuscitation equipment nearby.*

- Note antimicrobial therapy or chemotherapy on the laboratory request.
- Keep the container upright.
- Tell the laboratory if the suspected organism is *Corynebacterium diphtheriae* or *B. pertussis* because these need special growth media.
- Refrigerate a viral specimen according to your laboratory's procedure.
- If *B. pertussis* is suspected, Dacron or calcium alginate mini-tipped swabs should be used for collection.
- When specimens can't be directly placed onto growth media, the best media-based transport is one supplemented with antibiotics to reduce the growth of normal flora.

Normal findings

Flora commonly found in the nasopharynx include nonhemolytic streptococci, alpha-hemolytic streptococci, *Neisseria* species (except *N. meningitidis* and *N. gonorrhoeae*), coagulase-negative staphylococci such as *S. epidermidis* and, occasionally, the coagulase-positive *S. aureus.*

Abnormal findings

Pathogens include group A beta-hemolytic streptococci; occasionally groups B, C, and G beta-hemolytic streptococci; *B. pertussis, C. diphtheriae, S. aureus;* large numbers of pneumococci; *Haemophilus influenzae;* Myxovirus influenzae; paramyxoviruses; *Candida albicans;* mycoplasma species; and *M. tuberculosis.*

Interfering factors

- Recent antimicrobial therapy (decrease in bacterial growth)
- Failure to use proper collection technique
- Failure to place the specimen in transport medium
- Failure to keep a viral specimen cold
- Failure to send the specimen to the laboratory immediately

SPUTUM CULTURE

Bacteriologic examination of sputum (material raised from the lungs and bronchi) is an important aid to the management of lung disease. The usual method of specimen collection is deep coughing and expectoration, which may require ultrasonic nebulization, hydration, or chest physiotherapy; other methods include tracheal suctioning and bronchoscopy.

Purpose

- To isolate and identify the cause of pulmonary infection, thus aiding diagnosis of respiratory diseases (most commonly bronchitis, tuberculosis, lung abscess, and pneumonia)

Patient preparation

- Explain to the patient that this test is used to identify the organism causing respiratory tract infection.
- Tell him the test requires a sputum specimen and who will collect the specimen.
- If the suspected organism is *M. tuberculosis,* tell the patient that as many as three consecutive morning specimens may be required.
- If testing is for tuberculosis, explain that cultures for tuberculosis may take some time to develop; therefore, diagnosis of this disorder generally depends on clinical symptoms, a smear for acid-fast bacilli, a chest X-ray, and response to a purified protein derivative skin test.
- If the specimen is to be collected by expectoration, encourage fluid intake the night before collection to help sputum production, unless contraindicated by a fluid restriction. Teach the patient how to expectorate by taking three deep breaths and forcing a deep cough; emphasize that sputum isn't the same as saliva, which is unacceptable for culturing. Tell him to brush his teeth and gargle with water before the specimen collection to reduce contaminating oropharyngeal bacteria.
- If the specimen is to be collected by tracheal suctioning, tell the patient he'll experience discomfort as the catheter passes into the trachea.
- If the specimen is to be collected by bronchoscopy, instruct the patient to fast for 6 hours before the procedure. Make sure he or a responsible family member has signed an informed consent form. Tell him he'll receive a local anesthetic just before the test to minimize discomfort during passage of the tube.

Equipment

For expectoration: clean gloves, sterile, disposable, impermeable container with a tight-fitting cap; normal saline solution, acetylcysteine, propylene glycol, or sterile or distilled water aerosols to induce cough; leakproof bag

For tracheal suctioning: #16 or #18 French suction catheter, water-soluble lubricant, sterile gloves, sterile specimen container or in-line specimen trap, normal saline solution

For bronchoscopy: bronchoscope, local anesthetic, sterile needle and syringe, sterile specimen container, normal saline solution, bronchial brush, sterile gloves

Procedure and posttest care

Expectoration

- Put on gloves.
- Instruct the patient to cough deeply and expectorate into the container. If the cough is nonproductive, use chest physiotherapy or heated aerosol spray (nebulization) to induce sputum. Using sterile technique, close the container securely.
- Dispose of equipment properly; seal the container in a leakproof bag before sending it to the laboratory.

Tracheal suctioning

- Administer oxygen to the patient before and after the procedure if necessary.
- Attach the sputum trap to the suction catheter. Using sterile gloves, lubricate the catheter with normal saline solution, and pass it through the patient's

nostril without suction. (The patient will cough when the catheter passes through the larynx.) Advance the catheter into the trachea. Apply suction for no longer than 15 seconds to obtain the specimen.

■ Stop suction and gently remove the catheter. Discard the catheter and gloves in the proper receptacle. Then detach the in-line sputum trap from the suction apparatus, and cap the opening.

Bronchoscopy

■ After a local anesthetic is sprayed into the patient's throat or the patient gargles with a local anesthetic, the bronchoscope is inserted through the pharynx and trachea into the bronchus.

■ Secretions are then collected with a bronchial brush or aspirated through the inner channel of the scope, using an irrigating solution such as normal saline solution if necessary.

■ After the specimen is obtained, the bronchoscope is removed.

◆ CLINICAL ALERT *During and after bronchoscopy, observe the patient carefully for signs of hypoxemia (change in mental status), laryngospasm (laryngeal stridor), bronchospasm (paroxysms of coughing or wheezing), pneumothorax (dyspnea, cyanosis, pleural pain, tachycardia), perforation of the trachea or bronchus (subcutaneous crepitus), and trauma to respiratory structures (blood-tinged sputum, coughing up blood). Also, check for difficulty in breathing or swallowing. Don't give liquids until the gag reflex returns.*

All collection methods

■ Provide good mouth care.

■ Label the container with the patient's name. Include on the test request form the nature and origin of the specimen, the date and time of collection, the initial diagnosis, and any current antimicrobial therapy.

Precautions

■ Tracheal suctioning is contraindicated in patients with esophageal varices.

■ In a patient with asthma or chronic bronchitis, watch for aggravated bronchospasms with use of normal saline solution or acetylcysteine in an aerosol.

◆ CLINICAL ALERT *During tracheal suctioning, suction for only 5 to 10 seconds at a time. Never suction longer than 15 seconds. If the patient becomes hypoxic or cyanotic, remove the catheter immediately and administer oxygen.*

■ Wear gloves when performing the procedure and handling specimens.

■ Because the patient may cough violently during suctioning, wear gloves, a mask and, if necessary, a gown to avoid exposure to pathogens.

■ *Don't* use more than 20% propylene glycol with water as an inducer for a specimen scheduled for tuberculosis culturing because higher concentrations inhibit the growth of *M. tuberculosis.* (If propylene glycol isn't available, use 10% to 20% acetylcysteine with water or saline solution.)

■ Send the specimen to the laboratory immediately after collection.

Normal findings

Flora commonly found in the respiratory tract include alpha-hemolytic streptococci, *Neisseria* species, and diphtheroids. The presence of normal flora doesn't rule out infection.

Abnormal findings

Because sputum is invariably contaminated with normal oropharyngeal flora, a culture isolate must be interpreted in light of the patient's overall clinical condition. Isolation of *M. tuberculosis* is always a significant finding.

Interfering factors

- Failure to use proper collection technique
- Failure to report current or recent antimicrobial therapy on the laboratory request (possible false-negative)
- Collection over an extended period, which may cause pathogens to deteriorate or become overgrown by commensals (not accepted as a valid specimen by laboratories)

BLOOD CULTURE

A blood culture is performed to isolate and aid identification of the pathogens in bacteremia (bacterial invasion of the bloodstream) and septicemia (systemic spread of such infection). It requires inoculating a culture medium with a blood sample and incubating it.

Purpose

- To confirm bacteremia
- To identify the causative organism in bacteremia and septicemia

Patient preparation

- Explain to the patient that this procedure is used to help identify the organism causing his symptoms.
- Inform him that he need not restrict food or fluids before the test.
- Tell him how many samples the test will require and who will perform the venipunctures and when.
- Inform him that he may experience transient discomfort from the needle punctures and the tourniquet.

Equipment

Gloves; tourniquet; small adhesive bandages; alcohol swabs; povidone-iodine swabs; 10- to 20-ml syringe for an adult, 6-ml syringe for a child; three or four sterile needles; two blood culture bottles, one vented (aerobic) and one unvented (anaerobic), with nutritionally enriched broths and sodium polyethanol sulfonate added, or bottles with resin or a lysis-centrifugation tube

Procedure and posttest care

- Put on gloves.
- Clean the venipuncture site with an alcohol swab and then with an iodine swab, working in a circular motion from the site outward.
- Wait at least 1 minute for the skin to dry, and remove the residual iodine with an alcohol swab or remove the iodine after venipuncture.
- Apply the tourniquet.
- Perform a venipuncture; draw 10 to 20 ml of blood for an adult or 2 to 6 ml for a child.
- Clean the diaphragm tops of the culture bottles with alcohol or iodine, and change the needle on the syringe.
- If broth is used, add blood to each bottle until a 1:5 or 1:10 dilution is obtained. For example, add 10 ml of blood to a 100-ml bottle. (The size of the bottle varies, depending on facility procedure.)
- If a special resin is used, add blood to the resin in the bottles and invert them gently to mix.
- If you're using the lysis-centrifugation technique (Isolator), draw the blood directly into a special collection and processing tube.
- Indicate the tentative diagnosis on the laboratory request, and note current or recent antimicrobial therapy.
- Apply direct pressure to the venipuncture site until bleeding stops.
- If a hematoma develops at the venipuncture site, apply warm soaks.

Precautions

- Wear gloves when performing the procedure and handling specimens.

■ Send each specimen to the laboratory immediately after collection.
■ Don't draw blood from an existing I.V. catheter. Use a vein below an I.V. catheter or in the opposite arm.
■ Whenever possible, blood cultures should be collected prior to administration of antimicrobial agents.

Normal findings

Normally, blood cultures are negative for pathogens.

Abnormal findings

Positive blood cultures don't necessarily confirm pathologic septicemia. Mild, transient bacteremia may occur during the course of many infectious diseases or may complicate other disorders. Persistent, continuous, or recurrent bacteremia reliably confirms the presence of serious infection. To detect most causative agents, blood cultures are ideally drawn on 2 consecutive days.

Isolation of most organisms takes about 72 hours; negative cultures are held for 1 or more weeks before being reported negative.

Common blood pathogens include *Streptococcus pneumoniae* and other *Streptococcus* species, *H. influenzae, S. aureus, Pseudomonas aeruginosa, Bacteroides, Brucella,* Enterobacteriaceae, coliform bacilli, and *C. albicans.* Although 2% to 3% of cultured blood samples are contaminated by skin bacteria, such as *S. epidermidis,* diphtheroids, and *Propionibacterium,* these organisms may be clinically significant when isolated from multiple cultures or from immunocompromised patients. Debilitated or immunocompromised patients may have isolates of *C. albicans.* In patients with human immunodeficiency virus infection, *M. tuberculosis* and *M. avium* complex may be isolated as well as other mycobacterium species on a less frequent basis.

Interfering factors

■ Previous or current antimicrobial therapy on the laboratory request (possible false-negative)
■ Failure to use proper collection technique
■ Removal of culture bottle caps at the bedside (possible prevention of anaerobic growth)
■ Use of incorrect bottle and media (possible prevention of aerobic growth)

WOUND CULTURE

Performed to confirm infection, a wound culture is a microscopic analysis of a specimen from a lesion. Wound cultures may be aerobic, for detection of organisms that usually appear in a superficial wound, or anaerobic, for organisms that need little or no oxygen and appear in areas of poor tissue perfusion, such as postoperative wounds, ulcers, and compound fractures. Indications for wound culture include fever as well as inflammation and drainage in damaged tissue.

Purpose

■ To identify an infectious microbe in a wound

Patient preparation

■ Explain to the patient that this test is used to identify infectious microbes.
■ Describe the procedure, informing the patient that a drainage specimen from the wound is withdrawn by a syringe or removed on sterile cotton swabs.
■ Tell him who will collect the specimen.

Equipment

Sterile cotton swabs and sterile culture tube or commercial sterile collection

Anaerobic specimen collector

Some anaerobes die when exposed to oxygen. To facilitate anaerobic collection and culturing, tubes filled with carbon dioxide (CO_2) or nitrogen are used for oxygen-free transport.

The anaerobic specimen collector shown here consists of a rubber-stoppered tube filled with CO_2, a small inner tube, and a swab attached to a plastic plunger. The drawing on the left shows the tube before specimen collection. The small inner tube containing the swab is held in place by the rubber stopper.

After specimen collection (right), the swab is quickly replaced in the inner tube, and the plunger is depressed. This separates the inner tube from the stopper, forcing it into the larger tube and exposing the specimen to the CO_2-rich environment.

The tube should be kept upright.

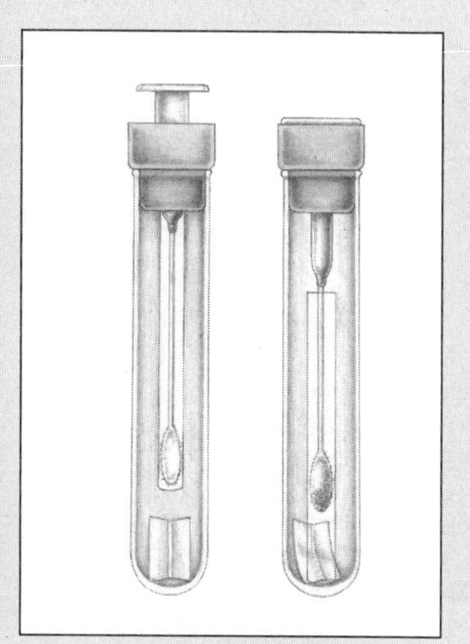

and transport system (for aerobic culture); sterile cotton swabs or sterile 10-ml syringe with 21G needle, and special culture tube containing carbon dioxide or nitrogen (for anaerobic culture); sterile gloves; alcohol pads; sterile gauze; povidone-iodine solution

Procedure and posttest care

- Put on gloves, prepare a sterile field, and clean the area around the wound with antiseptic solution.
- For an *aerobic culture,* express the wound and swab as much exudate as possible, or insert the swab deeply into the wound and gently rotate. Immediately place the swab in the aerobic culture tube.
- For an *anaerobic culture,* insert the swab deeply into the wound, gently rotate, and immediately place the swab in the anaerobic culture tube. (See *Anaerobic specimen collector.*) Or insert the needle into the wound, aspirate 1 to 5 ml of exudate into the syringe, and immediately inject the exudate into the anaerobic culture tube. If the needle is covered with a rubber stopper, the aspirate may be sent to the laboratory in the syringe.
- Record on the laboratory request recent antimicrobial therapy, the source of the specimen, and the suspected organism. Label the specimen container with the patient's name, the physician's name, the facility number, the wound site, and the time of collection.
- Dress the wound.

Precautions

- Clean the area around the wound thoroughly to limit contamination of the culture by normal skin flora, such as diphtheroids, *S. epidermidis,* and alpha-hemolytic streptococci. *Don't* clean the area around a perineal wound.

- Make sure no antiseptic enters the wound.
- Obtain exudate from the entire wound, using more than one swab if necessary.
- Because some anaerobes die in the presence of even a small amount of oxygen, place the specimen in the culture tube quickly, take care that no air enters the tube, and check that double stoppers are secure.
- Keep the specimen container upright, and send it to the laboratory within 15 minutes to prevent growth or deterioration of microbes.
- Wear gloves during the procedure and when handling the specimen, and take necessary isolation precautions when sending the specimen to the laboratory.

Normal findings

Normally, no pathogenic organisms are present in a clean wound.

Abnormal findings

The most common aerobic pathogens for wound infection include *S. aureus,* group A beta-hemolytic streptococci, *Proteus, E. coli* and other Enterobacteriaceae, and some *Pseudomonas* species; the most common anaerobic pathogens include some *Clostridium, Peptococcus, Bacteroides,* and *Streptococcus* species.

Interfering factors

- Failure to report recent or current antimicrobial therapy (possible false-negative)
- Failure to use proper collection technique
- Failure to use the proper transport medium, allowing the specimen to dry and the bacteria to deteriorate

GASTRIC CULTURE

A gastric culture requires aspiration of gastric contents and cultivation of any microbes present. Performed in conjunction with a chest X-ray and a purified protein derivative skin test, it's especially useful when a sputum specimen can't be obtained by expectoration or nebulization. Gastric aspiration also provides a specimen for rapid presumptive identification of bacteria (by Gram stain) in neonatal septicemia.

Purpose

- To aid diagnosis of mycobacterial infections
- To identify the infectious bacteria in neonatal septicemia

Patient preparation

- Explain to the patient (or parents if the patient is a child) that gastric culture helps diagnose tuberculosis.
- Instruct him to fast for 8 hours before the test.
- Tell him who will perform the procedure and that the same procedure may be performed on 3 consecutive mornings.
- Instruct him to remain in bed each morning until specimen collection has been completed to prevent premature emptying of stomach contents.
- Describe the procedure to the patient. Tell him that the nasogastric (NG) tube may make him gag but that it passes more easily if he relaxes and follows instructions about breathing and swallowing.
- Just before the procedure, obtain baseline oxygen saturation and heart rate and rhythm, and place the patient in high Fowler's position.

■ Inform the patient (or his parents) that test results may be prolonged because acid-fast bacteria is slow-growing.
■ Check the patient's history for recent antimicrobial therapy. Inform the physician of your findings; he may want to discontinue medications before the test.

Equipment

Water-soluble lubricating jelly; sterile water; #16 or #18 French disposable, plastic NG tube; 50-ml sterile syringe; sterile specimen container; sterile gloves; emesis basin; stethoscope; clamp (if necessary)

Procedure and posttest care

■ As soon as the patient awakens in the morning, put on gloves, perform NG insertion, confirming position, and obtain gastric washings.
■ Clamp the tube before quickly removing it from the patient.
■ Note recent antimicrobial therapy on the laboratory request, along with the site and time of collection.
■ Label the specimen container with the patient's name, the physician's name, and the facility number.
■ Resume administration of medications discontinued before the test as ordered.
■ Instruct the patient not to blow his nose for 4 hours to prevent bleeding.
■ Tell the patient that he may resume his normal diet.

Precautions

■ Gastric insertion is contraindicated in pregnancy, esophageal disorders (varices, stenosis, diverticula), malignant neoplasms, recent severe gastric hemorrhage, aortic aneurysm, heart failure, and myocardial infarction.
■ If possible, obtain the specimens before the start of antimicrobial therapy.
■ Watch for signs that the tube has entered the trachea, including coughing, cyanosis, decreasing oxygen saturation readings, and gasping.

◆ **CLINICAL ALERT** *Never inject water into an NG tube unless you're sure the tube is correctly placed in the patient's stomach. During lavage, use sterile distilled water to decrease the risk of contamination with saprophytic mycobacteria.*

■ Check the patient's pulse rate for irregularities during this procedure to detect arrhythmias and monitor for signs of hypoxia.
■ Wear gloves when performing the procedure and when handling specimens and the NG tube.
■ Put the specimen in a tightly capped container, wipe the outside of the container with disinfectant, and place it upright in a plastic bag.
■ Send the specimen to the laboratory immediately.
■ Dispose of all equipment carefully to prevent staff contamination.

Normal findings

Normally, the culture specimen is negative for pathogenic mycobacteria.

Abnormal findings

Isolation and identification of the organism *M. tuberculosis* indicates the presence of active tuberculosis; other species of *Mycobacterium,* such as *M. bovis, M. kansasii, and M. avium,* may cause pulmonary disease that's clinically indistinguishable from tuberculosis. Treatment of these mycobacterial infections may be difficult and commonly requires susceptibility studies to determine the most effective antimicrobial therapy. Pathogenic bacteria causing neonatal septicemia may also be identified through culture.

Interfering factors

- Failure to observe an 8-hour fast before the test (possible decrease)
- Drugs such as tetracycline and aminoglycosides (possible false-negative)
- Presence of saprophytic mycobacteria in gastric contents because these mycobacteria can't be microscopically distinguished from pathogenic mycobacteria (possible false-positive acid-fast smears)

DUODENAL CONTENTS CULTURE

A duodenal contents culture requires duodenal tube insertion, aspiration of duodenal contents, and cultivation of microbes to isolate and identify pathogens that may cause duodenitis, cholecystitis, and cholangitis. Occasionally, a specimen may be obtained during surgery.

Purpose

- To detect bacterial infection of the biliary tract and duodenum
- To differentiate between infection and gallstones
- To rule out bacterial infection as the cause of persistent GI symptoms (epigastric pain, nausea, vomiting, and diarrhea)

Patient preparation

- Explain to the patient that this test is used to determine the cause of his symptoms.
- Instruct him to restrict food and fluids for 12 hours before the test.
- Tell him who will perform the procedure and where it will be done.
- Describe the insertion procedure to the patient. Assure him that although this procedure is uncomfortable, it isn't dangerous; tell him that passage of the tube may cause gagging but that following the examiner's instructions about proper positioning, breathing, swallowing, and relaxing will minimize his discomfort.
- Suggest that he empty his bladder before the procedure to increase his general comfort.

Equipment

Gloves, double-lumen nasoenteric tube with olive tip, water-soluble jelly, 30-ml sterile syringe, emesis basin, sterile specimen container, ½" adhesive tape

Procedure and posttest care

- After the nasoenteric tube is inserted, place the patient in a left lateral decubitus position with his feet elevated to allow peristalsis to move the tube into the duodenum.
- Determine the pH of a small amount of aspirated fluid to ascertain tube position. If the tube is in the stomach, pH is lower than 7.0; if the tube is in the duodenum, pH is higher than 7.0.
- The position of the tube can also be confirmed by fluoroscopy.
- Aspirate duodenal contents.
- Occasionally, a specimen for culture of duodenal contents is obtained during duodenoscopy. (See "Esophagogastroduodenoscopy" in chapter 10, page 508.)
- Transfer the specimen to a sterile container, and label it with the patient's name, physician's name, date and time of collection, and collector's initials.
- After duodenal tube placement or duodenoscopy, observe the patient carefully for signs of perforation, such as dysphagia, epigastric or shoulder pain, dyspnea, and fever, from tube passage.
- After duodenoscopy, monitor vital signs until the patient is stable; keep the

side rails up, and enforce bed rest until the patient is fully alert.

■ Tell the patient that he may resume his normal diet as ordered.

Precautions

■ Wear gloves when assisting with this procedure and handling the specimen.

■ Duodenal tube insertion is contraindicated in pregnancy; acute pancreatitis or cholecystitis; esophageal varices, stenosis, and diverticular malignant neoplasms; recent severe gastric hemorrhage; aortic aneurysm; heart failure; and myocardial infarction.

■ Collect the specimen for culture before antimicrobial therapy begins.

■ Send the specimen to the laboratory immediately.

■ Withdraw the tube slowly (6″ to 8″ [15.5 to 20.5 cm] every 10 minutes) until it reaches the esophagus; then clamp the tube and remove it quickly. If you can't withdraw the tube easily, report the problem; *never* force the tube.

Normal findings

Normally, a duodenal contents culture contains small amounts of polymorphonuclear leukocytes and epithelial cells with no pathogens. The bacterial count is usually less than 100,000/ml of body fluid.

Abnormal findings

Generally, bacterial counts of 100,000/ml or more or the presence of pathogens in any number indicates infection. Susceptibility testing may be required.

Numerous polymorphonuclear leukocytes, copious mucus debris, and bile-stained epithelial cells in the bile fluid suggest inflammation of the biliary tract; many segmented neutrophils and exfoliated epithelial cells suggest inflammation of the pancreas, duodenum, or bile ducts. The presence of bile sand indicates cholelithiasis or calculi in the biliary tract. Differential diagnosis requires further testing.

Interfering factors

■ Failure to observe a 12-hour fast before the test (possible decrease)

■ Failure to use proper collection technique

GENITAL CULTURES

CULTURE FOR GONORRHEA

Gonorrhea almost always results from sexual transmission of *Neisseria gonorrhoeae.* A stained smear of genital exudate can confirm gonorrhea in 90% of males with characteristic symptoms, but a culture is usually necessary, especially in asymptomatic females. Possible culture sites include the urethra (usual site in males), endocervix (usual site in females), anal canal, and oropharynx.

Purpose

■ To confirm gonorrhea

Patient preparation

■ Describe the procedure to the patient. Explain that this test is used to confirm gonorrhea.

■ Inform the patient who will perform the test and when.

■ Instruct the female patient not to douche for 24 hours before the test.

■ Tell the male patient not to void during the hour preceding the test. Warn him that males sometimes experience nausea, sweating, weakness, and fainting due to stress or discomfort when the cotton swab or wire loop is introduced into the urethra.

Equipment

Sterile gloves, sterile cotton swabs, tongue blade, wire bacteriologic loop or thin urogenital alginate swabs (for male), vaginal speculum, modified Thayer-Martin medium in plates (or Transgrow medium in specimen bottles if laboratory isn't readily available), ring forceps, cotton balls

Procedure and posttest care

Endocervical culture

■ Place the patient in the lithotomy position, drape her appropriately, and instruct her to take deep breaths.

■ Using gloved hands, insert a vaginal speculum that has been lubricated only with warm water. Clean mucus from the cervix, using cotton balls in ring forceps.

■ Insert a dry, sterile cotton swab into the endocervical canal and rotate it from side to side. Leave the swab in place for several seconds for optimum absorption of organisms.

■ In cases of deep pelvic inflammatory disease, cultures of the endometrium or aspirations by laparoscopy or culdoscopy may be necessary. Endometrial specimens are obtained by inserting stents through a narrow-bore catheter introduced into the cervical canal.

Urethral culture

■ Place the patient in a supine position, and drape him appropriately.

■ Clean the urethral meatus with sterile gauze or a cotton swab; then insert a thin urogenital alginate swab or a wire bacteriologic loop ⅜″ to ¾″ (1 to 2 cm) into the urethra, and rotate the swab or loop from side to side. Leave it in place for several seconds for optimum absorption of organisms. If permitted, the patient may milk the urethra, bringing urethral secretions to the meatus for collection on a cotton swab.

Rectal culture

■ After obtaining an endocervical or a urethral specimen (while the patient is still on the examination table), insert a sterile cotton swab into the anal canal about 1″ (2.5 cm), move the swab from side to side, and leave it in place for several seconds for optimum absorption.

■ If the swab is contaminated with stool, discard it, and repeat the procedure with a clean swab.

Throat culture

■ Position the patient with his head tilted back.

■ Check his throat for inflamed areas, using a tongue blade. Rub a sterile swab from side to side over the tonsillar areas, including inflamed or purulent sites. Be careful not to touch the teeth, cheeks, or tongue with the swab.

After specimen collection

■ Roll the swab in a Z pattern in a plate containing modified Thayer-Martin medium. Then cross-streak the medium with a sterile wire loop or the tip of the swab, and cover the plate. (See *Culturing for* Neisseria gonorrhoeae.)

■ Label the specimen with the patient's name and room number (if applicable), the physician's name, and the date and time of collection.

■ Direct smears of obtained material should be made immediately to prepare the Gram stain. Remaining material must be quickly inoculated into selective culture media or into a transport system. A culturette transport tube or a swab transport medium containing charcoal can be used. Charcoal helps neutralize toxic materials in the specimen.

■ If laboratory facilities aren't readily available, do the following: Uncap the Transgrow medium specimen bottle just before inserting the swab of test material into the bottle. Keep the bottle upright to minimize loss of carbon dioxide. With the swab, absorb the ex-

Culturing for *Neisseria gonorrhoeae*

Culturing for *Neisseria gonorrhoeae* requires use of a modified Thayer-Martin (MTM) medium. If a laboratory isn't readily available, you may use Transgrow medium.

MODIFIED THAYER-MARTIN MEDIUM

MTM medium is a combination of hemoglobin, gonococcal growth-enhancing chemicals, and antimicrobial agents for culturing endocervical, urethral, and rectal specimens. To inoculate a culture plate treated with MTM medium and to spread organisms out of their associated mucus, take the following steps:

- ◆ Roll the swab in a Z pattern (illustration 1)
- ◆ Using the swab or a sterile wire loop, immediately cross-streak the plate (illustration 2). Incubate within 15 minutes of streaking.

Two-step method of streaking Thayer-Martin medium

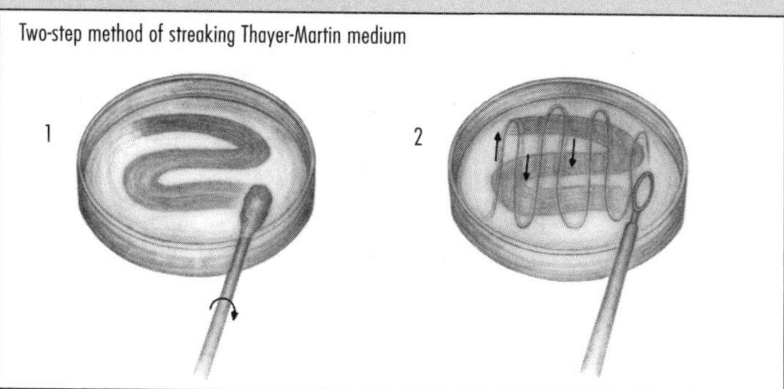

TRANSGROW MEDIUM

A modification of MTM medium, Transgrow is available in a screwcap bottle containing air and carbon dioxide. Transgrow bottles are used to transport suspect cultures when laboratory facilities aren't available at the site of specimen collection. Use the following procedure:

- ◆ To prevent loss of carbon dioxide, inoculate the specimen bottle while it's upright.
- ◆ After uncapping the bottle, immediately insert the swab and soak up all excess moisture.
- ◆ Starting at the bottom of the bottle, roll the swab from side to side across the medium.
- ◆ Recap the bottle, and send it to the laboratory immediately. Subculturing should begin within 24 to 48 hours.

One-step method of streaking Transgrow medium

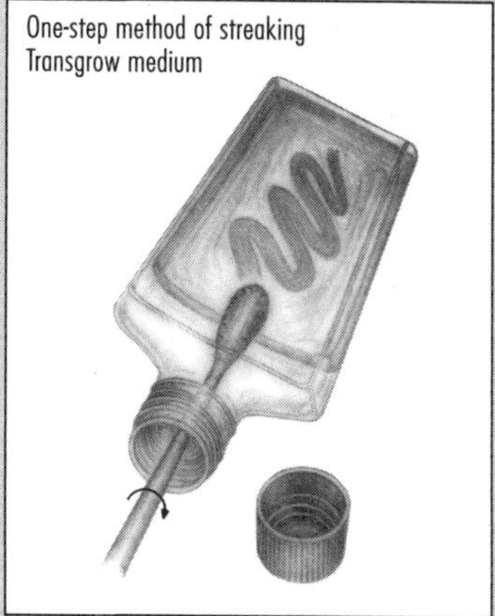

cess moisture within the bottle; then roll the swab across the Transgrow medium. Discard the swab. Place the lid on the bottle, and label the bottle appropriately.

- Advise the patient to avoid all sexual contact until test results are available.
- Explain that treatment usually begins after confirmation of a positive culture, except in a person who has symptoms of gonorrhea or who has had intercourse with someone known to have gonorrhea.
- Advise the patient that a repeat culture is required 1 week after completion of treatment to evaluate the effectiveness of therapy.
- Inform the patient that positive culture findings must be reported to the local health department.

Precautions

- Wear gloves when performing the procedures and handling the specimens.
- Place the male patient in the supine position to prevent falling if vasovagal syncope occurs when the cotton swab or wire loop is introduced into the urethra. Observe for profound hypotension, bradycardia, pallor, and sweating.
- Collect a urethral specimen at least 1 hour after the patient has voided to prevent loss of urethral secretions.
- After collecting the specimens, carefully dispose of gloves, swabs, and speculum to prevent staff exposure.
- Send the specimens to the laboratory immediately, or arrange for transport of the Transgrow bottle because the specimen must be subcultured within 24 to 48 hours.

Normal findings

Normally, no *N. gonorrhoeae* appears in the culture.

Abnormal findings

A positive culture confirms gonorrhea.

Interfering factors

- Pretest antimicrobial therapy
- Contamination due to fecal material in a rectal culture
- Improper collection technique (may provide a nonrepresentative or contaminated specimen)
- In males, voiding within 1 hour of specimen collection; in females, douching within 24 hours of specimen collection (fewer organisms available for culture)

CULTURE FOR HERPES SIMPLEX VIRUS

Herpes simplex virus (HSV) produces a wide spectrum of clinical manifestations, including keratitis, gingivostomatitis, and encephalitis. In immunocompromised individuals, it may lead to disseminated illness. The herpesvirus group includes Epstein-Barr virus, cytomegalovirus (CMV), varicella-zoster virus (VZV), human herpesvirus-6, herpesvirus-7, herpesvirus-8, and the two closely related serotypes of HSV—type 1 and type 2. Only CMV, VZV, and HSV replicate in the standard cell cultures used in diagnostic laboratories.

About 50% of the strains of HSV can be detected by characteristic cytopathic effects (CPE) within 24 hours after the laboratory receives the specimen; 5 to 7 days are required to detect the remaining HSV strains. (See *Rapid monoclonal test for cytomegalovirus.*)

Alternatively, early antigens of HSV can be detected by monoclonal antibodies in shell vial cell cultures within 16 hours after receipt of the specimen with the same sensitivity and specificity as standard tube cell cultures.

Rapid monoclonal test for cytomegalovirus

In the past, cytomegalovirus (CMV) infections were detected in the laboratory by recognizing the distinctive cytopathic effects (CPE) produced by the virus in conventional tube cell cultures. In this slow method of detecting CMV, CPE cultures grow in 9 days on average.

A FASTER TEST

The faster rapid monoclonal test (shell vial assay) is based on centrifugal inoculation of specimens onto cell monolayers grown on round cover slips in 1-dram shell vials. The immunologic detection of early products of viral replication with specific monoclonal antibodies usually occurs after 16 hours of incubation. This assay is based on the availability of a monoclonal antibody specific for the 72-kd protein of CMV synthesized during the immediate early stage of viral replication.

Through indirect immunofluorescence, CMV-infected fibroblasts are recognized by their dense, homogeneous staining confined to the nucleus of these cells. Because of the smooth, regular shape of the nucleus and the surrounding nuclear membrane, infected cells are readily differentiated from nonspecific background fluorescence, which may be present in some specimens.

This test is used to obtain rapid laboratory diagnosis of CMV infection, especially in immunocompromised patients who have or are at risk for developing systemic infections caused by this virus.

Specimen collection

Specimens should be collected during the prodromal and acute stages of clinical infection to ensure the best chance of detecting CMV. As required by the laboratory, collect a specimen for culture. Each type of specimen requires a specific collection device, as listed below:

- ◆ *Throat:* microbiologic transport swab
- ◆ *Urine, cerebrospinal fluid:* sterile screw-capped tube or vial
- ◆ Bronchoalveolar lavage tissue: sterile screw-capped jar
- ◆ *Blood:* sterile tube with anticoagulant (heparin)

CMV can be detected in urine and throat specimens from asymptomatic patients. The detection of CMV from these sites indicates active, asymptomatic infection, which may herald symptomatic involvement, especially in immunocompromised patients. Detection of CMV in specimens of blood, tissue, or bronchoalveolar lavage generally indicates systemic infection and disease.

Purpose

- To confirm diagnosis of HSV infection by culturing the virus from specimens

Patient preparation

- Explain to the patient that this test is performed to detect HSV infection.
- Explain to the patient that specimens will be collected from suspected lesions during the prodromal and acute stages of clinical infection.

Procedure and posttest care

- Collect a specimen for culture into the appropriate collection device. Vesicle fluid can be obtained with a 27-gauge needle on a tuberculin syringe. If the fluid is scant, the base of the ulcer can be scraped with a swab to remove cells.
- For the throat, skin, eye, or genital area, use a microbiologic transport swab.

■ For body fluids or other respiratory specimens (washings, lavage), use a sterile screw-capped jar.
■ Transport the specimen to the laboratory as soon as possible after collection. If the anticipated time between collection and inoculation of cell cultures is more than 3 hours, the specimen should be stored and transported at 39.2° F (4° C).

Precautions

■ Wear gloves when obtaining and handling all specimens.
■ Don't allow the specimen to dry up.

Normal findings

HSV is seldom recovered from immunocompetent patients who show no overt signs of disease.

Abnormal findings

HSV detected in specimens taken from dermal lesions, the eye, or cerebrospinal fluid is highly significant. Specimens from the upper respiratory tract may be associated with intermittent shedding of the virus, particularly in an immunocompromised patient.

Like other herpesviruses, HSV can be shed from immunocompromised patients intermittently in the absence of apparent disease. For epidemiologic purposes, HSV detected by CPE in standard tube cell cultures is confirmed and identified as type 1 or 2.

Interfering factors

■ Administration of antiviral drugs before specimen collection

CULTURE FOR CHLAMYDIA

The most common sexually transmitted disease in the United States, chlamydia is caused by the organism *Chlamydia trachomatis*. Identification of this parasite requires cultivation in the laboratory. After incubation, *Chlamydia*-infected cells can be detected by fluorescein isothiocyanate-conjugated monoclonal antibodies or by iodine stain. Detection in cell cultures of *C. psittaci* and *C. pneumoniae* requires specific technical manipulations and reagents; deoxyribonucleic acid detection may also be performed in women who may be susceptible to the infections, whether they have symptoms or not.

Culture is the detection method of choice, but rapid noncultural (antigen detection) procedures are also available.

Purpose

■ To confirm infections caused by *C. trachomatis*

Patient preparation

■ Explain the purpose of the test to the patient.
■ Describe the procedure for collecting a specimen for culture.
■ If the specimen will be collected from the patient's genital tract, instruct the patient not to urinate for 3 to 4 hours before the specimen is taken.
■ Tell a female patient not to douche for 24 hours before the test.
■ Tell a male patient that he may experience some burning and pressure as the culture is taken but that the discomfort will subside after a few minutes.

Equipment

Gloves, sterile cotton swabs, wire bacteriologic loop or thin urogenital alginate swabs (for male), vaginal speculum, sucrose phosphate (2SP) transport medium, microbiologic transport swab or cyrobrush.

Procedure and posttest care

- Obtain a specimen of the epithelial cells from the infected site. In adults, these sites may include the eye, urethra (rather than from the purulent exudate that may be present), endocervix, and rectum.
- Obtain a urethral specimen by inserting a cotton-tipped applicator ¾″ to 2″ (2 to 5 cm) into the urethra.
- To collect a specimen from the endocervix, use a microbiologic transport swab or cytobrush.
- Extract the specimen into 2SP transport medium.
- Specimens collected from the throat, eye, or nasopharynx and aspirates from infants should be extracted into 2SP transport medium. The specimens are sent to the laboratory at 39.2° F (4° C).
- If the anticipated time between specimen collection and inoculation into cell culture is more than 24 hours, freeze the 2SP transport medium and send it to the laboratory with dry ice.

♦ **CLINICAL ALERT** *In patients suspected of being sexually abused, be sure to process specimens by culture rather than by antigen detection methods.*

- Advise the patient to avoid all sexual contact until after test results are available.
- If the culture confirms infection, provide counseling for the patient regarding treatment of sexual partners.

Precautions

- Place the male patient in the supine position to prevent falling if vasovagal syncope occurs when the cotton swab or wire loop is introduced into the urethra. Observe for profound hypotension, bradycardia, pallor, and sweating.
- Wear gloves when performing the procedures and handling the specimens.
- Collect a urethral specimen at least 1 hour after the patient has voided to prevent loss of urethral secretions.
- After collecting the specimens, carefully dispose of gloves, swabs, and speculum to prevent staff exposure.

Normal findings

Normally, no *C. trachomatis* appears in the culture.

Abnormal findings

A positive culture confirms *C. trachomatis* infection.

Interfering factors

- Using an antimicrobial drug within a few days before specimen collection (possible inability to recover *C. trachomatis*)
- In males, voiding within 1 hour of specimen collection; in females, douching within 24 hours of specimen collection (fewer organisms available for culture)
- Failure to use proper collection technique
- Contamination of the specimen due to fecal material in a rectal culture

9

Biopsy

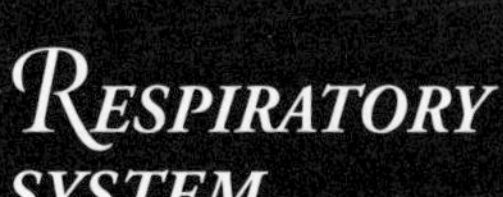

RESPIRATORY SYSTEM

LUNG BIOPSY

In lung biopsy, a specimen of pulmonary tissue is excised by closed or open technique for histologic examination. Closed technique, performed under local anesthesia, includes needle and transbronchial biopsies, transcatheter bronchial brushing, and video-assisted thoracotomy. Open technique, performed under general anesthesia in the operating room, includes limited and standard thoracotomies. Needle biopsy is appropriate when the lesion is readily accessible, originates in the lung parenchyma and is confined to it, or is affixed to the chest wall; it provides a much smaller specimen than the open technique. Transbronchial biopsy, the removal of multiple tissue specimens through a fiber-optic bronchoscope, may be used in patients with diffuse infiltrative pulmonary disease or tumors or when severe debilitation contraindicates open biopsy. Open biopsy is appropriate for the study of a well-circumscribed lesion that may require resection.

Generally, a biopsy of the lung is recommended after chest X-rays, computed tomography (CT) scan, and bronchoscopy have failed to identify the cause of diffuse parenchymal pulmonary disease or a pulmonary lesion. Complications of lung biopsy include bleeding, infection, and pneumothorax.

Purpose

- To confirm a diagnosis of diffuse parenchymal pulmonary disease and pulmonary lesions

Patient preparation

- Explain to the patient that this test is used to confirm or rule out a diagnostic finding in the lung.
- Describe the procedure to the patient, and answer questions.
- Tell the patient that a chest X-ray and blood studies (prothrombin time, activated partial thromboplastin time, and platelet count) will be performed before the biopsy.
- Tell him who will perform the biopsy and where it will be done.
- Instruct the patient to fast after midnight before the procedure. (Sometimes the patient is permitted to have clear liquids the morning of the test.)
- Make sure the patient or an appropriate family member has signed an informed consent form.
- Check the patient's history for hypersensitivity to the local anesthetic.
- Administer a mild sedative, as ordered, 30 minutes before the biopsy to help the patient relax. Tell him that he'll receive a local anesthetic but may experience a sharp, transient pain when the biopsy needle touches the lung.
- Reinforce that he'll need to lie still during the procedure because any movement or coughing can result in laceration of lung tissue by the biopsy needle.

Procedure and posttest care

- After the biopsy site is selected, lead markers are placed on the patient's skin, and X-rays are ordered to verify their correct placement.
- Position the patient in a sitting position with arms folded on a table in front of him; instruct him to maintain this position, remaining as still as possible, and to refrain from coughing.
- Prepare the skin over the biopsy site and drape the appropriate area.
- With a 25G needle, the local anesthetic is injected just above the rib be-

low the selected site to prevent damage to the intercostal nerves and vessels.

- Using a 22G needle, the examiner anesthetizes the intercostal muscles and parietal pleura, makes a small incision (2 to 3 mm) with a scalpel, and introduces the biopsy needle through the incision, chest wall, and pleura into the tumor or pulmonary tissue.
- If the intercostal space at the incision site is wide, the needle is inserted at a 90-degree angle; if the ribs overlap and the intercostal space is narrow, the needle is inserted at a 45-degree angle. When the needle is in the tumor or pulmonary tissue, the specimen is obtained and the needle is withdrawn.
- The specimen is divided immediately: The tissue for histology is placed in a properly labeled bottle containing 10% neutral buffered formalin solution; the tissue for microbiology is placed in a sterile container.
- Immediately following the procedure, exert pressure on the biopsy site to stop the bleeding, and apply a small bandage.

◆ **CLINICAL ALERT** *Check vital signs every 15 minutes for 1 hour, every 30 minutes for 2 hours, every hour for 4 hours, and then every 4 hours. Watch for bleeding, dyspnea, elevated pulse rate, diminished breath sounds on the biopsy side and, eventually, cyanosis. Complications include pneumothorax and bleeding. Make sure the chest X-ray is repeated as soon as the biopsy has been completed.*

- Inform the patient that he may resume his normal diet.

Precautions

- Needle biopsy is contraindicated in patients with a lesion that's separated from the chest wall or accompanied by emphysematous bullae, cysts, or gross emphysema and in patients with coagulopathy, hypoxia, pulmonary hypertension, or cardiac disease with cor pulmonale.
- During biopsy, observe for signs of respiratory distress — shortness of breath, elevated pulse rate, and cyanosis (late sign). If such signs develop, report them immediately.
- Because coughing and movement during biopsy can cause tearing of the lung by the biopsy needle, keep the patient calm and still.

Normal findings

Normal pulmonary tissue shows uniform texture of the alveolar ducts, alveolar walls, bronchioles, and small vessels.

Abnormal findings

Histologic examination of a pulmonary tissue specimen can reveal squamous cell or oat cell carcinoma and adenocarcinoma and supplements the results of microbiologic cultures, deep-cough sputum specimens, chest X-rays, bronchoscopy, and the patient's physical history in confirming cancer or parenchymal pulmonary disease.

Interfering factors

- Failure to obtain a representative tissue specimen
- Failure to store the specimen in the appropriate containers

PLEURAL BIOPSY

Pleural biopsy is the removal of pleural tissue by needle biopsy or open biopsy for histologic examination. Needle pleural biopsy is performed under local anesthesia. It generally follows or is done in conjunction with thoracentesis (aspiration of pleural fluid), which is performed when the cause of an effusion is unknown, but it can be performed separately.

Open pleural biopsy, performed in the absence of pleural effusion, permits direct visualization of the pleura and the underlying lung. It's performed in the operating room.

Purpose

- To differentiate between nonmalignant and malignant disease
- To diagnose viral, fungal, or parasitic disease and collagen vascular disease of the pleura

Patient preparation

- Describe the procedure to the patient, and answer questions.
- Explain that this test permits microscopic examination of pleural tissue.
- Tell him who will perform the biopsy, where it will be done, and that no fasting is required.
- Explain that blood studies will precede the biopsy, and chest X-rays will be taken before and after the biopsy.
- Make sure the patient or an appropriate family member has signed an informed consent form.
- Check the patient's history for hypersensitivity to the local anesthetic.
- Tell him he'll receive a local anesthetic and should experience little pain.
- Record vital signs just before the procedure.

Procedure and posttest care

- Seat the patient on the side of the bed, with his feet resting on a stool and his arms on the overbed table or supported by his upper body. Tell him to hold this position and remain still during the procedure.
- Prepare the skin and drape the area.
- The local anesthetic is then administered.
- In a *Vim-Silverman needle biopsy,* a needle is inserted through the appropriate intercostal space into the biopsy site, with the outer tip distal to the pleura and the central portion pushed in deeper and held in place. The outer case is inserted about 3/8" (1 cm), the entire assembly is rotated 360 degrees, and the needle and tissue specimen are withdrawn. In *Cope's needle biopsy,* a trocar is introduced through the appropriate intercostal space into the biopsy site. To obtain the specimen, a hooked stylet is inserted through the trocar. While the outer tube is held stationary, the inner tube is twisted to cut off the tissue specimen, and the assembly is withdrawn.
- After the specimens are obtained, additional parietal fluid may be removed to treat the effusion.
- Put the specimen immediately into a 10% neutral buffered formalin solution in a labeled specimen bottle, and send it to the laboratory immediately.
- Clean the skin around the biopsy site, and apply an adhesive bandage.
- Make sure the chest X-ray is repeated immediately after the biopsy.
- Check vital signs every 15 minutes for 1 hour and then every hour for 4 hours or until stable.

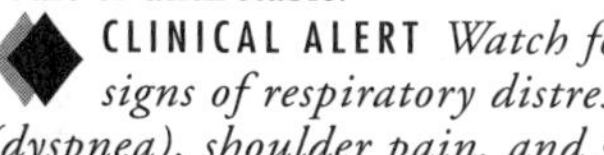

CLINICAL ALERT *Watch for signs of respiratory distress (dyspnea), shoulder pain, and such complications as pneumothorax (immediate), pneumonia (delayed), and hemorrhage.*

- Instruct the patient to lie on his unaffected side to promote healing of the biopsy site as indicated.

Precautions

- Pleural biopsy is contraindicated in patients with severe bleeding disorders.

Normal findings

The normal pleura consists primarily of mesothelial cells that are flattened in a uniform layer. Layers of areolar connective tissue that contain blood vessels, nerves, and lymphatics lie below.

Abnormal findings

Histologic examination of the tissue specimen can reveal malignant disease, tuberculosis, and viral, fungal, parasitic, or collagen vascular disease. Primary neoplasms of the pleura are generally fibrous and epithelial.

Interfering factors

- Failure to use the proper fixative or to obtain an adequate specimen
- Patient's inability to remain still, keep from coughing, or follow instructions, such as "Hold your breath," during the procedure

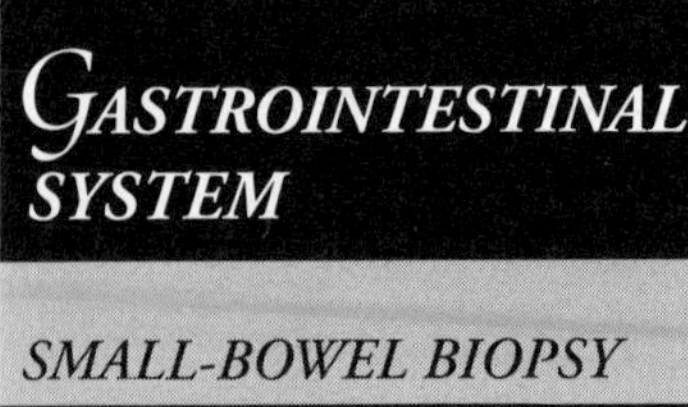

Small-bowel biopsy is used to evaluate diseases of the intestinal mucosa, which may cause malabsorption or diarrhea. It produces larger specimens than those produced by endoscopic biopsy and allows removal of tissue from areas beyond an endoscope's reach. (See *Endoscopic biopsy of the GI tract.*)

Several similar types of capsules are available for tissue collection. In each, a mercury-weighted bag is attached to one end of the capsule; a thin polyethylene tube about 5′ (1.5 m) long is attached to the other end. When the bag, capsule, and tube are in place in the small bowel, suction on the tube draws the mucosa into the capsule and closes it, cutting off the piece of tissue within. Although this is an invasive procedure, it causes little pain and rarely causes complications.

Small-bowel biopsy verifies diagnosis of some diseases, such as Whipple's disease, and may help confirm others, such as tropical sprue. Capsule biopsy is an invasive procedure, but it causes little pain and complications are rare.

Purpose

- To help diagnose diseases of the intestinal mucosa

Patient preparation

- Explain to the patient that this test is used to identify intestinal disorders.
- Describe the procedure to the patient, and answer questions.
- Instruct him to restrict food and fluids for at least 8 hours before the test.
- Tell him who will perform the biopsy and where it will be done.
- Make sure the patient or a responsible family member has signed an informed consent form.
- Ensure that coagulation tests have been performed and that the results are recorded on the patient's chart.
- Withhold aspirin and anticoagulants as ordered. If these drugs must be continued, note this on the laboratory request.

Procedure and posttest care

- Check the tubing and the mercury bag for leaks.
- Lightly lubricate the tube and capsule with a water-soluble lubricant, and moisten the mercury bag with water.
- Spray the back of the patient's throat with a local anesthetic to decrease gagging.
- Ask the patient to sit upright.
- The capsule is placed in his pharynx, and he's asked to flex his neck and swallow as the tube is advanced.

Endoscopic biopsy of the GI tract

Endoscopy allows direct visualization of the GI tract and any site that requires biopsy of tissue specimens for histologic analysis. This relatively painless procedure helps detect, support diagnosis of, or monitor GI tract disorders. Its complications, notably hemorrhage, perforation, and aspiration, are rare.

Endoscopic biopsy of the GI tract can be used to diagnose cancer, lymphoma, amyloidosis, candidiasis, and gastric ulcers; to support diagnosis of Crohn's disease, chronic ulcerative colitis, gastritis, esophagitis, and melanosis coli in laxative abuse; and to monitor progression of Barrett's esophagus, multiple gastric polyps, colon cancer and polyps, and chronic ulcerative colitis.

PATIENT PREPARATION

Careful patient preparation is vital for this procedure. Describe the procedure to the patient, and reassure him that he'll be able to breathe with the endoscope in place. Tell him to fast for at least 8 hours before the procedure. For lower GI biopsy, clean the bowel. Make sure the patient or a responsible family member has signed an informed consent form.

Just before the procedure, administer the prescribed sedative to the patient. He should be relaxed but not asleep because his cooperation is necessary to promote smooth passage of the endoscope. Spray the back of his throat with a local anesthetic to suppress his gag reflex. Have suction equipment and bipolar cauterizing electrodes available to prevent aspiration and excessive bleeding.

OBTAINING THE SAMPLE

After the endoscope is passed into the upper or lower GI tract and a lesion, node, or other abnormal area is visualized, a biopsy forceps is pushed through a channel in the endoscope until this, too, can be seen. The forceps are then opened, positioned at the biopsy site, and closed on the tissue. The closed forceps and tissue specimen are removed from the endoscope, and the tissue is taken from the forceps. Then the forceps may be used to cauterize any remaining abnormal tissue or stop bleeding.

The specimen is placed mucosal side up on fine-mesh gauze or filter paper and then placed in a labeled biopsy bottle containing fixative. When all specimens have been collected, the endoscope is removed. Specimens are sent to the laboratory immediately.

- If a local anesthetic is used to control the gag reflex, the patient must not receive any fluids to help him swallow the capsule.
- Place the patient on his right side; the tube is then advanced another 20″ (50.8 cm). The tube's position is checked by fluoroscopy or by instilling air through the tube and listening with a stethoscope for air to enter the stomach.
- Next, the tube is advanced 2″ to 4″ (5 to 10 cm) at a time to pass the capsule through the pylorus. (Talk to the patient about food to stimulate the pylorus and help the capsule pass.)
- When fluoroscopy confirms that the capsule has passed the pylorus, keep the patient on his right side to allow the capsule to move into the second and third portions of the small bowel.
- Tell the patient that he may hold the tube loosely to one side of his mouth if it makes him more comfortable.
- Capsule position is checked again by fluoroscopy. When the capsule is at or beyond the ligament of Treitz, the biopsy sample can be taken. (The physician will determine the biopsy site.)
- Place the patient in a supine position so that the capsule's position can be verified fluoroscopically. A 100-ml glass

syringe is placed on the end of the tube, and steady suction is applied to close the capsule and cut off a tissue specimen. Suction is maintained on the syringe as the tube and capsule are removed; then the suction is released. This opens the capsule and exposes the specimen, mucosal side down.

- The specimen is gently removed with forceps, placed mucosal side up on a piece of mesh, and then placed in a biopsy bottle with required fixative.
- As ordered, resume the patient's diet after confirming return of the gag reflex.
- Although complications are rare, watch for signs of hemorrhage, bacteremia with transient fever and pain, and bowel perforation. Tell the patient to report abdominal pain or bleeding.

Precautions

- Keep suction equipment nearby to prevent aspiration if the patient vomits.
- Don't allow the patient to bite the tubing.
- Handle the tissue carefully, and place it correctly on the slide.
- Send the specimen to the laboratory immediately.
- Biopsy is contraindicated in uncooperative patients, those taking aspirin or anticoagulants, and those with uncontrolled coagulation disorders.

Normal findings

A normal small-bowel biopsy specimen consists of fingerlike villi, crypts, columnar epithelial cells, and round cells.

Abnormal findings

Small-bowel tissue that reveals histologic changes in cell structure may indicate Whipple's disease, abetalipoproteinemia, lymphoma, lymphangiectasia, eosinophilic enteritis, and such parasitic infections as giardiasis and coccidiosis.

Abnormal specimens may also suggest celiac sprue, tropical sprue, infectious gastroenteritis, intraluminal bacterial overgrowth, folate and vitamin B_{12} deficiency, radiation enteritis, and malnutrition, but such disorders require further studies.

Interfering factors

- Failure to fast before biopsy (possible poor specimen or vomiting and aspiration)
- Mechanical failure of the biopsy capsule or hole in the tubing (possible difficulty in removing tissue specimen)
- Patient's inability to remain still or keep from coughing during the procedure
- Incorrect handling or positioning of the specimen or failure to place it in a fixative
- Delay in transporting the specimen to the laboratory

PERCUTANEOUS LIVER BIOPSY

Percutaneous biopsy of the liver is the needle aspiration of a core of liver tissue for histologic analysis. This procedure is performed under local or general anesthesia. Findings may help to identify hepatic disorders after ultrasonography, CT, and radionuclide studies have failed to detect them. Because many patients with hepatic disorders have clotting defects, testing for hemostasis should precede liver biopsy.

Purpose

- To diagnose hepatic parenchymal disease, malignant tumors, and granulomatous infections

Patient preparation

- Explain to the patient that this test is used to diagnose liver disorders.
- Describe the procedure to the patient, and answer questions.
- Instruct the patient to restrict food and fluids for 4 to 8 hours before the test.
- Tell him who will perform the biopsy and where it will be done.
- Make sure the patient or an appropriate family member has signed an informed consent form.
- Check the patient's history for hypersensitivity to the local anesthetic.
- Make sure coagulation studies (prothrombin time [PT], partial thromboplastin time [PTT], and platelet counts) have been performed and that the results are recorded on the patient's chart.
- A blood sample is usually drawn for baseline assessment of hematocrit.
- Just before the biopsy, tell the patient to void; then, record vital signs.
- Inform him that he'll receive a local anesthetic but may experience pain similar to that of a punch in his right shoulder as the biopsy needle passes the phrenic nerve.

Procedure and posttest care

- For aspiration biopsy using the Menghini needle, place the patient in a supine position with his right hand under his head. Instruct him to maintain this position and remain as still as possible during the procedure.
- The liver is palpated, the biopsy site is selected and marked, and the local anesthetic is then injected.
- The needle flange is set to control the depth of penetration, and 2 ml of sterile normal saline solution are drawn into the syringe.
- The syringe is attached to the biopsy needle, and the needle is introduced into the subcutaneous tissue through the right eighth or ninth intercostal space at the midaxillary line and advanced up to the pleura.
- Next, 1 ml of normal saline solution is injected to clear the needle and the plunger; then the plunger is drawn back to the 4-ml mark to create negative pressure.
- At this point in the procedure, ask the patient to take a deep breath, exhale, and hold his breath at the end of expiration to prevent movement of the chest wall.
- As the patient holds his breath, the biopsy needle is quickly inserted into the liver and withdrawn in 1 second.
- For patients who can't hold their breath, the biopsy needle is quickly inserted and withdrawn at the end of expiration.
- After the needle is withdrawn, tell the patient to resume normal respirations.
- The tissue specimen is then placed in a properly labeled specimen cup containing 10% formalin solution. This is done by releasing negative pressure while the point of the needle is in the formalin solution. Send the specimen to the laboratory immediately.
- Again, 1 ml of normal saline solution is injected to clear the needle of the tissue specimen.
- Apply pressure to the biopsy site to stop bleeding.
- Position the patient on his right side for 2 to 4 hours, with a small pillow or sandbag under the costal margin to provide extra pressure. Advise bed rest for at least 24 hours.
- Check the patient's vital signs every 15 minutes for 1 hour and then every 30 minutes for 4 hours, and every 4 hours thereafter for 24 hours. Throughout, observe carefully for signs of shock.

◆ **CLINICAL ALERT** *Immediately report bleeding or signs of bile peritonitis, such as tenderness and rigidity around the biopsy* *site. Be alert for symptoms of pneumothorax, such as rising respiratory rate, depressed breath sounds, dyspnea, persistent shoulder pain, and pleuritic chest pain. Report such complications promptly.*

- If the patient experiences pain, which may persist for several hours after the test, administer an analgesic.
- Inform the patient that he may resume his normal diet as ordered.

Precautions

- Percutaneous liver biopsy is contraindicated in a patient with a platelet count below 100,000/µl; PT time longer than 15 seconds; empyema of the lungs, pleurae, peritoneum, biliary tract, or liver; vascular tumor; hepatic angiomas; hydatid cyst; or tense ascites. If extrahepatic obstruction is suspected, ultrasonography or subcutaneous transhepatic cholangiography should rule out this condition before the biopsy is considered.
- Pain in the abdomen or dyspnea after the biopsy may indicate perforation of an abdominal organ or pneumothorax, respectively. In such cases, complete a thorough assessment and notify the physician at once.
- Instruct the patient to hold his breath while the needle is in place.

Normal findings

The normal liver consists of sheets of hepatocytes supported by a reticulin framework.

Abnormal findings

Examination of the hepatic tissue may reveal diffuse hepatic disease, such as cirrhosis or hepatitis, or granulomatous infections such as tuberculosis. Primary malignant tumors include hepatocellular carcinoma, cholangiocellular carcinoma, and angiosarcoma, but hepatic metastasis is more common.

Nonmalignant findings with a known focal lesion require further studies, such as laparotomy or laparoscopy with biopsy.

Interfering factors

- Failure to obtain a representative specimen
- Failure to place the specimen in the proper preservative
- Failure to send the specimen to the laboratory immediately
- Hemorrhage caused by inadvertent puncture of a liver blood vessel.

REPRODUCTIVE SYSTEM

BREAST BIOPSY

Breast biopsy is performed to confirm or rule out breast cancer after clinical examination, mammography, or thermography has identified a mass. Fine-needle biopsy or needle biopsy is usually done on a mass that has been identified by ultrasonography as being fluid-filled. Open biopsy provides complete tissue system, which can be sectioned to allow more accurate evaluation. Local anesthesia can usually be given to outpatients for these three techniques. Stereotactic breast biopsy immobilizes the breast and allows the computer to calculate the exact location of the mass based on X-rays from two angles.

An excisional biopsy may be done under general anesthesia. If sufficient tissue is obtained and the mass is found to be a malignant tumor, specimens are sent for estrogen and progesterone re-

BRCA testing

Recently, genetic researchers located two genes, BRCA1 and BRCA2, that have been linked to certain forms of breast cancer. BRCA testing can detect the presence of BRCA gene mutations, which may increase an individual's susceptibility to some breast cancers.

The test, performed on a blood sample, is available for women with a family history of breast cancer. Controversy continues over whether BRCA testing should be made available to the general public.

ceptor assays to assist in determining future therapy and the prognosis.

Because breast cancer remains the most prevalent cancer in women, genetic researchers are continually working to identify women at risk. (See *BRCA testing.*)

Purpose

- To differentiate between benign and malignant breast tumors

Patient preparation

- Describe the procedure to the patient, and explain that this test permits microscopic examination of a breast tissue specimen. Offer her emotional support, and assure her that breast masses don't always indicate cancer.
- If the patient is to receive a local anesthetic, tell her that she need not restrict food, fluids, or medication before the biopsy.
- If she'll receive a general anesthetic, advise her to fast from midnight before the test until after the biopsy.
- Tell her who will perform the biopsy and where it will be done.
- Explain that pretest studies, such as blood tests, urine tests, and chest X-rays, may be required.
- Make sure the patient or an appropriate family member has signed an informed consent form.
- Check the patient's history for hypersensitivity to anesthetics.

Procedure and posttest care

Needle biopsy

- Instruct the patient to undress to the waist, and guide her to a sitting or recumbent position with hands at her sides, reminding her to remain still.
- The biopsy site is prepared, a local anesthetic is administered, and the syringe (luer-lock syringe for aspiration, Vim-Silverman needle for tissue specimen) is introduced into the lesion.
- Fluid aspirated from the breast is expelled into a properly labeled, heparinized tub; the tissue specimen is placed in a labeled specimen bottle containing normal saline solution or formalin.
- With fine-needle aspiration, a slide is made for cytology and viewed immediately under a microscope.
- Pressure is exerted on the biopsy site and, after bleeding stops, an adhesive bandage is applied. Because breast fluid aspiration isn't considered diagnostically accurate, some physicians aspirate fluid only from cysts. If such fluid is clear yellow and the mass disappears, the aspiration procedure is diagnostic and therapeutic, and the aspirate is discarded. If aspiration yields no fluid or if the lesion recurs two or three times, an open biopsy is then considered appropriate.

Open biopsy

- After the patient receives a general or local anesthetic, an incision is made in the breast to expose the mass.

■ The examiner may then incise a portion of tissue or excise the entire mass. If the mass is smaller than ¾" (2 cm) in diameter and appears benign, it's usually excised; if it's larger or appears malignant, a specimen is usually incised before the mass is excised. Incisional biopsy generally provides an adequate specimen for histologic analysis.

■ The specimen is placed in a properly labeled specimen bottle containing 10% formalin solution. Tissue that appears malignant is sent for frozen section and receptor assays. Receptor assay specimens must not be placed in the formalin solution.

■ The wound is sutured, and an adhesive bandage applied.

All procedures

■ If the patient has received a general or local anesthetic, check vital signs, and provide medication for pain. If the patient has received a general anesthetic, check vital signs every 15 minutes for 1 hour, every 30 minutes for 2 hours, every hour for the next 4 hours, and then every 4 hours.

■ Administer an analgesic as ordered. An ice bag may provide comfort. Instruct the patient to wear a support bra at all times until healing is complete.

■ Watch for and report bleeding, tenderness, and redness at the biopsy site.

■ Provide emotional support to the patient who is awaiting diagnosis.

Precautions

■ Open breast biopsy is contraindicated in patients with conditions that preclude surgery.

■ Send the specimen to the laboratory immediately.

Normal findings

Normally, breast tissue consists of cellular and noncellular connective tissue, fat lobules, and various lactiferous ducts. It's pink, more fatty than fibrous, and shows no abnormal development of cells or tissue elements.

Abnormal findings

Abnormal breast tissue may exhibit a wide range of malignant or benign pathology. Breast tumors are common in women and account for 32% of female cancers; such tumors are rare in men (0.2% of male cancers). Benign tumors include fibrocystic disease, adenofibroma, intraductal papilloma, mammary fat necrosis, and plasma cell mastitis (mammary duct ectasia). Malignant tumors include adenocarcinoma, cystosarcoma, intraductal carcinoma, infiltrating carcinoma, inflammatory carcinoma, medullary or circumscribed carcinoma, colloid carcinoma, lobular carcinoma, sarcoma, and Paget's disease.

■ The receptor assays evaluate tumors for estrogen and progesterone protein and assign a positive or negative value to the estrogen and progesterone receptors. This positive or negative value assists in the prognosis and treatment of breast cancer.

Interfering factors

■ Failure to obtain an adequate tissue specimen

■ Failure to place the specimen in the proper solution and to send it to the laboratory immediately

PROSTATE GLAND BIOPSY

Prostate gland biopsy is the needle excision of a prostate tissue specimen for histologic examination. Indications include potentially malignant prostatic hypertrophy and prostatic nodules. A perineal, transrectal, or transurethral approach may be used—the transrectal approach is used for high prostatic lesions.

Purpose

- To confirm prostate cancer
- To determine the cause of prostatic hyperplasia

Patient preparation

- Describe the procedure to the patient, answer his questions, and tell him that the test provides a tissue specimen for microscopic study.
- Tell him who will perform the biopsy, where it will be done, and that he'll receive a local anesthetic.
- Make sure the patient or an appropriate family member has signed an informed consent form.
- Check the patient's history for hypersensitivity to the anesthetic or other drugs.
- For a transrectal approach, administer enemas until the return is clear and administer an antibacterial agent to minimize the risk of infection. This approach may be performed on outpatients without an anesthetic.
- Just before the biopsy, check vital signs and administer a sedative.
- Administer a prophylactic antibiotic as ordered.
- Instruct the patient to remain still during the procedure and to follow instructions.

Procedure and posttest care

Perineal approach

- Place the patient in the proper position (left lateral, knee-chest, or lithotomy), and clean the perineal skin.
- After the local anesthetic is administered, a 2-mm incision may be made into the perineum.
- The examiner immobilizes the prostate by inserting a finger into the rectum and introduces the biopsy needle into a prostate lobe. The needle is rotated gently, pulled out about 5 mm, and reinserted at another angle. The procedure is repeated at several areas.
- Pressure is exerted on the puncture site, which is then bandaged.

Transrectal approach

- Place the patient in the left lateral position.
- A digital rectal examination is performed before an ultrasound probe is inserted. A curved needle guide is attached to the finger palpating the rectum. The biopsy needle is pushed along the guide into the prostate that was localized by ultrasonography.
- As the needle enters the prostate, the patient may experience pain. The needle is rotated to cut off the tissue and is then withdrawn.
- An alternative method of transrectal detection is the automated cone biopsy, in which the physician uses a spring-powered device with an inner trocar needle to cut through prostatic tissue. This technique is quick and reportedly painless.

Transurethral approach

- An endoscopic instrument is passed through the urethra, permitting direct viewing of the prostate and passage of a cutting loop.
- The loop is rotated to obtain tissue and then withdrawn.

All approaches

- The specimen is placed immediately in a labeled specimen bottle containing 10% formalin solution and sent to the laboratory for analysis.
- Check vital signs immediately after the procedure, every 2 hours for 4 hours, and then every 4 hours.
- Observe the biopsy site for hematoma and for signs and symptoms of infection, such as redness, swelling, and pain. Watch for urine retention, urinary frequency, and hematuria.

Precautions

■ Complications may include transient, painless hematuria and bleeding into the prostatic urethra and bladder.

Normal findings

Normally, the prostate gland consists of a thin, fibrous capsule surrounding the stroma, which is made up of elastic and connective tissues and smooth-muscle fibers. The epithelial glands found in these tissues and muscle fibers drain into the chief excreting ducts.

Abnormal findings

Histologic examination can confirm cancer. Further tests — bone scans, bone marrow biopsy, tests for prostate-specific antigen, and serum acid phosphatase and prostatic acid phosphatase determinations — identify the extent of the cancer. Acid phosphatase levels usually rise in metastatic prostatic carcinoma; they tend to be low in carcinoma that's confined to the prostatic capsule.

Histologic examination can also be used to detect benign prostatic hyperplasia, prostatitis, tuberculosis, lymphomas, and rectal or bladder cancer.

Interfering factors

■ Failure to obtain an adequate tissue specimen
■ Failure to place the specimen in formalin

CERVICAL BIOPSY

Cervical biopsy (also known as cervical punch biopsy) is the excision by sharp forceps of a tissue specimen from the cervix for histologic examination. Generally, multiple biopsies are done to obtain specimens from all areas with abnormal tissue or from the squamocolumnar junction and other sites around the cervical circumference. The biopsy site is selected by direct visualization of the cervix with a colposcope or by Schiller's test, which stains normal squamous epithelium a dark mahogany but fails to color abnormal tissue. Other biopsies are done to detect other gynecological disorders. (See *Endometrial and ovarian biopsies.*) The biopsy is performed when the cervix is least vascular, usually 1 week after menses.

Purpose

■ To evaluate suspicious cervical lesions
■ To diagnose cervical cancer

Patient preparation

■ Describe the procedure to the patient, and explain that it provides a cervical tissue specimen for microscopic study.
■ Tell the patient who will perform the biopsy and where it will be done.
■ Tell the patient that she may experience mild discomfort during and after the biopsy.
■ Advise the outpatient to have someone accompany her home after the biopsy.
■ Make sure the patient or a responsible family member has signed an informed consent form.
■ Ask the patient to void just before the biopsy.

Procedure and posttest care

■ Place the patient in the lithotomy position, and tell her to relax as the unlubricated speculum is inserted.
■ *For direct visualization,* the colposcope is inserted through the speculum, the biopsy site is located, and the cervix is cleaned with a swab soaked in 3% acetic acid solution. The biopsy forceps are then inserted through the speculum or the colposcope, and tissue is removed from any lesion or from selected sites, starting from the posterior lip to avoid obscuring other sites with blood.

Endometrial and ovarian biopsies

The following list includes purposes and special considerations involved in endometrial and ovarian biopsies.

METHOD	PURPOSE	SPECIAL CONSIDERATIONS
Endometrial biopsy		
◆ Dilatation and curettage (D&C) ◆ Endometrial washing (by jet irrigation, aspiration, or brushing)	◆ To evaluate uterine bleeding ◆ To diagnose suspected endometrial cancer	◆ Time of menstrual cycle affects accuracy of biopsy results ◆ Type of specimen obtained depends on patient's age and disorder. ◆ D&C by endometrial washing may follow a negative biopsy. ◆ Specimens obtained by D&C may be processed as frozen sections.
Ovarian biopsy		
◆ Transrectal or transvaginal fine-needle biopsy ◆ Aspiration biopsy during laparoscopy	◆ To diagnose a missed abortion ◆ To detect an ovarian tumor ◆ To determine the spread of cancer	◆ Fine-needle biopsy may follow palpation, laparoscopy, or computed tomography that detects an abnormal ovary. ◆ Aspiration during laparoscopy is particularly useful for young women who are infertile or who have lesions that appear benign.

Each specimen is immediately put in 10% formalin solution in a labeled bottle. To control bleeding after biopsy, the cervix is swabbed with 5% silver nitrate solution (cautery or sutures may be used instead). If bleeding persists, the examiner may insert a tampon.

■ *For Schiller's test,* an applicator stick saturated with iodine solution is inserted through the speculum. This stains the cervix to identify lesions for biopsy.

■ Record the patient's and physician's names and the biopsy sites on the laboratory request.

■ Instruct the patient to avoid strenuous exercise for 24 hours after the biopsy. Encourage the outpatient to rest briefly before leaving the office.

■ If a tampon was inserted after the biopsy, tell the patient to leave it in place for 8 to 24 hours. Inform her that some bleeding may occur, but tell her to report heavy bleeding (heavier than menses). Warn the patient to avoid using tampons, which can irritate the cervix and provoke bleeding.

■ Tell the patient to avoid douching and intercourse for 2 weeks, or as directed, if she has undergone such treatments as cryotherapy or laser treatment during the procedure.

■ Tell the patient that a foul-smelling, gray-green vaginal discharge is normal for several days after the biopsy and may persist for 3 weeks.

Precautions

■ Send the specimens to the laboratory immediately.

Normal findings

Normal cervical tissue is composed of columnar and squamous epithelial cells, loose connective tissue, and smooth-muscle fibers with no dysplasia or abnormal cell growth.

Abnormal findings

Histologic examination of a cervical tissue specimen is used to identify abnormal cells and to differentiate the tissue as intraepithelial neoplasia or invasive cancer. If the cause of an abnormal Papanicolaou test isn't demonstrated by cervical biopsy or if the specimen shows advanced dysplasia or carcinoma in situ, a cone biopsy is performed under general anesthesia to obtain a larger tissue specimen and to allow a more accurate evaluation of dysplasia.

Interfering factors

■ Failure to obtain representative specimens

■ Failure to place the specimens in the preservative immediately

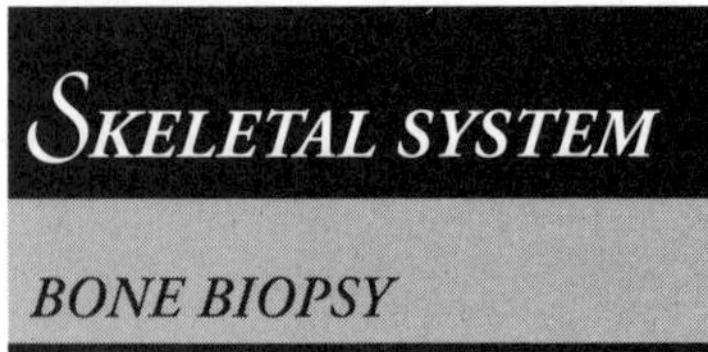

SKELETAL SYSTEM

BONE BIOPSY

Bone biopsy is the removal of a piece or a core of bone for histologic examination. It's performed either by using a special drill needle under local anesthesia or by surgical excision under general anesthesia.

Bone biopsy is indicated in patients with bone pain and tenderness after bone scan, CT scan, X-ray, or arteriography reveals a mass or deformity. Excision provides a larger specimen than drill biopsy and permits immediate surgical treatment if quick histologic analysis of the specimen reveals cancer.

Possible complications include bone fracture, damage to surrounding tissue, infection (osteomyelitis) and, possibly, contamination of normal tissue with tumor cells.

Purpose

■ To distinguish between benign and malignant bone tumors

Patient preparation

■ Describe the procedure to the patient, and answer questions.

■ Explain that this test permits microscopic examination of a bone specimen.

■ If the patient is to have a drill biopsy, he need not restrict food or fluids; if he's to have open biopsy, he must fast overnight before the test.

■ Tell the patient who will perform the biopsy and where it will be done.

■ Tell the patient that he'll receive a local anesthetic but will still experience discomfort and pressure when the biopsy needle enters the bone.

■ Explain that a special drill forces the needle into the bone; if possible, show him a photograph of the bone drill. Stress the importance of his cooperation during the biopsy.

■ Make sure the patient or a responsible family member has signed an informed consent form.

■ Check the patient's history for hypersensitivity to the local anesthetic.

Procedure and posttest care

Drill biopsy

■ The patient is properly positioned, and the biopsy site is shaved and prepared.

■ After the local anesthetic is injected, a small incision (usually about 3 mm) is made and the biopsy needle is pushed with a pointed trocar into the bone; then it's rotated about 180 degrees.

■ When the bone core is obtained, the trocar is withdrawn, and the specimen is placed in a properly labeled bottle containing 10% formalin solution. Then pressure is applied to the site with a sterile gauze pad.

■ When bleeding stops, apply a topical antiseptic (povidone-iodine ointment) and an adhesive bandage or other sterile covering to close the wound and prevent infection.

Open biopsy

■ The patient is anesthetized, and the biopsy site is shaved, cleaned with surgical soap, and disinfected with an iodine wash and alcohol.

■ An incision is made, and a piece of bone is removed and sent to the histology laboratory immediately for analysis. Further surgery can then be performed, depending on findings.

Both procedures

■ Check vital signs and the dressing at the biopsy site. Determine how much drainage is expected and report excessive drainage.

■ If the patient experiences pain, administer an analgesic.

■ For several days after the biopsy, watch for and report indications of bone infection: fever, headache, pain on movement, and redness or abscess near the biopsy site. Notify the physician if these symptoms develop.

■ Advise the patient that he may resume his usual diet.

Precautions

■ Bone biopsy should be performed cautiously in patients with coagulopathy.

■ Send the specimen to the laboratory immediately.

Normal findings

Normal bone tissue consists of fibers of collagen, osteocytes, and osteoblasts. It may be compact or cancellous. Compact bone has dense, concentric layers of mineral deposits, or lamellae. Cancellous bone has widely spaced lamellae, with osteocytes and red and yellow marrow between them.

Abnormal findings

Histologic examination of a bone specimen can reveal benign or malignant tumors. Benign tumors, generally well circumscribed and nonmetastasizing, include osteoid osteoma, osteoblastoma, osteochondroma, unicameral bone cyst, benign giant-cell tumor, and fibroma. Malignant tumors, which spread irregularly and rapidly, most commonly include multiple myeloma and osteosarcoma; the most lethal is Ewing's sarcoma. Most malignant tumors spread to the bone through the blood and lymphatic system from the breasts, lungs, prostate, thyroid, or kidneys.

Interfering factors

■ Failure to obtain a representative bone specimen

■ Failure to use the proper fixative

■ Failure to send the specimen to the laboratory immediately

BONE MARROW ASPIRATION AND BIOPSY

The histologic and hematologic examination of bone marrow provides reliable diagnostic information about blood disorders. Marrow may be removed by aspiration or needle biopsy under local anesthesia. In aspiration biopsy, a fluid specimen in which pustulae of marrow are suspended is removed from the bone marrow. In needle biopsy, a core of marrow cells (not fluid) is removed. These methods are typically used concurrently to obtain the best possible marrow specimens. Red marrow, which constitutes about 50% of an adult's marrow, actively produces stem cells that ultimately evolve into red blood cells, white blood cells, and platelets. Yellow marrow contains fat cells and connective tissue and is inactive, but it can become active in response to the body's needs.

Bleeding and infection may result from bone marrow biopsy at any site, but the most serious complications occur at the sternum. Such complications are rare but include puncture of the heart and major vessels, causing severe hemorrhage, and puncture of the mediastinum, causing mediastinitis or pneumomediastinum.

Purpose

- To diagnose thrombocytopenia, leukemias, and granulomas as well as aplastic, hypoplastic, and pernicious anemias
- To diagnose primary and metastatic tumors
- To determine the cause of infection
- To aid staging of disease such as Hodgkin's disease
- To evaluate the effectiveness of chemotherapy and monitor myelosuppression

Patient preparation

- Explain to the patient that the test permits microscopic examination of a bone marrow specimen.
- Describe the procedure to the patient, and answer questions.
- Inform the patient that he need not restrict food or fluids before the test.
- Tell him who will perform the biopsy and where it will be done.
- Inform him that more than one bone marrow specimen may be required and that a blood sample will be collected before biopsy for laboratory testing.
- Make sure the patient or a responsible family member has signed an informed consent form.
- Check the patient's history for hypersensitivity to the local anesthetic.
- Tell the patient which bone — the sternum, anterior or posterior iliac crest, vertebral spinous process, rib, or tibia — will be the biopsy site.
- Inform him that he'll receive a local anesthetic but will feel pressure on insertion of the biopsy needle and a brief, pulling pain on removal of the marrow. Administer a mild sedative 1 hour before the test.

Procedure and posttest care

- After positioning the patient, instruct him to remain as still as possible.
- Offer emotional support during the biopsy by talking quietly to the patient, describing what's being done, and answering questions.

Aspiration biopsy

- After the skin over the biopsy site is prepared and the area is draped, the local anesthetic is injected. With a twisting motion, the marrow aspiration needle is inserted through the skin, the subcutaneous tissue, and the cortex of the bone.

■ The stylet is removed from the needle, and a 10- to 20-ml syringe is attached. The examiner aspirates 0.2 to 0.5 ml of marrow and then withdraws the needle.

■ Apply pressure to the site for 5 minutes, while the marrow slides are being prepared. (If the patient has thrombocytopenia, apply pressure to the site for 10 to 15 minutes.)

■ The biopsy site is cleaned again, and a sterile adhesive bandage is applied.

■ If an adequate marrow specimen isn't obtained on the first attempt, the needle may be repositioned within the marrow cavity or removed and reinserted in another site within the anesthetized area. If the second attempt fails, a needle biopsy may be needed.

Needle biopsy

■ After preparing the biopsy site and draping the area, the examiner marks the skin at the site with an indelible pencil or marking pen.

■ A local anesthetic is then injected intradermally, subcutaneously, and at the bone's surface.

■ The biopsy needle is inserted into the periosteum, and the needle guard is set as indicated. The needle is advanced with a steady boring motion until the outer needle passes through the bone's cortex.

■ The inner needle with trephine tip is inserted into the outer needle. By alternately rotating the inner needle clockwise and counterclockwise, the examiner directs the needle into the marrow cavity and then removes a tissue plug.

■ The needle assembly is withdrawn, and the marrow is expelled into a labeled bottle containing Zenker's acetic acid solution.

■ After the biopsy site is cleaned, a sterile adhesive bandage or a pressure dressing is applied.

Both procedures

■ Check the biopsy site for bleeding and inflammation.

■ Observe the patient for signs of hemorrhage and infection, such as rapid pulse rate, low blood pressure, and fever.

Precautions

■ Bone marrow biopsy is contraindicated in patients with severe bleeding disorders.

■ Send the tissue specimen or slides to the laboratory immediately.

Normal findings

Yellow marrow contains fat cells and connective tissue; red marrow contains hematopoietic cells, fat cells, and connective tissue.

In addition, special stains that are used to detect hematologic disorders produce these normal findings: The iron stain, which is used to measure hemosiderin (storage iron), has a +2 level; the Sudan black B (SBB) fat stain, which shows granulocytes, is negative; and the periodic acid–Schiff (PAS) stain, which is used to detect glycogen reactions, is negative.

Abnormal findings

Histologic examination of a bone marrow specimen can be used to detect myelofibrosis, granulomas, lymphoma, and cancer. Hematologic analysis, including the differential count and myeloid-erythroid ratio, can implicate a wide range of disorders. (See *Bone marrow: Normal values and implications of abnormal findings,* pages 488 and 489.)

In an iron stain, decreased hemosiderin levels may indicate a true iron deficiency. Increased levels may accompany other types of anemias and blood disorders. A positive SBB stain can differentiate acute granulocytic leukemia from acute lymphocytic leukemia

Bone marrow: Normal values and implications of abnormal findings

CELL TYPES	NORMAL MEAN VALUES			CLINICAL IMPLICATIONS
	Adults	Children	Infants	
Normoblasts, total	25.6%	23.1%	8.0%	*Elevated values:* polycythemia vera *Depressed values:* vitamin B_{12} or folic acid deficiency; hypoplastic or aplastic anemia
Pronormoblasts	0.2% to 1.3%	0.5%	0.1%	
Basophilic	0.5% to 2.4%	1.7%	0.34%	
Polychromatic	17.9% to 29.2%	18.2%	6.9%	
Orthochromatic	0.4% to 4.6%	2.7%	0.54%	
Neutrophils, total	56.5%	57.1%	32.4%	*Elevated values:* acute myeloblastic or chronic myeloid leukemia *Depressed values:* lymphoblastic, lymphatic, or monocytic leukemia; aplastic anemia
Myeloblasts	0.2% to 1.5%	1.2%	0.62%	
Promyelocytes	2.1% to 4.1%	1.4%	0.76%	
Myelocytes	8.2% to 15.7%	18.3%	2.5%	
Metamyelocytes	9.6% to 24.6%	23.3%	11.3%	
Bands	9.5% to 15.3%	0	14.1%	
Segmented	6.0% to 12.0%	12.9%	3.6%	
Eosinophils	3.1%	3.6%	2.6%	*Elevated values:* bone marrow carcinoma, lymphadenoma, myeloid leukemia, eosinophilic leukemia, pernicious anemia (in relapse)
Plasma cells	1.3%	0.4%	0.02%	*Elevated values:* myeloma, collagen disease, infection, antigen sensitivity, malignancy

Bone marrow: Normal values and implications of abnormal findings *(continued)*

CELL TYPES	NORMAL MEAN VALUES			CLINICAL IMPLICATIONS
	Adults	Children	Infants	
Basophils	0.01%	0.06%	0.07%	*Elevated values:* no relation between basophil count and symptoms *Depressed values:* no relation between basophil count and symptoms
Lymphocytes	16.2%	16.0%	49.0%	*Elevated values:* B- and T-cell chronic lymphocytic leukemia, other lymphatic leukemias, lymphoma, mononucleosis, aplastic anemia, macroglobulinemia
Plasma cells	1.3%	0.4%	0.02%	*Elevated values:* Myeloma, collagen disease, infection, antigen sensitivity, malignancy.
Megakaryocytes	0.1%	0.1%	0.05%	*Elevated values:* old age, chronic myeloid leukemia, polycythemia vera, megakaryocytic myelosis, infection, idiopathic thrombocytopenic purpura, thrombocytopenia *Depressed values:* pernicious anemia
Myeloiderythroid ratio	2:1 to 4:1	2.9:1	4.4:1	*Elevated values:* myeloid leukemia, infection, leukemoid reactions, depressed hematopoiesis *Depressed values:* agranulocytosis, hematopoiesis after hemorrhage or hemolysis, iron deficiency anemia, polycythemia vera

(SBB-negative) or may indicate granulation in myeloblasts. A positive PAS stain may indicate acute or chronic lymphocytic leukemia, amyloidosis, thalassemia, lymphomas, infectious mononucleosis, iron deficiency anemia, or sideroblastic anemia.

Interfering factors

- Failure to obtain a representative specimen
- Failure to use a fixative for histologic analysis
- Failure to send the specimen to the laboratory immediately

SYNOVIAL MEMBRANE BIOPSY

Biopsy of the synovial membrane is needle excision of a tissue specimen for histologic examination of the thin epithelium lining the diarthrodial joint capsules. In a large joint, such as the knee, preliminary arthroscopy can aid selection of the biopsy site. Synovial membrane biopsy is performed when analysis of synovial fluid — a viscous, lubricating fluid contained within the synovial membrane — proves nondiagnostic or when the fluid is absent.

Purpose

- To diagnose gout, pseudogout, bacterial infections and lesions, and granulomatous infections
- To aid diagnosis of systemic lupus erythematosus (SLE), rheumatoid arthritis, or Reiter's disease
- To monitor joint pathology

Patient preparation

- Explain to the patient that this test provides a tissue specimen from the membrane that lines the affected joint.
- Describe the procedure to the patient, and answer questions.
- Advise him that he need not restrict food or fluids.
- Tell him who will perform the procedure and where it will be done.
- Inform the patient that complications include infection and bleeding into the joint, but they are rare.
- Advise him that he'll receive a local anesthetic to minimize discomfort but will experience pain when the needle enters the joint.
- Make sure the patient or an appropriate family member has signed an informed consent form.
- Check the patient's history for hypersensitivity to the local anesthetic.
- Inform the patient which site — knee (most common), elbow, wrist, ankle, or shoulder — has been chosen for this biopsy (usually, the most symptomatic joint is selected).
- Administer a sedative to help him relax.

Procedure and posttest care

- Place the patient in the proper position, clean the biopsy site, and drape the area.
- The local anesthetic is injected into the joint space; then the trocar is forcefully thrust into the joint space.
- The biopsy needle is inserted through the trocar. The hooked notch side of the biopsy needle is positioned against the synovium, and suction is applied with a 50-ml luer-lock syringe.
- While the trocar is held stationary, the biopsy needle is twisted to cut off a tissue segment.
- The biopsy needle is withdrawn, and the specimen is placed in a properly labeled sterile container or a specimen bottle containing absolute ethyl alcohol as indicated.

■ By changing the angle of the biopsy needle, several specimens can be obtained without reinserting the trocar.
■ The trocar is then removed, the biopsy site is cleaned, and a pressure bandage is applied.
■ Watch for signs of bleeding into the joint (swelling and tenderness) every hour for 4 hours and then every 4 hours for 12 hours.
■ Administer an analgesic as ordered if the patient experiences pain.
■ Tell the patient to rest the joint for 1 day before resuming normal activity.

Precautions
■ Send a specimen in a container with absolute ethyl alcohol to the histology laboratory immediately or send one in a sterile container to the microbiology laboratory.

Normal findings
The synovial membrane contains cells that are identical to those found in other connective tissue. The membrane surface is relatively smooth, except for villi, folds, and fat pads that project into the joint cavity. The membrane tissue produces synovial fluid and contains a capillary network, lymphatic vessels, and a few nerve fibers. A pathologic condition of the synovial membrane also affects the synovial fluid's cellular composition.

Abnormal findings
Histologic examination of synovial tissue can diagnose coccidioidomycosis, gout, pseudogout, hemochromatosis, tuberculosis, sarcoidosis, amyloidosis, pigmented villonodular synovitis, synovial tumors, and synovial cancer (rare). Such examination can also aid diagnosis of rheumatoid arthritis, SLE, and Reiter's disease.

Interfering factors
■ Failure to obtain several biopsy specimens
■ Failure to obtain the specimens away from the anesthetic's infiltration site
■ Failure to store the specimens in the appropriate solution or to send them to the laboratory immediately

Other organ-specific biopsies

Thyroid biopsy

Thyroid biopsy is the excision of a thyroid tissue specimen for histologic examination. This procedure is indicated in patients with thyroid enlargement or nodules, breathing and swallowing difficulties, vocal cord paralysis, weight loss, hemoptysis, and a sensation of fullness in the neck. It's commonly performed when noninvasive tests, such as thyroid ultrasonography and scans, are abnormal or inconclusive. Coagulation studies should always precede thyroid biopsy.

Thyroid tissue may be obtained with a hollow needle under local anesthesia or during open (surgical) biopsy under general anesthesia. Fine-needle aspiration with a cytologic smear examination can aid in diagnosis and replace an open biopsy. Open biopsy, performed in the operating room, provides more information than needle biopsy; it also permits direct examination and immediate excision of suspicious tissue.

Purpose
■ To differentiate between benign and malignant thyroid disease

■ To help diagnose Hashimoto's disease, hyperthyroidism, and nontoxic nodular goiter

Patient preparation

■ Describe the procedure to the patient, and answer questions.
■ Explain that this test permits microscopic examination of a thyroid tissue specimen.
■ Inform the patient that he need not restrict food or fluids (unless he receives a general anesthetic).
■ Tell him who will perform the biopsy and where it will be done.
■ Make sure the patient or an appropriate family member has signed an informed consent form.
■ Check the patient's history for hypersensitivity to anesthetics or analgesics.
■ Tell the patient he'll receive a local anesthetic to minimize pain during the procedure but may experience some pressure when the tissue specimen is procured.
■ Check the results of the patient's coagulation studies, and make sure they're in his chart.
■ Advise him that he may have a sore throat the day after the test.
■ Administer a sedative to the patient 15 minutes before biopsy.

Procedure and posttest care

■ For needle biopsy, place the patient in the supine position, with a pillow under his shoulder blades. (This position pushes the trachea and thyroid forward and allows the neck veins to fall backward.)
■ Prepare the skin over the biopsy site.
■ As the examiner prepares to inject the local anesthetic, warn the patient not to swallow.
■ After the anesthetic is injected, the carotid artery is palpated and the biopsy needle is inserted parallel to the thyroid cartilage to prevent damage to the deep structures and the larynx.
■ When the specimen is obtained, the needle is removed and the specimen is placed in formalin immediately.
■ Apply pressure to the biopsy site to stop bleeding. If bleeding continues for more than a few minutes, press on the site for up to an additional 15 minutes. Apply an adhesive bandage. (Bleeding may persist in a patient with prolonged PT or prolonged PTT or in a patient with a large, vascular thyroid with distended veins.)
■ To make the patient more comfortable, place him in the semi-Fowler position; tell him to avoid straining the biopsy site by putting both hands behind his neck when he sits up.
■ Watch for tenderness or redness, and report signs of bleeding at the biopsy site immediately. Check the back of the neck and the patient's pillow for bleeding every hour for 8 hours. Observe for difficult breathing due to edema or hematoma, with resultant tracheal collapse.
■ Keep the biopsy site clean and dry.

Precautions

■ Thyroid biopsy should be used cautiously in patients with coagulation defects, as indicated by prolonged PT or PTT.
■ The specimen must be placed immediately in formalin solution because cell breakdown in the tissue specimen begins immediately after excision.

Normal findings

Histologic examination of normal tissue shows fibrous networks dividing the gland into pseudolobules that are made up of follicles and capillaries. Cuboidal epithelium lines the follicle walls and contains the protein thyroglobulin, which stores T_4 and T_3.

Abnormal findings

Malignant tumors appear as well-encapsulated, solitary nodules of uniform but abnormal structure. Papillary carcinoma is the most common thyroid cancer. Follicular carcinoma, a less common form, strongly resembles normal cells.

Benign tumors, such as nontoxic nodular goiter, demonstrate hypertrophy, hyperplasia, and hypervascularity. Distinct histologic patterns characterize subacute granulomatous thyroiditis, Hashimoto's thyroiditis, and hyperthyroidism.

Because thyroid tumors are usually multicentric and small, a negative histologic report doesn't rule out cancer.

Interfering factors

- Failure to obtain a representative tissue specimen
- Failure to place the specimen in formalin solution immediately

LYMPH NODE BIOPSY

Lymph node biopsy is the surgical excision of an active lymph node or the needle aspiration of a nodal specimen for histologic examination. Both techniques usually use a local anesthetic and sample the superficial nodes in the cervical, supraclavicular, axillary, or inguinal region. Excision is preferred because it yields a larger specimen.

Although lymph nodes swell during infection, biopsy is indicated when nodal enlargement is prolonged and accompanied by backache, leg edema, breathing and swallowing difficulties and, later, weight loss, weakness, severe itching, fever, night sweats, cough, hemoptysis, and hoarseness. Generalized or localized lymph node enlargement is typical of such diseases as chronic lymphatic leukemia, Hodgkin's disease, infectious mononucleosis, and rheumatoid arthritis.

Complete blood count, liver function studies, liver and spleen scans, and X-rays should precede this test.

Purpose

- To determine the cause of lymph node enlargement
- To distinguish between benign and malignant lymph node processes
- To stage metastatic cancer

Patient preparation

- Explain to the patient that this test allows microscopic study of lymph node tissue.
- Describe the procedure to the patient, and answer questions.
- For excisional biopsy, instruct the patient to restrict food after midnight and to drink only clear liquids on the morning of the test (if general anesthesia is needed for deeper nodes, he must also restrict fluids).
- For needle biopsy, inform him that he need not restrict food or fluids. Tell him who will perform the biopsy and where it will be done.
- Make sure the patient or a responsible family member has signed an informed consent form.
- Check the patient's history for hypersensitivity to the anesthetic.
- If the patient will receive a local anesthetic, explain that he may experience discomfort during the injection.
- Record baseline vital signs just before the biopsy.

Procedure and posttest care

Excisional biopsy

- After the skin over the biopsy site is prepared and draped, the local anesthetic is administered.

- The examiner makes an incision, removes an entire node, and places it in a properly labeled bottle containing normal saline solution.
- The wound is sutured and a sterile dressing applied.

Needle biopsy

- After preparing the biopsy site and administering a local anesthetic, the examiner grasps the node between his thumb and forefinger, inserts the needle directly into the node, and obtains a small core specimen.
- The needle is removed, and the specimen is placed in a properly labeled bottle containing normal saline solution.
- Pressure is exerted at the biopsy site to control bleeding, and an adhesive bandage is applied.

Both procedures

- Check vital signs, and watch for bleeding, tenderness, and redness at the site.
- Inform the patient that he may resume his usual diet.

Precautions

- Storing the tissue specimen in normal saline solution instead of 10% formalin solution allows part of the specimen to be used for cytologic impression smears, which are studied along with the biopsy specimen.

Normal findings

The normal lymph node is encapsulated by collagenous connective tissue and divided into smaller lobes by tissue strands called trabeculae. It has an outer cortex, composed of lymphoid cells and nodules or follicles containing lymphocytes, and an inner medulla, composed of reticular phagocytic cells that collect and drain fluid.

Abnormal findings

Histologic examination of the tissue specimen distinguishes between malignant and nonmalignant causes of lymph node enlargement. Lymphatic cancer accounts for up to 5% of all cancers and is slightly more prevalent in males than in females. Hodgkin's disease, a lymphoma affecting the entire lymph system, is the leading cancer affecting adolescents and young adults. Lymph node cancer may also result from metastatic cancer.

When histologic results aren't clear or nodular material isn't involved, mediastinoscopy or laparotomy can provide another nodal specimen. Occasionally, lymphangiography can furnish additional diagnostic information.

Interfering factors

- Failure to obtain a representative tissue specimen
- Improper specimen storage
- Inability to differentiate nodal pathology

SENTINEL LYMPH NODE BIOPSY

Sentinel lymph node biopsy is considered experimental for breast cancer patients but has become part of the standard of care for melanoma patients. A sentinel lymph node is defined as the first node in the lymphatic basin into which a primary tumor site drains. Hypothetically, the histology of the sentinel node will reflect the histology of the rest of the nodes in that basin. Hence, if that sentinel node is identified and found to be negative for tumor invasion, it's hypothesized that the rest of the nodes are also negative for tumor. In breast cancer, if the hypothesis is proven true, axillary lymph node dissections and their resulting morbidity could be avoided.

Sentinel lymph node biopsy is performed using one of two techniques; the techniques are usually combined to increase the likelihood of identifying the sentinel node. One technique is lymphoscintigraphy, performed in nuclear medicine using injected technetium-99m (^{99m}Tc), a radioactive isotope. The second technique uses the injection of blue dye.

Purpose

- To identify the sentinel lymph node and evaluate it for the presence or absence of tumor cells indicating nodal metastasis

Patient preparation

- Explain to the patient that this test evaluates a particular lymph node to determine if cancer has spread into the lymph system. Tell her that it's usually done in conjunction with lumpectomy or mastectomy.
- Tell the patient that a radioactive substance will be injected under the skin. Assure her that she won't be radioactive and that the amount of radiation exposure will be less than that of a routine chest X-ray.

Procedure and posttest care

- The patient is positioned on the table in the nuclear medicine suite.
- A standard dose of ^{99m}Tc is injected circumferentially around the margins of a palpable mass using a 25G needle. For a nonpalpable mass, injections are guided with ultrasound or mammographic techniques. If the tumor has already been excised, the injections are made around the tumor bed.
- Images of the axilla are taken with a gamma camera. The location of the sentinel node is marked on the skin in indelible ink and noted on a data sheet.
- The patient is then transported to the operating room and placed under appropriate anesthesia.
- Blue dye is injected circumferentially in the tissue immediately surrounding the biopsy site using a 25G needle.
- Within 10 to 15 minutes of the dye injection, a small incision is made in the axilla over the suspected location of the sentinel lymph node. The surgeon follows the trail of stained lymphatics to the sentinel lymph node. The node is identified by the blue dye and by using an intraoperative gamma probe that measures radioactivity; the node having the highest radioactivity is deemed the sentinel node and removed.
- The axilla is then checked for remaining radioactivity; if none is noted, the surgical procedure concludes.
- Because of the radioactivity, the sentinel lymph node is maintained in formalin for 24 to 48 hours before it can be processed.
- Other than routine postoperative care, no special posttest care is required for this procedure.

Precautions

- Because ^{99m}Tc is a radioactive substance, all radiation precautions must be implemented. Staff members need to be monitored for radiation exposure. Radiation levels need to be determined in the nuclear medicine suite and the operating room postsurgically.
- Rare cases of allergy to the ^{99m}Tc or blue dye have been noted; patients should be observed for signs of allergic reaction (skin changes and respiratory difficulties).

Normal findings

Normal findings are the same as for a normal lymph node biopsy.

Abnormal findings

Sentinel lymph node biopsy is performed only in breast cancer and melanoma, so abnormal findings mean the identification of melanoma or breast cancer cells. Their presence indicates lymph node metastasis and guides the prognosis and treatment.

Interfering factors

- Allergy to radioactive substance
- Inability to raise arm to allow access to axilla
- Inability to obtain adequate specimen
- Improper specimen storage

SKIN BIOPSY

Skin biopsy is the removal of a small piece of tissue under local anesthesia from a lesion suspected of being malignant or from other dermatoses. One of three techniques may be used: shave biopsy, punch biopsy, or excisional biopsy. Shave biopsy uses a scalpel to slice a superficial specimen from the site. Punch biopsy removes an oval core from the center of a lesion down to the dermis or subcutaneous tissue. Excisional biopsy removes the entire lesion with a small border of normal skin.

Lesions suspected of being malignant usually have changed color, size, or appearance or have failed to heal properly after injury. Fully developed lesions should be selected for biopsy whenever possible because they provide more diagnostic information than lesions that are resolving or in early developing stages.

Purpose

- To provide differential diagnosis among basal cell carcinoma, squamous cell carcinoma, malignant melanoma, and benign growths
- To diagnose chronic bacterial or fungal skin infections

Patient preparation

- Explain to the patient that the biopsy provides a specimen for microscopic study.
- Describe the procedure to the patient, and answer questions.
- Inform him that he need not restrict food or fluids.
- Tell him who will perform the procedure and where it will be done.
- Tell him he'll receive a local anesthetic to minimize pain during the procedure.
- Have the patient or a responsible family member sign an informed consent form.
- Check the patient's history for hypersensitivity to the local anesthetic.

Procedure and posttest care

- Position the patient comfortably, and clean the biopsy site before the local anesthetic is administered.

Shave biopsy

- The protruding growth is cut off at the skin line with a #15 scalpel and the tissue is placed immediately in a properly labeled specimen bottle containing 10% formalin solution.
- Apply pressure to the area to stop the bleeding.

Punch biopsy

- The skin surrounding the lesion is pulled taut, and the punch is firmly introduced into the lesion and rotated to obtain a tissue specimen. The plug is lifted with forceps or a needle and severed as deeply into the fat layer as possible.
- The specimen is placed in a properly labeled specimen bottle containing 10% formalin solution or in a sterile container if indicated.

- Closing the wound depends on the size of the punch: A 3-mm punch requires only an adhesive bandage, a 4-mm punch requires one suture, and a 6-mm punch requires two sutures.

Excisional biopsy

- A #15 scalpel is used to excise the entire lesion; the elliptical incision is made as wide and as deep as necessary.
- The tissue specimen is removed and placed immediately in a properly labeled specimen bottle containing 10% formalin solution.
- Apply pressure to the site to stop the bleeding.
- The wound is closed using 4-0 suture. If the incision is large, skin graft may be required.

All procedures

- Check the biopsy site for bleeding.
- If the patient experiences pain, administer an analgesic as ordered.
- Advise the patient with sutures to keep the area as clean and dry as possible. Facial sutures are removed in 3 to 5 days; trunk sutures, in 7 to 14 days. Tell the patient with adhesive strips to leave them in place for 14 to 21 days or until they fall off.

Precautions

- Send the specimen to the laboratory immediately.

Normal findings

Normal skin consists of squamous epithelium (epidermis) and fibrous connective tissue (dermis).

Abnormal findings

Histologic examination of the tissue specimen may reveal a benign or malignant lesion. Benign growths include cysts, seborrheic keratoses, warts, pigmented nevi (moles), keloids, dermatofibromas, and multiple neurofibromas.

Malignant tumors include basal cell carcinoma, squamous cell carcinoma, and malignant melanoma. Basal cell carcinoma occurs on hair-bearing skin; the most common location is the face, including the nose and its folds. Squamous cell carcinoma most commonly appears on the lips, mouth, and genitalia. Malignant melanoma, the deadliest skin cancer, can spread through the body by way of the lymphatic system and blood vessels.

Cultures can be used to detect chronic bacterial and fungal infections in which flora are relatively sparse.

Interfering factors

- Improper selection of the biopsy site
- Failure to use the appropriate fixative or a sterile container

PERCUTANEOUS RENAL BIOPSY

Percutaneous renal biopsy is the needle excision of a core of kidney tissue for histologic examination. This biopsy may help assess histologic changes caused by acute or chronic glomerulonephritis, pyelonephritis, renal vein thrombosis, amyloid infiltration, and systemic lupus erythematosus. In the case of a mass, results can differentiate a primary renal cancer from a metastatic lesion.

Complications of percutaneous biopsy include bleeding, hematoma, arteriovenous fistula, and infection. This procedure is safer than open biopsy, which is the preferred method for sampling a solid lesion, but noninvasive procedures, especially renal ultrasonography and computed tomography, have replaced percutaneous renal biopsy in many hospitals. (See *Urinary tract brush biopsy,* page 498.)

Urinary tract brush biopsy

Retrograde brush biopsy of the urinary tract may be used to obtain a renal tissue specimen when X-rays show a lesion in the renal pelvis or calyx. It can also be used to obtain specimens from other areas of the urinary tract. Retrograde brush biopsy is contraindicated in patients with acute urinary tract infection or an obstruction at or below the biopsy site.

PATIENT PREPARATION

To prepare the patient for brush biopsy, describe the procedure, and tell him that he may experience some discomfort. Inform him who will perform the biopsy and when. Reassure the patient that the procedure will take only 30 to 60 minutes.

Make sure the patient or a responsible family member has signed an informed consent form. Because this procedure requires use of a contrast medium and a general, local, or spinal anesthetic, check the patient's history for hypersensitivity to anesthetics, contrast media, or iodine-containing foods such as shellfish. Just before the biopsy procedure, administer a sedative to the patient.

OBTAINING THE BIOPSY

After the patient has received a sedative and an anesthetic, place him in the lithotomy position. Using a cystoscope, a guide wire is passed up the ureter and a urethral catheter is passed over the guide wire. Contrast medium is instilled through the catheter, which is positioned next to the lesion under fluoroscopic guidance. The contrast medium is washed out with normal saline solution to prevent cell distortions from the dye. A nylon or steel brush is passed up the catheter and the lesion is brushed. This procedure is repeated at least six times, using a new brush each time.

As each brush is removed from the catheter, a smear is made for Papanicolaou staining and the brush tip is cut off and placed in formalin solution for 1 hour. The biopsy material is then removed from the brush tip for histologic examination. When the last brush is withdrawn, the catheter is irrigated with normal saline solution to remove additional cells. These cells are also sent for histologic examination.

Results differentiate between malignant and benign lesions, which may appear the same on X-rays.

POSTTEST CARE

Because brush biopsy may cause complications, such as perforation, hemorrhage, sepsis, and contrast medium extravasation, carefully monitor the patient's vital signs. Be sure to record the time, color, and amount of voiding, being alert for hematuria and abdominal or flank pain. Report abnormal findings immediately, and administer analgesics and antibiotics as ordered.

Purpose

- To aid diagnosis of renal parenchymal disease
- To monitor the progression of renal disease and assess the effectiveness of therapy

Patient preparation

- Explain to the patient that this test is used to diagnose kidney disorders.
- Describe the procedure to the patient, and answer questions.
- Instruct the patient to restrict food and fluids for 8 hours before the test.
- Tell him who will perform the biopsy and where it will be done.
- Ensure that blood samples and urine specimens are collected and tested before the biopsy and that results of other tests to determine the biopsy site, such

as excretory urography, ultrasonography, and an erect film of the abdomen, are available.

■ Make sure the patient or a responsible family member has signed an informed consent form.

■ Check the patient's history for hemorrhagic tendencies and hypersensitivity to the local anesthetic.

■ Administer a mild sedative 30 minutes to 1 hour before the biopsy to help the patient relax, as ordered.

■ Inform the patient that he'll receive a local anesthetic but may experience a pinching pain when the needle is inserted through the back into the kidney.

■ Check vital signs, and tell the patient to void just before the test.

Procedure and posttest care

■ Place the patient in a prone position on a firm surface with a sandbag beneath his abdomen.

■ Tell him to take a deep breath while his kidney is being palpated.

■ A 7″ 20G needle is used to inject the local anesthetic into the skin at the biopsy site. Instruct the patient to hold his breath and remain still as the needle is inserted through the back muscles, the deep lumbar fascia, the perinephric fat, and the kidney capsule. After the needle is inserted, tell the patient to take several deep breaths. If the needle swings smoothly during deep breathing, it has penetrated the kidney capsule. After the penetration depth is marked on the needle shaft, instruct the patient to hold his breath and remain as still as possible while the needle is withdrawn.

■ After a small incision is made in the anesthetized skin, instruct the patient to hold his breath and remain still while the Vim-Silverman needle with stylet is inserted to the measured depth.

■ Tell the patient to breathe deeply. Then tell him to remain still while the tissue specimen is obtained.

■ The tissue is examined immediately under a hand lens to ensure that the specimen contains tissue from cortex and medulla. Then it's placed on a saline-soaked gauze pad and placed in a properly labeled container.

■ If an adequate tissue specimen hasn't been obtained, the procedure is repeated immediately.

■ After an adequate specimen is secured, apply pressure to the biopsy site for 3 to 5 minutes to stop superficial bleeding. Then apply a pressure dressing.

■ Instruct the patient to lie flat on his back without moving for at least 12 hours to prevent bleeding. Check vital signs every 15 minutes for 4 hours, then every 30 minutes for 4 hours, then every hour for 4 hours and, finally, every 4 hours. Report any changes.

■ Examine urine for blood; small amounts may be present after the biopsy but should disappear within 8 hours. Hematocrit may be monitored after the procedure to screen for internal bleeding.

■ Encourage fluid ingestion to minimize colic and obstruction from blood clotting within the renal pelvis.

■ Inform the patient that he may resume his normal diet.

■ Discourage the patient from engaging in strenuous activities for several days after the procedure to prevent possible bleeding.

Precautions

■ Percutaneous renal biopsy is contraindicated in a patient with a severe bleeding disorder, markedly reduced plasma or blood volume, severe hypertension, hydronephrosis, perinephric abscess, advanced renal failure with uremia, or only one kidney.

- Instruct the patient to hold his breath and remain still whenever the needle or prongs are advanced into or retracted from the kidney.
- Send the specimen to the laboratory immediately.

Normal findings

Usually, a section of kidney tissue shows Bowman's capsule — the area between two layers of flat epithelial cells — the glomerular tuft, and the capillary lumen. The tubule sections differ, depending on the area of tubule involved. The proximal tubule is one layer of epithelial cells with microvilli that form a brush border. The descending loop of Henle has flat squamous epithelial cells. The ascending, distal convoluted, and collecting tubules are lined with squamous epithelial cells.

Abnormal findings

Histologic examination of renal tissue can reveal cancer or renal disease. Malignant tumors include Wilms' tumor, which is usually present in early childhood, and renal cell carcinoma, which is most prevalent in people over age 40. Diseases indicated by characteristic histologic changes include disseminated lupus erythematosus, amyloid infiltration, acute or chronic glomerulonephritis, renal vein thrombosis, and pyelonephritis.

Interfering factors

- Failure to obtain an adequate tissue specimen
- Failure to store the specimen properly
- Failure to send the specimen to the laboratory immediately

10

Endoscopy

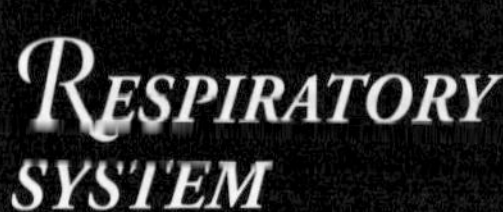

Respiratory System

DIRECT LARYNGOSCOPY

Direct laryngoscopy allows visualization of the larynx by the use of a fiber-optic endoscope or laryngoscope passed through the mouth and pharynx to the larynx. It's indicated for children, patients with strong gag reflexes due to anatomic abnormalities, and those who have had no response to short-term therapy for symptoms of pharyngeal or laryngeal disease, such as stridor and hemoptysis. Secretions or tissue may be removed during this procedure for further study. The test is usually contraindicated in patients with epiglottiditis but may be performed on them in an operating room with resuscitative equipment available.

Purpose

- To detect lesions, strictures, or foreign bodies
- To remove benign lesions or foreign bodies from the larynx
- To aid diagnosis of laryngeal cancer
- To examine the larynx when indirect laryngoscopy is inadequate

Patient preparation

- Explain to the patient that this test is used to detect laryngeal abnormalities.
- Instruct the patient to fast for 6 to 8 hours before the test.
- Tell him who will perform the procedure and where it will be done.
- Inform the patient that he'll receive a sedative to help him relax, medication to reduce secretions and, during the procedure, a general or local anesthetic. Reassure him that this procedure won't obstruct his airway.
- Make sure the patient or a responsible family member has signed an informed consent form.
- Check the patient's history for hypersensitivity to the anesthetic.
- Obtain baseline vital signs.
- Administer the sedative and other medication (usually 30 minutes to 1 hour before the test) as ordered.
- Instruct the patient to remove dentures, contact lenses, and jewelry, and to void before giving him a sedative.

Equipment

Laryngoscope, sedative, atropine, local anesthetic (spray or jelly) or general anesthetic, sterile container for microbiology specimen, sterile gloves, Coplin jar with 95% ethyl alcohol for cytology smears, container with 10% formalin solution for histology specimen, forceps for biopsy, emesis basin, suction and resuscitation equipment

Procedure and posttest care

- Place the patient in the supine position.
- Encourage him to breathe through his nose and to relax with his arms at his sides.
- A general anesthetic is administered, or the patient's mouth and throat are sprayed with a local anesthetic.
- A laryngoscope is introduced through the patient's mouth, the larynx is examined for abnormalities, and a specimen or secretions may be removed for further study; minor surgery, such as removal of polyps or nodules, may be performed at this time.
- Place the specimens in their respective containers. Collection of specimen should be done in accordance with laboratory and pathology guidelines.
- Place the conscious patient in semi-Fowler's position; place the unconscious

patient on his side with his head slightly elevated to prevent aspiration.

- Check vital signs according to facility protocol, or every 15 minutes until the patient is stable and then every 30 minutes for 2 hours, every hour for the next 4 hours, and then every 4 hours for 24 hours. Immediately report to the physician any adverse reaction to the anesthetic or sedative (tachycardia, palpitations, hypertension, euphoria, excitation, and rapid, deep respirations).
- Apply an ice collar to minimize laryngeal edema.
- Provide an emesis basin, and instruct the patient to spit out saliva rather than swallow it. Observe sputum for blood, and report excessive bleeding immediately.
- Instruct the patient to refrain from clearing his throat and coughing to prevent hemorrhaging at the biopsy site.
- Advise the patient to avoid smoking until vital signs are stable and there's no evidence of complications.
- Immediately report subcutaneous crepitus around the patient's face and neck, which may indicate tracheal perforation.
- Listen to the patient's neck with a stethoscope for signs of stridor and airway obstruction.

CLINICAL ALERT *Observe the patient with epiglottiditis for signs of airway obstruction, and immediately report signs of respiratory difficulty. Keep emergency resuscitation equipment available; keep a tracheotomy tray nearby for 24 hours.*

- Restrict food and fluids to avoid aspiration until the gag reflex returns (usually within 2 hours). Then the patient may resume his usual diet, beginning with sips of water.
- Reassure the patient that voice loss, hoarseness, and sore throat are temporary. Provide throat lozenges or a soothing liquid gargle when his gag reflex returns.

Precautions

- Send the specimens to the laboratory immediately.

Normal findings

A normal larynx shows no evidence of inflammation, lesions, strictures, or foreign bodies.

Abnormal findings

The combined results of direct laryngoscopy, biopsy, and radiography may indicate laryngeal carcinoma. Direct laryngoscopy also may show benign lesions, strictures, or foreign bodies and, with a biopsy, may distinguish laryngeal edema from a radiation reaction or a tumor. It can also determine vocal cord dysfunction.

Interfering factors

- Failure to place the specimens in appropriate containers or to send them to the laboratory immediately

BRONCHOSCOPY

Bronchoscopy allows direct visualization of the larynx, trachea, and bronchi through a flexible fiber-optic bronchoscope or a rigid metal bronchoscope. Although a flexible fiber-optic bronchoscope allows a wider view and is used more often, the rigid metal bronchoscope is required to remove foreign objects, excise endobronchial lesions, and control massive hemoptysis. A brush, biopsy forceps, or catheter may be passed through the bronchoscope to obtain specimens for cytologic examination.

Purpose

- To visually examine a tumor, an obstruction, secretions, bleeding, or a foreign body in the tracheobronchial tree
- To help diagnose bronchogenic carcinoma, tuberculosis, interstitial pulmonary disease, and fungal or parasitic pulmonary infection by obtaining a specimen for bacteriologic and cytologic examination
- To remove foreign bodies, malignant or benign tumors, mucus plugs, and excessive secretions from the tracheobronchial tree

Patient preparation

- Explain to the patient that this test is used to examine the lower airways.
- Describe the procedure, and instruct the patient to fast for 6 to 12 hours before the test.
- Tell him who will perform the test, where it will be done, and that the room will be darkened.
- Tell the patient that a chest X-ray and blood studies will be performed before the bronchoscopy and afterward if appropriate.
- Advise him that he may receive a sedative I.V. to help him relax.
- If the procedure isn't being performed under general anesthesia, inform the patient that a local anesthetic will be sprayed into his nose and mouth to suppress the gag reflex. Warn him that the spray has an unpleasant taste and that he may experience discomfort during the procedure.
- Reassure him that his airway won't be blocked during the procedure and that oxygen will be administered through the bronchoscope.
- Make sure the patient or a responsible family member has signed a consent form.
- Check the patient's history for hypersensitivity to the anesthetic.
- Obtain baseline vital signs.
- Administer the preoperative sedative.
- Have the patient remove his dentures, if appropriate, before he receives a sedative.

Equipment

Flexible fiber-optic bronchoscope, sedative, local anesthetic (spray, jelly, or liquid), sterile gloves, sterile container for microbiology specimen, container with 10% formalin solution for histology specimen, Coplin jar with 95% ethyl alcohol for cytology smears, six glass slides (frosted, if possible, or with frosted tips), emesis basin, handheld resuscitation bag with face mask, oral and endotracheal airways, continuous suction equipment, laryngoscope, oxygen delivery equipment, ventilating bronchoscope for a patient requiring controlled mechanical ventilation

Procedure and posttest care

- Place the patient in the supine position, or have him sit upright in a chair.
- Tell him to remain relaxed with his arms at his sides and to breathe through his nose.
- Provide supplemental oxygen by nasal cannula if necessary.
- After the local anesthetic is sprayed into the patient's throat and takes effect, a bronchoscope is introduced through the patient's mouth or nose. When the scope is just above the vocal cords, about 3 to 4 ml of 2% to 4% lidocaine is flushed through the inner channel of the scope to the vocal cords to anesthetize deeper areas. The physician inspects the anatomic structure of the trachea and bronchi, observes the color of the mucosal lining, and notes masses or inflamed areas.
- Biopsy forceps may be used to remove a tissue specimen from a suspect area, a bronchial brush may be used to obtain cells from the surface of a lesion, and a suction apparatus may be used to

remove foreign bodies or mucus plugs. Bronchoalveolar lavage may be performed to diagnose the infectious causes of infiltrates in immunocompromised patients or to remove thickened secretions.

- After collection, place the specimens in their respective, properly labeled containers in accordance with laboratory and pathology guidelines and send them to the laboratory at once.
- Bronchoscopy may require fluoroscopic guidance for distal evaluation of lesions for a transbronchial biopsy in alveolar areas.
- Check vital signs as per facility policy, or at least every 15 minutes until the patient is stable and then every 30 minutes for 4 hours, every hour for the next 4 hours, and then every 4 hours for 24 hours. Immediately notify the physician of adverse reactions to the anesthetic or sedative.
- Place the conscious patient in semi-Fowler's position; place the unconscious patient on his side with his head slightly elevated to prevent aspiration.
- Provide an emesis basin, and instruct the patient to spit out saliva rather than swallow it. Observe sputum for blood, and report excessive bleeding immediately.
- Tell the patient who has had a biopsy to refrain from clearing his throat and coughing, which may dislodge the clot at the biopsy site and cause hemorrhaging.
- Immediately report subcutaneous crepitus around the patient's face and neck because this may indicate tracheal or bronchial perforation.

◆ CLINICAL ALERT *Watch for, listen for, and immediately report symptoms of respiratory difficulty resulting from laryngeal edema or laryngospasm, such as laryngeal stridor and dyspnea. Observe for signs of hypoxemia, pneumothorax, bronchospasm, and bleeding.*

- Restrict food and fluids to avoid aspiration until the gag reflex returns (usually in 1 to 2 hours). Then the patient may resume his usual diet, beginning with sips of clear liquid or ice chips.
- Reassure the patient that hoarseness, loss of voice, and sore throat are temporary. Provide lozenges or a soothing liquid gargle to ease discomfort when his gag reflex returns.

Precautions

- A patient with respiratory failure who can't breathe adequately by himself should be placed on a ventilator before bronchoscopy.
- Send the specimens to the laboratory immediately.

Normal findings

The trachea normally consists of smooth muscle containing C-shaped rings of cartilage at regular intervals, and it's lined with ciliated mucosa. The bronchi appear structurally similar to the trachea; the right bronchus is slightly larger and more vertical than the left. Smaller segmental bronchi branch off the main bronchi.

Abnormal findings

Bronchial wall abnormalities include inflammation, swelling, protruding cartilage, ulceration, enlargement of the mucous gland orifices or submucosal lymph nodes, and tumors. Endotracheal abnormalities include stenosis, compression, ectasia (dilation of tubular vessel), irregular bronchial branching, and abnormal bifurcation due to diverticulum.

Abnormal substances in the trachea or bronchi include blood, secretions, calculi, and foreign bodies.

Results of tissue and cell studies may indicate interstitial pulmonary disease, bronchogenic carcinoma, tuberculosis, or other pulmonary infections. Correlation of radiographic, bronchoscopic, and cytologic findings with clinical signs and symptoms is essential.

Interfering factors

- Failure to observe pretest restrictions may result in aspiration
- Failure to place specimens in the appropriate containers or to send them to the laboratory immediately

MEDIASTINOSCOPY

Using an exploring speculum with built-in fiber light and side slit, mediastinoscopy allows direct viewing of mediastinal structures. It also permits palpation and biopsy of paratracheal and carinal lymph nodes. This surgical procedure is indicated when other tests, such as sputum cytology, lung scans, radiography, and bronchoscopic biopsy, fail to confirm the diagnosis.

Scarring of the area from previous mediastinoscopy contraindicates this procedure.

Purpose

- To detect bronchogenic carcinoma, lymphoma (including Hodgkin's disease), and sarcoidosis
- To determine stages of lung cancer

Patient preparation

- Explain to the patient that this test is used to evaluate the lymph nodes and other structures in the chest. Review the patient's history for previous mediastinoscopy because scarring from a previous mediastinoscopy contraindicates the test.
- Describe the procedure, and answer questions.
- Instruct the patient to fast after midnight before the test.
- Tell him who will perform the procedure, where it will be done, that he'll be given general anesthesia, and that the procedure takes about 1 hour.
- Tell him that he may have temporary chest pain, tenderness at the incision site, or a sore throat (from intubation).
- Reassure him that complications are rare with this procedure.
- Make sure the patient or a responsible family member has signed a consent form.
- Check the patient's history for hypersensitivity to the anesthetic.
- Give a sedative the night before the test and again before the procedure, as ordered.

Procedure and posttest care

- After the endotracheal tube is in place, a small transverse suprasternal incision is made.
- Using finger dissection, the surgeon forms a channel and palpates the lymph nodes.
- The mediastinoscope is inserted, and tissue specimens are collected and sent to the laboratory for frozen section examination.
- If analysis confirms malignancy of a resectable tumor, thoracotomy and pneumonectomy may follow immediately.
- Monitor postoperative vital signs and check dressings for bleeding and fluid drainage.
- Observe for the following complications: fever (a sign of mediastinitis); crepitus (a sign of subcutaneous emphysema); dyspnea, cyanosis, and diminished breath sounds on the affected side (signs of pneumothorax); tachycardia and hypotension (signs of hemorrhage).

- Administer the prescribed analgesic as needed.

Precautions

- Immediately send collected specimens to the laboratory.

Normal findings

Lymph nodes appear as small, smooth, flat oval bodies of lymphoid tissue.

Abnormal findings

Malignant lymph nodes usually indicate inoperable, but not always untreatable, lung or esophageal cancer or lymphomas (such as Hodgkin's disease). Staging of lung cancer helps determine the therapeutic regimen. (For example, multiple nodular involvement can contraindicate surgery.)

Interfering factors

- Previous mediastinoscopy with scarring (makes dissection of nodes difficult or impossible)

THORACOSCOPY

In thoracoscopy, an endoscope is inserted directly into the chest wall to view the pleural space, thoracic walls, mediastinum, and pericardium. It's used for both diagnostic and therapeutic purposes and can sometimes replace traditional thoracotomy. Thoracoscopy reduces morbidity (by reducing the use of open chest surgery) and postoperative pain, decreases surgical and anesthesia time, and allows faster recovery.

Purpose

- To diagnose pleural disease
- To obtain biopsy specimens
- To treat pleural conditions, such as cysts, blebs, and effusions
- To perform wedge resections

Patient preparation

- Explain to the patient that this procedure permits visual examination of the chest wall to view the pleural space, thoracic wall, mediastinum, and pericardium.
- Describe the procedure. Caution the patient that an open thoracotomy may still be needed for diagnosis or treatment and that general anesthesia may be required.
- Instruct the patient not to eat or drink for 10 to 12 hours before the procedure.
- Make sure the appropriate preoperative tests (such as pulmonary function and coagulation tests, electrocardiography [ECG], and chest X-ray) have been performed and that a consent form has been signed.
- Tell the patient that he'll have a chest tube and drainage system in place after surgery. Reassure him that analgesics will be available and that complications are rare.

Equipment

Monitors, videocassette recorder, camera, light source, insufflator, cautery, suction and irrigation equipment, trocars, endostaplers, endosutures

Procedure and posttest care

- The patient is anesthetized, and a double-lumen endobronchial tube is inserted.
- The lung on the operative side is collapsed, and a small intercostal incision is made, through which a trocar is inserted.
- A lens is then inserted to view the area and assess thoracoscopy access.
- Two or three more small incisions are made, and trocars are placed for insertion of suction and dissection instruments.

- The camera lens and instruments are moved from site to site as needed.
- After thoracoscopy, the lung is reexpanded, a chest tube is placed through one incision site, and a water-sealed drainage system is attached. The other incisions are closed with adhesive strips and dressed.
- Monitor postoperative vital signs as per facility policy or every 15 minutes for 1 hour, every 30 minutes for 2 hours, every hour for 2 hours, and then every 4 hours.
- Assess respiratory status and the patency of the chest drainage system.
- Give analgesics as needed for pain and monitor for effect.

Precautions

- Send specimens to the laboratory immediately.
- Thoracoscopy is contraindicated in patients who have coagulopathies or lesions near major blood vessels, who have had previous thoracic surgery, or who can't be adequately oxygenated with one lung.
- Complications, although rare, include hemorrhage, nerve injury, perforation of the diaphragm, air emboli, and tension pneumothorax.

Normal findings

A normal pleural cavity contains a small amount of lubricating fluid that facilitates movement of the lung and chest wall. The parietal and visceral layers are lesion-free and can separate from each other.

Abnormal findings

Lesions, such as tumors, ulcers, and bleeding sites, adjacent to or involving the pleura or mediastinum can be seen and biopsies can be taken. Diagnosis may include carcinoma, empyema, pleural effusion, tuberculosis, or an inflammatory process. Areas of blebs can be removed by wedge resection to reduce the risk of repeat episodes of spontaneous pneumothorax.

Interfering factors

- Extensive disease or inaccessibility (may prevent thoracoscopy)
- Excessive bleeding during the procedure (may require open thoracotomy)

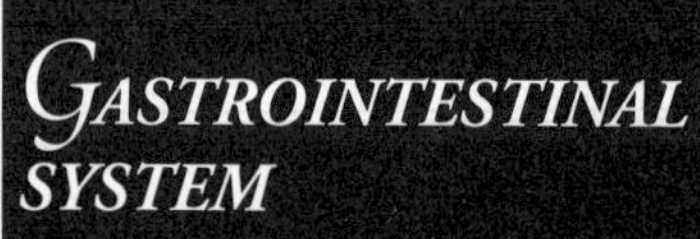

GASTROINTESTINAL SYSTEM

ESOPHAGOGASTRODUODENOSCOPY

Esophagogastroduodenoscopy (EGD) permits visual examination of the lining of the esophagus, stomach, and upper duodenum using a flexible fiber-optic or video endoscope. It's indicated for patients with GI bleeding, hematemesis, melena, substernal or epigastric pain, gastroesophageal reflux disease, dysphagia, anemia, strictures, or peptic ulcer disease; those requiring foreign body retrieval; and postoperative patients with recurrent or new symptoms.

EGD eliminates the need for extensive exploratory surgery and can be used to detect small or surface lesions missed by radiography. Because the scope provides a channel for biopsy forceps or a cytology brush, it permits laboratory evaluation of abnormalities detected by radiography. Similarly, it allows removal of foreign bodies by suction (for small, soft objects) or by electrocautery snare or forceps (for large, hard objects).

Purpose

- To diagnose inflammatory disease, malignant and benign tumors, ulcers, Mallory-Weiss syndrome and structural abnormalities
- To evaluate the stomach and duodenum postoperatively
- To obtain emergency diagnosis of duodenal ulcer or esophageal injury such as that caused by ingestion of chemicals

Patient preparation

- Explain to the patient that this procedure permits visual examination of the lining of the esophagus, stomach, and upper duodenum.
- Check the patient's medical history for allergies, medications, and information pertinent to the current complaint. Check for hypersensitivity to the medications and anesthetics ordered for the test.
- Instruct him to fast for 6 to 12 hours before the test.
- Tell him that a flexible instrument with a camera on the end will be passed through his mouth; explain who will perform this procedure, where it will be done, and that it takes about 30 minutes.
- If an emergency EGD is to be performed, tell the patient that stomach contents may be aspirated through a nasogastric tube.
- Inform the patient that a bitter-tasting local anesthetic will be sprayed into his mouth and throat to calm the gag reflex and that his tongue and throat may feel swollen, making swallowing seem difficult. Advise him to let the saliva drain from the side of his mouth; a suction machine may be used to remove saliva if necessary.
- Explain that a mouth guard will be inserted to protect his teeth and the endoscope; assure him that this won't obstruct his breathing.
- Inform him that an I.V. line will be started and a sedative will be administered before the endoscope is inserted to help him relax. If the procedure is being done on an outpatient basis, advise the patient to arrange for someone to drive him home because he may feel drowsy from the sedative. Drugs that retard peristalsis of the upper GI tract may be administered in some circumstances.
- Tell the patient that he may experience pressure in the stomach as the endoscope is moved about and a feeling of fullness when air or carbon dioxide is insufflated. If the patient is apprehensive, administer meperidine or another analgesic I.M. about 30 minutes before the test as ordered; also administer atropine sulfate subcutaneously at this time as ordered to decrease gastric secretions, which would interfere with test results.
- Make sure the patient or a responsible family member has signed an informed consent form.
- Just before the procedure, instruct the patient to remove dentures, eyeglasses, and constricting undergarments.

Procedure and posttest care

- Obtain baseline vital signs, and leave the blood pressure cuff in place for monitoring throughout the procedure.
- If the patient has known cardiac disease, continuous ECG monitoring should be instituted. Continuous or periodic pulse oximetry is advisable, particularly in patients with pulmonary compromise.
- Ask the patient to hold his breath while his mouth and throat are sprayed with a local anesthetic, if requested by the physician.
- Remind the patient to let saliva drain from the side of his mouth. Provide an emesis basin to spit out saliva and tissues to wipe saliva from his mouth, or use oropharyngeal suction as needed.

- The patient is placed in a left lateral position, his head is bent forward, and he's asked to open his mouth.
- The examiner guides the tip of the endoscope to the back of the throat and downward. As the endoscope passes through the posterior pharynx and the cricopharyngeal sphincter, the patient's neck is slowly extended. The patient's chin must be kept at midline. The endoscope is then passed along the esophagus under direct vision.
- When the endoscope is well into the esophagus (about 12″ [30 cm]), the patient's head is positioned with his chin toward the table so that saliva can drain out of his mouth.
- After examination of the esophagus and the cardiac sphincter, the endoscope is rotated clockwise and advanced to allow examination of the stomach and duodenum. During the examination, air or water may be introduced through the endoscope to aid visualization, and suction may be applied to remove insufflated air and secretions.
- A camera may be attached to the endoscope to photograph areas for later study, or a measuring tube may be passed through the endoscope to determine the size of a lesion.
- Biopsy forceps or a cytology brush may be passed through the scope to obtain specimens for histologic or cytologic study.
- The endoscope is slowly withdrawn, and suspicious-looking areas of the gastric and esophageal lining are reexamined.
- Specimens should be collected in accordance with laboratory and pathology guidelines. Place tissue specimens immediately in a specimen bottle containing 10% formalin solution; cell specimens are smeared on glass slides and placed in a Coplin jar containing 95% ethyl alcohol.

CLINICAL ALERT *Observe the patient for possible perforation. Perforation in the cervical area of the esophagus produces pain on swallowing and with neck movement; thoracic perforation causes substernal or epigastric pain that increases with breathing or movement of the trunk; diaphragmatic perforation produces shoulder pain and dyspnea; gastric perforation causes abdominal or back pain, cyanosis, fever, and pleural effusion.*

- Observe the patient for evidence of aspiration of gastric contents, which could precipitate aspiration pneumonia.
- Monitor vital signs, and document according to the facility's policy.
- Test the gag reflex by touching the back of the throat with a tongue blade. Withhold food and fluids until the gag reflex returns (usually in 1 hour), and then allow fluids and a light meal.
- Tell the patient that he may burp some insufflated air and have a sore throat for 3 to 4 days. Throat lozenges and warm saline gargles may ease his discomfort.
- If the patient experiences soreness at the I.V. site, apply warm soaks.
- Because of sedation, outpatients should avoid alcohol for 24 hours and shouldn't drive for 12 hours. Make sure these patients have transportation home.
- Instruct the patient to notify the physician immediately if he experiences persistent difficulty with swallowing, pain, fever, black stools, or bloody vomitus.

Precautions

- If tissue or cell specimens are obtained during the procedure, label and send them to the appropriate laboratory immediately.
- This procedure is generally safe but can cause perforation of the esophagus,

stomach, or duodenum, especially if the patient is restless or uncooperative.

- EGD is usually contraindicated in patients with Zenker's diverticulum, a large aortic aneurysm, recent ulcer perforation, known as suspected viscus perforation, and unstable cardiac or pulmonary condition.
- EGD shouldn't be performed within 2 days after an upper GI series.
- Patients requiring dental prophylaxis may also require antibiotics before this procedure.

CLINICAL ALERT *Observe closely for adverse effects of the sedative: respiratory depression, apnea, hypotension, excessive diaphoresis, bradycardia, and laryngospasm. Have available emergency resuscitation equipment and a narcotic antagonist such as naloxone. Be prepared to intervene as necessary.*

Normal findings

The smooth mucosa of the esophagus is normally yellow-pink and marked by a fine vascular network. A pulsation on the anterior wall of the esophagus between 8″ and 10″ (20.5 and 25.5 cm) from the incisor teeth represents the aortic arch. The orange-red mucosa of the stomach begins at the "Z" line, an irregular transition line slightly above the esophagogastric junction.

Unlike the esophagus, the stomach has rugal folds, and its blood vessels aren't visible beneath the gastric mucosa. The reddish mucosa of the duodenal bulb is marked by a few shallow longitudinal folds. The mucosa of the distal duodenum has prominent circular folds, is lined with villi, and appears velvety.

Abnormal findings

EGD, coupled with the results of histologic and cytologic tests, may indicate acute or chronic ulcers, benign or malignant tumors, and inflammatory disease, including esophagitis, gastritis, and duodenitis. This test may demonstrate diverticula, varices, Mallory-Weiss syndrome, esophageal rings, esophageal and pyloric stenoses, and esophageal hiatal hernia. Although EGD can evaluate gross abnormalities of esophageal motility, as occur in achalasia, manometric studies are more accurate.

Interfering factors

- Patients taking anticoagulants (increased risk of bleeding)
- Failure of the patient to adhere to pretest restrictions
- Failure to send specimens to the laboratory immediately
- Patient's inability to cooperate, preventing optimal visualization

COLONOSCOPY

Colonoscopy uses a flexible fiber-optic video endoscope to permit visual examination of the lining of the large intestine. It's indicated for patients with a history of constipation or diarrhea, persistent rectal bleeding, and lower abdominal pain when the results of proctosigmoidoscopy and a barium enema test are negative or inconclusive.

Purpose

- To detect or evaluate inflammatory and ulcerative bowel disease
- To locate the origin of lower GI bleeding
- To aid diagnosis of colonic strictures and benign or malignant lesions
- To evaluate the colon postoperatively for recurrence of polyps and malignant lesions

Patient preparation

- Tell the patient that this test permits examination of the lining of the large intestine.
- Instruct him to maintain a clear liquid diet for 24 to 48 hours before the test and to take nothing by mouth after midnight the night before the procedure.
- Describe the procedure, and tell the patient who will perform it and where it will be done.
- Explain that the large intestine must be thoroughly cleaned to be clearly visible. Instruct the patient to take a laxative, as ordered, or a gallon of GoLYTELY solution in the evening (drinking the chilled solutions at 8 oz [236.6 ml] every 10 minutes until the entire gallon is consumed).
- If fecal results aren't clear, the patient will receive a laxative, suppository, or tap-water enema. Don't administer a soapsuds enema because this irritates the mucosa and stimulates mucus secretions that may hinder the examination.
- Inform the patient that an I.V. line will be started before the procedure and that a sedative will be administered just before the procedure. Advise him to arrange for someone to drive him home if he receives sedation.
- Assure him that the colonoscope is well lubricated to ease its insertion, that it initially feels cool, and that he may feel an urge to defecate when it's inserted and advanced.
- Explain that air may be introduced through the colonoscope to distend the intestinal wall and to facilitate viewing the lining and advancing the instrument. Tell him that flatus normally escapes around the instrument because of air insufflation and that he shouldn't attempt to control it.
- Tell him that suction may be used to remove blood or liquid stools that obscure vision but that this won't cause discomfort.
- Check the patient's medical history for allergies, medications, and information pertinent to the current complaint.
- Make sure the patient or a responsible family member has signed an informed consent form.

Procedure and posttest care

- Place the patient on his left side with his knees flexed, and drape him.
- Obtain baseline vital signs. Be prepared to monitor vital signs through the procedure. If the patient has known cardiac disease, continuous ECG monitoring should be instituted. Continuous or periodic pulse oximetry is advisable, particularly in high-risk patients with possible respiratory depression secondary to sedation.
- Place the patient on his left side, with knees flexed, and drape him.
- Instruct the patient to breathe deeply and slowly through his mouth as the physician palpates the mucosa of the anus and rectum and inserts the colonoscope.
- The physician inserts the lubricated colonoscope through the patient's anus into the sigmoid colon under direct vision.
- A small amount of air is insufflated to locate the bowel lumen. The scope is advanced through the rectum.
- When the instrument reaches the descending sigmoid junction, assist the patient to a supine position to aid the scope advance if necessary. After passing the splenic flexure, the scope is advanced through the transverse colon, through the hepatic flexure, and into the ascending colon and cecum.
- Abdominal palpation or fluoroscopy may be used to help guide the colonoscope through the large intestine.

Virtual colonoscopy

Virtual colonoscopy combines computed tomography (CT) scanning and X-ray images with sophisticated image processing computers to generate three-dimensional (3-D) images of the patient's colon. These images are interpreted by a skilled radiologist to recreate and evaluate the colon's inner surface. Although this procedure isn't as accurate as a routine colonoscopy, it's less invasive and is useful in screening patients with very small polyps. The colon must be free from residue and fecal material. Bowel preparation consists of following a clear liquid diet for 24 hours prior to the procedure; also, GoLYTELY bowel preparation is performed the evening before, and a rectal suppository is taken on the morning of the test.

While in the CT, a thin red rectal tube is placed, and air is introduced into the colon to distend the bowel. This may produce mild cramping. The CT is done with the patient in the supine position and again while prone to obtain images. The CT is then shipped over a network to a 3-D image-processing computer, and a radiologist evaluates the images obtained. If polyps are identified, a colonoscopy may be scheduled to remove them.

- Suction may be used to remove blood and secretions that obscure vision.
- Biopsy forceps or a cytology brush may be passed through the colonoscope to obtain specimens for histologic or cytologic examination; an electrocautery snare may be used to remove polyps.
- If the examiner removes a tissue specimen, immediately place it in a specimen bottle containing 10% formalin; immediately place cytology smears in a Coplin jar containing 95% ethyl alcohol. Send specimens to the laboratory immediately. Specimens should be collected in accordance with laboratory and pathology guidelines.
- Observe the patient closely for signs of bowel perforation. Report such signs immediately.
- Check vital signs, and document them according to facility policy.
- After the patient has recovered from sedation, he may resume his usual diet unless the physician orders otherwise.
- Provide privacy while the patient rests after the test; tell him that he may pass large amounts of flatus after insufflation.
- If a polyp has been removed, inform the patient that his stool may contain some blood, but excessive bleeding should be reported immediately.

Precautions

- Although it's usually a safe procedure, colonoscopy can cause perforation of the large intestine, excessive bleeding, and retroperitoneal emphysema.
- This procedure is contraindicated in pregnant women near term, patients who have had recent acute myocardial infarction or abdominal surgery, those who have ischemic bowel disease, acute diverticulitis, peritonitis, fulminant granulomatous colitis, perforated viscus, or fulminant ulcerative colitis. For these patients or for screening purposes, a virtual colonoscopy may be an option to help visualize polyps early before they became concerns. (See *Virtual colonoscopy.*)

◆ **CLINICAL ALERT** *Watch closely for adverse effects of the sedative. Have available emergency resuscitation equipment and a narcotic antagonist such as*

naloxone for I.V. use if necessary.
- If a polyp is removed but not retrieved during the examination, give enemas and strain stools to retrieve it if the physician requests it.

Normal findings

Normally, the mucosa of the large intestine beyond the sigmoid colon appears light pink-orange and is marked by semilunar folds and deep tubular pits. Blood vessels are visible beneath the intestinal mucosa, which glistens from mucus secretions.

Abnormal findings

Visual examination of the large intestine, coupled with histologic and cytologic test results, may indicate proctitis, granulomatous or ulcerative colitis, Crohn's disease, and malignant or benign lesions. Diverticular disease or the site of lower GI bleeding can be detected through colonoscopy alone.

Interfering factors

- Fixation of the sigmoid colon due to inflammatory bowel disease, surgery, or radiation therapy (may hinder passage of the colonoscope)
- Blood from acute colonic hemorrhage (hinders visualization)
- Insufficient bowel preparation or barium retained in the intestine from previous diagnostic studies (makes accurate visual examination impossible)
- Failure to place histologic or cytologic specimens in the appropriate preservative or to send the specimens to the laboratory immediately

PROCTO-SIGMOIDOSCOPY

Proctosigmoidoscopy uses a proctoscope, sigmoidoscope, and digital examination to evaluate the lining of the distal sigmoid colon, rectum, and anal canal. It's indicated in patients with recent changes in bowel habits, lower abdominal and perineal pain, prolapse on defecation, pruritus, and passage of mucus, blood, or pus in the stool. Specimens may be obtained from suspicious areas of the mucosa by biopsy, lavage or cytology brush, or culture swab.

Possible complications of this procedure include rectal bleeding and, rarely, bowel perforation.

Purpose

- To aid diagnosis of inflammatory, infectious, and ulcerative bowel disease
- To detect hemorrhoids, hypertrophic anal papilla, polyps, fissures, fistulas, and abscesses in the rectum and anal canal

Patient preparation

- Explain to the patient that this procedure allows visual examination of the lining of the distal sigmoid colon, rectum, and anal canal.
- Tell him that the test requires passage of two special instruments through the anus, and tell him who will perform the procedure and where it will be done.
- Check the patient's history for allergies, medications, and information pertinent to the current complaint. Find out if he has had a barium test within the past week because barium in the colon hinders accurate examination.
- Because dietary and bowel preparations for this procedure vary according to the physician's preference, follow the

orders carefully. If a special bowel preparation is ordered, explain to the patient that this clears the intestine to ensure a better view.

■ Instruct the patient to maintain a clear liquid diet for 24 to 48 hours before the test, to avoid eating fruits and vegetables before the procedure and to fast the morning of the procedure, according to the physician's preference.

■ Describe the position the patient will be asked to assume, and assure him that he'll be adequately draped.

■ As ordered, administer a warm tap-water or sodium biphosphate enema 3 to 4 hours before the procedure. The procedure may be started without bowel preparation because enemas can alter intestinal markings and traumatize mucous membranes. For this reason, irritating soapsuds enemas are inappropriate before this test. If the examination is hindered by excessive fecal matter, an enema may be ordered before the examination proceeds.

■ Tell him that he may be secured to a tilting table that rotates into horizontal and vertical positions.

■ Tell the patient that the examiner's finger and the instrument are well lubricated to ease insertion, that the instrument initially feels cool, and that he may experience the urge to defecate when the instrument is inserted and advanced.

■ Inform him that the instrument may stretch the intestinal wall and cause transient muscle spasms or colicky lower abdominal pain.

■ Instruct the patient to breathe deeply and slowly through his mouth to relax the abdominal muscles; this reduces the urge to defecate and eases discomfort.

■ Explain to the patient that air may be introduced through the endoscope into the intestine to distend its walls. Tell him that this causes flatus to escape around the endoscope and that he shouldn't attempt to control it.

■ Inform him that a suction machine may remove blood, mucus, or liquid stool that obscures vision but that it won't cause discomfort.

■ Inform the patient that an I.V. line may be started if an I.V. sedative is to be used. If the procedure is being done on an outpatient basis, advise him to arrange for someone to drive him home.

■ Make sure the patient or a responsible family member has signed a consent form.

■ If the patient has rectal inflammation, provide a local anesthetic about 15 to 20 minutes before the procedure to minimize discomfort.

Procedure and posttest care

■ Obtain baseline vital signs and monitor the patient throughout the procedure.

■ Place the patient in a knee-chest or left lateral position with knees flexed, and drape him.

■ If a left lateral position is used, a sandbag may be placed under the patient's left hip so that the buttocks project over the edge of the table. The right buttock is gently raised, and the anus and perianal region are examined under good lighting.

■ Instruct the patient to breathe deeply and slowly through his mouth as the examiner palpates the anal canal, rectum, and rectal mucosa for induration and tenderness; the examiner then withdraws his finger and checks for the presence of blood, mucus, or stool.

■ The sigmoidoscope is lubricated, and the patient is told that the instrument is about to be inserted. The right buttock is raised, and the sigmoidoscope is inserted into the anus. As the scope is passed with steady pressure through the anal sphincters, instruct the patient to bear down as though defecating to aid its passage. The sigmoidoscope is advanced through the anal canal into the rectum.

- At the rectosigmoid junction, a small amount of air may be insufflated to open the bowel lumen. The scope is then gently advanced to its full length into the distal sigmoid colon.
- As the sigmoidoscope is slowly withdrawn, air is carefully insufflated, and the intestinal mucosa is thoroughly examined.
- If stool obscures vision, the eyepiece on the scope is removed, a cotton swab is inserted through the scope, and the bowel lumen is swabbed. A suction machine may remove blood, excessive secretions, or liquid feces.
- To obtain specimens from suspicious areas of the intestinal mucosa, a biopsy forceps, cytology brush, or culture swab is passed through the sigmoidoscope.
- Polyps may be removed for histologic examination by inserting an electrocautery snare through the sigmoidoscope.
- Specimens are collected in accordance with laboratory and pathology guidelines and immediately placed in a specimen bottle containing 10% formalin; cytology slides are placed in a Coplin jar containing 95% ethyl alcohol; culture swabs are placed in a culture tube.
- After the sigmoidoscope is withdrawn, the proctoscope is lubricated and the patient is told that it's about to be inserted. Assure him that he'll experience less discomfort during passage of the proctoscope.
- The right buttock is raised, and the proctoscope is inserted through the anus and gently advanced to its full length.
- The obturator is removed, and the light source is inserted through the proctoscope handle.
- As the instrument is slowly withdrawn, the rectal and anal mucosa are carefully examined. Specimens may be obtained from suspicious areas of the intestinal mucosa.
- If a biopsy of the anal canal is required, a local anesthetic may be administered first.
- After the examination is completed, the proctoscope is withdrawn.
- If the patient has been examined in a knee-chest position, instruct him to rest in a supine position for several minutes before standing to prevent orthostatic hypotension.
- Observe the patient closely for signs of bowel perforation and for vasovagal attack due to emotional stress. Report such signs immediately.
- Allow the patient nothing by mouth until he's alert.
- Monitor vital signs as per facility protocol until the patient is alert.
- If air was introduced into the intestine, tell the patient that he may pass large amounts of flatus. Provide privacy while he rests after the test.
- If a biopsy or polypectomy was performed, inform the patient that blood may appear in his stool.

Precautions

- If a tissue specimen or culture swab has been obtained, label it and send it to the appropriate laboratory immediately.
- In general, anticoagulant therapy isn't contraindicated, however, it may increase the risk of bleeding.
- If the patient received sedation, he should avoid alcohol for 24 hours and shouldn't drive for 12 hours, so make sure he has transportation home.

Normal findings

The mucosa of the sigmoid colon appears light pink-orange and is marked by semilunar folds and deep tubular pits. The rectal mucosa is redder due to its rich vascular network, deepens to a purple hue at the pectinate line (the anatomic division between the rectum and anus), and has three distinct valves. The lower two-thirds of the anus (anoderm) is lined with smooth gray-tan skin and joins with the hair-fringed perianal skin.

Abnormal findings

Visual examination and palpation demonstrate abnormalities of the anal canal and rectum, including internal and external hemorrhoids, hypertrophic anal papilla, anal fissures, anal fistulas, and anorectal abscesses. The examination may also reveal inflammatory bowel diseases, polyps, cancer, and other tumors. Biopsy, culture, and other laboratory tests are typically necessary to detect various disorders.

Interfering factors

- Barium in the intestine from previous diagnostic studies (hinders visualization)
- Large amounts of stool in the intestine (hinders visual examination and advancement of the endoscope)
- Failure to place histologic or cytologic specimens in the appropriate preservative or to send the specimens to the laboratory immediately

ENDOSCOPIC ULTRASONOGRAPHY

Endoscopic ultrasonography (EUS) combines ultrasonography and endoscopy to visualize the GI wall and adjacent structures. The incorporation of the ultrasound probe at the distal end of the ultrasonic endoscope allows ultrasound imaging with high resolution.

Purpose

- To evaluate or stage lesions of the esophagus, stomach, duodenum, pancreas, ampulla, biliary ducts, and rectum
- To evaluate submucosal tumors and large folds
- To localize endocrine tumors

Patient preparation

- Explain to the patient that this procedure permits visual examination of tumors and large folds in the GI tract.
- Check the patient's medical history for allergies, medications, and information pertinent to the current complaint.
- Instruct the patient to fast for 6 to 8 hours before the test.
- Describe the procedure to the patient. Tell him who will perform it and where it will be done.
- For an esophagogastroduodenoscopy (EGD) EUS, explain that a flexible instrument will be passed through the mouth and into the esophagus, as in an EGD.
- If a sigmoid EUS is to be performed, tell the patient that the scope is well lubricated to ease its insertion through the anus, that it initially feels cool, and that he may feel an urge to defecate when it's inserted and advanced.
- For the sigmoid EUS, the patient may have to take a laxative the evening before if ordered.
- Inform the patient that he may receive an I.V. sedative to help him relax before the endoscope is inserted. If the procedure is being done on an outpatient basis, advise the patient to arrange for someone to drive him home because conscious sedation may affect his reaction time and reflexes, even though he may feel fine.
- Make sure the patient or a responsible family member has signed an informed consent form.

Procedure and posttest care

- Obtain baseline vital signs and monitor the patient throughout the procedure, according to facility policy.
- Follow the procedures for EGD or sigmoidoscopy, depending on which type of EUS is to be performed.

Precautions

- This procedure is generally safe but can cause perforation of the esophagus, stomach, or duodenum, as in EGD, or of the intestine, as in sigmoidoscopy or colonoscopy.

Normal findings

EUS usually reveals normal anatomy with no evidence of tumor.

Abnormal findings

Refer to the abnormal findings for EGD, colonoscopy, endoscopy, and sigmoidoscopy.

Interfering factors

- Esophageal stricture (hinders passage of the endoscope)
- All interfering factors listed under EGD — endoscopy, colonoscopy, and sigmoidoscopy

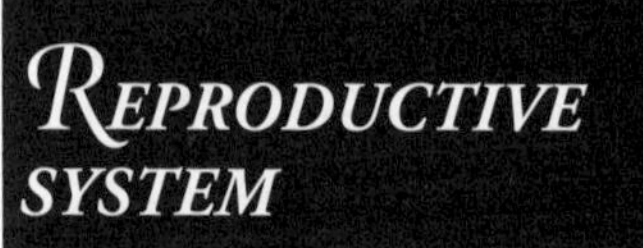

COLPOSCOPY

In colposcopy, the cervix and vagina are visually examined by an instrument containing a magnifying lens and a light (colposcope). This test is primarily used to evaluate abnormal cytology or grossly suspicious lesions and to examine the cervix and vagina after a positive Papanicolaou (Pap) test.

During the examination, a biopsy may be performed and photographs taken of suspicious lesions with the colposcope and its attachments. Risks of biopsy include bleeding (especially during pregnancy) and infection.

Purpose

- To help confirm cervical intraepithelial neoplasia or invasive carcinoma after a positive Pap test
- To evaluate vaginal or cervical lesions
- To monitor conservatively treated cervical intraepithelial neoplasia
- To monitor patients whose mothers received diethylstilbestrol during pregnancy

Patient preparation

- Explain to the patient that this test magnifies the image of the vagina and cervix, providing more information than a routine vaginal examination.
- Inform the patient that she need not restrict food or fluids.
- Tell her who will perform the examination, where it will be done, and that it's safe and painless.
- Tell the patient that a biopsy may be performed during colposcopy and that this may cause minimal but easily controlled bleeding and mild cramping.
- Make sure the patient or a responsible family member has signed an informed consent form.

Equipment

Colposcopy: gloves, colposcope, vaginal speculum, 5% acetic acid solution, swabs

Biopsy: gloves, biopsy forceps, endocervical curette, forceps for uterine dressing, tenaculum, ring forceps, Monsel's (ferric subsulfate) solution, biopsy bottle and preservative, sterile cotton balls, Pap test equipment (glass slide, wooden spatula, swabs, and fixative)

Procedure and posttest care

- The examiner puts on gloves. With the patient in the lithotomy position, the examiner inserts the speculum and, if indicated, performs a Pap test. Help the patient relax during insertion by telling her to breathe through her mouth and concentrate on relaxing her abdominal muscles.
- The cervix is gently swabbed with acetic acid solution to remove mucus.
- After the cervix and vagina are examined, biopsy is performed on areas that appear abnormal.
- Bleeding is stopped by applying pressure, hemostatic solutions, or by cautery.
- After a biopsy, instruct the patient to abstain from intercourse and to avoid inserting anything in her vagina (including a tampon) until healing of the biopsy site is confirmed (in approximately 10 days).

Normal findings

Surface contour of the cervical vessels should be smooth and pink; columnar epithelium appears grapelike. Different tissue types are sharply demarcated.

Abnormal findings

Abnormal colposcopy findings include white epithelium (leukoplakia) or punctate and mosaic patterns, which may indicate underlying cervical intraepithelial neoplasia; keratinization in the transformation zone, which may indicate cervical intraepithelial neoplasia or invasive carcinoma; and atypical vessels, which may indicate invasive carcinoma.

Other abnormalities visible on colposcopic examination include inflammatory changes (usually from infection), atrophic changes (usually from aging or, less commonly, the use of oral contraceptives), erosion (probably from increased pathogenicity of vaginal flora due to changes in vaginal pH), and papilloma and condyloma (possibly from viruses).

Histologic study of the biopsy specimen confirms colposcopic findings. If the results of the examination and biopsy are inconsistent with the results of the Pap test and biopsy of the squamocolumnar junction, conization of the cervix for biopsy may be indicated.

Interfering factors

- Failure to clean the cervix of menstrual blood or foreign materials, such as creams and medications (possible obstruction to visualization)

GYNECOLOGIC LAPAROSCOPY

Gynecologic laparoscopy permits visualization of the peritoneal cavity by the insertion of a small fiber-optic telescope (laparoscope) through the anterior abdominal wall. This surgical technique may be used diagnostically to detect abnormalities, such as cysts, adhesions, fibroids, and infection. It can also be used therapeutically to perform procedures such as lysis of adhesions; ovarian biopsy; tubal sterilization; removal of ectopic pregnancies, fibroids, hydrosalpinx, and foreign bodies; and fulguration of endometriotic implants.

Although laparoscopy has largely replaced laparotomy, the latter is usually preferred when extensive surgery is indicated. Potential risks of laparoscopy include a punctured visceral organ, causing bleeding or spilling of intestinal contents into the peritoneum.

Purpose

- To identify the cause of pelvic pain
- To help detect endometriosis, ectopic pregnancy, and pelvic inflammatory disease (PID)
- To evaluate pelvic masses or the fallopian tubes of infertile patients
- To stage carcinoma

Patient preparation

- Explain the procedure to the patient, and tell her that the test is used to detect abnormalities of the uterus, fallopian tubes, and ovaries.
- Instruct her to fast for at least 8 hours before surgery.
- Tell her who will perform the procedure and where it will be done.
- Tell the patient whether she'll receive a local or general anesthetic and whether the procedure will require an outpatient visit or overnight hospitalization.
- Warn her that she may experience pain at the puncture site and in the shoulder.
- Make sure the patient or a responsible family member has signed an informed consent form.
- Check the patient's history for hypersensitivity to the anesthetic.
- Make sure laboratory work is completed and results are reported before the test.
- Instruct the patient to empty her bladder just before the test.

Equipment

Indwelling urinary or straight catheter; sterile tray with scalpel, hemostats, needle holder, suture, and suture scissors; Veress needle; gas insufflator; laparoscope; fiber-optic light source and cable; laparoscope sheath and trocar; electrosurgical generator; tenaculum and intrauterine manipulator; probes, scissors, or forceps; adhesive bandages

Procedure and posttest care

- The patient is anesthetized and placed in the lithotomy position.
- The examiner catheterizes the bladder and then performs a bimanual examination of the pelvic area to detect abnormalities that may contraindicate the test and to ensure that the bladder is empty.
- The tenaculum is placed on the cervix and a uterine manipulator is inserted; an incision is made at the inferior rim of the umbilicus.
- The Veress needle is inserted into the peritoneal cavity, and 2 to 3 L of carbon dioxide or nitrous oxide is insufflated to distend the abdominal wall and provide an organ-free space for trocar insertion; the needle is removed and a trocar and sheath are inserted into the peritoneal cavity; another trocar may be inserted at the pubic hairline to allow other instruments.
- After removal of the trocar, the laparoscope is inserted through the sheath to examine the pelvis and abdomen.
- To evaluate tubal patency, the examiner infuses a dye through the cervix and observes the tubes for spillage.
- After the examination, minor surgical procedures such as ovarian biopsy may be performed.
- Monitor vital signs and urine output. Report sudden changes immediately; they may indicate complications.
- Monitor the patient for adverse or allergic reactions. After administration of a general anesthetic, monitor electrolyte balance, hemoglobin level, and hematocrit. Help the patient ambulate after recovery.
- Tell the patient that she may resume her usual diet.
- Instruct her to restrict activity for 2 to 7 days as necessary.
- Reassure the patient that some abdominal and shoulder pain is normal and should disappear within 24 to 36

hours. Provide analgesics as ordered and monitor for effect.

Precautions

- Laparoscopy is contraindicated in patients with advanced abdominal wall cancer, advanced pulmonary or cardiovascular disease, intestinal obstruction, palpable abdominal mass, large abdominal hernia, chronic tuberculosis, or a history of peritonitis.
- During the procedure, check for proper drainage of the catheter.

Normal findings

The uterus and fallopian tubes are of normal size and shape, free from adhesions, and mobile. The ovaries are of normal size and shape; cysts and endometriosis are absent. Dye injected through the cervix flows freely from the fimbria.

Abnormal findings

An ovarian cyst appears as a bubble on the surface of the ovary. The cyst may be clear if filled with follicular fluid or serous or mucous material, or it may be red, blue, or brown if filled with blood. Adhesions may appear as thick and fibrous tissue or as almost transparent strands of tissue.

Endometriosis resembles small, blue powder burns on the peritoneum or the serosa of any pelvic or abdominal structure. Fibroids appear as lumps on the uterus; hydrosalpinx as an enlarged fallopian tube; and ectopic pregnancy as an enlarged or ruptured fallopian tube. In PID, infection or abscess is evident.

Interfering factors

- Adhesions or marked obesity (possible obstruction to visualization)
- Tissue or fluid becoming attached to the lens (possible obstruction to visualization)

SKELETAL SYSTEM

ARTHROSCOPY

Arthroscopy is the visual examination of the interior of a joint (most commonly a major joint, such as a shoulder, hip, or knee) with a specially designed fiber-optic endoscope that's inserted through a cannula in the joint cavity. It usually follows and confirms a diagnosis made through physical examination, radiography, and arthrography.

Arthroscopy may be performed under local anesthesia, but it's usually performed under a spinal or general anesthesia, particularly when surgery is anticipated. A camera may be attached to the arthroscope to photograph areas for later study. (See *Arthroscopy of the knee,* page 522.)

Complications associated with arthroscopy are rare and may include infection, hemarthrosis, swelling, thrombophlebitis, and joint injury.

Purpose

- To detect and diagnose meniscal, patellar, condylar, extrasynovial, and synovial diseases
- To monitor disease progression
- To perform joint surgery
- To monitor effectiveness of therapy

Patient preparation

- Explain to the patient that this test is used to examine the interior of the joint, to evaluate joint disease, or to monitor his response to therapy as appropriate.
- Describe the procedure to the patient, and answer questions.
- If surgery or another treatment is anticipated, explain that this may be accomplished during arthroscopy.

Arthroscopy of the knee

With the patient's knee flexed about 40 degrees, the arthroscope is introduced into the joint. The examiner flexes, extends, and rotates the knee to view the joint space. Counterclockwise from the top right, these illustrations show a normal patellofemoral joint with smooth joint surfaces; the articular surface of the patella, showing chondromalacia; and a tear in the anterior cruciate ligament.

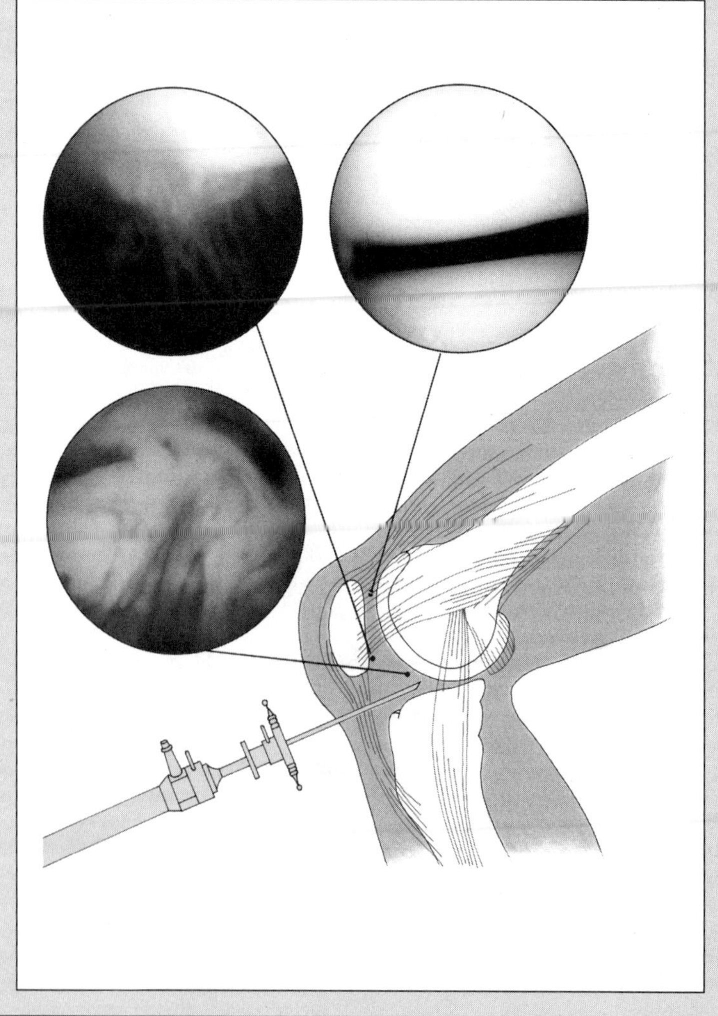

■ Instruct the patient to fast after midnight before the procedure.
■ Tell him who will perform this procedure and where it will be done.
■ If local anesthesia is to be used, tell the patient that he may experience transient discomfort from the injection of the local anesthetic and the pressure of the tourniquet on his leg. The patient will also feel a thumping sensation as the cannula is inserted in the joint capsule.
■ Make sure the patient or a responsible family member has signed an informed consent form.
■ Check the patient's history for hypersensitivity to the anesthetic.
■ The surgical site is prepared by shaving the area 5″ (12.7 cm) above and below the joint and a sedative is administered as ordered. The patient is positioned and draped according to the facility's policies.

Equipment

Skin antiseptic (povidone-iodine solution), arthroscope and accessory equipment, pointed scalpel, sterile gloves, local anesthetic, sterile needle, 12- and 60-ml syringes, waterproof stockinette, elastic bandages, pneumatic tourniquet, epinephrine (1:100,000 in 1% lidocaine solution), 500-ml sterile normal saline solution, continuous drainage system, sponges, 2″ × 2″ sterile gauze pads, sterile drapes, small adhesive bandages

Procedure and posttest care

Arthroscopic techniques vary, depending on the surgeon and the type of arthroscope used.
■ The patient's leg is elevated and wrapped with an elastic bandage to drain as much blood from the leg as possible, or a mixture of lidocaine with epinephrine and normal saline is instilled into the patient's knee to distend the knee and help reduce bleeding.
■ The local anesthetic is administered, a small incision is made, and a cannula is passed through the incision and positioned in the joint cavity.
■ The arthroscope is then inserted, and the knee structures are visually examined and photographed for further study.
■ After visual examination, a synovial biopsy or appropriate surgery is performed as indicated.
■ When the examination is completed, the arthroscope is removed, the joint is irrigated, the cannula is removed, and an adhesive strip and compression dressing are applied over the incision site.
■ Watch for fever, swelling, increased pain, and localized inflammation at the incision site. If the patient reports discomfort, provide an analgesic as ordered.
■ Monitor the patient's circulation and sensation in his leg.
■ Advise the patient to elevate the leg and apply ice for the first 24 hours.
■ Instruct the patient to report fever, bleeding, drainage, or increased swelling or pain in the joint.
■ Advise the patient to bear only partial weight, using crutches, a walker, or a cane for 48 hours.
■ If an immobilizer is ordered, teach the patient how to apply it.
■ Tell the patient that showering is permitted after 48 hours, but a tub bath should be avoided until after the postoperative visit.
■ Tell the patient that usual diet may be resumed as ordered.

Precautions

■ Arthroscopy is contraindicated in a patient with fibrous ankylosis with flexion of less than 50 degrees.

- The procedure is contraindicated when a patient with local skin or wound infections has a risk of subsequent joint involvement.

Normal findings

The knee is a typical diarthrodial joint surrounded by muscles, ligaments, cartilage, and tendons and lined with synovial membrane. In children, the menisci are smooth and opaque, with their thick outer edges attached to the joint capsule and their inner edges lying snugly against the condylar surfaces, unattached. Articular cartilage appears smooth and white; ligaments and tendons appear cablelike and silvery. The synovium is smooth and marked by a fine vascular network. Degenerative changes begin during adolescence.

Abnormal findings

Arthroscopic examination can reveal meniscal disease, such as a torn medial or lateral meniscus or other meniscal injuries; patellar disease, such as chondromalacia, dislocation, subluxation, parapatellar synovitis or fracture; condylar disease, such as degenerative articular cartilage, osteochondritis dissecans and loose bodies; extrasynovial disease, such as torn anterior cruciate or tibial collateral ligaments, Baker's cyst, and ganglionic cyst; and synovial disease, such as synovitis, rheumatoid and degenerative arthritis, and foreign bodies associated with gout, pseudogout, and osteochondromatasis.

Depending on test findings, appropriate treatment or surgery can follow arthroscopy. If arthroscopic surgery can't be performed, arthrotomy is the procedure of choice.

Interfering factors

- Failure to use the arthroscope properly

11

Ultrasonography

CARDIOVASCULAR SYSTEM

ECHOCARDIOGRAPHY

Echocardiography is a noninvasive test that shows the size, shape, and motion of cardiac structures. It's useful for evaluating patients with chest pain, enlarged cardiac silhouettes on X-ray films, electrocardiographic changes unrelated to coronary artery disease, and abnormal heart sounds on auscultation.

In this test, a transducer directs ultra-high-frequency sound waves toward cardiac structures, which reflect these waves. The echoes are converted to images that are displayed on a monitor and recorded on a strip chart or videotape. Results are correlated with clinical history, physical examination, and findings from additional tests.

The techniques most commonly used in echocardiography are M-mode (motion-mode), for recording the motion and dimensions of intracardiac structures, and two-dimensional (cross-sectional), for recording lateral motion and providing the correct spatial relationship between cardiac structures. (See *M-mode echocardiograms.*)

Purpose

- To diagnose and evaluate valvular abnormalities
- To measure the size of the heart's chambers
- To evaluate chambers and valves in congenital heart disorders
- To aid diagnosis of hypertrophic and related cardiomyopathies
- To detect atrial tumors
- To evaluate cardiac function or wall motion after myocardial infarction
- To detect pericardial effusion
- To detect mucal thrombi

Patient preparation

- Explain to the patient that this test is used to evaluate the size, shape, and motion of various cardiac structures.
- Inform the patient that he need not restrict food or fluids before the test.
- Tell the patient who will perform the test, where it will take place, and that it's safe, painless, and noninvasive.
- Explain that the room may be darkened slightly to aid visualization on the monitor screen, and that other procedures (electrocardiography and phonocardiography) may be performed simultaneously to time events in the cardiac cycle.
- Describe the procedure and instruct the patient to remain still during the test because movement may distort results.
- Tell the patient that conductive gel will be applied to his chest and a quarter-sized transducer will be placed directly over it. Warn the patient he may feel minor discomfort because pressure is exerted to keep the transducer in contact with the skin.
- Explain that the transducer is angled to observe different parts of the heart and that he may be repositioned on his left side during the procedure.
- Inform the patient that he may be asked to inhale a gas with a slightly sweet odor (amyl nitrite) while changes in heart function are recorded; describe the possible adverse effects of amyl nitrite (dizziness, flushing, and tachycardia), but assure the patient that such symptoms quickly subside.

Procedure and posttest care

- The patient is placed in a supine position.
- Conductive gel is applied to the third or fourth intercostal space to the left

M-mode echocardiograms

In the normal motion-mode echocardiogram of the mitral valve shown below (top), valve movement appears as a characteristic lopsided M-shaped tracing. The anterior and posterior mitral valve leaflets separate (D) in early diastole, quickly reach maximum separation (E), then close during rapid ventricular filling (E-F).

Leaflet separation varies during mid-diastole, and the valve opens widely again (A) following atrial contraction. The valve starts to close with atrial relaxation (A-B) and is completely closed during the start of ventricular systole (C). The steepness of the E-F slope indirectly shows the speed of ventricular filling, which is normally rapid.

NORMAL ECHOCARDIOGRAM

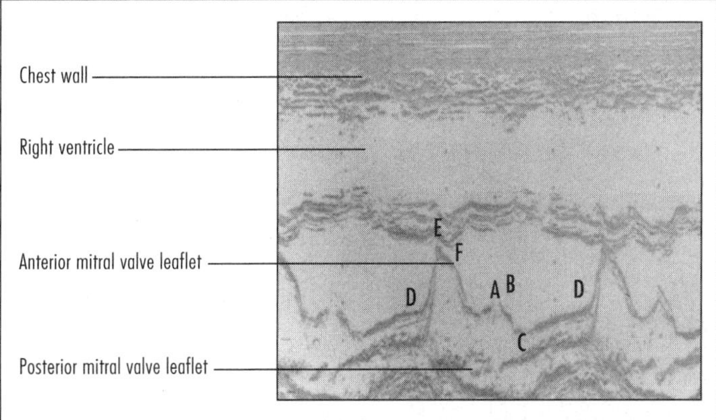

ABNORMAL ECHOCARDIOGRAM

Mitral stenosis is evident in the abnormal echocardiogram shown at right. The E-F slope (dashed line) is very shallow, indicating slowed left ventricular filling.

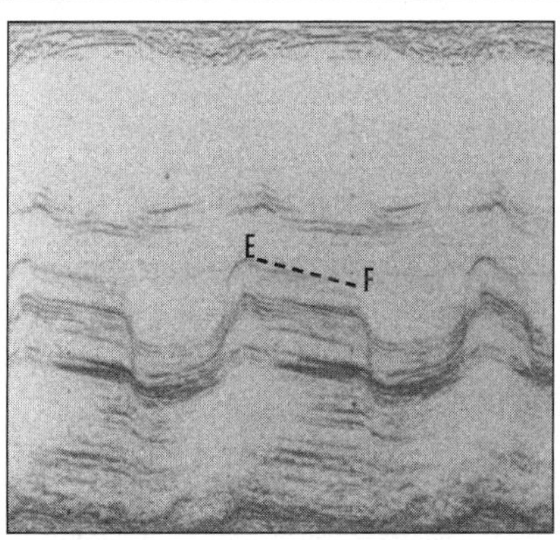

of the sternum, and the transducer is placed directly over it.

- The transducer is systematically angled to direct ultrasonic waves at specific parts of the patient's heart.
- During the test, the oscilloscope screen, which displays the returning echoes, is observed.
- Significant findings are recorded on a strip chart recorder (M-mode echocardiography) or on a videotape recorder (two-dimensional echocardiography).
- For a different view of the heart, the transducer is placed beneath the xiphoid process or directly above the sternum.
- For a left lateral view, the patient may be positioned on his left side.
- To record heart function under various conditions, the patient is asked to inhale and exhale slowly, to hold his breath, or to inhale amyl nitrite.
- Doppler echocardiography may be used in this examination to assess speed and direction of blood flow. The sound of blood flow may be heard as the continuous-wave and pulsed-wave Doppler sampling of cardiac valves is performed. This technique is used primarily to assess heart sounds and murmurs as they relate to cardiac hemodynamics.
- Remove the conductive gel from the patient's skin.

Normal findings

An echocardiogram can reveal both the motion pattern and structure of the four cardiac valves. Anterior and posterior mitral valve leaflets normally separate in early diastole, with the anterior leaflet moving toward the chest wall and the posterior leaflet moving away from it. The leaflets attain maximum excursion rapidly, then move toward each other during ventricular diastole; after atrial contraction, they come together and remain so during ventricular systole. On an M-mode echocardiogram, the leaflets appear as two fine lines within the echo-free, blood-filled left ventricular cavity.

The aortic valve cusps lie between the parallel walls of the aortic root, which move anteriorly during systole and posteriorly during diastole. During ventricular systole, these cusps separate and appear as a boxlike configuration on an M-mode echocardiogram. They remain open throughout systole and normally demonstrate a characteristic fine fluttering motion. During diastole, the cusps come together and appear as a single or double line within the aortic root on an M-mode echocardiogram.

The motion of the tricuspid valve resembles that of the mitral valve. The motion of the pulmonic valve — particularly the posterior cusp — is different: During diastole, this cusp gradually moves posteriorly; during atrial systole, it's displaced posteriorly; during ventricular systole, it quickly moves posteriorly; and during right ventricular ejection, the cusp moves anteriorly, attaining its most anterior position during diastole.

The left ventricular cavity normally appears as an echo-free space between the interventricular septum and the posterior left ventricular wall. Echoes produced by the chordae tendineae and the mitral leaflet appear within this cavity. The right ventricular cavity normally appears as an echo-free space between the anterior chest wall and the interventricular septum.

Abnormal findings

Valvular abnormalities readily appear on the echocardiogram. In mitral stenosis, the valve narrows abnormally due to the leaflets' thickening and disordered motion. Instead of moving in opposite directions during diastole, both mitral valve leaflets move anteriorly. In mitral valve prolapse, one or both leaflets balloon into the left atrium during systole.

Aortic valve abnormalities—especially aortic insufficiency—can also affect the mitral valve because the anterior mitral leaflet is just below the aortic cusps. When blood regurgitates through the aortic valve during diastole, it strikes this leaflet, causing the flutter seen in M-mode. Although the aortic valve may appear normal, this characteristic fluttering confirms aortic insufficiency. In stenosis, due to conditions such as rheumatic fever or bacterial endocarditis, the aortic valve thickens and thus generates more echoes. However, in rheumatic fever, the valve may thicken slightly and allow normal motion during systole, or it may thicken severely and curtail motion. In bacterial endocarditis, valve motion is disrupted, and shaggy or fuzzy echoes usually appear on or near the valve.

Other chamber or valve abnormalities may indicate a congenital heart disorder, such as aortic stenosis, which may require further tests. A large chamber size may indicate cardiomyopathy, valvular disorders, or heart failure; a small chamber, restrictive pericarditis.

Idiopathic hypertrophic subaortic stenosis can also be identified by the echocardiogram, with systolic anterior motion of the mitral valve and asymmetric septal hypertrophy.

Left atrial tumors are usually on a pedicle and can thus shift in and out of the mitral opening. During diastole, the tumor appears as a mass of echoes against the anterior mitral valve leaflet. During ventricular systole, these echoes shift back into the body of the atrium.

In coronary artery disease, ischemia or infarction may cause absent or paradoxical motion in ventricular walls that normally move together and thicken during systole. These affected areas may also fail to thicken or may become thinner, particularly if scar tissue is present.

The echocardiogram is especially sensitive in detecting pericardial effusion. Normally, the epicardium and pericardium are continuous membranes, and thus produce a single or near-single echo. When fluid accumulates between these membranes, it causes an abnormal echo-free space to appear. In large effusions, pressure exerted by excess fluid can restrict pericardial motion.

An echocardiogram should be correlated with the patients' history, physical examination findings, and results of additional tests. For patients with suboptimal echocardiogram, an agent composed of human albumin microspheres filled with perfluorocarbon gas (Optison) can be used. This agent can enhance the contrast of the ultrasound scans to opacify the left ventricle and improve the delineation of the left ventricular endocardial borders.

Interfering factors

- Incorrect transducer placement and excessive movement
- Thick chest or chest wall abnormalities, or chronic obstructive pulmonary disease (possible poor imaging)

TRANSESOPHAGEAL ECHOCARDIOGRAPHY

Transesophageal echocardiography combines ultrasound with endoscopy to give a better view of the heart's structures. In this procedure, a small transducer is attached to the end of a gastroscope and inserted into the esophagus, allowing images to be taken from the posterior aspect of the heart. This causes less tissue penetration and interference from chest wall structures and produces high-quality images of the thoracic aorta, except for the superior ascending aorta, which is shadowed by the trachea.

This test is appropriate for both inpatients and outpatients, for patients under general anesthesia, and for critically ill, intubated patients.

Purpose

To visualize and evaluate:

- thoracic and aortic disorders, such as dissection and aneurysm
- valvular disease, especially in the mitral valve and in prosthetic devices
- endocarditis
- congenital heart disease
- intracardiac thrombi
- cardiac tumors
- valvular repairs

Patient preparation

- Explain to the patient that this test allows visual examination of heart function and structures.
- Tell the patient who will perform the test, when it's scheduled, and that he'll need to fast for 6 hours beforehand.
- Review the patient's medical history for possible contraindications to the test, such as esophageal obstruction or varices, GI bleeding, previous mediastinal radiation therapy, or severe cervical arthritis.
- Ask the patient about any allergies and note them on the chart.
- Before the test, have the patient remove any dentures or oral prostheses, and note any loose teeth.
- Explain that his throat will be sprayed with a topical anesthetic and that he may gag when the tube is inserted.
- Tell the patient that an I.V. line will be inserted to administer sedation before the procedure and that he may feel some discomfort from the needle puncture and the pressure of the tourniquet. Reassure him that he'll be made as comfortable as possible during the procedure and that his blood pressure and heart rate will be monitored continuously.
- Make sure the patient or a responsible family member has signed an informed consent form, if required.

Equipment

Cardiac monitor, sedative, topical anesthetic, bite block, gastroscope, ultrasonography equipment, suction equipment, resuscitation equipment

Procedure and posttest care

- Connect the patient to a cardiac monitor, the automated blood pressure cuff, and pulse oximetry probe so that all parameters can be assessed during the procedure.
- Help the patient lie down on his left side, and administer the prescribed sedative.
- The back of the patient's throat is sprayed with a topical anesthetic.
- A bite block is placed in his mouth, and he's instructed to close his lips around it.
- A gastroscope is introduced and advanced 12″ to 14″ (30 to 35 cm) to the level of the right atrium. To visualize the left ventricle, the scope is advanced 16″ to 18″ (40 to 45 cm).
- Ultrasound images are recorded and then reviewed after the procedure.
- Monitor the patient's vital signs and oxygen levels for any changes.
- Keep the patient in a supine position until the sedative wears off.
- Encourage the patient to cough after the procedure while lying on his side or sitting upright.
- Don't give food or water until the gag response returns.
- If the procedure is done on an outpatient basis, make sure someone is available to drive the patient home.

■ Treat sore throat symptomatically.

Precautions

■ Keep resuscitation equipment readily available.
■ Have suction equipment nearby to avoid aspiration if vomiting occurs.
■ Vasovagal responses may occur with gagging, so observe the cardiac monitor closely.
■ Use pulse oximetry to detect hypoxia.
■ If bleeding occurs, stop the procedure immediately.
■ Laryngospasm, arrhythmias, or bleeding increase the risk of complications. If any of these occurs, postpone the test.

Normal findings

Transesophageal echocardiography should reveal no cardiac problems.

Abnormal findings

This test can reveal thoracic and aortic disorders, endocarditis, congenital heart disease, intracardiac thrombi, or tumors, and it can evaluate valvular disease or repairs. Findings may include aortic dissection or aneurysm, mitral valve disease, or congenital defects such as patent ductus arteriosus.

Interfering factors

■ Uncooperative patient
■ Transesophageal approach (restricted visualization of the left atrial appendage and ascending or descending aorta)
■ Hyperinflation of lungs due to such causes as chronic obstructive pulmonary disease or mechanical ventilation (possible poor imaging)

DOPPLER ULTRASONOGRAPHY

Doppler ultrasonography is a noninvasive test used to evaluate blood flow in the major veins and arteries of the arms and legs and in the extracranial cerebrovascular system. An alternative to arteriography and venography, it's safer, less costly, and faster than invasive tests.

In Doppler ultrasonography, a handheld transducer directs high-frequency sound waves to the artery or vein being tested. The sound waves strike moving red blood cells and are reflected back to the transducer, allowing direct listening and graphic recording of blood flow.

Measurement of systolic pressure during this test is used to detect the presence, location, and extent of peripheral arterial occlusive disease. Changes in sound wave frequency during respiration are observed to detect venous occlusive disease. Compression maneuvers detect occlusion of the veins and occlusion or stenosis of carotid arteries.

Pulse volume recorder testing may be performed with Doppler ultrasonography to record changes in blood volume or flow in an extremity or organ.

Purpose

■ To aid diagnosis of venous insufficiency and superficial and deep vein thromboses (popliteal, femoral, iliac)
■ To aid diagnosis of peripheral artery disease and arterial occlusion
■ To monitor patients who have had arterial reconstruction and bypass grafts
■ To detect abnormalities of carotid artery blood flow associated with conditions such as aortic stenosis
■ To evaluate possible arterial trauma

Patient preparation

- Explain to the patient that this test is used to evaluate blood flow in the arms and legs or neck.
- Tell the patient who will perform the test.
- Reassure the patient that the test doesn't involve risk or discomfort.
- Tell the patient that he'll be asked to move his arms to different positions and to perform breathing exercises as measurements are taken. A small ultrasonic probe resembling a microphone is placed at various sites along veins or arteries, and blood pressure is checked at several sites.
- Check with the vascular laboratory about special equipment or instructions.

Procedure and posttest care

- Water-soluble conductive gel is applied to the tip of the transducer.

Peripheral arterial evaluation

- This test is always performed bilaterally. The usual test sites in each leg are the common femoral, superficial femoral, popliteal, posterior tibial, and dorsalis pedis arteries; in each arm the test sites are usually the subclavian, brachial, radial, ulnar and, occasionally, the palmar arch and digital arteries.
- The patient is instructed to remove all clothing above or below the waist, depending on the test site, and he's placed in a supine position on the examining table or bed, with his arms at his sides.
- Brachial blood pressure is measured, and the transducer is placed at various points along the test arteries.
- The signals are monitored and the waveforms recorded for later analysis.
- Segmental limb blood pressure is obtained to localize arterial occlusive disease.
- During lower extremity tests, a blood pressure cuff is wrapped around the calf, pressure readings are obtained, and waveforms are recorded from the dorsalis pedis and posterior tibial arteries. Then the cuff is wrapped around the thigh, and waveforms are recorded at the popliteal artery.
- In upper extremity tests, examination is performed on one arm, with the patient first placed in a supine position and then sitting; it's then repeated on the other arm. A blood pressure cuff is wrapped around the forearm, pressure readings are taken, and waveforms are recorded over both the radial and ulnar arteries. Then, the cuff is wrapped around the upper arm, pressure readings are taken, and waveforms are recorded with the transducer over the brachial artery.
- Blood pressure readings and waveform recordings are repeated with the arm in extreme hyperextension and hyperabduction to check for possible compression factors that may interfere with arterial blood flow. The upper extremity examination is performed on one arm, with the patient first placed in a supine position, then sitting; it's then repeated on the other arm.

Peripheral venous evaluation

- Usual test sites include the popliteal, superficial femoral, and common femoral veins in the leg and the posterior tibial vein at the ankle; the brachial, axillary, and subclavian veins in the arm; jugular veins; and, occasionally, the inferior and superior vena cava.
- The patient is instructed to remove all clothing above or below the waist, depending on the test site.
- He's placed in a supine position and instructed to breathe normally.
- The transducer is placed over the appropriate vein, waveforms and compressibility are recorded, and respiratory modulations noted.
- Proximal limb compression maneuvers are performed and augmentation

noted after release of compression, to evaluate venous valve competency.

- Changes in respiration are monitored.
- During lower extremity tests, the patient is asked to perform Valsalva's maneuver, and venous blood flow is recorded.
- The procedure is repeated for the other arm or leg.

Extracranial cerebrovascular evaluation

- Usual test sites include the supraorbital, common carotid, external carotid, internal carotid, and vertebral arteries.
- The patient is placed in a supine position on the examining table or bed, with a pillow beneath his head for support.
- Brachial blood pressure is then recorded using the Doppler probe.
- The transducer is positioned over the test artery, and blood flow velocity is monitored and recorded.
- The influence of compression maneuvers on blood flow velocity is measured, and the procedure is repeated on the opposite side. (See *How to detect thrombi with a Doppler probe,* page 534.)

All procedures

- Remove the conductive gel from the patient's skin.

Precautions

- Don't place the Doppler probe over an open or draining lesion.

Normal findings

Arterial waveforms of the arms and legs are triphasic, with a prominent systolic component and one or more diastolic sounds. The ankle-arm pressure index — the ratio between ankle systolic pressure and brachial systolic pressure — is normally equal to or greater than 1. (The ankle-arm pressure index is also known as arterial ischemia index, the ankle-brachial index, or the pedal-brachial index.) Proximal thigh pressure is normally 20 to 30 mm Hg higher than arm pressure, but pressure measurements at adjacent sites are similar. In the arms, pressure readings should remain unchanged despite postural changes.

Venous blood flow velocity is normally phasic with respiration, and is of a lower pitch than arterial flow. Distal compression or release of proximal limb compression increases blood flow velocity. In the legs, abdominal compression eliminates respiratory variations, but release increases blood flow; Valsalva's maneuver also interrupts venous flow velocity.

In cerebrovascular testing, a strong velocity signal is present. In the common carotid artery, blood flow velocity increases during diastole due to low peripheral vascular resistance of the brain. The direction of periorbital arterial flow is normally anterograde out of the orbit.

Abnormal findings

Arterial stenosis or occlusion diminishes the blood flow velocity signal, with no diastolic sound and a less prominent systolic component distal to the lesion. At the lesion, the signal is high-pitched and, occasionally, turbulent. If complete occlusion is present and collateral circulation has not taken over, the velocity signal may be absent.

A pressure gradient exceeding 20 mm Hg at adjacent sites of measurement in the leg may indicate occlusive disease. Specifically, low proximal thigh pressure signifies common femoral or aortoiliac occlusive disease. An abnormal gradient between the proximal thigh and the above- or below-knee cuffs indicates superficial femoral or popliteal artery occlusive disease; an abnormal gradient between the below-knee and ankle cuffs indicates tibiofibular disease. Abnormal gra-

How to detect thrombi with a Doppler probe

The Doppler probe is typically used to detect venous thrombi by first positioning the transducer and then occluding the blood vessel by compression (as illustrated with the normal leg at right). Water-soluble conductive gel is applied to the tip of the transducer to provide coupling between the skin and the transducer.

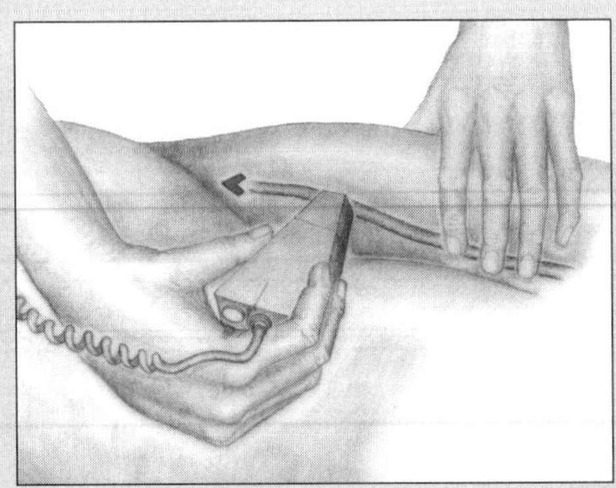

When pressure is released, allowing blood flow to resume, the transducer picks up the sudden augmentation of the flow sound and permits graphic recording of blood flow. If a thrombus is present, a compression maneuver fails to produce the augmented flow sound because the blood flow (as shown at right in the femoral vein) is significantly impaired.

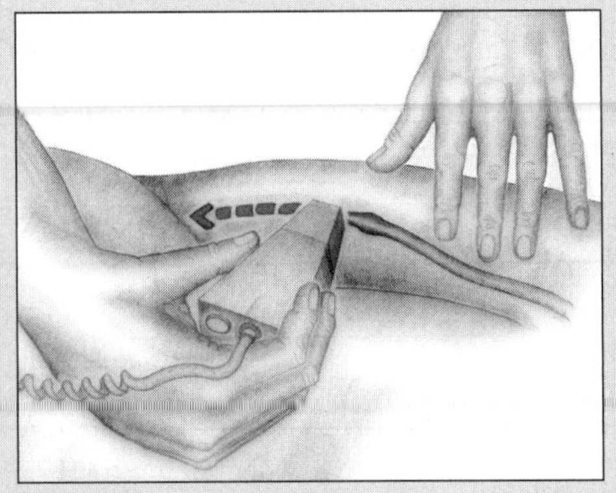

dients of arm and forearm pressure readings may indicate brachial artery occlusion.

An abnormal ankle-arm pressure index is directly proportional to the degree of circulatory impairment: mild ischemia, 1 to 0.75; claudication, 0.75 to 0.50; pain at rest, 0.50 to 0.25; and pregangrene, 0.25 to 0.

If venous blood flow velocity is unchanged by respirations, doesn't increase in response to compression or Valsalva's maneuver, or is absent, venous thrombosis is indicated. In chronic venous insufficiency and varicose veins, the flow velocity signal may be reversed. Confirmation of results may require venography.

Inability to identify Doppler signals during cerebrovascular examination implies total arterial occlusion. Reversed periorbital arterial flow indicates significant arterial occlusive disease of the extracranial internal carotid artery. In addition, the audible signal may take on the acoustic characteristics of a normal peripheral artery. Stenosis of the internal carotid artery causes turbulent signals.

Collateral circulation can be assessed by compression maneuvers.

Oculoplethysmography, carotid phonoangiography, or carotid imaging can further evaluate cerebrovascular disease. Retrograde blood velocity in the vertebral artery can indicate subclavian steal syndrome. A weak velocity signal on comparison of contralateral vertebral arteries can indicate diffuse vertebral artery disease.

Interfering factors

- Uncooperative patient

ULTRASONOGRAPHY OF THE ABDOMINAL AORTA

In ultrasonography of the abdominal aorta, a transducer directs high-frequency sound waves into the abdomen over a wide area from the xiphoid process to the umbilical region. The echoing sound waves are displayed on a monitor to indicate internal organs, the vertebral column, and the size and course of the abdominal aorta and other major vessels.

Purpose

- To detect and measure a suspected abdominal aortic aneurysm (findings may be supported and refined by angiography or computed tomography angiography)
- To detect and measure expansion of a known abdominal aortic aneurysm

Patient preparation

- Explain to the patient that this test allows examination of the abdominal aorta.
- Instruct the patient to fast for 12 hours before the test to minimize bowel gas and motility.
- Tell the patient who will perform the test, where it will take place, that the lights may be lowered, and that he'll feel only slight pressure.
- Describe the procedure. Tell the patient that mineral oil or a gel, which may feel cool, will be applied to his abdomen.
- Explain that a transducer will pass over his skin, from the costal margins to the umbilicus or slightly below, directing safe, painless, and inaudible sound waves into the abdominal vessels and organs.
- Reassure the patient with a known aneurysm that the sound waves won't cause rupture.
- Instruct the patient to remain still during scanning and to hold his breath when requested.
- If ordered, give simethicone to reduce bowel gas.

Procedure and posttest care

- The patient is placed in a supine position, and conductive gel or mineral oil is applied to his abdomen.
- Longitudinal scans are made at 1/8″ to 3/8″ (0.5- to 1-cm) intervals left and right of the midline until the entire abdominal aorta is outlined; transverse scans are made at 3/8″ to 3/4″ (1- to 2-cm) intervals from the xiphoid to the bifurcation at the common iliac arteries.
- The patient may be placed in right and left lateral positions.
- Appropriate views are photographed or videotaped.
- Remove the conductive gel from the patient's skin.
- Instruct the patient to resume his usual diet and medications.

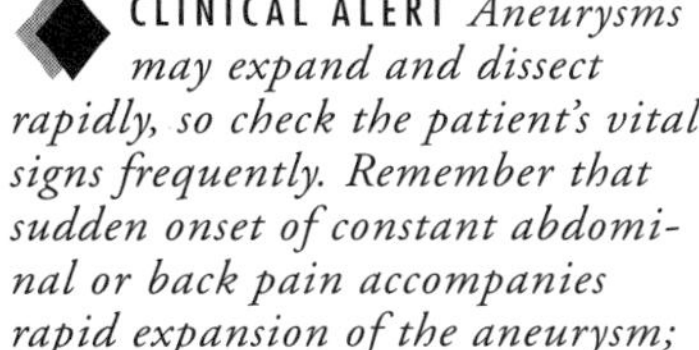

CLINICAL ALERT *Aneurysms may expand and dissect rapidly, so check the patient's vital signs frequently. Remember that sudden onset of constant abdominal or back pain accompanies rapid expansion of the aneurysm;*

sudden, excruciating pain with weakness, sweating, tachycardia, and hypotension signals rupture.

Normal findings

In adults, the normal abdominal aorta tapers from about 2.5 to 1.5 cm in diameter along its length from the diaphragm to the bifurcation. It descends through the retroperitoneal space, anterior to the vertebral column and slightly left of the midline. Four of its major branches are usually well visualized: the celiac trunk, the renal arteries, the superior mesenteric artery, and the common iliac arteries.

Abnormal findings

Luminal diameter of the abdominal aorta greater than 1½″ (3.8 cm) suggests aneurysm; greater than 2¾″ (7 cm) suggests aneurysm with high risk of rupture.

Interfering factors

The following factors may hinder imaging:

- Bowel gas and motility, excessive body movement, surgical wounds, and severe dyspnea
- Residual barium from GI contrast studies within past 24 hours
- Air introduced during endoscopy within past 12 to 24 hours
- Mesenteric fat in obese patients

GASTROINTESTINAL SYSTEM

ULTRASONOGRAPHY OF THE GALLBLADDER AND BILIARY SYSTEM

In ultrasonography of the gallbladder and biliary system, a focused beam of high-frequency sound waves passes into the right upper quadrant of the abdomen, creating echoes that vary with changes in tissue density. These echoes are converted to images on a screen, indicating the size, shape, and position of the gallbladder and biliary system.

Purpose

- To confirm diagnosis of cholelithiasis
- To diagnose acute cholecystitis
- To distinguish between obstructive and nonobstructive jaundice

Patient preparation

- Explain to the patient that this procedure allows examination of the gallbladder and the biliary system.
- Instruct the patient to eat a fat-free meal in the evening and then to fast for 8 to 12 hours before the procedure, if possible; this promotes accumulation of bile in the gallbladder and enhances ultrasonic visualization.
- Tell the patient who will perform the procedure and where.
- Tell the patient that the room may be darkened slightly to aid visualization on the screen.
- Describe the procedure. Tell the patient that a transducer will pass smoothly over his abdomen in direct contact with his skin, but assure him that he'll feel only mild pressure.

■ Instruct the patient to remain as still as possible during the procedure and to hold his breath when requested to ensure that the gallbladder is in the same position for each scan.

Procedure and posttest care

■ The patient is placed in a supine position.
■ A water-soluble conductive gel is applied to the face of the transducer.
■ Transverse and longitudinal oblique scans of the gallbladder are taken at ⅜″ (1-cm) intervals, starting at the level of the xiphoid and moving laterally to the right subcostal area. Longitudinal oblique scans are taken at 5-mm intervals parallel to the long axis of the gallbladder marked on the patient's skin, beginning medial to the gallbladder and continuing through to its lateral border.
■ During each scan, the patient is asked to inhale deeply and to hold his breath. (If the gallbladder is positioned deeply under the right costal margin, a scan may be taken through the intercostal spaces while the patient holds his breath.)
■ The patient is then placed in a left lateral decubitus position and is scanned beneath the right costal margin. (This position and scanning angle may displace and allow detection of stones lodged in the gallbladder neck and the cystic duct region.)
■ Scanning with the patient erect helps demonstrate mobility or fixity of suspicious echogenic areas. Views may be photographed for later study.
■ Remove the conductive gel from the patient's skin.
■ Inform the patient that he may resume his usual diet.

Precautions

■ Keep the patient in a fasting state to prevent the excretion of bile in the gallbladder. Even smelling greasy foods, such as popcorn, can cause the gallbladder to empty.

Normal findings

The normal gallbladder is sonolucent; it appears circular on transverse scans and pear-shaped on longitudinal scans. Although the size of the gallbladder varies, its outer walls normally appear sharp and smooth. Intrahepatic radicles seldom appear because the flow of sonolucent bile is very fine. The cystic duct may also be indistinct — the result of folds known as Heister's valves that line the cystic duct lumen. When visualized, the cystic duct has a serpentine appearance. The common bile duct, in contrast, has a linear appearance but is sometimes obscured by overlying bowel gas.

Abnormal findings

Gallstones within the gallbladder lumen or the biliary system typically appear as mobile, echogenic areas, usually associated with an acoustic shadow. The size of gallstones generally parallels the size of their shadows; gallstones 5 mm or larger usually produce shadows. However, if the gallbladder is distended with bile, gallstones as small as 1 mm can be detected because of the acoustic contrast between liquid bile and solid gallstones. Detecting stones in the biliary ducts, which contain little bile, may be difficult. When the gallbladder is shrunken or fully impacted with gallstones, inadequate bile may likewise make gallstone detection difficult, and the gallbladder itself might not be detectable. In this case, an acoustic shadow in the gallbladder fossa indicates cholelithiasis; the presence of such a shadow in the cystic and common bile ducts can also indicate cholelithiasis.

Polyps and carcinoma within the gallbladder lumen are distinguished from gallstones by their fixity. Polyps usually appear as sharply defined, echogenic areas; carcinoma appears as a poorly defined mass, often associated with a thickened gallbladder wall.

Biliary sludge within the gallbladder lumen appears as a fine layer of echoes that slowly gravitates to the dependent portion of the gallbladder as the patient changes position. Although biliary sludge may arise without accompanying pathology, it may also result from obstruction and can predispose to gallstone formation.

Acute cholecystitis is indicated by an enlarged gallbladder with thickened, double-rimmed walls, usually with gallstones within the lumen. There may also be precholecystic fluid. In chronic cholecystitis, the walls of the gallbladder appear thickened; the organ itself, however, is generally contracted. In obstructive jaundice, ultrasonography readily demonstrates a dilated biliary system and, usually, a dilated gallbladder. Dilated intrahepatic radicles appear tortuous and irregular; a dilated gallbladder usually loses its characteristic pear shape, becoming spherical.

Biliary obstruction may result from intrinsic factors, such as a gallstone or small carcinoma within the biliary system. (Ultrasonography cannot distinguish between these two echogenic masses.) Or, it may result from extrinsic factors, such as a mass in the hepatic portal that compresses the cystic duct and interferes with bile drainage from the intrahepatic radicles, or from pathology in the head of the pancreas that obstructs the common bile duct. Such pathology includes carcinoma and pancreatitis, although ultrasonography cannot distinguish between the two. When ultrasonography fails to clearly define the site of biliary obstruction, percutaneous transhepatic cholangiography or endoscopic retrograde cholangiopancreatography should be performed.

Interfering factors

- Failure to observe pretest dietary restrictions
- Overlying bowel gas or retained barium from a previous test (possible poor imaging)
- Deficiency of body fluids in a dehydrated patient, obscuring boundaries between organs and tissue structures (possible poor imaging)

ULTRASONOGRAPHY OF THE LIVER

Ultrasonography of the liver produces images by channeling high-frequency sound waves into the right upper quadrant of the abdomen. Resultant echoes are converted to cross-sectional images on a monitor; different shades of gray depict various tissue densities. Ultrasonography can show intrahepatic structures and organ size, shape, and position.

This procedure is indicated in patients with jaundice of unknown etiology, with unexplained hepatomegaly and abnormal biochemical test results, with suspected metastatic tumors and elevated serum alkaline phosphatase levels, and with recent abdominal trauma.

When used with liver-spleen scanning, ultrasonography can define cold spots (focal defects that fail to pick up the radionuclide) as tumors, abscesses, or cysts; it also provides better views of the periportal and perihepatic spaces than liver-spleen scanning. If ultrasonography fails to provide definitive diagnosis, computed tomography, gallium scanning, or liver biopsy may yield more information.

Purpose

- To distinguish between obstructive and nonobstructive jaundice
- To screen for hepatocellular disease
- To detect hepatic metastases and hematoma
- To define cold spots as tumors, abscesses, or cysts

Patient preparation

- Explain to the patient that this procedure allows examination of the liver. Tell him who will perform the test and where it will take place.
- Instruct the patient to fast for 8 to 12 hours before the test to reduce bowel gas, which hinders transmission of ultrasound.
- Describe the procedure. Tell the patient a transducer will pass smoothly over his abdomen, channeling sound waves into the liver, but assure him that he'll feel only mild pressure.
- Instruct him to remain as still as possible during the procedure and to hold his breath when requested.

Procedure and posttest care

- The patient is placed in a supine position.
- A water-soluble conductive gel is applied to the face of the transducer.
- Transverse scans are taken at ⅜″ (1-cm) intervals, using a single-sweep technique between the costal margins. Although this technique demonstrates the left lobe of the liver and part of the right lobe, sector scans through the intercostal spaces are used to view the remainder of the right lobe.
- Scans are taken longitudinally from the right border of the liver to the left.
- For better demonstration of the right lateral dome, oblique cephalad-angled scans may be taken beneath the right costal margin.
- Scans are then taken parallel to the hepatic portal, at a 45-degree angle toward the superior right lateral dome, to examine the peripheral anatomy, portal venous system, common bile duct, and biliary tree. Clear images are photographed for later study.
- During each scan, ask the patient to hold his breath briefly in deep inspiration to displace the liver caudally from the costal margin and the ribs, to aid visualization.
- Remove the conductive gel from the patient's skin.
- Inform the patient that he may resume his usual diet.

Normal findings

The liver normally demonstrates a homogeneous, low-level echo pattern, interrupted only by the different echo patterns of its portal and hepatic veins, the aorta, and the inferior vena cava. Hepatic veins appear completely sonolucent; portal veins have margins that are highly echogenic.

Abnormal findings

In obstructive jaundice, ultrasonography shows dilated intrahepatic biliary radicles and extrahepatic ducts. Conversely, in nonobstructive jaundice, ultrasonography shows a biliary tree of normal diameter.

Ultrasonographic characteristics of hepatocellular disease are generally nonspecific, and disorders in early stages can escape detection; liver-spleen scanning is a more sensitive diagnostic tool. In cirrhosis, ultrasonography may demonstrate variable liver size; dilated, tortuous portal branches associated with portal hypertension; and an irregular echo pattern with increased echo amplitude, causing overall increased attenuation. Demonstration of splenomegaly by spleen ultrasonography or liver-spleen scanning aids diagnosis. In fatty infiltration of the liver, ultrasonography may show hepatomegaly and a regular echo pattern that, although greater in echo amplitude than that of normal parenchyma, doesn't alter attenuation.

Ultrasonographic characteristics of metastases in the liver vary widely; metastases may appear either hypoechoic or echogenic, poorly defined or well defined. For example, metastatic lymphomas and sarcomas are generally hypoechoic; mucin-secreting adenocarcinoma of the colon is highly echogenic. Liver biopsy is necessary to confirm tumor type. Serial ultrasonography may be used to monitor the effectiveness of therapy.

Primary hepatic tumors also present a varied appearance and may mimic metastases, requiring angiography and liver biopsy for definitive diagnosis. Hepatomas are the most common malignant tumors in adults; hepatoblastomas are most common in children. Benign tumors are far less common than malignant ones.

Abscesses usually appear as sonolucent masses with ill-defined, slightly thickened borders and accentuated posterior wall transmission; scattered internal echoes, caused by necrotic debris, may also be present. Because they produce similar echo patterns, intrahepatic abscesses are occasionally mistaken for hematomas, necrotic metastases, or hemorrhagic cysts. Gas-containing intrahepatic abscesses, which may be echogenic, are sometimes confused with solid intrahepatic lesions. Subphrenic abscesses occur between the diaphragm and the liver; subhepatic abscesses appear inferior to the liver and anterior to the upper pole of the right kidney. Ascitic fluid resembles a subhepatic abscess, but lacks internal echoes and has a more regular border.

Cysts usually appear as spherical, sonolucent areas with well-defined borders and accentuated posterior wall transmission. When a cyst cannot be distinguished from an abscess or necrotic metastases, gallium scanning, computed tomography, and angiography should be performed.

Hematomas—either intrahepatic or subcapsular—usually result from trauma. Intrahepatic hematomas appear as poorly defined, relatively sonolucent masses and may have scattered internal echoes due to clotting; serial ultrasonography can differentiate between a hematoma and a cyst or tumor as the hematoma becomes smaller. Subcapsular hematoma may appear as a focal, sonolucent mass on the periphery of the liver or as a diffuse, sonolucent area surrounding part of the liver.

Interfering factors

- Overlying ribs and gas or residual barium in the stomach or colon (possible misleading results)
- Deficiency of body fluids in a dehydrated patient, obscuring boundaries between organs and tissue structures (possible misleading results)

ULTRASONOGRAPHY OF THE SPLEEN

In ultrasonography of the spleen, a focused beam of high-frequency sound waves passes into the left upper quadrant of the abdomen, creating echoes that vary with changes in tissue density. These are displayed on a monitor as real-time images that indicate the size, shape, and position of the spleen and surrounding viscera.

Ultrasonography is indicated in patients with an upper left quadrant mass of unknown origin; with known splenomegaly, to evaluate changes in splenic size; with left upper quadrant pain and local tenderness; and with recent abdominal trauma.

Purpose

- To demonstrate splenomegaly
- To monitor progression of primary and secondary splenic disease and to evaluate effectiveness of therapy
- To evaluate the spleen after abdominal trauma
- To help detect splenic cysts and subphrenic abscess

Patient preparation

- Explain to the patient that this procedure allows examination of the spleen.
- Tell the patient who will perform this test and where and that the room may be darkened slightly to aid visualization on the monitor.
- Instruct the patient to fast for 8 to 12 hours before the procedure, if possible; this reduces the amount of gas in the bowel, improving the transmission of sound waves.
- Describe the procedure. Tell the patient a transducer will pass smoothly over his abdomen in direct contact with his skin, but assure him that he'll feel only mild pressure.
- Instruct the patient to remain as still as possible during the procedure and to hold his breath when requested, to aid visualization.

Procedure and posttest care

- Because the procedure for ultrasonography varies, depending on the size of the spleen and the patient's physique, the patient is usually repositioned several times; the transducer scanning angle or path is also changed.
- Generally, the patient is first placed in a supine position, with his chest uncovered.
- A water-soluble conductive gel is applied to the face of the transducer, and transverse scans of the spleen are taken at 3⁄8″ to 3⁄4″ (1- to 2-cm) intervals, beginning at the level of the diaphragm and moving posteriorly, while the transducer is angled anteromedially.
- The patient is then placed in a right lateral decubitus position, and transverse scans are taken through the intercostal spaces using a sectoring motion.
- A pillow may be placed under the patient's right side to help separate the intercostal spaces, making it easier to position the transducer face between them.
- Longitudinal scans are taken from the axilla toward the iliac crest.
- To prevent rib artifacts and to obtain the best view of the splenic parenchyma, oblique scans are taken by passing the transducer face along the intercostal spaces.
- During each scan, the patient may be asked to hold his breath briefly at various stages of inspiration.
- Good views are photographed for later study.
- Remove the conductive gel from the patient's skin.
- Inform the patient that he may resume his usual diet.

Normal findings

The splenic parenchyma normally demonstrates a homogeneous, low-level echo pattern; its individual vascular channels aren't usually apparent. The superior and lateral splenic borders are clearly defined, each having a convex margin. The undersurface and medial borders, in contrast, show indentations from surrounding organs (stomach, left kidney, and pancreas). The hilar region, where the vascular pedicle enters the spleen, commonly produces an area of highly reflective echoes. The medial surface is generally concave, which helps differentiate between left upper quadrant masses and an enlarged spleen.

Even when splenomegaly is present, the spleen generally remains concave medially unless a space-occupying lesion distorts this contour.

Abnormal findings

Ultrasonography can show splenomegaly, but it usually doesn't indicate the cause; a computed tomography (CT) scan can provide more specific information. Splenomegaly is generally accompanied by increased echogenicity. Enlarged vascular channels are commonly visible, especially in the hilar region. If space-occupying lesions distort the splenic contour, liver-spleen scanning should be performed to confirm splenomegaly.

Abdominal trauma may result in splenic rupture or subcapsular hematoma. In splenic rupture, ultrasonography demonstrates splenomegaly and an irregular, sonolucent area (the presence of free intraperitoneal fluid); however, these findings must be confirmed by arteriography. In subcapsular hematoma, ultrasonography shows splenomegaly as well as a double contour, altered splenic position, and a relatively sonolucent area on the periphery of the spleen. The double contour results from blood accumulation between the splenic parenchyma and the intact splenic capsule. As the spleen enlarges, a transverse section shows its anterior margin extending more anteriorly than the aorta. Ultrasonography may be difficult and painful after abdominal trauma because the transducer may have to pass across fractured ribs and contusions; CT scanning, which differentiates blood and fluid in the peritoneal space, should be used instead.

In subphrenic abscess, ultrasonography shows a sonolucent area beneath the diaphragm. Clinical findings may differentiate between abscess and blood or fluid accumulation.

Used with liver-spleen scanning, ultrasonography differentiates cold spots as cystic or solid lesions. It shows cysts as spherical, sonolucent areas with well-defined, regular margins with acoustic enhancement behind them. When ultrasonography fails to identify a cyst as splenic or extrasplenic—especially if the cyst is located in the upper pole of the left kidney and the adrenal gland, or in the tail of the pancreas—a CT scan and arteriography are used. Ultrasonography can readily clarify cystic cold spots, but using a CT scan with a contrast medium is superior for evaluating primary and metastatic tumors. Ultrasonography usually fails to identify tumors associated with lymphoma and chronic leukemias because these resemble tumors of the splenic parenchyma.

Interfering factors

- Overlying ribs, aerated left lung, gas or residual barium in the colon or the stomach (possible poor imaging)
- Deficiency of body fluids in a dehydrated patient, obscuring boundaries between organs and tissue structures (possible poor imaging)
- Body physique affecting the spleen's shape or adjacent masses displacing the spleen (possible poor imaging, may be mistaken for splenomegaly)
- Patient with splenic trauma (possible difficulty in tolerating the procedure)

ULTRASONOGRAPHY OF THE PANCREAS

In ultrasonography of the pancreas, cross-sectional images of the pancreas are produced by channeling high-frequency sound waves into the epigastric region and converting the resultant echoes to real-time images, which are displayed on a monitor. The pattern varies with tissue density and indicates the size, shape, and position of the pancreas and surrounding viscera.

Purpose

- To aid diagnosis of pancreatitis, pseudocysts, and pancreatic carcinoma

Patient preparation

- Explain to the patient that this procedure permits examination of the pancreas.
- Instruct the patient to fast for 8 to 12 hours before the procedure to reduce bowel gas.
- Tell the patient who will perform the procedure, where it will take place, and that the room may be darkened slightly to aid visualization on the monitor.
- If the patient is a smoker, ask him to abstain before the test; this eliminates the risk of swallowing air while inhaling, which interferes with test results.
- Describe the procedure. Tell the patient a transducer will pass smoothly over his epigastric region, channeling sound waves into the pancreas, but assure him that he'll only feel mild pressure.
- Tell the patient he'll be asked to inhale deeply during scanning, and instruct him to remain still during the procedure.

Procedure and posttest care

- The patient is placed in a supine position.
- A water-soluble conductive gel or mineral oil is applied to the abdomen and, with the patient at full inspiration, transverse scans are taken at 1-cm intervals, starting from the xiphoid and moving caudally; longitudinal scans are taken to view the head, body, and tail of the pancreas in sequence; scanning the right anterior oblique view allows imaging of the head and body of the pancreas; oblique sagittal scans are used to view the portal vein; and scanning from the sagittal view images the vena cava.
- When good ultrasonography views are obtained they're photographed for later study.
- Remove the conductive gel from the patient's skin.
- Inform the patient that he may resume his usual diet.

Normal findings

The pancreas normally demonstrates a coarse, uniform echo pattern and usually appears more echogenic than the adjacent liver.

Abnormal findings

Alterations in the size, contour, and parenchymal texture of the pancreas characterize pancreatic disease. An enlarged pancreas with decreased echogenicity and distinct borders suggests pancreatitis; a well-defined mass with an essentially echo-free interior indicates pseudocyst; an ill-defined mass with scattered internal echoes or a mass in the head of the pancreas (obstructing the common bile duct) and a large noncontracting gallbladder suggest pancreatic carcinoma.

Subsequent computed tomography scan and biopsy of the pancreas may be necessary to confirm a diagnosis.

Interfering factors

- Gas or residual barium in the stomach and intestine (possible poor imaging)
- Deficiency of body fluids in a dehydrated patient, obscuring boundaries between organs and tissue structures (possible poor imaging)
- Obesity (possible poor imaging)
- Fatty infiltration of pancreas (possible poor imaging)

Miscellaneous Tests

Thyroid Ultrasonography

In thyroid ultrasonography, high-frequency sound waves emitted from a transducer are directed at the thyroid gland and reflected back to produce structural images on a monitor.

When a mass is located by palpation or by thyroid imaging, thyroid ultrasonography can differentiate between a cyst and a tumor larger than ⅜″ (1 cm) with a high degree of accuracy. This test is also used to evaluate thyroid nodules during pregnancy because it doesn't require use of radioactive iodine.

Purpose

- To evaluate thyroid structure
- To differentiate between a cyst and a solid tumor
- To monitor the size of the thyroid gland during suppressive therapy

Patient preparation

- Describe the procedure to the patient, and explain that this test defines the size and shape of the thyroid gland.
- Inform the patient that he need not restrict food or fluids before the test.
- Tell the patient who will perform the procedure, where it will take place, and that it's painless and safe.

Procedure and posttest care

- The patient is placed in a supine position with a pillow under his shoulder blades to hyperextend his neck.
- His neck is coated with water-soluble conductive gel.
- The transducer then scans the thyroid, projecting its echographic image on the oscilloscope screen.
- The image on the monitor is photographed for subsequent examination.
- Accurate visualization of the anterior portion of the thyroid requires use of a short-focused transducer.
- Thoroughly clean the patient's neck to remove the conductive gel.

Normal findings

Thyroid ultrasonography exhibits a uniform echo pattern throughout the gland.

Abnormal findings

Cysts appear as smooth-bordered, echo-free areas with enhanced sound transmission; adenomas and carcinomas appear either solid and well demarcated with identical echo patterns or, less frequently, solid with cystic areas. Carcinoma infiltrating the gland may not be well demarcated.

Identification of a tumor is generally followed up by fine needle aspiration or an excisional biopsy to determine malignancy.

Interfering factors

- None significant

Pelvic Ultrasonography

In pelvic ultrasonography, high-frequency sound waves are reflected to a transducer to provide images of the interior pelvic area on a monitor. Techniques of sound imaging include A-mode (amplitude modulation, recorded as spikes), B-mode (brightness modulation), gray scale (a representation of organ texture in shades of gray), and real-time imaging (instantaneous images of the tissues in motion, similar to fluoroscopic examination). Selected views may be photographed for later examination and a permanent record of the test.

Purpose

- To detect foreign bodies and distinguish between cystic and solid masses (tumors)
- To measure organ size
- To evaluate fetal viability, position, gestational age, and growth rate
- To detect multiple pregnancy
- To confirm fetal abnormalities and maternal abnormalities
- To guide amniocentesis by determining placental location and fetal position

Patient preparation

- Describe the test to the patient, and tell her the reason it's being performed.
- Assure the patient that this procedure is safe, noninvasive, and painless.
- Because this test requires a full bladder as a landmark to define pelvic organs, instruct the patient to drink liquids and not to void before the test.
- Tell the patient who will perform the procedure and where.
- Explain that a water enema may be necessary to produce a better outline of the large intestine.
- Reassure the patient that the test won't harm the fetus, and provide emotional support throughout.

Procedure and posttest care

- With the patient in a supine position, the pelvic area is coated with mineral oil or water-soluble conductive gel to increase sound wave conduction.
- The transducer is guided over the area, images are observed on the monitor, and good images are photographed.
- Remove the conductive gel from the patient's skin.
- Allow the patient to immediately empty her bladder after the test.

Normal findings

The uterus is normal in size and shape. The ovaries' size, shape, and sonographic density are normal. The body of the uterus lies on the superior surface of the bladder; the uterine tubes are attached laterally. The ovaries are located on the lateral pelvic walls, with the external iliac vessels above the ureter posteroinferiorly and covered by the fimbria of the uterine tubes medially. No other masses are visible. If the patient is pregnant, the gestational sac and fetus are of normal size in relation to gestational age.

Abnormal findings

Both cystic and solid masses have homogeneous densities, but solid masses (such as fibroids) appear denser. Inappropriate fetal size may indicate miscalculated conception or delivery date, fetal anomalies, or a dead fetus. Abnormal echo patterns may indicate foreign bodies (such as an intrauterine device), multiple pregnancy, maternal abnormalities (such as placenta previa or abruptio placentae), fetal abnormalities (such as molar pregnancy or abnormalities of the arms and legs, spine, heart, head, kidneys, and abdomen), fetal malpresentation (such as breech or shoulder presentation), and cephalopelvic disproportion.

Interfering factors

- Failure to fill the bladder, obesity, or fetal head deep in the pelvis (possible poor imaging)

RENAL ULTRASONOGRAPHY

In renal ultrasonography, high-frequency sound waves are transmitted from a transducer to the kidneys and perirenal structures. The resulting echoes are displayed on a monitor as anatomic images.

Renal ultrasonography can be used to detect abnormalities or clarify those detected by other tests. It's especially useful in cases in which excretory urography is ruled out. Unlike excretory urography, this test isn't dependent on renal function and therefore may be useful in patients with renal failure. Ultrasonography of the ureter, bladder, and gonads also may be used to evaluate urologic disorders.

Purpose

- To determine the size, shape, and position of the kidneys, their internal structures, and perirenal tissues
- To evaluate and localize urinary obstruction and abnormal fluid accumulation
- To assess and diagnose complications after kidney transplantation
- To detect renal or perirenal masses
- To differentiate between renal cysts and solid masses
- To verify placement of a nephrostomy tube

Patient preparation

- Explain to the patient that this test is used to detect kidney abnormalities.
- Inform the patient that he need not restrict food or fluids before the test.
- Tell the patient who will perform the test and where and that it's safe and painless.

Procedure and posttest care

- The patient is placed in prone position, the area to be scanned is exposed, and conductive gel is applied to the area.
- The longitudinal axis of the kidneys is located by using measurements from excretory urography or by performing transverse scans through the upper and lower renal poles.
- These points are marked on the skin and connected with straight lines. Sectional images ⅜″ to ¾″ (1 to 2 cm) apart can then be obtained by moving the transducer longitudinally, transversely, or at any other angle required.
- During the test, the patient may be asked to breathe deeply to visualize upper portions of the kidney.
- Remove the conductive gel from the patient's skin.
- If bladder abnormalities are found, prepare the patient for further testing.
- If rejection of a transplanted kidney is suspected or diagnosed, monitor intake and output, blood pressure, blood urea nitrogen and creatinine levels, and vital signs. In addition, monitor for adrenal dysfunction (hypotension, decreased urine output, and electrolyte imbalances) if a tumor is detected on the gland.
- If ultrasonography is used as a guide for nephrostomy tube placement or drainage of an abscess, monitor the amount and characteristics of drainage and tube patency.

Normal findings

The kidneys are located between the superior iliac crests and the diaphragm. The renal capsule should be outlined sharply; the cortex should produce more echoes than the medulla. In the center of each kidney, the renal collecting systems appear as irregular areas of higher density than surrounding tissue. The renal veins and, depending on the scanner, some internal structures can be visualized. If the bladder is also being evaluated, its size, shape, position, and urine content can be determined.

Abnormal findings

Cysts are usually fluid-filled, circular structures that don't reflect sound waves. Tumors produce multiple echoes and appear as irregular shapes. Abscesses found within or around the kidneys usually echo sound waves poorly; their boundaries are slightly more irregular than those of cysts. A perirenal abscess may displace the kidney anteriorly.

Generally, acute pyelonephritis and glomerulonephritis aren't detectable unless the renal parenchyma is significantly scarred and atrophied. In such patients, the renal capsule appears irregular and the kidney may appear smaller than normal; also, an increased number of echoes may arise from the parenchyma due to fibrosis.

In patients with hydronephrosis, renal ultrasonography may show a large, echo-free, central mass that compresses the renal cortex. Calyceal echoes are usually circularly diffused and the pelvis significantly enlarged. This test can also be used to detect congenital anomalies, such as horseshoe, ectopic, or duplicated kidneys. Ultrasonography clearly detects renal hypertrophy.

Following renal transplantation, compensatory hypertrophy of the transplanted kidney is normal but an acute increase in size indicates rejection.

This test allows identification of abnormal accumulations of fluid within or around the kidneys that sometimes arise from an obstruction. It also allows evaluation of perirenal structures and can identify abnormalities of the adrenal glands, such as tumors, cysts, and adrenal dysfunction. However, a normal adrenal gland is difficult to define ultrasonically because of its small size.

Renal ultrasonography can be used to detect changes in the shape of the bladder that result from masses and can assess urine volume. Increased urine volume or residual urine post-voiding may indicate bladder outlet obstruction.

Interfering factors

- Retained barium from a previous test, obesity (possible poor imaging)

TRANSCRANIAL DOPPLER STUDIES

Transcranial Doppler studies provide information about the presence, quality, and changing nature of circulation to an area of the brain by measuring the velocity of blood flow through cerebral arteries. Narrowed blood vessels produce high velocities, indicating possible stenosis or vasospasm. High velocities may also indicate an arteriovenous malformation.

Purpose

- To measure the velocity of blood flow through certain cerebral vessels
- To detect and monitor the progression of cerebral vasospasm
- To determine whether collateral blood flow exists before surgical ligation or radiologic occlusion of diseased vessels

Patient preparation

- Explain the purpose of the study to the patient (or to his family).
- Tell the patient that the test will be done while he lies on a bed or stretcher or sits in a reclining chair (or it can be performed at the bedside if he's too ill to be moved to the laboratory).
- Describe the procedure. Explain that a small amount of gel will be applied to his skin and that a probe will be used to

transmit a signal to the artery being studied. Tell the patient that it usually takes less than 1 hour, depending on the number of vessels to be examined and any interfering factors.
■ Tell the patient that fasting isn't required before the test.

Equipment
Transcranial Doppler unit, probe, conductive gel

Procedure and posttest care
■ The patient reclines in a chair or on a stretcher or bed.
■ A small amount of conductive gel is applied to the transcranial window (an area where bone is thin enough to allow the Doppler signal to enter and be detected); the most common approaches are temporal, transorbital, and through the foramen magnum.
■ The technician directs the signal toward the artery being studied and records the velocities detected. In a complete study, the middle cerebral arteries, anterior cerebral arteries, posterior cerebral arteries, ophthalmic arteries, carotid siphon, vertebral arteries, and basilar artery are studied.
■ The Doppler signal waveforms may be printed for later analysis and can be transmitted to varying depths (measured in millimeters).
■ When the study is completed, wipe away the conductive gel.

Precautions
■ Be sure to remove turban head dressings or thick dressings over the test site.

Normal findings
The type of waveforms and velocities obtained indicate whether pathology exists.

Abnormal findings
Although this test often isn't definitive, high velocities are typically abnormal and suggest that blood flow is too turbulent or the vessel is too narrow.

After the transcranial Doppler study and before surgery, the patient may undergo cerebral angiography to further define cerebral blood flow patterns and locate the exact vascular abnormality.

Interfering factors
■ Failure to remove dressings over the test site (possible poor imaging)

VAGINAL ULTRASONOGRAPHY

In vaginal ultrasonography, a probe inserted into the vagina reflects high-frequency sound waves to a transducer, forming an image of the pelvic structures. This study allows better evaluation of pelvic anatomy and earlier diagnosis of pregnancy. It also circumvents the poor visualization encountered with obese patients.

Purpose
■ To establish pregnancy with fetal heart motion as early as the 5th to 6th week of gestation
■ To determine ectopic pregnancy
■ To evaluate abnormal pregnancy
■ To diagnose fetal abnormalities and placental location
■ To visualize retained products of conception
■ To evaluate adnexal pathology, such as tubo-ovarian abscess, hydrosalpinx, and ovarian masses

- To evaluate the uterine lining (in cases of dysfunctional uterine bleeding and postmenopausal bleeding)
- To monitor follicular growth during infertility treatment

Patient preparation

- Describe the procedure to the patient, and explain the reason for the test.
- Assure the patient that the procedure is safe.

Procedure and posttest care

- The patient is placed in the lithotomy position. If the sonographer is a male, a female assistant should be present during the examination.
- Water-soluble conductive gel is placed on the transducer tip to allow better sound transmission, and a protective sheath is placed over the transducer.
- Place more lubricant on the sheathed transducer tip to allow for its gentle insertion into the vagina by the patient or the sonographer. Allowing the patient to introduce the probe may decrease her anxiety.
- To observe the pelvic structures, rotate the probe 90 degrees to one side and then the other.

Normal findings

If the patient is not pregnant, the uterus and ovaries are normal in size and shape. The body of the uterus lies on the superior surface of the bladder; the uterine tubes are attached laterally. The ovaries are located on the lateral pelvic walls, with the external iliac vessels above the ureter posteroinferiorly and covered by the fimbria of the uterine tubes medially. If the patient is pregnant, the gestational sac and fetus are of normal size for the gestational dates.

Abnormal findings

Vaginal ultrasonography may reveal an empty uterus if the patient was pregnant. Free peritoneal fluid may be visible in the pelvic cavity, indicating possible peritonitis. Ectopic pregnancies may also be visible in the pelvic cavity.

Interfering factors

- Mistaking the bowel for the ovaries
- Small tubal mass (possible difficulty in detecting ectopic pregnancies)

12

Radiography

GENITOURINARY SYSTEM 599

REPRODUCTIVE SYSTEM 621

SKELETAL SYSTEM 624

MISCELLANEOUS TESTS 629

Neurologic System

Skull Radiography

Although skull radiography is of limited value in assessing patients with head injuries, skull X-rays are extremely valuable for studying abnormalities of the base of the skull and the cranial vault, congenital and perinatal anomalies, and systemic diseases that produce bone defects of the skull. For more accurate assessment of head injuries as well as of skull and head abnormalities, nonenhanced computed tomography studies of the head are done.

Skull radiography evaluates the three groups of bones that comprise the skull: the calvaria (vault), the mandible (jaw bone), and the facial bones. The calvaria and the facial bones are closely connected by immovable joints with irregular serrated edges called sutures. The bones of the skull form an anatomic structure so complex that a complete skull examination requires several radiologic views of each area.

Purpose

- To detect fractures in patients with head trauma
- To aid diagnosis of pituitary tumors
- To detect congenital anomalies
- To detect metabolic and endocrinologic disorders

Patient preparation

- Explain to the patient that his head will be immobilized and that several X-rays of his skull will be taken from various angles.
- Tell the patient that this test helps determine the presence of anomalies and helps establish a diagnosis.
- Tell the patient who will perform the test and where it will take place.
- Explain to the patient that he need not restrict food or fluid before the test and that the test will cause no discomfort.
- Tell the patient to remove glasses, dentures, jewelry, or any metallic objects that would be in the X-ray field.

Procedure and posttest care

- Have the patient recline on the X-ray table or sit in a chair.
- Tell the patient to remain still during the procedure.
- Use foam pads, sandbags, or a headband to immobilize the patient's head and increase comfort.
- Five views of the skull are routinely taken: left and right lateral, anteroposterior Townes, posteroanterior Caldwell, and axial (or base).
- Films are developed and checked for quality before the patient leaves the area.

Normal findings

A radiologist interprets the X-rays, evaluating the size, shape, thickness, and position of the cranial bones as well as the vascular markings, sinuses, and sutures. All should be normal for the patient's age.

Abnormal findings

Skull radiography is often used to diagnose fractures of the vault or base, although basilar fractures may not show on the film if the bone is dense. This test may confirm congenital anomalies and may show erosion, enlargement, or decalcification of the sella turcica that result from increased intracranial pressure (ICP). A marked rise in ICP may cause the brain to expand and press against the inner bony table of the skull, yielding visible marks or impressions.

In conditions such as osteomyelitis (with possible calcification of the skull itself) and chronic subdural hematomas, X-rays may show abnormal areas of calcification. The X-rays can detect neoplasms within brain substance that contains calcium (such as oligodendrogliomas or meningiomas) or the midline shifting of a calcified pineal gland caused by a space-occupying lesion.

Radiography may also detect other changes in bone structure, for example, those that arise from metabolic disorders such as acromegaly or Paget's disease.

Interfering factors

- Improper positioning of the patient and excessive head movement (possible poor imaging)
- Failure to remove radiopaque objects from the X-ray field (possible poor imaging)

CEREBRAL ANGIOGRAPHY

Cerebral angiography involves injecting a contrast medium to allow radiographic examination of the cerebral vasculature. Possible injection sites include the femoral, carotid, and brachial arteries. Because it allows visualization of four vessels (the carotid and the vertebral arteries), the femoral artery is used most commonly.

Usually, this test is performed on patients with suspected abnormality of the cerebral vasculature; abnormalities may be suggested by intracranial computed tomography, lumbar puncture, magnetic resonance imaging, or magnetic resonance angiography.

Purpose

- To detect cerebrovascular abnormalities, such as aneurysm or arteriovenous malformation, thrombosis, narrowing, or occlusion
- To study vascular displacement caused by tumor, hematoma, edema, herniation, vasospasm, increased intracranial pressure (ICP), or hydrocephalus
- To locate clips applied to blood vessels during surgery and to evaluate the postoperative status of affected vessels

Patient preparation

- Explain to the patient that this test shows blood circulation in the brain.
- Describe the test, including who will administer it and where it will take place.
- Tell the patient to fast for 8 to 10 hours before the test.
- Ensure any pretest blood work results are on the chart to determine bleeding tendency or kidney function.
- Explain to the patient that he'll wear a gown and that he must remove all jewelry, dentures, hairpins, and other metallic objects in the radiographic field.
- If ordered, administer a sedative and an anticholinergic drug 30 to 45 minutes before the test.
- Make sure the patient voids before leaving his room.
- Tell the patient that he'll be positioned on an X-ray table, with his head immobilized, and that he should remain still.
- Explain that a local anesthetic will be administered (some patients — especially children — receive a general anesthetic).
- Explain to the patient that he'll feel a transient burning sensation as the

medium is injected; a warm, flushed feeling; transient headache; a salty or metallic taste in his mouth; or nausea and vomiting after the dye is injected.

- Make sure the patient or a responsible family member has signed an informed consent form, if required.

◆ **CLINICAL ALERT** *Check the patient's history for hypersensitivity to iodine, iodine-containing substances (such as shellfish), or other contrast media. Note any hypersensitivities on his chart and report them as appropriate.*

Equipment

Contrast medium, automatic contrast injector, radiograph machine with rapid biplane cassette changes, arterial needles (18G or 19G, 2½" needle for adults; 20G, 1½" needle for children), femoral arterial catheters for femoral injection

Procedure and posttest care

- Have the patient recline on an X-ray table and instruct him to lie still with his arms at his sides.
- Shave the injection site (femoral, carotid, or brachial artery) and clean it with alcohol and povidone-iodine.
- A local anesthetic is injected. Then the artery is punctured with the appropriate needle and catheterized.
- In the femoral artery approach, a catheter is threaded to the aortic arch.
- In the brachial artery approach (least common), a blood pressure cuff is placed distal to the puncture site and inflated before injection to prevent the contrast medium from flowing into the forearm and hand.
- After X-rays or fluoroscopy verifies placement of the needle or catheter, the contrast medium is injected. Observe the patient for an adverse reaction, such as hives, flushing, or laryngeal stridor.
- An initial series of lateral and anteroposterior X-rays is taken, developed, and reviewed. Depending on the results, more contrast medium may be injected and another series taken.
- During the test, maintain arterial catheter patency by continuous or periodic flushing. Monitor vital and neurologic signs.
- When a satisfactory series of X rays is obtained, the needle (or catheter) is withdrawn. Apply firm pressure to the puncture site for 15 minutes.
- After the test, observe the patient for bleeding, check distal pulses, and apply a pressure bandage.
- Typically, the patient will be on bed rest for 6 to 8 hours. Administer prescribed pain medications and monitor his vital signs and neurologic status for 6 hours. The patient is usually discharged the same day.
- Observe the puncture site for signs of extravasation (redness, swelling) and apply an ice bag to ease the patient's discomfort and minimize swelling. If bleeding occurs, apply firm pressure to the puncture site and inform the physician.
- If the femoral approach was used, keep the affected leg straight for 6 hours or longer and routinely check pulses distal to the site (dorsalis pedis, popliteal). Monitor the leg for temperature, color, and sensation. Thrombosis or hematoma can occlude blood flow; extravasation can also impede the flow of blood by exerting pressure on the artery.
- Monitor for disorientation and weakness or numbness in the extremities (signs of thrombosis or hematoma) and for arterial spasms, which may produce symptoms of transient ischemic attacks.
- If the brachial approach was used, immobilize the affected arm for 6 hours or longer and routinely check the radial pulse.

- Place a sign near the patient's bed warning personnel not to take blood pressure readings from the affected arm.
- Observe the patient's arm and hand for any changes in color, temperature, or sensation. If they become pale, cool, or numb, report these changes at once.
- After the test, tell the patient he may resume his usual diet. Encourage him to drink fluids to help him pass the contrast medium.

Precautions

- Cerebral angiography is contraindicated in patients with hepatic, renal, or thyroid disease.
- This test is also contraindicated in patients with hypersensitivity to iodine or contrast media.
- If the patient has been receiving aspirin or other anticoagulants daily, take extra care when compressing the puncture site. Anticoagulants may need to be discontinued for 3 days prior to testing.

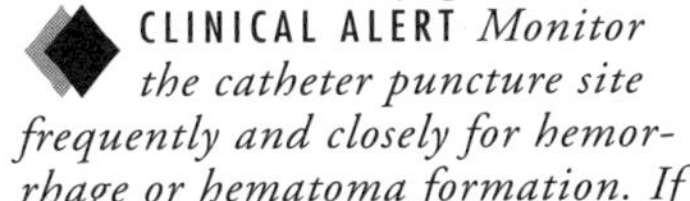

CLINICAL ALERT *Monitor the catheter puncture site frequently and closely for hemorrhage or hematoma formation. If either occurs, notify the physician immediately.*

Normal findings

During the arterial phase of perfusion, the contrast medium fills and opacities superficial and deep arteries and arterioles; it opacities superficial and deep veins during the venous phase. The finding of apparently normal (symmetrical) cerebral vasculature must be correlated with the patient's history and clinical status.

Abnormal findings

Changes in the caliber of vessel lumina suggest vascular disease, possibly due to spasms, plaques, fistulas, arteriovenous malformation, or arteriosclerosis. Diminished blood flow to vessels may be related to increased ICP.

Vessel displacement may reflect the presence and size of a tumor, areas of edema, or obstruction of the cerebrospinal fluid pathway. Cerebral angiography may also show circulation within a tumor, usually giving precise information on the tumor's position and nature. Meningeal blood supply originating in the external carotid artery may indicate an extracerebral tumor but usually designates a meningioma. Such a tumor may arise outside the brain substance, but it may still be within the cerebral hemisphere.

Interfering factors

- Head movement during the test (possible poor imaging)
- Failure to remove metallic objects from the X-ray field (possible poor imaging)

MYELOGRAPHY

Myelography uses fluoroscopy and radiography to evaluate the spinal subarachnoid space after injection of a contrast medium. Because the contrast medium is heavier than cerebrospinal fluid (CSF), it flows through the subarachnoid space to the dependent area when the patient, lying prone on a fluoroscopic table, is tilted up or down. The fluoroscope allows the physician to see the flow of the contrast medium and the outline of the subarachnoid space. X-rays are taken to provide a permanent record.

Purpose

- To evaluate and determine the cause of neurologic symptoms (numbness, pain, weakness)

- To identify lesions, such as tumors and herniated intervertebral disks that partially or totally block the flow of CSF in the subarachnoid space
- To help detect arachnoiditis, spinal nerve root injury, or tumors in the posterior fossa of the skull

Patient preparation

- Explain to the patient that this test reveals obstructions in the spinal cord.
- Tell the patient that his food and fluid intake will be restricted for 8 hours before the test. If the test is scheduled for the afternoon, and facility policy permits, the patient may have clear liquids before the test.
- Describe the test, including who will administer it and where it will take place.
- Explain to the patient that he may feel a transient burning sensation as the contrast medium is injected; a warm, flushed feeling; transient headache; a salty taste; or nausea and vomiting after the dye is injected. Explain that he may feel some pain caused by his positioning, needle insertion and, in some cases, removal of the contrast medium.
- Make sure the patient or a responsible family member has signed an informed consent form.

◆ **CLINICAL ALERT** *Check the patient's history for hypersensitivity to iodine and iodine-containing substances (for example, shellfish), radiographic contrast media, and associated medications. Notify the radiologist if the patient has a history of epilepsy or phenothiazine use. If metrizamide is to be used as a contrast medium, discontinue phenothiazine 48 hours before the test.*

- Tell the patient to remove all jewelry and other metallic objects in the X-ray field.
- Tell the patient that the head of his bed must be elevated for 6 to 8 hours after the test and that he'll remain on bed rest for an additional 6 to 8 hours. If an oil-based contrast agent is used, inform the patient that it will be manually removed after the test and that he'll need to remain flat in bed for 6 to 24 hours.
- Perform pretest procedures and administer prescribed medications. If the puncture is to be performed in the lumbar region, an enema may be prescribed. A sedative and anticholinergic (such as atropine sulfate) may be prescribed to reduce swallowing during the procedure. Ensure pretest laboratory work (may include coagulation and kidney function studies) is present in the chart.

Equipment

Alcohol, 1% lidocaine solution, lumbar puncture tray, contrast medium (iophendylate or metrizamide sodium), two 10-ml syringes, spinal needle (18G for iophendylate or 11G for metrizamide), X-ray machine capable of fluoroscopy, povidone-iodine solution, sterile gloves, small adhesive bandage

Procedure and posttest care

- Position the patient on his side at the edge of the table, with his chin on his chest and his knees drawn up to his abdomen. (If the patient has lumbar deformity or infection at the puncture site, cisternal puncture may be done.)
- After the lumbar puncture is performed, the fluoroscope is used to verify proper positioning of the needle in the subarachnoid space. Some CSF may be removed for routine laboratory analysis.
- Turn the patient to the prone position and secure him with straps across his upper back, under his arms, and across his ankles. Hyperextend his chin

to prevent the contrast medium from flowing into the cranium; place a towel or sponge under his chin for comfort.

- If the patient complains of a headache or difficulty swallowing or reports that he isn't breathing deeply enough, provide reassurance and explain that he can rest periodically during the procedure.
- The contrast medium is injected and the table tilted so that the dye flows through the subarachnoid space. (In rare circumstances, air is used as a negative contrast medium; however, this is typically reserved for patients with suspected congenital abnormalities such as syringomyelia.)
- The flow of the contrast medium is observed by fluoroscope and X-rays are taken. If an obstruction in the subarachnoid space blocks the upward flow of the contrast medium, a cisternal puncture may be performed.
- The contrast medium is withdrawn, if necessary, after satisfactory X-rays are obtained, and the needle is removed. Clean the puncture site with povidone-iodine solution and apply a small adhesive bandage.
- Based on the contrast medium used during the test, position the patient as follows: If metrizamide was used, tell him to stay in bed for the next 12 to 16 hours. Keep the head of his bed elevated for at least 8 hours. If an oil-based contrast medium was used, tell him to remain flat in bed for 24 hours.
- Monitor vital signs and neurologic status at least every 15 minutes for the first hour, every 30 minutes for the next 2 hours, then every 4 hours for 24 hours. The patient may be discharged the same day.
- Encourage the patient to drink extra fluids. He should void within 8 hours after returning to his room.
- If there are no complications or adverse reactions, tell the patient that he may resume his usual diet and activities the day after the test.
- Monitor for radicular pain, fever, back pain, or signs of meningeal irritation, such as headache, irritability, or stiff neck. If these signs or symptoms occur, keep the room quiet and dark and administer an analgesic or antipyretic as needed.

Precautions

- Generally, myelography is contraindicated for patients with increased intracranial pressure, hypersensitivity to iodine or contrast media, or an infection at the puncture site.
- Improper positioning after the test may affect recovery.

Normal findings

Normally, the contrast medium flows freely through the subarachnoid space, showing no obstruction or structural abnormalities.

Abnormal findings

Myelography can identify and localize lesions within or surrounding the spinal cord or subarachnoid space. Examples of common extradural lesions include herniated intervertebral disks and metastatic tumors. Neurofibromas and meningiomas are common lesions within the subarachnoid space, and ependymomas and astrocytomas are common within the spinal cord.

If the test confirms a spinal tumor, the patient may be taken directly to the operating room. Immediate surgery may also be necessary if the contrast medium causes a total block of the subarachnoid space.

Myelography may help locate or confirm a ruptured or herniated disk, spinal stenosis, or abscess and, occasionally, confirm the need for surgery. This test may also detect syringomyelia (a congenital abnormality marked by fluid-filled cavities within the spinal cord and widening of the cord itself), arachnoiditis, spinal nerve root injury, and tumors in the posterior fossa of the skull. Other findings may include fractures, dislocations, thinning of bones (osteoporosis), deformities in the curvature of the spine, bone spurs, and vertebral degeneration. Test results must be correlated with the patient's history and clinical status.

Interfering factors

- Incorrect needle placement
- Uncooperative patient

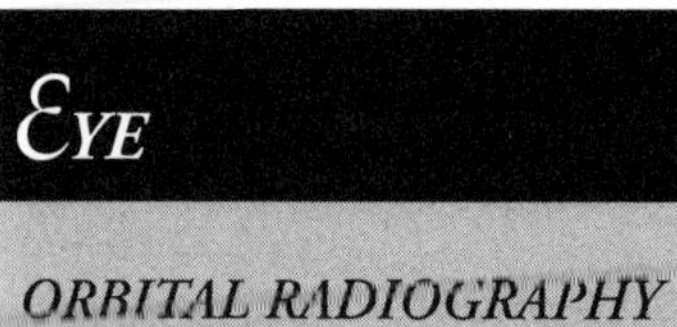

Orbital radiography evaluates the orbit, the bony cavity that houses the eye and the lacrimal glands, as well as blood vessels, nerves, muscles, and fat. Because portions of the orbit are composed of thin bone that fractures easily, X-rays are commonly taken following facial trauma. They're also useful in diagnosing ocular and orbital pathologies. Special radiographic techniques can reveal foreign bodies in the orbit or eye that are invisible to an ophthalmoscope. In some cases, radiography is used in conjunction with computed tomography (CT) scans and ultrasonography to better define an abnormality.

Purpose

- To aid in diagnosis of orbital fractures and pathologies
- To help locate intraorbital or intraocular foreign bodies

Patient preparation

- Explain that this test involves taking several X-rays to assess the condition of the bones around the eye.
- Describe the test, including who will perform it and where it will take place.
- Reassure the patient that the procedure is usually painless unless he has suffered facial trauma, in which case positioning may cause some discomfort. Explain that he'll be asked to turn his head from side to side and to flex or extend his neck.
- Instruct the patient to remove all jewelry and other metallic objects from the X-ray field.

Procedure and posttest care

- Have the patient recline on the X-ray table or sit in a chair.
- Instruct the patient to remain still while the X-rays are taken.
- Usually, a series of orbital X-rays includes a lateral view, posteroanterior view, submentovertical (base) view, stereo Waters' views (views from both sides), Towne's (half-axial) projection, and optic canal projections. If enlargement of the superior orbital fissure is suspected, apical views are obtained.
- The films are developed and inspected before the patient leaves the radiography department.

Normal findings

Each orbit is composed of a roof, a floor, and medial and lateral walls. The bones of the roof and floor are very thin (the floor can be less than 1 mm thick). The medial walls, which parallel each other, are slightly thicker, except for the portion formed by the ethmoid bone. The lateral walls are the thickest part of the orbit and are strongest at the orbital rim.

The superior orbital fissure, at the back of the orbit between the lateral wall and the roof, is actually a gap between the greater and lesser wings of the sphenoid bone. The optic canal, which carries the optic nerve and ophthalmic artery, is an opening in the lesser wing of the sphenoid bone located at the apex of the orbit.

Abnormal findings

Orbital fractures associated with facial trauma are most common in the thin structures of the floor and ethmoid bone. Abnormalities are detected by comparing the size and shape of orbital structures on the affected side with those on the opposite side.

Generally, orbit enlargement indicates the presence of a lesion that has caused proptosis due to increased intraorbital pressure. Any growing tumor can produce these changes. Superior orbital fissure enlargement can result from orbital meningioma, from intracranial conditions such as pituitary tumors or, more characteristically, from vascular anomalies. Optic canal enlargement may result from extraocular extension of a retinoblastoma or, in children, from an optic nerve glioma. In adults, only prolonged pathology can increase orbital size; however, in children, even a rapidly growing lesion can cause orbital enlargement because orbital bones aren't fully developed. A decrease in the size of the orbit may follow childhood enucleation of the eye or conditions such as congenital microphthalmia.

Destruction of the orbital walls may indicate a malignant neoplasm or an infection. A benign tumor or cyst produces a clear-cut local indentation of the orbital wall. Lesions of adjacent structures may also produce radiographic changes due to enlargement and erosion of the orbit.

Increased bone density may be seen in conditions, such as osteoblastic metastasis, sphenoid ridge meningioma, or Paget's disease. To confirm orbital pathology, however, radiographic findings must be supplemented with results from other appropriate tests and procedures.

Interfering factors

- None significant

FLUORESCEIN ANGIOGRAPHY

In fluorescein angiography, a special camera takes rapid-sequence photographs of the fundus following I.V. injection of sodium fluorescein (a contrast medium), thereby recording the appearance of blood vessels within the eye. This technique provides enhanced visibility of the microvascular structures of the retina and choroid, which permits evaluation of the entire retinal vascular bed, including retinal circulation.

Purpose

- To document retinal circulation when evaluating intraocular abnormalities, such as retinopathy, tumors, and circulatory or inflammatory disorders

Patient preparation

- Explain that this procedure takes about 30 minutes and evaluates the small blood vessels in the eyes.
- Make sure the patient or an appropriate family member has signed an informed consent form.
- Check the patient's history for glaucoma and hypersensitivity reactions or allergies, especially to contrast media and dilating eyedrops. If necessary, tell a patient with glaucoma not to use miotic eyedrops on the day of the test.
- Explain that eyedrops will be instilled to dilate his pupils and that a dye

will be injected into his arm. Tell him that his eyes will be photographed with a special camera before and after the injection. Stress that these are photographs, not X-rays.

■ Warn the patient that his skin may be discolored and his urine may appear orange for 24 to 48 hours after the procedure.

Equipment

Fundus camera and film, mydriatic eyedrops, alcohol swabs, tourniquet, 21G scalp-vein needle, 5- to 10-ml syringe, 2 ml of 25% sodium fluorescein or 5 ml of 10% sodium fluorescein, small sterile dressing, emesis basin, emergency resuscitation kit

Procedure and posttest care

■ Administer mydriatic eyedrops. Usually, two instillations are necessary to achieve maximum mydriasis within 15 to 40 minutes.

■ Following mydriasis, seat the patient comfortably in the examining chair, facing the camera.

■ Have the patient loosen or remove any restrictive clothing around his neck.

■ Tell the patient to place his chin in the chin rest and his forehead against the bar. Tell him to open his eyes wide and stare straight ahead, while keeping his teeth together and maintaining normal breathing and blinking.

■ The antecubital vein is prepared and punctured; however, dye isn't injected yet. At this time, a few photographs may be taken. Make sure the patient keeps his arm extended; if necessary, use an arm board.

■ Warn the patient that the dye will be injected rapidly. Remind him to maintain his position and to continue to stare straight ahead; then inject the dye.

■ The patient may experience nausea and a feeling of warmth. Provide reassurance and observe for hypersensitivity reactions, such as vomiting, dry mouth, metallic taste, suddenly increased salivation, sneezing, light-headedness, fainting, or hives. In rare instances, anaphylactic shock may occur.

■ As the dye is injected, 25 to 30 photographs are taken in rapid sequence. Each photograph is taken 1 second after the other.

■ The needle and syringe are removed carefully; pressure and a dressing are applied to the injection site.

■ If late-phase photographs are needed, tell the patient to sit and relax for 20 minutes, then reposition him for 5 to 10 photographs. If necessary, photographs may be taken up to 1 hour after the injection.

■ Remind the patient that his skin and urine will be slightly discolored for 24 to 48 hours after the test. Encourage the patient to drink increased amounts of fluids to help excrete the dye.

■ Explain that his near vision will be blurred for up to 12 hours and that he should avoid direct sunlight and refrain from driving during this time.

Precautions

■ Don't leave the patient unattended. He may experience mild adverse reactions, such as nausea, vomiting, sneezing, paresthesia of the tongue, and dizziness.

◆ **CLINICAL ALERT** *Have emergency resuscitation equipment at hand. Serious adverse effects (laryngeal edema, bronchospasm, and respiratory arrest) are possible. If a reaction occurs, note it on the patient's allergy history.*

■ The needle must be placed in the vein correctly; extravasation of dye around the injection site is painful.

Normal findings

After rapid injection into the antecubital vein, sodium fluorescein reaches the retina in 12 to 15 seconds (filling phase). As the choroidal vessels and choriocapillaries fill, the background of the retina fluoresces, taking on an evenly mottled appearance known as the choroidal flush. Then the dye fills the arteries (arterial phase). The arteriovenous phase lasts from the complete filling of the arteries and capillaries to the earliest evidence of dye in the veins. The time the arteries begin to empty to the time the veins fill and empty is known as the venous phase. Finally, the recirculation phase occurs 30 to 60 minutes after the injection, when the fluorescein — if at all present — is barely detectable in the retinal vessels. Normally, there is no leakage from the retinal vessels.

Abnormal findings

The varying and complex findings after fluorescein angiography require interpretation by a highly skilled ophthalmologist with extensive experience in the diagnosis of retinal disorders.

Abnormalities detected in the early filling phase may include microaneurysms, arteriovenous shunts, and neovascularization. The test may identify arterial occlusion by showing delayed or absent flow of the dye through the arteries, stenosis, and prolonged venous drainage. Venous occlusion may be associated with dilation of the vessels and fluorescein leakage. Chronic obstruction may produce recanalization and collateral circulation.

In hypertensive retinopathy, abnormalities may include areas of increased vascular tortuosity, microaneurysms around zones of capillary nonperfusion, and generalized suffusion of the dye in the retina. Aneurysms and capillary hemangiomas may leak fluorescein and are typically surrounded by hard yellow exudate. Tumors exhibit variable fluorescein patterns, depending on histologic type. Retinal edema or inflammation and fibrous tissue may show variable degrees of fluorescence. Papilledema produces vascular leakage in the disk area.

Interfering factors

- Inadequate view of the fundus due to insufficient pupillary dilation (possible poor imaging)
- Cataract, media opacity, or inability to keep eyes open and to maintain fixation (possible poor imaging)

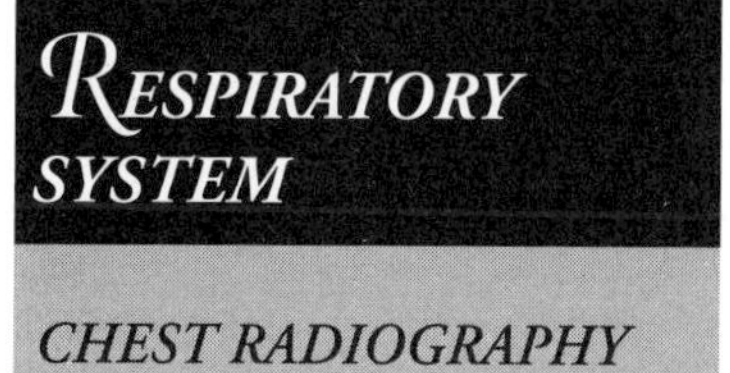

RESPIRATORY SYSTEM

CHEST RADIOGRAPHY

In chest radiography, X-rays or electromagnetic waves penetrate the chest and cause an image to form on specially sensitized film. Normal pulmonary tissue is radiolucent, whereas abnormalities — such as infiltrates, foreign bodies, fluids, and tumors — appear as densities on the film. A chest X-ray is most useful when compared with prior films to detect changes. (See *Selected clinical implications of chest X-ray films,* page 562.)

Purpose

- To detect pulmonary disorders, such as pneumonia, atelectasis, pneumothorax, pulmonary bullae, pleurisy, and tumors
- To detect mediastinal abnormalities such as tumors, and cardiac disease such as heart failure

(Text continues on page 564.)

Selected clinical implications of chest X-ray films

NORMAL ANATOMIC LOCATION AND APPEARANCE	POSSIBLE ABNORMALITY	IMPLICATIONS
Trachea Visible midline in the anterior mediastinal cavity; translucent tubelike appearance	◆ Deviation from midline	◆ Tension pneumothorax, atelectasis, pleural effusion, consolidation, mediastinal nodes or, in children, enlarged thymus
	◆ Narrowing with hourglass appearance and deviation to one side	◆ Substernal thyroid or stenosis secondary to trauma
Heart Visible in the anterior left mediastinal cavity; solid appearance due to blood contents; edges may be clear in contrast with surrounding air density of the lung	◆ Shift ◆ Hypertrophy of right heart ◆ Cardiac borders obscured by stringy densities ("shaggy heart")	◆ Atelectasis, pneumothorax ◆ Cor pulmonale, heart failure ◆ Cystic fibrosis
Aortic knob Visible as water density; formed by the arch of the aorta	◆ Solid densities, possibly indicating calcifications ◆ Tortuous shape	◆ Atherosclerosis ◆ Atherosclerosis
Mediastinum (mediastinal shadow) Visible as the space between the lungs; shadowy appearance that widens at the hilum of the lungs	◆ Deviation to nondiseased side; deviation to diseased side by traction ◆ Gross widening	◆ Pleural effusion or tumor, fibrosis or collapsed lung ◆ Neoplasms of esophagus, bronchi, lungs, thyroid, thymus, peripheral nerves, lymphoid tissue; aortic aneurysm; mediastinitis; cor pulmonale
Ribs Visible as thoracic cavity encasement	◆ Break or misalignment ◆ Widening of intercostal spaces	◆ Fractured sternum or ribs ◆ Emphysema
Spine Visible midline in the posterior chest; straight bony structure	◆ Spinal curvature ◆ Break or misalignment	◆ Scoliosis, kyphosis ◆ Fractures

Selected clinical implications of chest X-ray films *(continued)*

NORMAL ANATOMIC LOCATION AND APPEARANCE	POSSIBLE ABNORMALITY	IMPLICATIONS
Clavicles Visible in upper thorax; intact and equidistant in properly centered X-ray films	◆ Break or misalignment	◆ Fractures
Hila (lung roots) Visible above the heart, where pulmonary vessels, bronchi, and lymph nodes join the lungs; appear as small, white, bilateral densities	◆ Shift to one side ◆ Accentuated shadows	◆ Atelectasis ◆ Pneumothorax, emphysema, pulmonary abscess, tumor, enlarged lymph nodes
Mainstem bronchus Visible; part of the hila with translucent tubelike appearance	◆ Spherical or oval density	◆ Bronchogenic cyst
Bronchi Usually not visible	◆ Visible	◆ Bronchial pneumonia
Lung fields Usually not visible throughout, except for the blood vessels	◆ Visible ◆ Irregular	◆ Atelectasis ◆ Resolving pneumonia, infiltrates, silicosis, fibrosis, metastatic neoplasm
Hemidiaphragm Rounded, visible; right side 3/8" to 3/4" (1 to 2 cm)	◆ Elevation of diaphragm (difference in elevation can be measured on inspiration and expiration to detect movement) ◆ Flattening of diaphragm ◆ Unilateral elevation of either side ◆ Unilateral elevation of left side only	◆ Active tuberculosis, pneumonia, pleurisy, acute bronchitis, active disease of the abdominal viscera, bilateral phrenic nerve involvement, atelectasis ◆ Asthma, emphysema ◆ Possible unilateral phrenic nerve paresis ◆ Perforated ulcer (rare), gas distention of stomach or splenic flexure of colon, free air in abdomen

- To determine correct placement of pulmonary catheters, endotracheal tubes, and other chest tubes
- To determine the location and size of lesions or foreign bodies (coins, broken central lines) that were swallowed or aspirated
- To help assess pulmonary status
- To evaluate response to interventions

Patient preparation

- Explain that this test assesses respiratory status.
- Tell the patient he need not restrict food or fluids.
- Describe the test, including who will perform it and when it will take place.
- Provide a gown without snaps and instruct the patient to remove jewelry and other metallic objects that may be in the X-ray field.
- Explain to the patient that he'll be asked to take a deep breath and to hold it momentarily while the film is being taken to provide a clearer view of pulmonary structures.

Procedure and posttest care

- If a stationary X-ray machine is used, the patient stands or sits in front of the machine so films can be taken of the posteroanterior and left lateral views.
- If a portable X-ray machine is used at the patient's bedside, the patient is moved to the top of the bed, if his tolerance permits. The head of the bed is elevated for maximum upright positioning.
- Move cardiac monitoring lead wires, I.V. tubing from central lines, pulmonary artery catheter lines, and safety pins as far from the X-ray field as possible.

Precautions

- Chest radiography is usually contraindicated during the first trimester of pregnancy; however, when radiography is absolutely necessary, a lead apron placed over the patient's abdomen can shield the fetus.
- If the patient is intubated, check that no tubes have been dislodged during positioning.
- To avoid exposure to radiation, leave the room or the immediate area while the films are being taken. If you must stay in the area, wear a lead-lined apron or protective clothing.

Findings

For an overview of normal and abnormal chest radiography findings, see the accompanying chart. For an accurate diagnosis, radiography findings must be correlated with the results of additional radiologic and pulmonary tests as well as physical assessment findings. For example, pulmonary hyperinflation with low diaphragm and generalized increased radiolucency may suggest emphysema but may also occur in a healthy person.

Interfering factors

- Portable chest X-rays (possibly lower quality image than stationary X-rays)
- Portable chest X-rays taken in the anteroposterior position (may show larger cardiac shadowing than other X-rays due to shorter distance between beam and anterior structures)
- Patient in a supine position (hides fluid levels that are visible in decubitus views)
- Age and sex of the patient (may influence findings)
- Patient's inability to take a full inspiration
- Underexposure or overexposure of films
- Incorrect view of the area (for example, lateral film views reveal infiltrates [pneumonia, atelectasis] that may not be seen in anteroposterior views or pos-

teroanterior views because of heart obstruction)

PARANASAL SINUS RADIOGRAPHY

The paranasal sinuses — air-filled cavities lined with mucous membrane — lie within the maxillary, ethmoid, sphenoid, and frontal bones. Sinus abnormalities resulting from inflammation, trauma, cysts, mucoceles, granulomatosis, and other conditions may include distorted bony sinus walls, altered mucous membranes, and fluid or masses within the cavities. In paranasal sinus radiography, X-rays or electromagnetic waves penetrate the paranasal sinuses and react on specially sensitized film, forming a film image that differentiates sinus structures.

When surrounding facial structures that are superimposed on the paranasal sinuses interfere with visualization of relevant areas, computed tomography scanning may be performed to provide further information.

Purpose

- To detect unilateral or bilateral abnormalities, possibly indicating trauma or disease
- To confirm diagnosis of neoplastic or inflammatory paranasal sinus disease
- To determine the location and size of a malignant neoplasm

Patient preparation

- Explain that this test helps evaluate abnormalities of the paranasal sinuses.
- Describe the test, including who will perform it and where it will take place.
- Tell the patient that his head may be immobilized in a foam vise during the test to help him maintain the correct position but that the vise doesn't hurt.
- Explain to the patient that he'll be asked to sit upright and avoid moving while the X-rays are being taken to prevent blurring of the image and to allow visualization of air-fluid levels, if present. Emphasize the importance of his cooperation.
- Instruct the patient to remove dentures, all jewelry, and metallic objects in the X-ray field.

Procedure and posttest care

- Have the patient sit upright (his head may be placed in a foam vise) between the X-ray tube and a film cassette.
- During the test, the X-ray tube is positioned at specific angles and the patient's head is placed in various standard positions, while his paranasal sinuses are filmed from different angles. If necessary, assist with positioning the patient.

Precautions

- Paranasal sinus radiography is usually contraindicated during pregnancy; however, when it's absolutely necessary, a lead-lined apron placed over the patient's abdomen can shield the fetus.
- To avoid exposure to radiation, leave the room or the immediate area during the test; if you must stay in the area, wear a lead-lined apron.

Normal findings

Normal paranasal sinuses are radiolucent and filled with air, which appears black on films.

Abnormal findings

See *Abnormal findings in paranasal sinus radiography,* page 566.

Interfering factors

- Presence of dentures, jewelry, or other metallic objects in X-ray field, or

Abnormal findings in paranasal sinus radiography

This chart lists abnormal radiographic findings associated with various sinus disorders.

DISORDER	ABNORMAL FINDINGS
Paranasal sinus trauma or fracture	◆ Edema or hemorrhage in mucous membrane lining or sinus cavity ◆ Clouded sinus air cells ◆ Air-fluid level ◆ Radiolucent, linear bone defects ◆ Irregular, overriding bone edges ◆ Depression or displacement of bone fragments ◆ Foreign bodies
Acute sinusitis	◆ Swollen, inflamed mucous membrane ◆ Inflammatory exudate ◆ Hazy to opaque sinus air cells ◆ Air-fluid level
Chronic sinusitis	◆ Thickened mucous membrane ◆ Hazy to opaque sinus air cells ◆ Air-fluid level ◆ Thickening or sclerosis of bony wall of affected sinus
Wegener's granulomatosis	◆ Clouded to opaque sinus air cells ◆ Destruction of bony sinus wall
Malignant neoplasm	◆ Rounded or lobulated soft-tissue mass, projecting into sinus ◆ Destruction of bony sinus wall
Benign bone tumor	◆ Distortion of bony sinus wall in specific patterns
Cyst, polyp, or benign tumor	◆ Rounded or lobulated soft-tissue mass, projecting into sinus
Mucocele	◆ Clouded sinus air cells ◆ Destruction of bony sinus wall resulting in various degrees of radiolucency

presence of numerous metallic foreign bodies around paranasal sinuses (possible poor imaging)

■ Patient movement (possible poor imaging)

■ Patient unable to sit upright (may require supine position, reducing diagnostic value of test)

■ Superimposition of the surrounding facial structures on the film (obscures paranasal sinuses)

FLUOROSCOPY

In fluoroscopy, a continuous stream of X-rays passes through the patient, casting shadows of the heart, lungs, and diaphragm on a fluorescent screen, which allows moving structures to be studied. Because fluoroscopy reveals less detail than standard chest radiography, it's indicated only when diagnosis requires visualization of physiologic or pathologic motion of thoracic contents — for example, to rule out paralysis in patients with diaphragmatic elevation.

Purpose

- To assess lung expansion and contraction during quiet breathing, deep breathing, and coughing
- To assess movement and paralysis of the diaphragm (sniff test) or digestive tract
- To detect bronchial obstructions and pulmonary disease
- To assist with the placement of tubes or catheters, such as a pulmonary artery (PA) catheter or a central venous catheter

Patient preparation

- Explain to the patient that this test assesses respiratory structures and their motion.
- Describe the test, including who will perform it and where it will take place.
- Tell the patient that he'll be asked to follow specific instructions — for example, to breathe deeply and cough — while X-ray images depict his breathing.
- Instruct the patient to remove all jewelry and other metallic objects within the X-ray field.

Procedure and posttest care

- If necessary, assist with positioning the patient.
- Move cardiac monitoring cables, I.V. tubing from subclavian lines, PA catheter lines, and safety pins as far from the X-ray field as possible.
- During the test, the patient's cardiopulmonary or digestive motion is observed on a screen. Special equipment may be used to intensify the images, or a videotape recording of the fluoroscopy may be made for later study.

Precautions

- Fluoroscopy is contraindicated during pregnancy.
- If the patient is intubated, check that no tubes have been dislodged during positioning.
- To avoid exposure to radiation, leave the room or the immediate area during the test; if you must stay in the area, wear a lead-lined apron.

Normal findings

Normal diaphragmatic movement is synchronous and symmetrical. Normal diaphragmatic excursion ranges from ¾″ to 1⅝″ (2 to 4 cm).

Abnormal findings

Diminished diaphragmatic movement may indicate pulmonary disease. Increased lung translucency may indicate loss of elasticity or bronchial obstruction. In elderly patients, the lowest part of the trachea may be displaced to the right by an elongated aorta.

Diminished or paradoxical diaphragmatic movement may indicate paralysis of the diaphragm; however, fluoroscopy may not detect such paralysis in patients who compensate for diminished diaphragm function by forcefully contracting their abdominal muscles to aid expiration.

Gaps in the stomach or small intestine may indicate ulcers or poor peristalsis.

Interfering factors

■ Failure to remove all metallic objects within the X-ray field (possible poor imaging)

CHEST TOMOGRAPHY

Also called laminagraphy, planigraphy, stratigraphy, or body section roentgenography, chest tomography provides clearly focused radiographic images of selected body sections otherwise obscured by shadows of overlying or underlying structures. In this procedure, the X-ray tube and film move around the patient in opposite directions (a motion called the linear tube sweep), producing exposures in which a selected body plane appears sharply defined and the areas above and below it are blurred. Some facilities have spiral CT available. (See *Spiral CT.*) It's used to further evaluate chest lesions when other tests are inconclusive. In more modern facilities, computer tomography has superseded plain film tomography.

Purpose

■ To demonstrate pulmonary densities (for cavitation, calcification, and presence of fat), tumors (especially those obstructing the bronchial lumen), or lesions (especially those located deep within the mediastinum such as at lymph nodes at the hilum)

■ To evaluate severity of disease such as emphysema

Patient preparation

■ Explain to the patient that this test helps evaluate lesions inside the chest.

■ Describe the test, including who will perform it and where it will take place.

■ Tell the patient that he need not restrict food or fluids.

■ Warn the patient that the equipment is noisy because of rapidly moving metal-on-metal parts and that the X-ray tube swings overhead.

■ Advise the patient to breathe normally during the test but to remain immobile; tell him that foam wedges will be used to help him maintain a comfortable, motionless position.

■ Tell the patient to close his eyes to prevent involuntary movement.

■ Instruct the patient to remove all jewelry and metallic objects within the X-ray field.

Procedure and posttest care

■ The patient is placed in a supine position or in different degrees of lateral rotation on the X-ray table. The X-ray tube then swings over the patient, taking numerous films from different angles.

■ For lung tomography, the X-ray tube is usually moved in a linear direction but may be moved in a hypocycloid, circular, elliptic, trispiral, or figure-eight pattern. Multidirectional films aid diagnosis of mediastinal lesions or tumors.

Precautions

■ Tomography is contraindicated during pregnancy.

■ To avoid exposure to radiation, leave the room or the immediate area during the test; if you must stay in the area, wear a lead-lined apron.

Normal findings

A normal chest tomogram shows structures equivalent to those seen on a normal chest radiograph film.

Abnormal findings

Central calcification in a nodule suggests a benign lesion; an irregularly bordered tumor suggests malignancy; a sharply defined tumor suggests granuloma or nonmalignancy. Evaluation of the hilum can help differentiate blood

Spiral CT

The spiral (helical) computed tomography (CT) scan is produced while the X-ray tube rotates continuously around the patient, forming a spiral path through the patient. This path represents a contiguous volumetric data set, covering a specific volume of the patient's anatomy with no spatial or temporal gaps. The patient continuously moves through the slip-ring gantry, and no two data points are taken in exactly the same plane.

Benefits include increased speed (spiral CT is typically 8 to 10 times faster than conventional CT), improved image quality and diagnostic accuracy, and reduced radiation exposure. The improved speed — the scan can usually be obtained during a single breath hold — is especially beneficial for the elderly, pediatric, and critically ill populations, in which scanning commonly proves difficult.

There are disadvantages. Spiral CT delivers a limited amount of milliamperes, which can result in a grainier image than conventional CT (more common in larger patients). In addition, artifacts ("pseudothrombi") can be created in the infrahepatic inferior vena cava by the admixture of unopacified blood and contrast medium flowing in from the renal veins. These disadvantages are being resolved with improved equipment and technique.

vessels from nodes, detect tumor extension into the hilar lung area, and identify bronchial dilation, stenosis, and endobronchial lesions. Tomography can also identify extension of a mediastinal lesion to the ribs or spine.

Interfering factors

- Failure to remove all metallic objects within the X-ray field (possible poor imaging)
- Uncooperative patient

BRONCHOGRAPHY

Bronchography is X-ray examination of the tracheobronchial tree after instillation of a radiopaque iodine contrast agent through a catheter into the lumens of the trachea and bronchi. The contrast agent coats the bronchial tree, permitting visualization of any anatomic deviations. Bronchography of a localized lung area may be accomplished by instilling contrast dye through a fiberoptic bronchoscope placed in the area to be filmed.

Since the development of computed tomography scanning, bronchography is used less frequently. It may be performed using a local anesthetic instilled through the catheter or bronchoscope, although a general anesthetic may be necessary for children or during a concurrent bronchoscopy.

Purpose

- To help detect bronchiectasis and map its location for surgical resection
- To detect bronchial obstruction, pulmonary tumors, cysts, and cavities and, indirectly, to pinpoint the cause of hemoptysis
- To provide permanent films of pathologic findings
- To guide procedures such as bronchoscopy

Patient preparation

- Explain to the patient that this test helps evaluate abnormalities of the bronchial structures.
- Instruct the patient to fast for 12 hours before the test.
- Tell the patient to perform good oral hygiene the night before and the morning of the test.
- Explain who will perform the test and where and when it will take place.
- Make sure the patient or a responsible family member has signed an informed consent form.
- Check the patient's history for hypersensitivity to anesthetics, iodine, or contrast media.
- If the patient has a productive cough, administer a prescribed expectorant and perform postural drainage 1 to 3 days before the test.
- If the procedure is to be performed under a local anesthetic, tell the patient he'll receive a sedative to help him relax and to suppress the gag reflex. Prepare him for the unpleasant taste of the anesthetic spray. Warn him that he may experience some difficulty breathing during the procedure, but reassure him that his airway won't be blocked and that he'll receive enough oxygen. Tell him the catheter or bronchoscope will pass more easily if he relaxes.
- If bronchography is to be performed under a general anesthetic, inform the patient that he'll receive a sedative before the test to help him relax.
- Just before the test, instruct the patient to remove his dentures (if present) and to void.

Equipment

Radiograph machine, tilting table, sedative, anesthetic, catheter or bronchoscope, radiopaque oils or water-soluble contrast agent, emergency resuscitation equipment

Procedure and posttest care

- After a local anesthetic is sprayed into the patient's mouth and throat, a bronchoscope or catheter is passed into the trachea, and the anesthetic and contrast medium are instilled.
- The patient is placed in various positions during the test to promote movement of the contrast medium into different areas of the bronchial tree. After X-rays are taken, the contrast medium is removed through postural drainage and by having the patient cough it up.

◆ **CLINICAL ALERT** *Watch for signs of laryngeal spasms (dyspnea) or edema (hoarseness, dyspnea, laryngeal stridor) secondary to traumatic intubation.*

◆ **CLINICAL ALERT** *Immediately report signs of allergic reaction to the contrast medium or anesthetic, such as itching, dyspnea, tachycardia, palpitations, excitation, hypotension, hypertension, or euphoria.*

- Withhold food, fluids, and oral medications until the gag reflex returns (usually in 2 hours). Fluid intake before the gag reflex returns may cause aspiration.
- Encourage gentle coughing and postural drainage to facilitate clearing of the contrast medium. A postdrainage film is usually done in 24 to 48 hours.
- Watch for signs of chemical or secondary bacterial pneumonia — fever, dyspnea, crackles, or rhonchi — the result of incomplete expectoration of the contrast medium.
- If the patient has a sore throat, reassure him that it's only temporary and provide throat lozenges or a liquid gargle when his gag reflex returns.
- Advise the outpatient not to resume his usual activities until the next day.

Precautions

- Bronchography is contraindicated during pregnancy, in people with hypersensitivity to iodine or contrast media, and usually in people with respiratory insufficiency.
- Observe the patient with asthma for laryngeal spasm (such as dyspnea) secondary to the instillation of the contrast medium.
- Observe the patient with chronic obstructive pulmonary disease for airway occlusion secondary to the instillation of the contrast medium.

Normal findings

The right mainstem bronchus is shorter, wider, and more vertical than the left bronchus. Successive branches of the bronchi become smaller in diameter and are free of obstruction or lesions.

Abnormal findings

Bronchography may demonstrate bronchiectasis or bronchial obstruction due to tumors, cysts, cavities, or foreign objects. Findings must be correlated with physical examination, patient history, and perhaps other pulmonary studies.

Interfering factors

- Presence of secretions or improper patient positioning (possible poor imaging due to inadequate filling of bronchial tree)
- Inability to suppress coughing (interferes with bronchial filling and retention of the contrast medium)

PULMONARY ANGIOGRAPHY

Also called pulmonary arteriography, pulmonary angiography is the radiographic examination of the pulmonary circulation following injection of a radiopaque iodine contrast agent into the pulmonary artery or one of its branches.

Possible complications include arterial occlusion, myocardial perforation or rupture, ventricular arrhythmias from myocardial irritation, and acute renal failure from hypersensitivity to the contrast agent.

Purpose

- To detect pulmonary embolism in a patient who is equivocal
- To evaluate pulmonary circulation abnormalities
- To evaluate pulmonary circulation preoperatively in the patient with congenital heart disease
- To locate a large embolus before surgical removal

Patient preparation

- Describe the procedure to the patient. Explain that this test permits evaluation of the blood vessels to help identify the cause of his symptoms.
- Instruct the patient to fast for 8 hours before the test or as prescribed. Tell him who will perform the test, where it will take place, and that laboratory work for kidney function and coagulation may precede the test.
- Tell the patient a small puncture will be made in the blood vessel of his right arm where blood samples are usually drawn, or in the right groin at the femoral vein, and that a local anesthetic will be used to numb the area. Inform him that a small catheter will then be inserted into the blood vessel and passed into the right side of the heart and then to the pulmonary artery.
- Tell the patient the contrast medium will then be injected into this artery. Warn him that he may feel flushed, experience an urge to cough, or experi-

ence a salty taste for approximately 3 to 5 minutes after the injection.

■ Inform the patient that his heart rate will be monitored continuously during the procedure and that he should tell the physician or nurse if he's having any concerns.

■ Make sure the patient or a responsible family member has signed an informed consent form. Check the patient's history for hypersensitivity to anesthetics, iodine, seafood, or radiographic contrast agents.

■ Obtain or check laboratory tests (including prothrombin time, partial thromboplastin time, platelet count, and blood urea nitrogen [BUN] and serum creatinine levels), and notify the radiologist of any abnormal results. IV hydration may need to be considered, depending on the patient's renal and cardiac status. The radiologist may want to discontinue a heparin drip 3 to 4 hours before the test.

Equipment

Angiography tray, 50 ml of contrast medium, imaging equipment, angiography catheters and guide wires, monitoring equipment (electrocardiogram, arterial oxygen saturation, blood pressure, pulmonary artery pressure), emergency resuscitation equipment

Procedure and posttest care

■ After the patient is placed in a supine position, the local anesthetic is injected and the cardiac monitor is attached to the patient. Blood pressure and pulse oximeter are monitored as per facility protocol.

■ A puncture is made at the procedure site and a catheter is introduced into the antecubital or femoral vein. As the catheter passes through the right atrium, the right ventricle, and the pulmonary artery, pressures are measured and blood samples are drawn from various regions of the pulmonary circulation.

■ The contrast medium is injected and circulates through the pulmonary artery and lung capillaries while X-rays are taken.

■ Apply pressure over the catheter insertion site for 15 to 20 minutes or until bleeding stops.

■ Maintain bed rest for about 6 hours.

■ Observe the site for bleeding and swelling. If either occur, maintain pressure at the insertion site for 10 minutes and notify the radiologist.

■ Check blood pressure, pulse rate, and the catheter insertion site (arm or groin) every 15 minutes for 1 hour, then every hour for 4 hours, then every 4 hours for 16 hours.

■ Observe for signs of myocardial perforation or rupture by monitoring vital signs.

■ Be alert for signs of acute renal failure, such as sudden onset of oliguria, nausea, and vomiting. Check BUN and serum creatinine levels.

■ Check the catheter insertion site for inflammation or hematoma formation and report symptoms of a delayed hypersensitivity response to the contrast agent or to the local anesthetic (dyspnea, itching, tachycardia, palpitations, hypotension or hypertension, excitation, or euphoria).

■ Advise the patient about any restriction of activity. Tell him that he may resume his usual diet after the test (encourage him to drink lots of fluids), or administer I.V. fluids as ordered to flush the contrast agent from his body.

Precautions

◆ CLINICAL ALERT *Pulmonary angiography is contraindicated during pregnancy.*

■ Monitor for ventricular arrhythmias due to myocardial irritation from passage of the catheter through the heart chambers.

- Observe for signs of hypersensitivity to the contrast agent, such as dyspnea, nausea, vomiting, sweating, increased heart rate, and numbness of extremities.
- Keep emergency equipment available in case of a hypersensitivity reaction to the contrast agent.
- Measure pulmonary artery pressures. Right ventricular end-diastolic pressure is usually less than or equal to 20 mm Hg, and pulmonary artery systolic pressure is usually less than or equal to 70 mm Hg. Pressures greater than this increase the risk of mortality associated with this procedure.

Normal findings

Normally, the contrast agent flows symmetrically and without interruption through the pulmonary circulatory system.

Abnormal findings

Interruption of blood flow may result from emboli and from other types of pulmonary vascular abnormalities or tumors.

Interfering factors

- None significant

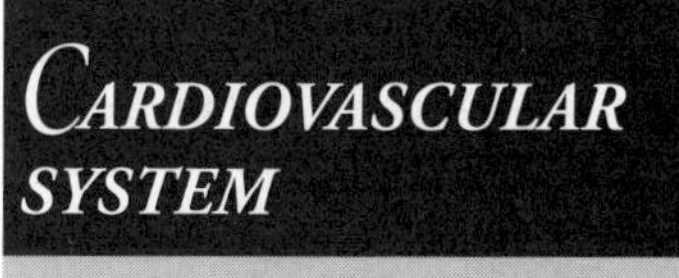

Among the most frequently used tests for evaluating cardiac disease and its effects on the pulmonary vasculature, cardiac radiography provides images of the thorax, mediastinum, heart, and lungs. In a routine evaluation, posteroanterior and left lateral views are taken. The posteroanterior view is preferable to the anteroposterior view because it places the heart slightly closer to the plane of the film, providing a sharper, less distorted image. Cardiac radiography may be performed on a bedridden patient using portable equipment, but such equipment can provide only anteroposterior views.

Purpose

- To help detect cardiac disease and abnormalities that change the size, shape, or appearance of the heart and lungs
- To ensure correct positioning of pulmonary artery and cardiac catheters and of pacemaker wires

Patient preparation

- Explain to the patient that this test reveals the size and shape of the heart. Tell him who will perform the test and where it will take place. Reassure him that the test uses little radiation and is harmless.
- Instruct the patient to remove jewelry, other metallic objects, and clothing above his waist and to put on a gown that has ties instead of metal snaps.

Procedure and posttest care

Posteroanterior view

- The patient stands erect about 6′ (2 m) from the X-ray machine with his back to the machine and his chin resting on top of the film cassette holder.
- The holder is adjusted to slightly hyperextend the patient's neck. The patient places his hands on his hips, with his shoulders touching the holder, and centers his chest against it.
- The patient is asked to take a deep breath and hold it during the X-ray film exposure.

Left lateral view

■ The patient is positioned with his arms extended over his head and his left torso flush against the cassette and centered.

■ The patient is asked to take a deep breath and hold it during the X-ray film exposure.

Anteroposterior view of a bedridden patient

■ The head of the bed is elevated as much as possible.

■ The patient is assisted to an upright position to reduce visceral pressure on the diaphragm and other thoracic structures.

■ The film cassette is centered under the patient's back. Although the distance between the patient and the X-ray machine may vary a little, the path between the two should be clear.

■ The patient is instructed to take a deep breath and hold it during the X-ray film exposure.

Precautions

■ Cardiac radiography is usually contraindicated during the first trimester of pregnancy. If it's performed during pregnancy, a lead shield or apron should cover the patient's abdomen and pelvic area during the X-ray exposure.

■ When testing an ambulatory patient, make sure the radiographic order stipulates a posteroanterior view and not an anteroposterior view. Include on the order any pertinent findings from previous cardiac radiographs as well as the indication for this test.

■ When testing a bedridden patient, make sure anyone else in the room is protected from X-rays by a lead shield, a room divider, or sufficient distance.

Normal findings

Normally, in the posteroanterior view, the thoracic cage appears at least twice as wide as the heart. However, in the anteroposterior view, relative heart size and position may look different, and the cardiac silhouette and vascular markings may increase.

If cardiac radiography is performed to evaluate the position of cardiac catheters and pacemakers, the films should confirm accurate placement.

Abnormal findings

Cardiac X-ray films must be evaluated in light of the patient's history, physical examination, electrocardiography results, and results of previous radiographic tests for cardiac abnormalities.

An abnormal cardiac silhouette usually reflects left or right ventricular or left atrial enlargement, or even a multichamber enlargement. In left ventricular enlargement, the posteroanterior view shows the border of the left side of the heart to be rounded and convex, with lateral extension of the lower left border; the lateral view shows posterior bulging of the left ventricle. In right ventricular enlargement, the posteroanterior view shows secondary prominence of the pulmonary artery segment at the border of the left side of the heart; the lateral view shows anterior bulging in the region of the right ventricular outflow tract.

In left atrial enlargement, the posteroanterior view shows double density of the enlarged left atrium, straightening of the border of the left side of the heart, elevation of the left mainstem bronchus and, rarely, lateral extension of the border of the right side of the heart superior to the right ventricle; the lateral view shows a posterior bulge at the level of the left atrium.

In the posteroanterior view, dilation of pulmonary venous shadows in the superior lateral aspect of the hilus and vascular shadows horizontally and inferiorly along the margin of the right side of the heart may be the first signs of pulmonary vascular congestion. Chronic pulmonary venous hypertension produces an antler pattern, caused by dilated superior pulmonary veins and normal or constricted inferior pulmonary veins. Acute alveolar edema may produce a butterfly appearance, with increased densities in central lung fields; interstitial pulmonary edema, a cloudy or cotton-puff appearance.

Interfering factors

- Patient's failure to maintain inspiration or to remain motionless
- Patient's chest off-center on the film cassette (may hinder viewing of costophrenic angle on X-ray)
- Thoracic deformity such as scoliosis (possible misleading results)
- Underexposure or overexposure of films

LOWER LIMB VENOGRAPHY

Lower limb venography, or ascending contrast phlebography, is the radiographic examination of a vein. Commonly used to assess the condition of the deep leg veins after injection of a contrast medium, it's the definitive test for deep vein thrombosis (DVT). Venography shouldn't be used for routine screening because it exposes the patient to relatively high doses of radiation and can cause complications, such as phlebitis, local tissue damage and, occasionally, DVT itself.

Venography is also expensive and not easily repeated. A combination of three noninvasive tests — Doppler ultrasonography, impedance plethysmography, and ^{125}I fibrinogen scan — is an acceptable though less accurate alternative to venography. Radionuclide tests, such as the ^{125}I fibrinogen scan, are used to screen for DVT or to attempt to detect the disorder in a patient who is too ill for venography or is hypersensitive to the contrast medium.

Purpose

- To confirm a diagnosis of DVT
- To distinguish clot formation from venous obstruction (a large tumor of the pelvis impinging on the venous system, for example)
- To evaluate congenital venous abnormalities
- To assess deep vein valvular competence (especially helpful in identifying underlying causes of leg edema)
- To locate a suitable vein for arterial bypass grafting

Patient preparation

- Explain to the patient that this test helps detect abnormal conditions in the veins of the legs.
- Instruct the patient to restrict food and to drink only clear liquids for 4 hours before the test.
- Describe the test, including who will perform it and where it will take place. Tell the patient pretest blood work for coagulation and kidney function may be needed.
- Warn the patient that he may feel a burning sensation in his leg on injection of the contrast medium and some discomfort during the procedure.
- Make sure the patient or a responsible family member has signed an informed consent form.
- Check the patient's history for hypersensitivity to iodine or iodine-containing foods or to contrast media. Mark any sensitivities on the chart and notify the physician.
- Reassure the patient that contrast media complications are rare, but tell him to report nausea, severe burning or itching, constriction in the throat or

chest, or dyspnea immediately. Restrict anticoagulant therapy, if ordered.

■ Just before the test, instruct the patient to void, to remove all clothing below the waist, and to put on a gown.

■ If ordered, administer a prescribed sedative to an anxious or uncooperative patient.

Procedure and posttest care

■ The patient is positioned on a tilting radiographic table so that the leg being tested doesn't bear any weight. He's instructed to relax this leg and keep it still; a tourniquet may be tied around the ankle to expedite venous filling.

■ A superficial vein in the dorsum of the patient's foot is injected with normal saline solution.

■ When needle placement is correct, 100 to 150 ml of the contrast medium is slowly injected over 90 seconds to 3 minutes and the presence of extravasation is checked.

■ If a suitable superficial vein can't be found (due to edema), a surgical cutdown of the vein may be performed.

■ Using a fluoroscope, the distribution of the contrast medium is monitored and spot films are taken from the anteroposterior and oblique projections and over the thigh and femoroiliac regions. Then, overhead films are taken of the calf, knee, thigh, and femoral area.

■ After filming, the patient is repositioned horizontally, the leg is quickly elevated and normal saline solution infused to flush the contrast medium from the veins.

■ The fluoroscope is checked to confirm complete emptying. Then the needle is removed.

■ Apply an adhesive bandage to the injection site.

■ Monitor vital signs until stable; check the pulse rate and quality on the dorsalis pedis, popliteal, and femoral arteries.

■ Administer prescribed analgesics, as ordered, to counteract the irritating effects of the contrast medium.

■ Watch for an allergic reaction to the contrast medium, hematoma, redness, bleeding, or infection (especially if a cutdown of the vein was performed) at the puncture site, and replace the dressing when necessary. Notify the physician if complications develop.

■ If the venogram indicates DVT, initiate prescribed therapy (heparin infusion, bed rest, leg elevation or support, or blood chemistry tests).

■ Tell the patient he may resume his usual diet and medications as ordered.

■ Observe for signs and symptoms of latent reaction to the dye. Encourage fluids to flush dye from the kidneys.

Precautions

◆ CLINICAL ALERT *Most allergic reactions to the contrast medium occur within 30 minutes of injection. Carefully observe for signs of anaphylaxis (flushing, urticaria, laryngeal stridor).*

Normal findings

A normal venogram shows steady opacification of the superficial and deep vasculature with no filling defects.

Abnormal findings

A venogram that shows consistent filling defects on repeat views, abrupt termination of a column of contrast material, unfilled major deep veins, or diversion of flow (through collaterals, for example) is diagnostic of DVT.

Interfering factors

■ Patient placing weight on the leg being tested (possible filling of leg veins with contract medium)

■ Movement of the leg being tested

■ Excessive tourniquet constriction

- Insufficient injection or dilution of contrast medium
- Delay between injection and radiography
- Previous thrombosis, severe edema or obesity, or cellulitis may limit visualization of the deep venous system

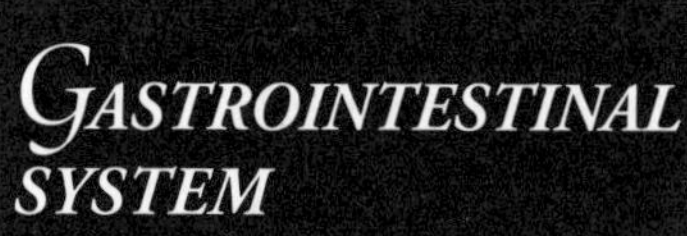

Barium swallow (esophagography) is the cineradiographic, radiographic, or fluoroscopic examination of the pharynx and the fluoroscopic examination of the esophagus after ingestion of thick and thin mixtures of barium sulfate. This test, most commonly performed as part of the upper GI series, is indicated in patients with histories of dysphagia and regurgitation. Further testing is usually required for definitive diagnosis. (See *Gastroesophageal reflux scanning.*)

Cholangiography and the barium enema test, if necessary, should precede the barium swallow because ingested barium may obscure anatomic detail on the X-rays.

Purpose

- To diagnose hiatal hernia, diverticula, and varices
- To detect strictures, ulcers, tumors, polyps, and motility disorders

Patient preparation

- Explain to the patient that this test evaluates the function of the pharynx and esophagus.
- Instruct the patient to fast after midnight the night before the test. (If the patient is an infant, delay feeding to ensure complete digestion of barium.) He may also be given a restricted diet for 2 to 3 days before the test.
- Describe the test, including who will perform it and where it will take place.
- Describe the milk shake consistency and chalky taste of the barium preparation the patient is required to ingest. Although it's flavored, he may find it unpleasant to swallow. Tell the patient he'll first receive a thick mixture, then a

Gastroesophageal reflux scanning

When the results of a barium swallow are inconclusive, gastroesophageal reflux scanning may be conducted to evaluate esophageal function and detect reflux. This test delivers less radiation than a barium swallow and is a much more sensitive indicator of reflux. It also allows reflux to be measured without insertion of an esophageal tube, an important consideration in testing infants, small children, and other patients for whom intubation is contraindicated.

The patient is instructed to fast beginning at midnight the day of the test. As the test begins, the patient is placed in a supine or upright position and asked to swallow a solution containing a radiopharmaceutical such as technetium 99m sulfur colloid. A gamma counter placed over the patient's chest records its passage through the esophagus into the stomach to determine transit time and evaluate esophageal function.

If reflux is suspected, the patient is repositioned as his stomach distends, and continuous recordings visualize reflux and estimate its quantity. In reflux, radioactivity may be detected in the esophagus.

thin one, and that he must drink 12 to 14 oz (355 to 414 ml) during the examination.

■ Inform the patient that he'll be placed in various positions on a tilting X-ray table and that X-rays will be taken. Reassure him that safety precautions will be maintained.

■ Withhold antacids, histamine-2 blockers, and proton pump inhibitors, as ordered, if gastric reflux is suspected.

■ Just before the procedure, instruct the patient to put on a gown without snap closures and to remove jewelry, dentures, hair clips, or other radiopaque objects from the X-ray field.

Procedure and posttest care

■ The patient is placed in an upright position behind the fluoroscopic screen and his heart, lungs, and abdomen are examined.

■ He is then instructed to take one swallow of the thick barium mixture, and the pharyngeal action is recorded using cineradiography. (This action occurs too rapidly for adequate fluoroscopic evaluation.)

■ The patient is then told to take several swallows of the thin barium mixture. The passage of the barium is examined fluoroscopically and spot films of the esophageal region are taken from lateral angles and from right and left posteroanterior angles. Esophageal strictures and obstruction of the esophageal lumen by the lower esophageal ring are best detected when the patient is upright. To accentuate small strictures or demonstrate dysphagia, the patient may be requested to swallow a special "barium marshmallow" (soft white bread that has been soaked in barium) or a barium pill.

■ The patient is then secured to the X-ray table and is rotated to the Trendelenburg position to evaluate esophageal peristalsis or demonstrate hiatal hernia and gastric reflux.

■ The patient is instructed to take several swallows of barium while the esophagus is examined fluoroscopically, and spot films of significant findings are taken when indicated. After the table is rotated to a horizontal position, the patient is told to take several swallows of barium so that the esophagogastric junction and peristalsis may be evaluated. The passage of the barium is fluoroscopically observed, and spot films of significant findings are taken with the patient in the supine and prone positions.

■ During fluoroscopic examination of the esophagus, the cardiac and fundus of the patient's stomach are also carefully studied because neoplasms in these areas may invade the esophagus and cause obstruction.

■ Check that additional spot films and repeat fluoroscopic evaluation haven't been ordered before allowing the patient to resume his usual diet.

■ Instruct the patient to drink plenty of fluids, unless contraindicated, to help eliminate the barium.

■ Administer a cathartic, if prescribed.

■ Inform the patient that stools will be chalky and light colored for 24 to 72 hours. Record description of all stools passed by the patient in the hospital.

■ Barium retained in the intestine may harden, causing obstruction or fecal impaction. Notify the physician if the patient fails to expel barium in 2 or 3 days.

■ Check the patient for abdominal distention and absent bowel sounds, which are associated with constipation and may suggest barium impaction.

Precautions

■ Barium swallow is usually contraindicated in a patient with intestinal

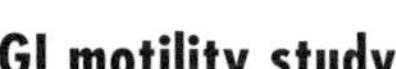

GI motility study

A GI motility study evaluates the intestinal motility and integrity of the mucosal lining by recording the passage of barium through the lower digestive tract. About 6 hours after the patient ingests the barium, the head of the barium column is usually in the hepatic flexure and the tail is in the terminal ileum; 24 hours after ingestion, the barium has completely opacified the large intestine. Spot films taken 24, 48, or 72 hours after ingestion are inferior to barium enema because the amount of barium passing through the large intestine isn't sufficient to fully extend the lumen. However, when spot films suggest intestinal abnormalities, barium enema and colonoscopy can provide more specific results and confirm diagnostic information.

obstruction as well as in patients who are pregnant because of radiation's possible teratogenic effects.

Normal findings

After the barium sulfate is swallowed, the bolus pours over the base of the tongue into the pharynx. A peristaltic wave propels the bolus through the entire length of the esophagus in about 2 seconds. When the peristaltic wave reaches the base of the esophagus, the cardiac sphincter opens, allowing the bolus to enter the stomach. After passage of the bolus, the cardiac sphincter closes. Normally, the bolus evenly fills and distends the lumen of the pharynx and esophagus, and the mucosa appears smooth and regular.

Abnormal findings

Barium swallow may reveal hiatus hernia, diverticula, and varices. Aspiration into the lungs will also be revealed. Although strictures, tumors, polyps, ulcers, and motility disorders (pharyngeal muscular disorders, esophageal spasms, and achalasia) may be detected, definitive diagnosis commonly requires endoscopic biopsy or, for motility disorders, manometric studies. (See *GI motility study.*)

Interfering factors

- Aspiration of barium into lungs due to poor swallowing reflex

UPPER GI AND SMALL-BOWEL SERIES

The upper GI and small-bowel series is the fluoroscopic examination of the esophagus, stomach, and small intestine after the patient ingests barium sulfate, a contrast agent. As the barium passes through the digestive tract, fluoroscopy outlines peristalsis and the mucosal contours of the respective organs, and spot films record significant findings. This test is indicated in patients who have upper GI symptoms (difficulty swallowing, regurgitation, burning or gnawing epigastric pain), signs of small-bowel disease (diarrhea, weight loss), and signs of GI bleeding (hematemesis, melena).

Although this test can detect various mucosal abnormalities, subsequent biopsy is typically necessary to rule out malignancy or distinguish specific inflammatory diseases. Oral cholecystography, barium enema, and routine X-rays should always precede this test because retained barium clouds anatomic detail on X-ray films.

Purpose

- To detect hiatus hernia, diverticula, and varices
- To aid diagnosis of strictures, blockages, ulcers, tumors, regional enteritis, and malabsorption syndrome
- To help detect motility disorders

Patient preparation

- Explain to the patient that this procedure uses ingested barium and X-ray films to examine the esophagus, stomach, and small intestine.
- Tell the patient to consume a low-residue diet for 2 or 3 days before the test and then to fast and avoid smoking after midnight the night before the test.
- Describe the test, including who will perform it and where it will take place.
- Encourage the patient to bring reading material.
- Inform the patient that he'll be placed on an X-ray table that rotates into vertical, semivertical, and horizontal positions.
- Explain to the patient that he'll be adequately secured and assisted to the supine, prone, and side-lying positions.
- Describe the milk shake consistency and chalky taste of the barium mixture. Although it's flavored, the patient may find its taste unpleasant, but tell him he must drink 16 to 20 oz (475 to 590 ml) for a complete examination.
- Inform the patient that his abdomen may be compressed to ensure proper coating of the stomach or intestinal walls with barium, or to separate overlapping bowel loops.
- As ordered, withhold most oral medications after midnight and anticholinergics and narcotics for 24 hours because these drugs affect small intestinal motility. Antacids, histamine-2-receptor antagonists, and proton pump inhibitors are also sometimes withheld for several hours if gastric reflux is suspected.
- Just before the procedure, instruct the patient to put on a gown without snap closures and to remove jewelry, dentures, hair clips, or other objects that might obscure anatomic detail on the X-ray films.

Procedure and posttest care

- After the patient is secured in a supine position on the X-ray table, the table is tilted until the patient is erect, and the heart, lungs, and abdomen are examined fluoroscopically.
- The patient is instructed to take several swallows of the barium suspension, and its passage through the esophagus is observed. (Occasionally, the patient is given a thick barium suspension, especially when esophageal pathology is strongly suspected.)
- During fluoroscopic examination, spot films of the esophagus are taken from lateral angles and from right and left posteroanterior angles.
- When barium enters the stomach, the patient's abdomen is palpated or compressed to ensure adequate coating of the gastric mucosa with barium.
- To perform a double-contrast examination, the patient is instructed to sip the barium through a perforated straw. As he does so, a small amount of air is also introduced into the stomach; this permits detailed examination of the gastric rugae, and spot films of significant findings are taken. The patient is then instructed to ingest the remaining barium suspension and the filling of the stomach and emptying into the duodenum are observed fluoroscopically.
- Two series of spot films of the stomach and duodenum are taken from posteroanterior, anteroposterior, lateral, and oblique angles, with the patient erect and then in a supine position.

- The passage of barium into the remainder of the small intestine is then observed fluoroscopically, and spot films are taken at 30- to 60-minute intervals until the barium reaches the region of the ileocecal valve. If abnormalities in the small intestine are detected, the area is palpated and compressed to help clarify the defect, and a spot film is taken. The examination ends when the barium enters the cecum.
- Make sure additional X-rays haven't been ordered before allowing the patient food, fluids, and oral medications (if applicable).
- Tell the patient to drink plenty of fluid (unless contraindicated) to help eliminate the barium.
- Administer a cathartic or enema to the patient. Tell the patient his stool will be light colored for 24 to 72 hours. Record and describe any stool passed by the patient in the hospital. Retention of barium in the intestine may cause obstruction or fecal impaction, so notify the physician if the patient doesn't pass the barium within 2 to 3 days. Also, barium retention may affect scheduling of other GI tests.
- Instruct the patient to tell the physician of abdominal fullness or pain or a delay in return to brown stools.

Precautions

- The upper GI and small-bowel series may be contraindicated in patients with obstruction or perforation of the digestive tract. Barium may intensify the obstruction or seep into the abdominal cavity. Sometimes a small-bowel series is performed to find a "transition zone." If a perforation is suspected, Gastrografin (a water-soluble contrast medium) rather than barium may be used.
- The test is contraindicated in pregnant patients because of the radiation's possible teratogenic effects.

Normal findings

After the barium suspension is swallowed, it pours over the base of the tongue into the pharynx and is propelled by a peristaltic wave through the entire length of the esophagus in about 2 seconds. The bolus evenly fills and distends the lumen of the pharynx and esophagus, and the mucosa appears smooth and regular. When the peristaltic wave reaches the base of the esophagus, the cardiac sphincter opens, allowing the bolus to enter the stomach. After passage of the bolus, the cardiac sphincter closes.

As barium enters the stomach, it outlines the characteristic longitudinal folds called rugae, which are best observed using the double-contrast technique. When the stomach is completely filled with barium, its outer contour appears smooth and regular without evidence of flattened, rigid areas suggestive of intrinsic or extrinsic lesions.

After barium enters the stomach, it quickly empties into the duodenal bulb through relaxation of the pyloric sphincter. Although the mucosa of the duodenal bulb is relatively smooth, circular folds become apparent as barium enters the duodenal loop. These folds deepen and become more numerous in the jejunum. The barium temporarily lodges between these folds, producing a speckled pattern on the X-ray film. As barium enters the ileum, the circular folds become less prominent and, except for their broadness, resemble those in the duodenum. The film also shows that the diameter of the small intestine tapers gradually from the duodenum to the ileum.

Abnormal findings

X-ray studies of the esophagus may reveal strictures, tumors, hiatus hernia, diverticula, varices, and ulcers (particularly in the distal esophagus). Benign strictures usually dilate the esophagus, whereas malignant ones cause erosive changes in the mucosa. Tumors produce filling defects in the column of barium, but only malignant ones change the mucosal contour. Nevertheless, biopsy is necessary for definitive diagnosis of both esophageal strictures and tumors.

Motility disorders, such as esophageal spasm, are usually difficult to detect because spasms are erratic and transient; manometry, which measures the length and pressure of peristaltic contractions and evaluates the function of the cardiac sphincter, is generally performed to detect such disorders. However, achalasia (cardiospasm) is strongly suggested when the distal esophagus has a beaking appearance. Gastric reflux appears as a backflow of barium from the stomach into the esophagus.

X-ray studies of the stomach may reveal tumors and ulcers. Malignant tumors, usually adenocarcinomas, appear as filling defects on the X-ray film and usually disrupt peristalsis. Benign tumors, such as adenomatous polyps and leiomyomas, appear as outpouchings of the gastric mucosa and generally don't affect peristalsis. Ulcers occur most commonly in the stomach and duodenum (particularly in the duodenal bulb), and these two areas are thus examined together. Benign ulcers usually demonstrate evidence of partial or complete healing and are characterized by radiating folds extending to the edge of the ulcer crater. Malignant ulcers, usually associated with a suspicious mass, generally have radiating folds that extend beyond the ulcer crater to the edge of the mass. However, biopsy is necessary for definitive diagnosis of both tumors and ulcers.

Occasionally, this test detects signs that suggest pancreatitis or pancreatic carcinoma. Such signs include edematous changes in the mucosa of the antrum or duodenal loop or dilation of the duodenal loop. These findings mandate further studies for pancreatic disease, such as endoscopic retrograde cholangiopancreatography, abdominal ultrasonography, or computed tomography scanning.

X-ray studies of the small intestine may reveal regional enteritis, malabsorption syndrome, and tumors. Although regional enteritis may not be detected in its early stages, small ulcerations and edematous changes develop in the mucosa as the disease progresses. Edematous changes, segmentation of the barium column, and flocculation characterize malabsorption syndrome. Filling defects occur with Hodgkin's disease and lymphosarcoma.

Interfering factors

- Failure to observe diet, smoking, and medication restrictions (may invalidate results)
- Excess air in the small bowel (possible poor imaging)
- Failure to remove metallic objects in the X-ray field (possible poor imaging)

BARIUM ENEMA

Also called lower GI examination, barium enema is the radiographic examination of the large intestine after rectal instillation of barium sulfate (single-contrast technique) or barium sulfate and air (double-contrast technique). It's indicated in patients with histories of altered bowel habits, lower abdominal pain, or the passage of blood, mucus, or pus in the stool. It may also be indicated after colostomy or ileostomy; in these patients, barium (or barium and air) is instilled through the stoma.

Complications include perforation of the colon, water intoxication, barium granulomas and, rarely, intraperitoneal and extraperitoneal extravasation of barium and barium embolism.

The single-contrast technique provides a profile view of the large intestine; the double-contrast technique provides profile and frontal views. The latter technique best detects small intraluminal tumors (especially polyps), the early mucosal changes of inflammatory disease, and the subtle intestinal bleeding caused by ulcerated polyps or the shallow ulcerations of inflammatory disease.

Although barium enema clearly outlines most of the large intestine, proctosigmoidoscopy provides the best view of the rectosigmoid region. Barium enema should precede the barium swallow and upper GI and small-bowel series because barium ingested in the latter procedure may take several days to pass through the GI tract and thus may interfere with subsequent X-ray studies.

Purpose

- To aid diagnosis of colorectal cancer and inflammatory disease
- To detect polyps, diverticula, and structural changes in the large intestine

Patient preparation

- Explain to the patient that this test permits examination of the large intestine through X-ray films taken after a barium enema.
- Describe the test, including who will perform it and where it will take place.
- Because residual fecal material in the colon obscures normal anatomy on X-rays, instruct the patient to carefully follow the prescribed bowel preparation, which may include diet, laxatives, or an enema. However, in certain conditions, such as ulcerative colitis and active GI bleeding, their use may be prohibited.
- Stress that accurate test results depend on the patient's cooperation with prescribed dietary restrictions and bowel preparation. A common bowel preparation technique includes restricted intake of dairy products and maintenance of a liquid diet for 24 hours before the test. The patient is encouraged to drink five 8-oz glasses of water or clear liquids 12 to 24 hours before the test. Administer a bowel preparation supplied by the radiography department (a GoLYTELY preparation isn't recommended because it leaves the bowel too wet and the barium won't coat the walls of the bowel).
- Advise the patient to administer prescribed enemas until return is clear.
- Tell the patient not to eat breakfast before the procedure; if the test is scheduled for late afternoon (or delayed), he may have clear liquids.
- Tell the patient that he'll be placed on a tilting X-ray table and adequately draped. Assure him that he'll be secured to the table and will be assisted to various positions.
- Tell the patient that he may experience cramping pains or the urge to defecate as the barium or air is introduced into the intestine. Instruct him to breathe deeply and slowly through his mouth to ease this discomfort.
- Tell the patient to keep his anal sphincter tightly contracted against the rectal tube; this holds the tube in position and helps prevent leakage of barium. Stress the importance of retaining the barium enema; if the intestinal walls aren't adequately coated with barium, test results may be inaccurate.
- Assure the patient that the barium enema is fairly easy to retain because of its cool temperature.

Procedure and posttest care

- After the patient is in a supine position on a tilting X-ray table, scout films of the abdomen are taken.
- The patient is assisted to Sims' position and a well-lubricated rectal tube is inserted through the anus. If the patient has anal sphincter atony or severe mental or physical debilitation, a rectal tube with a retaining balloon may be inserted.
- The barium is administered slowly and the filling process is monitored fluoroscopically. To aid filling, the table may be tilted or the patient assisted to supine, prone, and lateral decubitus positions.
- As the flow of barium is observed, spot films are taken of significant findings. When the intestine is filled with barium, overhead films of the abdomen are taken. The rectal tube is withdrawn and the patient is escorted to the toilet or provided with a bedpan and is instructed to expel as much barium as possible.
- After evacuation, an additional overhead film is taken to record the mucosal pattern of the intestine and to evaluate the efficiency of colonic emptying.
- A double-contrast barium enema may directly follow this examination or may be performed separately. If it's performed immediately, a thin film of barium remains in the patient's intestine, coating the mucosa and air is carefully injected to distend the bowel lumen.
- When the double-contrast technique is performed separately, a colloidal barium suspension is instilled, filling the patient's intestine to either the splenic flexure or the middle of the transverse colon. The suspension is then aspirated and air is forcefully injected into the intestine. If the intestine is filled to the lower descending colon, air is forcefully injected without prior aspiration of the suspension.
- The patient is then assisted to erect, prone, supine, and lateral decubitus positions in sequence. Barium filling is monitored fluoroscopically and spot films are taken of significant findings. After the required films are taken, the patient is escorted to the toilet or provided with a bedpan.
- Make sure further studies haven't been ordered before allowing the patient food and fluids. Encourage extra fluid intake because bowel preparation and the test itself can cause dehydration.
- Encourage rest because this test and the bowel preparation that precedes it exhaust most patients.
- Because retention of barium after this test can cause intestinal obstruction or fecal impaction, administer a mild cathartic or an enema. Tell the patient his stool will be light colored for 24 to 72 hours. Record and describe any stool passed by the patient in the hospital.

Precautions

- Barium enema is contraindicated in patients with tachycardia, fulminant ulcerative colitis associated with systemic toxicity and megacolon, toxic megacolon, or suspected perforation.
- This test should be performed cautiously in patients with obstruction, acute inflammatory conditions (such as ulcerative colitis and diverticulitis), acute vascular insufficiency of the bowel, acute fulminant bloody diarrhea, and suspected pneumatosis cystoides intestinalis.
- Barium enema is contraindicated in a patient who is pregnant because of radiation's possible teratogenic effects.

Normal findings

In the single-contrast enema, the intestine is uniformly filled with barium, and colonic haustral markings are clearly apparent. The intestinal walls collapse as the barium is expelled and the mucosa has a regular, feathery appearance on the postevacuation film. In the double-contrast enema, the intestine is uniformly distended with air and has a thin layer of barium providing excellent detail of the mucosal pattern. As the patient is assisted to various positions, the barium collects on the dependent walls of the intestine by the force of gravity.

Abnormal findings

Although most colonic cancers occur in the rectosigmoid region and are best detected by proctosigmoidoscopy, X-ray films may reveal adenocarcinoma and, rarely, sarcomas occurring higher in the intestine. Carcinoma usually appears as a localized filling defect, with a sharp transition between the normal and the necrotic mucosa. If it's circumferential, it will have an "apple core" appearance. These characteristics help distinguish carcinoma from the more diffuse lesions of inflammatory disease, but endoscopic biopsy may be necessary to confirm the diagnosis.

X-ray studies demonstrate and define the extent of inflammatory disease, such as diverticulitis, ulcerative colitis, and granulomatous colitis. Ulcerative colitis usually originates in the anal region and ascends through the intestine; granulomatous colitis usually originates in the cecum and terminal ileum, and then descends through the intestine. However, biopsy may be necessary to confirm diagnosis.

Barium X-ray films may also reveal saccular adenomatous polyps, broad-based villous polyps, structural changes in the intestine (such as intussusception, telescoping of the bowel, sigmoid volvulus [360-degree turn or greater], and sigmoid torsion [up to 180-degree turn]), gastroenteritis, irritable colon, vascular injury due to arterial occlusion, and selected cases of acute appendicitis.

Interfering factors

- Inadequate bowel preparation (possible poor imaging)
- Barium retained from previous studies (possible poor imaging)
- Patient's inability to retain barium enema

HYPOTONIC DUODENOGRAPHY

Hypotonic duodenography is the fluoroscopic examination of the duodenum after instillation of barium sulfate and air through an intestinal catheter. This test is indicated in patients with symptoms of duodenal or pancreatic pathology such as persistent upper abdominal pain.

After the catheter is passed through the patient's nose into the duodenum, I.V. infusion of glucagon or I.M. injection of propantheline bromide (or other anticholinergic) induces duodenal atony. Instillation of barium and air distends the relaxed duodenum, flattening its deep circular folds; spot films then record the precise delineation of the duodenal anatomy. Although these films readily demonstrate small duodenal lesions and tumors of the head of the pancreas that impinge on the duodenal wall, differential diagnosis requires further studies.

Purpose

- To detect small postbulbar duodenal lesions, tumors of the head of the pancreas, and tumors of the ampulla of Vater
- To aid diagnosis of chronic pancreatitis

Patient preparation

- Explain to the patient that this test permits examination of the duodenum and pancreas after the instillation of barium and air.
- Instruct the patient to fast after midnight the night before the test.
- Describe the test, including who will perform it and where it will take place.
- Inform the patient that a tube will be passed through his nose into the duodenum to serve as a channel for the barium and air.
- Tell the patient that he may experience a cramping pain as air is introduced into the duodenum. Instruct him to breathe deeply and slowly through his mouth if he experiences this pain to help relax the abdominal muscles.
- If glucagon or an anticholinergic is to be administered during the procedure, describe the possible adverse effects of glucagon (nausea, vomiting, hives, and flushing) or of anticholinergics (dry mouth, thirst, tachycardia, urine retention, and blurred vision). If an anticholinergic is administered to an outpatient, advise him to have someone accompany him home.
- Just before the test, tell the patient to remove dentures, glasses, necklaces, hairpins, combs, and constricting undergarments.
- Instruct the patient to void.

Procedure and posttest care

- While the patient is in a sitting position, a catheter is passed through his nose into the stomach. He's then placed in a supine position on an X-ray table and the catheter is advanced into the duodenum, under fluoroscopic guidance.
- Glucagon I.V. is administered, which quickly induces duodenal atony for approximately 20 minutes, or an anticholinergic is injected I.M.
- Barium is instilled through the catheter and spot films are taken of the duodenum.
- Some of the barium is then withdrawn and air is instilled; then additional spot films are taken.
- When the required films have been obtained, the catheter is removed.
- After the procedure, encourage the patient to drink extra fluids (unless contraindicated) to help eliminate the barium.
- Throughout the procedure, observe the patient for adverse reactions. Be aware that such reactions may follow administration of glucagon or an anticholinergic. If an anticholinergic was given, make sure the patient voids within a few hours after the test. Advise the outpatient to rest in a waiting area until his vision clears (about 2 hours) unless someone can take him home.
- Administer a cathartic as prescribed.
- Tell the patient he may burp instilled air or pass flatus, and that the barium colors the stool chalky white for 24 to 72 hours. Extra fluid may be ordered to aid barium elimination.
- Record description of any stool passed by the patient in the hospital and notify the physician if the patient hasn't expelled the barium after 2 to 3 days.

Precautions

Anticholinergics are contraindicated in patients with severe cardiac disorders or glaucoma.

Glucagon is contraindicated in patients with uncontrolled diabetes and should be used cautiously in patients with type 1 diabetes mellitus.

- Patients with strictures in the upper GI tract, particularly those associated with ulcerations or large masses, shouldn't undergo this procedure.
- Monitor elderly or very ill patients for gastric reflux.

■ This test is contraindicated in patients who are pregnant because of radiation's possible teratogenic effects.

Normal findings

When barium and air distend the atonic duodenum, the mucosa normally appears smooth and even. The regular contour of the head of the pancreas also appears on the duodenal wall.

Abnormal findings

Irregular nodules or masses on the duodenal wall could mean duodenal lesions, tumors of the ampulla of Vater, tumors of the head of the pancreas, or chronic pancreatitis. Differential diagnosis requires further tests, such as endoscopic retrograde cholangiopancreatography, serum and urine amylase determinations, ultrasonography of the pancreas, and computed tomography of the pancreas.

Interfering factors

■ Failure to fast may interfere with accurate test results

ORAL CHOLECYSTOGRAPHY

Oral cholecystography is the radiographic examination of the gallbladder after administration of a contrast medium. This test is now commonly replaced by nuclear medicine ^{99}technetium-labeled scan, ultrasound, and computerized tomography. It's indicated in patients with symptoms of biliary tract disease, such as right upper quadrant epigastric pain, fat intolerance, and jaundice, and is most commonly performed to confirm gallbladder disease.

After the contrast medium is ingested, it's absorbed by the small intestine, filtered by the liver, excreted in the bile, and then concentrated and stored in the gallbladder. Full gallbladder opacification usually occurs 12 to 14 hours after ingestion, and a series of X-ray films then records gallbladder appearance. Additional information is obtained by giving the patient a fat stimulus, causing the gallbladder to contract and empty the contrast-laden bile into the common bile duct and small intestine. Films are then taken to record this emptying and to evaluate patency of the common bile duct.

Oral cholecystography should precede barium studies because retained barium may cloud subsequent X-ray films.

Purpose

■ To detect gallstones
■ To aid diagnosis of inflammatory disease and tumors of the gallbladder

Patient preparation

■ Explain to the patient that this procedure permits examination of the gallbladder through X-ray films taken after ingestion of a contrast medium.
■ Describe the test, including who will perform it and where it will take place.
■ Instruct the patient to eat a normal meal at noon the day before the test and a fat-free meal in the evening. The former stimulates release of bile from the gallbladder, preparing it to receive the contrast-laden bile; the latter inhibits gallbladder contraction, promoting accumulation of bile.
■ After the evening meal, instruct the patient to restrict food and fluids, except water.
■ Give the patient six tablets (3 g) of iopanoic acid 2 or 3 hours after the evening meal, as necessary. (Other commercial contrast agents are available, such as sodium ipodate, but iopanoic acid is most commonly used.) Have the

patient swallow the tablets one at a time at 5-minute intervals, with one or two mouthfuls of water for a total of 8 oz (240 ml) of water. Thereafter, withhold water, cigarettes, and gum.

- Tell the patient he'll be placed on an X-ray table and that films will be taken of his gallbladder.
- Check the patient's history for hypersensitivity to iodine, seafood, or contrast media used for other diagnostic tests.
- Inform the patient that the possible adverse effects of dye ingestion include diarrhea (common) and, rarely, nausea, vomiting, abdominal cramps, and dysuria. Tell him to report such symptoms immediately if they develop.
- Examine any vomitus or diarrhea for undigested tablets. If any tablets were expelled, notify the X-ray department.
- Administer an enema the morning of the test, if prescribed. This clears the GI tract of interfering shadows that may obscure the gallbladder.

Procedure and posttest care

- After the patient is in a prone position on the radiographic table, the abdomen is examined fluoroscopically to evaluate gallbladder opacification, and films are taken of significant findings.
- The patient is then examined while in left lateral decubitus and erect positions to detect possible layering or mobility of any filling defects, and additional films are taken.
- The patient may then be given a fat stimulus, such as a high-fat meal or a synthetic fat-containing agent (such as sincalide).
- Fluoroscopy is used to observe the emptying of the gallbladder in response to the fat stimulus, and spot films are taken at 15- and 30-minute intervals to visualize the common bile duct. If the gallbladder empties slowly or not at all, these films are also taken at 60 minutes.
- If the test results are normal, tell the patient he may resume his usual diet.
- If gallstones are discovered during opacification, the patient will need an appropriate diet — usually one that restricts fat intake — to help prevent acute attacks.
- Nonopacification and repeat cholecystography require continuation of a low-fat diet until definitive diagnosis can be made.

Precautions

- Oral cholecystography is contraindicated in patients with severe renal or hepatic damage and in those with a hypersensitivity to iodine, seafood, or contrast media.
- This test is also contraindicated in patients who are pregnant because of radiation's possible teratogenic effects.

Normal findings

The gallbladder is normally opacified and appears pear-shaped, with smooth, thin walls. Although its size is variable, its basic structure — neck, infundibulum, body, and fundus — is clearly outlined on film.

Abnormal findings

When the gallbladder is opacified, filling defects (typically appearing within the lumen as negative shadows that show mobility) indicate the presence of gallstones. Fixed defects, on the other hand, may indicate the presence of cholesterol polyps or a benign tumor such as an adenomyoma.

When the gallbladder fails to opacify or when only faint opacification occurs, inflammatory disease such as cholecystitis — with or without gallstone formation — may be present. Gallstones may obstruct the cystic duct and prevent the contrast medium from entering the gallbladder; inflammation may impair the concentrating ability of the gallbladder mucosa and prevent or diminish opacification.

When the gallbladder fails to contract following stimulation by a fatty meal, cholecystitis or common bile duct obstruction may be present. If the X-ray films are inconclusive, oral cholecystography will have to be repeated the following day.

Interfering factors

- Patient movement during the procedure
- Failure to follow dietary restrictions
- Failure to ingest the full dose of contrast medium or partial loss of contrast medium through emesis or diarrhea (may invalidate test results)
- Inadequate absorption of the contrast medium in the small intestine or barium retained from previous studies (may invalidate test results)
- Decreased excretion of the contrast medium into the bile due to impaired hepatic function and moderate jaundice (possible poor imaging)

PERCUTANEOUS TRANSHEPATIC CHOLANGIOGRAPHY

Percutaneous transhepatic cholangiography is the fluoroscopic examination of the biliary ducts after injection of an iodinated contrast medium directly into a biliary radicle. This test is especially useful for evaluating patients with persistent upper abdominal pain after cholecystectomy and for evaluating patients with severe jaundice.

Although computed tomography scan or ultrasonography is usually performed first when obstructive jaundice is suspected, percutaneous transhepatic cholangiography may provide the most detailed view of the obstruction; however, this invasive procedure carries a potential risk of complications that include bleeding, septicemia, bile peritonitis, extravasation of the contrast medium into the peritoneal cavity, and subcapsular injection.

Purpose

- To determine the cause of upper abdominal pain following cholecystectomy
- To distinguish between obstructive and nonobstructive jaundice
- To determine the location, the extent, and commonly the cause of mechanical obstruction

Patient preparation

- Explain to the patient that this procedure allows examination of the biliary ducts through X-ray films taken after a contrast medium is injected into the liver.
- Instruct the patient to fast for 8 hours before the test.
- Describe the test, including who will perform it and where it will take place.
- Inform the patient that he may receive a laxative the night before and an enema the morning of the test.
- Inform the patient that he'll be placed on a tilting X-ray table that rotates into vertical and horizontal positions during the procedure.
- Assure the patient that he'll be adequately secured to the table and assisted to supine and side-lying positions throughout the procedure.
- Warn the patient that injection of the local anesthetic may sting the skin and produce transient pain when it punctures the liver capsule.
- Advise the patient that injection of the contrast medium may produce a sensation of pressure and epigastric fullness and may cause transient upper back pain on his right side.

■ Tell the patient that he must rest for at least 6 hours after the procedure.
■ Make sure the patient or a responsible family member has signed an informed consent form.
■ Check the patient's history for hypersensitivity to iodine, seafood, contrast media used in other diagnostic tests, and the local anesthetic. Advise him of possible adverse effects of contrast medium administration, such as nausea, vomiting, excessive salivation, flushing, urticaria, sweating and, rarely, anaphylaxis; tachycardia and fever may accompany intraductal injection.
■ Check the patient's history for normal bleeding, clotting, and prothrombin times, and a normal platelet count. If prescribed, administer 1 g of ampicillin I.V. every 4 to 6 hours for 24 hours before the procedure.
■ Just before the procedure, administer a sedative, if prescribed.

Procedure and posttest care

■ After the patient is placed in a supine position on the X-ray table and is adequately secured, the right upper quadrant of the abdomen is cleaned and draped; the skin, subcutaneous tissue, and liver capsule are infiltrated with a local anesthetic.
■ While the patient holds his breath at the end of expiration, the flexible needle is inserted under fluoroscopic guidance through the 10th or 11th intercostal space at the right midclavicular line.
■ The needle is aimed toward the xiphoid process and is advanced through the liver parenchyma. It's then slowly withdrawn, injecting the contrast medium to locate a biliary radicle. When fluoroscopy reveals placement in a radicle, the needle is held in position and the remaining contrast medium is injected.
■ Using a fluoroscope and television monitor, the opacification of the biliary ducts is observed, and spot films of significant findings are taken with the patient in supine and lateral recumbent positions. When the required films have been taken, the needle is removed.
■ Apply a sterile dressing to the puncture site.
■ Check the patient's vital signs until they're stable.
■ Enforce bed rest for at least 6 hours after the test, preferably with the patient lying on his right side, to help prevent hemorrhage.
■ Check the injection site for bleeding, swelling, and tenderness. Watch for signs of peritonitis: chills, temperature of 102° to 103° F (38.8° to 39.4° C), and abdominal pain, tenderness, and distention. Notify the physician immediately if such complications develop.
■ Tell the patient that he may resume his usual diet.

Precautions

■ Percutaneous transhepatic cholangiography is contraindicated in patients with cholangitis, massive ascites, uncorrectable coagulopathy, or hypersensitivity to iodine as well as in patients who are pregnant because of radiation's possible teratogenic effects.

Normal findings

The biliary ducts are of normal diameter and appear as regular channels homogeneously filled with contrast medium.

Abnormal findings

Distinguishing between obstructive and nonobstructive jaundice hinges on whether biliary ducts are dilated or of normal size. Obstructive jaundice is associated with dilated ducts; nonobstructive jaundice, with normal-sized ducts. When ducts are dilated, the obstruction site may be defined. Obstruction may result from cholelithiasis, biliary tract carcinoma, or carcinoma of the pancreas or papilla of Vater that impinges on the common bile duct, causing deviation or stricture.

When ducts are of normal size and intrahepatic cholestasis is indicated, liver biopsy may be performed to distinguish among hepatitis, cirrhosis, and granulomatous disease. If ducts are dilated as a result of obstruction, a drainage tube may be inserted to allow percutaneous drainage of bile into a collection bag.

Interfering factors

- Marked obesity or gas overlying the biliary ducts (possible poor imaging)

POSTOPERATIVE CHOLANGIOGRAPHY

During cholecystectomy or common bile duct exploration, a T-shaped rubber tube may be inserted into the common bile duct to facilitate drainage. Postoperative cholangiography — radiographic and fluoroscopic examination of the biliary ducts — may be performed 7 to 10 days after surgery.

This procedure requires injection of contrast medium through the T-tube. The contrast medium flows through the biliary ducts and outlines the size and patency of the ducts, revealing any obstruction overlooked during surgery.

Purpose

- To detect calculi, strictures, neoplasms, and fistulae in the biliary ducts

Patient preparation

- Explain to the patient that this procedure permits examination of the biliary ducts through X-ray films taken after the injection of a contrast medium.
- Describe the test, including who will perform it and where it will take place.
- Warn the patient that he may feel a bloating sensation (not pain) in the right upper quadrant as the contrast medium is injected.
- Clamp the T-tube the day before the procedure, if necessary. Because bile fills the tube after clamping, this helps prevent air bubbles from entering the ducts.
- Withhold the meal just before the test and administer an enema about 1 hour before the procedure.
- Make sure the patient or a responsible family member has signed an informed consent form.
- Check the patient's history for hypersensitivity to iodine, seafood, or contrast media used in other diagnostic tests. Tell the patient that the adverse effects of intraductal administration may include nausea, vomiting, excessive salivation, flushing, urticaria, sweating and, rarely, anaphylaxis.

Procedure and posttest care

- After the patient is in a supine position on the X-ray table, the injection area of the T-tube is cleaned with sponges soaked with povidone-iodine solution. The T-tube is held in a vertical position, which allows trapped air to surface, and a needle attached to a long transparent catheter is carefully inserted into the end of the T-tube. Care must be taken to avoid injecting air into the biliary tree because air bubbles may affect the clarity of the X-ray films.
- Approximately 5 ml of contrast medium (usually sodium diatrizoate) is injected under fluoroscopic guidance, and a spot film is taken in the anteroposterior position. Additional injections are then administered and spot films and plain films are taken with the patient in

supine and right lateral decubitus positions.

- The T-tube is then clamped and the patient is assisted to an erect position for additional films; in this position, air bubbles may be distinguished from calculi or other pathology.
- A final film is taken 15 minutes after contrast injection to record the emptying of contrast-laden bile into the duodenum. If emptying is delayed, additional films may be taken at 15 or 30 minutes intervals until this action is demonstrated.
- If a sterile dressing is applied after removal of the T-tube, observe and record any drainage. Change the dressing, as necessary.
- If the T-tube is left in place, attach it to the drainage system.
- Tell the patient that he may resume his normal diet and return to pretest activity as directed.

Precautions

- Postoperative cholangiography is contraindicated in patients who are hypersensitive to iodine, seafood, or contrast media used in other tests.

Normal findings

Biliary ducts demonstrate homogeneous filling with contrast medium and are normal in diameter. When Oddi's sphincter is functioning properly and the ducts are patent, the contrast flows unimpeded into the duodenum.

Abnormal findings

Negative shadows or filling defects within the biliary ducts associated with dilation may indicate calculi or neoplasms overlooked during surgery. Abnormal channels of contrast medium departing from the biliary ducts indicate fistulae.

Interfering factors

- Marked obesity or gas overlying the biliary ducts (possible poor imaging)

ENDOSCOPIC RETROGRADE CHOLANGIO-PANCREATOGRAPHY

Endoscopic retrograde cholangiopancreatography (ERCP) is the radiographic examination of the pancreatic ducts and hepatobiliary tree after injection of a contrast medium into the duodenal papilla. It's indicated in patients with confirmed or suspected pancreatic disease or obstructive jaundice of unknown etiology. Complications may include cholangitis and pancreatitis.

Purpose

- To evaluate obstructive jaundice
- To diagnose cancer of the duodenal papilla, the pancreas, and the biliary ducts
- To locate calculi and stenosis in the pancreatic ducts and hepatobiliary tree
- To identify leaks from trauma or surgery

Patient preparation

- Explain to the patient that this procedure permits examination of the liver, the gallbladder, and the pancreas through X-ray films taken after injection of a contrast medium.
- Instruct the patient to fast after midnight before the test.
- Describe the test, including who will perform it and where it will take place.
- Inform the patient that a local anesthetic will be sprayed into his mouth to calm the gag reflex. Warn him that the spray has an unpleasant taste and makes

the tongue and throat feel swollen, causing difficulty swallowing.

■ Instruct the patient to let saliva drain from the side of his mouth, and tell him that suction may be used to remove saliva. Tell him a mouth guard will be inserted to protect his teeth and the endoscope; assure him that it won't obstruct his breathing.

■ Tell the patient that he'll receive a sedative before insertion of the endoscope to help him relax, but that he'll remain conscious.

■ Tell the patient that he'll also receive an anticholinergic or glucagon I.V. after insertion of the endoscope. Describe the possible adverse effects of anticholinergics (dry mouth, thirst, tachycardia, urine retention, and blurred vision) or of glucagon (nausea, vomiting, urticaria, and flushing).

■ Warn the patient that he may experience transient flushing on injection of the contrast medium. Advise him that he may have a sore throat for 3 or 4 days after the examination.

■ Make sure the patient or responsible family member has signed an informed consent form.

■ Check the patient's history for hypersensitivity to iodine, seafood, or contrast media used for other diagnostic procedures and inform the physician of sensitivities.

■ Just before the procedure, obtain baseline vital signs. Instruct the patient to remove all metallic or other radiopaque objects and constricting undergarments. Then tell him to void, to minimize the discomfort of urine retention that may follow the procedure.

Procedure and posttest care

■ An I.V. infusion is started with 150 ml of normal saline solution. The local anesthetic is then administered and usually takes effect in about 10 minutes.

■ If a spray is used, ask the patient to hold his breath while his mouth and throat are sprayed.

■ Place the patient in a left lateral position and give him an emesis basin; provide tissues. Because the anesthetic causes the patient to lose some control of his secretions and thus increases the risk of aspiration, encourage him to allow saliva to drain from the side of his mouth.

■ Insert the mouth guard.

■ While the patient remains in the left lateral position, 5 to 20 mg of diazepam or midazolam is administered I.V. as well as a narcotic analgesic if needed.

■ When ptosis or dysarthria develops, the patient's head is bent forward and he's asked to open his mouth.

■ The examiner inserts his left index finger in the patient's mouth and guides the tip of the endoscope along his finger to the back of the patient's throat. The scope is then deflected downward with the left index finger and advanced. As the endoscope passes through the posterior pharynx and cricopharyngeal sphincter, the patient's head is slowly extended to assist the advance of the endoscope. The patient's chin must be kept midline. When the endoscope has passed the cricopharyngeal sphincter, the scope is advanced under direct vision. When it's well into the esophagus, the patient's chin is moved toward the table so saliva can drain from the mouth. The endoscope is advanced through the remainder of the esophagus and into the stomach under direct vision.

■ When the pylorus is located, a small amount of air is insufflated, and the tip of the endoscope is angled upward and passed into the duodenal bulb.

■ After the endoscope is rotated clockwise to enter the descending duodenum, the patient is assisted to a prone position.

■ An anticholinergic or glucagon I.V. is administered to induce duodenal atony and to relax the ampullary sphincter.
■ A small amount of air is insufflated, and the endoscope is manipulated until the optic lies opposite the duodenal papilla. Then the cannula filled with contrast medium is passed through the biopsy channel of the endoscope, the duodenal papilla, and into the ampulla of Vater.
■ The pancreatic duct is visualized first under fluoroscopic guidance with injection of contrast medium.
■ The cannula is repositioned at a more cephalad angle, and the hepatobiliary tree is visualized with injection of contrast medium.
■ After each injection, rapid-sequence X-ray films are taken.
■ Instruct the patient to remain prone while the films are developed and reviewed. If necessary, additional films may be taken.
■ When the required radiographs have been obtained, the cannula is removed. Before the endoscope is withdrawn, a tissue specimen may be obtained or fluid aspirated for histologic and cytologic examination, respectively.
■ Observe closely for signs of cholangitis and pancreatitis. Hyperbilirubinemia, fever, and chills are the immediate signs of cholangitis; hypotension associated with gram-negative septicemia may develop later. Left upper quadrant pain and tenderness, elevated serum amylase levels, and transient hyperbilirubinemia are the usual signs of pancreatitis. Draw blood samples for amylase and bilirubin determinations, if necessary, but remember that these levels usually rise after ERCP.
■ Observe the patient for signs of perforation, such as abdominal pain, bleeding, and fever.
■ Tell the patient that he may experience a feeling of fullness, some cramping, and passage of flatus several hours after the test.
■ Continue to watch for signs of respiratory depression, apnea, hypotension, excessive diaphoresis, bradycardia, and laryngospasm. Check vital signs every 15 minutes for 1 hour, then every 30 minutes for 2 hours, then every hour for 4 hours, and then every 4 hours for 48 hours.
■ Withhold food and fluids until the gag reflex returns. Test the gag reflex by touching the back of the throat with a tongue blade. When the gag reflex returns, allow fluids and a light meal.
■ Discontinue or maintain the I.V. infusion as ordered.
■ Check for signs of urine retention. Notify the physician if the patient hasn't voided within 8 hours.
■ If the patient has a sore throat, provide soothing lozenges and warm saline gargles to ease discomfort.
■ If a tissue biopsy or polypectomy occurred, a small amount of blood in the patient's first stool is normal. Report excessive bleeding immediately.
■ If this test is performed on an outpatient basis, be sure that transportation is available. Patients who have undergone anesthesia or sedation shouldn't operate an automobile for at least 12 hours postprocedure. Alcohol should be avoided for 24 hours.

Precautions

■ ERCP is contraindicated in patients who are patients because of the risk of fetal harm secondary to radiation exposure.
■ ERCP is contraindicated in patients with infectious disease, pancreatic pseudocysts, stricture or obstruction of the esophagus or duodenum, and acute pancreatitis, cholangitis, or cardiorespiratory disease.
■ Patients receiving anticoagulants have an increased risk of bleeding.

■ Monitor vital signs and airway patency throughout the procedure. Watch for signs of respiratory depression, apnea, hypotension, excessive diaphoresis, bradycardia, and laryngospasm. Be sure to have available emergency resuscitation equipment and a narcotic antagonist, such as naloxone.
■ If the patient has known cardiac disease, continuous ECG monitoring should be instituted. Continuing periodic pulse oximetry is advisable, particularly in patients with pulmonary compromise.

Normal findings

The duodenal papilla appears as a small red (or sometimes pale) erosion protruding into the lumen. Its orifice is commonly bordered by a fringe of white mucosa, and a longitudinal fold running perpendicular to the deep circular folds of the duodenum helps mark its location. Although the pancreatic and hepatobiliary ducts usually unite in the ampulla of Vater and empty through the duodenal papilla, separate orifices are sometimes present.

The contrast medium uniformly fills the pancreatic duct, the hepatobiliary tree, and the gallbladder.

Abnormal findings

Obstructive jaundice may result from various abnormalities of the hepatobiliary tree and pancreatic duct. Examination of the hepatobiliary tree may reveal stones, strictures, or irregular deviations that suggest biliary cirrhosis, primary sclerosing cholangitis, or carcinoma of the bile ducts.

Examination of the pancreatic ducts may also show stones, strictures, and irregular deviations that may indicate pancreatic cysts and pseudocysts, pancreatic tumor, carcinoma of the head of the pancreas, chronic pancreatitis, pancreatic fibrosis, carcinoma of the duodenal papilla, and papillary stenosis.

Depending on test findings, a definitive diagnosis may require further studies. In addition, certain interventions, such as the placement of a stent to allow drainage or a papillotomy to decrease scar tissue and allow light drainage, may be indicated.

Interfering factors

■ Barium in GI tract from previous studies (possible poor imaging)

CELIAC AND MESENTERIC ARTERIOGRAPHY

Celiac and mesenteric arteriography involves the radiographic examination of the abdominal vasculature after intra-arterial injection of contrast medium through a catheter. Most commonly, the catheter is passed through the femoral artery into the aorta and then, using fluoroscopy, is positioned in the celiac, superior mesenteric, or inferior mesenteric artery. Injection of contrast medium into one or more of these arteries provides a map of abdominal vasculature; injection into specific arterial branches, called superselective angiography, permits detailed visualization of a particular area. As the contrast medium flows through the abdominal vasculature, serial radiographs outline abdominal vessels in the arterial, capillary, and venous phases of perfusion.

Celiac and mesenteric arteriography is indicated when endoscopy is unable to locate the source of GI bleeding or when barium studies, ultrasonography, and nuclear medicine or computed tomography scanning prove inconclusive in evaluating neoplasms. It's also used to evaluate cirrhosis and portal hypertension (especially when a portacaval shunt is being considered); to evaluate vascular damage, particularly in the spleen and liver, after abdominal trauma; and to detect vascular abnormalities. Because arteriography can demonstrate the portal vein even when portal venous flow is reversed, it's used more often than splenoportography.

Complications associated with this test include hemorrhage, venous and intracardiac thrombosis, cardiac arrhythmia, and emboli caused by dislodging atherosclerotic plaques.

Purpose

- To locate the source of GI bleeding
- To help distinguish between benign and malignant neoplasms
- To evaluate cirrhosis and portal hypertension
- To evaluate vascular damage after abdominal trauma
- To detect vascular abnormalities

Patient preparation

- Explain to the patient that this test permits examination of the abdominal blood vessels after injection of a contrast medium.
- Instruct the patient to fast for 8 hours before the test.
- Tell the patient that he'll receive I.V. conscious sedation and a local anesthetic and that he may feel a brief, stinging sensation as the anesthetic is injected. He may also feel pressure when the femoral artery is palpated, but the local anesthetic will minimize the pain when the needle is introduced into the artery.
- Tell the patient he may feel a transient burning as the contrast medium is injected.
- Tell the patient that the X-ray equipment makes a loud, clacking sound as the films are taken.
- Instruct the patient to lie still during the test to avoid blurring the films, and inform him that restraints may be used to help him remain still.
- Warn the patient that he may feel some temporary stiffness after the test from lying still on the hard X-ray table.
- Tell the patient who will perform the test, where it will take place, and that it takes 30 minutes to 3 hours, depending on the number of vessels studied.
- Make sure the patient or a responsible family member has signed an informed consent form, if required.
- Check the patient's history for hypersensitivity to iodine, shellfish, or the contrast medium.
- Make sure blood studies (hemoglobin and hematocrit levels; clotting, prothrombin, and activated partial thromboplastin times; and platelet count) have been completed.
- Just before the procedure, instruct the patient to put on a gown and to remove jewelry and other objects that might obscure anatomic detail on X-ray films.
- Tell the patient to void; then record baseline vital signs.
- Administer a sedative, if prescribed.

Procedure and posttest care

- After the patient is placed in a supine position on the X-ray table, an I.V. infusion is started to maintain hydration and to permit emergency administration of medication. The patient is attached to a heart monitor and pulse oximeter and his blood pressure is monitored according to facility policy.
- Scout films of the patient's abdomen are taken and the peripheral pulses are palpated and marked.
- The puncture site is cleaned with soap and water; the area is shaved, cleaned with povidone-iodine preparation, and surrounded by sterile drapes.
- The local anesthetic is injected and the femoral artery is located by palpa-

tion. The needle is gently inserted until a pulsing blood flow is obtained.

- A guide wire is passed through the needle into the aorta; then the needle is removed, leaving the guide wire in place.
- The angiocath is inserted over the guide wire; the guide wire is withdrawn to inject the contrast medium to check for catheter placement. The guide wire is again inserted into the selected artery for fluoroscopic guidance.
- When the wire is in position, the catheter is advanced over it into the artery. The wire is then removed and placement verified by hand injection of contrast medium.
- The automatic injector is then attached to the catheter. As the contrast medium is injected, a series of films is taken in rapid sequence.
- After injecting into one or more major arteries, superselective catheterization may be performed. Using fluoroscopy, the catheter is repositioned in a specific branch of a major artery, contrast medium is injected, and rapid-sequence films are taken. If necessary, several specific branches may be catheterized.
- If an occlusion is detected, balloon angioplasty is performed.
- After filming, the catheter is withdrawn and firm pressure is applied to the puncture site for about 15 minutes.
- Observe the puncture site for hematoma formation, and check peripheral pulses.
- Inform the patient that he'll be on bed rest for 4 to 6 hours and that he must keep the leg with the puncture site straight. Don't raise the bed further than 30 degrees. He'll be able to logroll and may use the unaffected leg to reposition himself to use the bedpan.
- Monitor vital signs until stable and check peripheral pulses. Note the color and temperature of the leg that was used for the test.
- Check the puncture site for bleeding and hematoma. If bleeding develops, apply pressure to the site. If a hematoma develops, apply warm soaks.
- Confirm whether the patient can resume his usual diet. If the patient isn't receiving I.V. infusions, encourage intake of fluids to speed excretion of the contrast medium.

Precautions

- Celiac and mesenteric arteriography should be performed cautiously in patients with coagulopathy.

◆ **CLINICAL ALERT** *Most reactions to the contrast medium occur within a half-hour. Watch carefully for cardiovascular shock or arrest, flushing, laryngeal stridor, or urticaria.*

- This test is contraindicated in patients who are pregnant because of radiation's possible teratogenic effects.

Normal findings

X-ray films show the three phases of perfusion — arterial, capillary, and venous. The arteries normally taper regularly, becoming gradually smaller with subsequent divisions. The contrast medium then spreads evenly within the sinusoids. The portal vein appears 10 to 20 seconds after the injection, as the contrast medium empties from the spleen into the splenic vein or from the intestine into the superior mesenteric vein and further into the portal vein.

Abnormal findings

GI hemorrhage appears on the angiogram as the extravasation of contrast medium from the damaged vessels. Upper GI hemorrhage can result from conditions such as Mallory-Weiss syndrome, gastric or peptic ulcer, hemorrhagic gastritis, and eroded hiatal hernia. Esophageal hemorrhage rarely appears on the angiogram because the contrast medium usually fails to fill the esophageal vein. Lower GI hemorrhage can result from conditions such as bleeding diverticula, carcinoma, and angiodysplasia.

Abdominal neoplasms — carcinoid tumors, adenomas, leiomyomas, angiomas, and adenocarcinomas — can disrupt the normal vasculature in several ways. Neoplasms can invade or encase nearby arteries and veins, distorting their regular channel-like appearance and, in late stages, displacing them. Vessels within the neoplasm, known as neovasculature, appear as abnormal vascular areas. Areas of necrosis appear as puddles of contrast medium. Contrast medium may also remain in the neoplasm longer during capillary perfusion, producing a tumor blush or stain on the angiogram. Arteriovenous shunting may also be present, depending on the size and location of the tumor. Because these characteristics aren't uniformly present in all neoplasms, combinations of these characteristics can often distinguish between benign and malignant neoplasms.

In early or mild cirrhosis, portal venous flow to the liver remains relatively unaffected, and the hepatic artery and its branches appear normal. As this disease progresses, portal venous flow diminishes, the hepatic artery and its branches become dilated and tortuous, and collateral veins develop. In advanced cirrhosis, portal venous flow reverses. However, the portal vein still appears on the X-ray film, which may also show thrombi.

Abdominal trauma commonly causes splenic injury; less commonly, hepatic injury. Splenic rupture usually displaces intrasplenic arterial branches, causing contrast medium to leak from splenic arteries into the splenic pulp. When rupture occurs without subcapsular hematoma, the spleen usually maintains its normal size. However, in subcapsular hematoma, the spleen enlarges to displace the splenic artery and vein; the subcapsular hematoma itself appears as a large, avascular mass that stretches intrasplenic arteries and compresses the splenic pulp away from the capsule.

Hepatic injury causes similar vascular distortion, such as displacement of the common hepatic artery and extrahepatic branches. Intrahepatic and subcapsular hematomas displace and stretch intrahepatic arteries. As the hepatic vascular supply is disrupted, an arteriovenous fistula may develop between the hepatic artery and the portal vein.

Various abnormalities affecting the diameter and course of an artery may appear on the angiogram. Atherosclerotic plaques or atheromas — lipid deposits on the intima — narrow the arterial lumen and may even occlude it, resulting in formation of collaterals. Other identifiable vascular abnormalities include aneurysms, thrombi, and emboli.

Interfering factors

- Patient's inability to remain still during the procedure
- Barium, gas, or stool from a previous procedure (possible poor imaging)
- Presence of an atherosclerotic lesion in the vessel to be cannulated (prevents entry and passage of catheter)

GENITOURINARY SYSTEM

KIDNEY-URETER-BLADDER RADIOGRAPHY

Usually the first step in diagnostic testing of the urinary system, kidney-ureter-bladder (KUB) radiography surveys the abdomen to determine the position of the kidneys, ureters, and bladder, and to detect gross abnormalities.

This test doesn't require intact renal function and may aid differential diagnosis of urologic and GI diseases, which often produce similar signs and symptoms. However, KUB radiography has many limitations and nearly always must be followed by more elaborate tests, such as excretory urography or renal computed tomography. KUB radiography should not follow recent instillation of barium.

Purpose

- To evaluate the size, structure, and position of the kidneys
- To screen for abnormalities, such as calcifications, in the region of the kidneys, ureters, and bladder

Patient preparation

- Explain to the patient that this test helps detect urinary system abnormalities.
- Inform the patient that he need not restrict food or fluids. Tell him who will perform the test, where it will take place, and that it takes only a few minutes.

Procedure and posttest care

- The patient is placed in a supine position in correct body alignment on an X-ray table. His arms are extended overhead, and the iliac crests are checked for symmetrical positioning.
- If the patient can't extend his arms or stand, he may lie on his left side with his right arm up.
- A single X-ray is taken.

Precautions

- Male patients should have gonadal shielding to prevent irradiation of the testes. Female patients' ovaries can't be shielded because they're too close to the kidneys, ureters, and bladder.

Normal findings

The shadows of the kidneys appear bilaterally, the right slightly lower than the left. Both kidneys should be approximately the same size, with the superior poles tilted slightly toward the vertebral column, paralleling the shadows (or stripes) produced by the psoas muscles. The ureters are only visible when an abnormality such as calcification is present. Visualization of the bladder depends on the density of its muscular wall and on the amount of urine in it. Generally, the bladder's shadow can be seen but not as clearly as the kidneys' shadows.

Abnormal findings

Bilateral renal enlargement may result from polycystic disease, multiple myeloma, lymphoma, amyloidosis, diabetes, hydronephrosis, or compensatory hypertrophy. Tumor, cyst, or hydronephrosis may cause unilateral enlargement. Abnormally small kidneys may suggest end-stage glomerulonephritis or bilateral atrophic pyelonephritis. An apparent decrease in the size of one kidney suggests possible congenital hypoplasia, atrophic pyelonephritis, or ischemia. Renal displacement may be due to a retroperitoneal tumor, such as an adrenal tumor. Obliteration or bulging of a portion of the psoas muscle stripe may result from tumor, abscess, or hematoma.

Congenital anomalies, such as abnormal location or absence of a kidney, may be detected. Horseshoe kidney may be suggested by renal axes that parallel the vertebral column, especially if the inferior poles of the kidneys can't be clearly distinguished. A lobulated edge or border may suggest polycystic kidney disease or patchy atrophic pyelonephritis.

Opaque bodies may reflect calculi or vascular calcification due to aneurysm or atheroma; opacification may also suggest cystic tumors, fecaliths, foreign bodies, or abnormal fluid collection. Calcifications may appear anywhere in the urinary system, but positive identification requires further testing. The lone exception is staghorn calculus, which forms a perfect cast of the renal pelvis and calyces.

Interfering factors

- Gas, stool, contrast medium, or foreign bodies in the intestine (possible poor imaging)
- Calcified uterine fibromas or ovarian lesions
- Obesity or ascites (possible poor imaging)

NEPHROTOMOGRAPHY

In nephrotomography, special films are exposed before and after opacification of the renal arterial network and parenchyma with contrast medium. The resulting tomographic slices clearly delineate various linear layers of the kidneys, while blurring structures in front of and behind these selected planes.

Nephrotomography can be performed as a separate procedure or as an adjunct to excretory urography. Nephrotomography is particularly helpful in visualizing space-occupying lesions suggested by excretory urography or retrograde ureteropyelography. Additional films are exposed to define the thickness of the wall of the mass and its interior. Other tests that may resolve nephrotomographic findings include renal angiography and radionuclide renal imaging.

Purpose

- To differentiate between a simple renal cyst and a solid neoplasm
- To assess renal lacerations as well as posttraumatic nonperfused areas of the kidneys
- To localize adrenal tumors when laboratory tests indicate their presence

Patient preparation

- Explain to the patient that this test provides images of sections or layers of the kidney tissues and blood vessels.
- Instruct the patient to fast for 8 hours before the test. Tell him who will perform the test and where it will take place.
- Tell the patient that he'll be positioned on an X-ray table and that he may hear loud, clacking sounds as the films are exposed. Tell him that he may experience transient adverse effects from the injection of the contrast medium — usually a burning or stinging sensation at the injection site, flushing, and a metallic taste.
- Make sure the patient or a responsible family member has signed an informed consent form, if required.
- Check the patient's history for hypersensitivity to iodine or iodine-containing foods or to contrast media used in other diagnostic tests. If he has a history of sensitivity, provide antiallergenic

prophylaxis (such as diphenhydramine) or use a non–iodine-containing contrast medium, as necessary.

■ Elderly and dehydrated patients are at increased risk for contrast-induced renal failure. Check serum creatinine levels, and inform the physician if they are elevated. I.V. fluids may be ordered before the test to ensure hydration and decrease nephrotoxic potential.

Procedure and posttest care

■ The test may be performed using either the infusion method or the bolus method. Complications resulting from either technique are minor and infrequent.

■ A plain film of the kidneys is exposed to provide general information about their position, size, and shape, and preliminary anteroposterior tomograms are made to determine tomographic levels. Posterior oblique tomograms are made to rule out the presence of radiopaque renal calculi, which would be masked by the contrast medium.

Infusion method

■ After test tomograms are reviewed, five vertical slices of renal parenchyma 1 cm apart are selected for filming.

■ Contrast medium is then administered through the antecubital vein — the first half in 4 to 5 minutes (rapid phase) and the second half in the following 8 to 10 minutes (slow phase). Serial tomograms are made as soon as the slow phase begins.

Bolus method

■ After test tomograms are reviewed, circulation time from arm to tongue is determined by injecting a bolus of a bitter-tasting agent (dehydrocholic acid or sodium dehydrocholate) into the antecubital vein. Arm-to-tongue circulation time is close to arm-to-kidney circulation time.

■ With the needle still in place, a loading dose of a conventional urographic contrast medium is injected to perform excretory urography.

■ Five minutes after this injection, a loading dose of a contrast medium is quickly injected to ensure a high concentration of the contrast medium in the kidneys. A multifilm tomographic cassette, exposed at the predetermined arm-to-kidney circulation time, visualizes the main renal vessels and possible vessels within tumors.

■ A series of individual tomograms measuring 1 cm are then made in rapid succession through the opacified kidneys.

■ If the exposures are poor, this method requires a second infusion of contrast medium because normal kidneys quickly clear the substance.

Both methods

■ If a hematoma develops at the injection site, apply warm soaks.

■ Monitor vital signs and urine output for 24 hours after the test.

■ Ensure adequate hydration (unless contraindicated) and monitor serum creatinine levels because of the risk of contrast-induced renal failure.

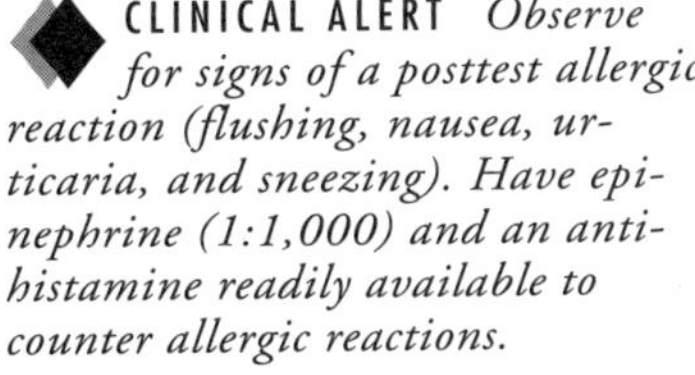

CLINICAL ALERT *Observe for signs of a posttest allergic reaction (flushing, nausea, urticaria, and sneezing). Have epinephrine (1:1,000) and an antihistamine readily available to counter allergic reactions.*

Precautions

■ Nephrotomography should be performed with extreme caution in patients with hypersensitivity to iodine-based compounds, cardiovascular disease, or multiple myeloma, and in elderly and dehydrated patients with impaired renal function, as evidenced by elevated serum creatinine.

Normal findings

The size, shape, and position of the kidneys appear within normal range,

Simple cyst or solid tumor: Differential diagnosis in nephrotomography

FEATURE	CYST	TUMOR
Consistency	Homogeneous	Irregular
Contact with healthy renal tissue	Sharply distinct	Poorly resolved
Density	Radiolucent	Variable radiolucent patches (or same as normal renal parenchyma)
Shape	Spherical	Variable
Wall of lesion	Thin and well defined	Thick and irregular

with no space-occupying lesions or other abnormalities.

Abnormal findings

Among the abnormalities detectable through nephrotomography are simple cysts and solid tumors, renal sinus–related lesions, ectopic renal lobes, adrenal tumors, areas of nonperfusion, and renal lacerations following trauma. (See *Simple cyst or solid tumor: Differential diagnosis in nephrotomography.*)

Interfering factors

- Residual barium from a recent enema or other GI studies (possible poor imaging)

RETROGRADE URETHROGRAPHY

Used almost exclusively in men, retrograde urethrography requires instillation or injection of a contrast medium into the urethra and permits visualization of its membranous, bulbar, and penile portions.

Although visualization of the anterior portion of the urethra is excellent with this test alone, the posterior portion is more effectively outlined by retrograde urethrography in tandem with voiding cystourethrography.

Purpose

- To diagnose urethral strictures, diverticula, and congenital anomalies
- To assess urethral lacerations or other trauma
- To assist with follow-up examination after surgical repair of the urethra

Patient preparation

- Explain to the patient that this test diagnoses urethral structural problems. Inform him that he need not restrict food or fluids.
- Describe the test, including who will perform it and where it will take place.
- Inform the patient that he may experience some discomfort when the cathe-

ter is inserted and when the contrast medium is instilled through the catheter.

■ Tell the patient that he may hear loud, clacking sounds as the X-ray films are made.

■ Make sure the patient or a responsible family member has signed a consent form, if required.

■ Check the patient's history for hypersensitivity to iodine-containing foods, such as shellfish, or contrast media.

■ Just before the procedure, administer any prescribed sedatives and instruct the patient to void before leaving the unit.

Equipment

Radiograph machine and table, penile clamp, 50-ml syringe with tapered universal adapter, indwelling urinary catheter, 1″ (2.5 cm) roller gauze, contrast medium (half-strength preparation)

Procedure and posttest care

For men

■ The patient is placed in a recumbent position on the examining table. Anteroposterior exposures of the bladder and urethra are made, and the resulting films studied for radiopaque densities, foreign bodies, or stones.

■ The glans and meatus are cleaned with an antiseptic solution. The catheter is filled with the contrast medium before insertion to eliminate air bubbles.

■ Although no lubricant should be used, the tip of the catheter may be dipped in sterile water to facilitate insertion.

■ The catheter is inserted until the balloon portion is inside the meatus; the balloon is then inflated with 1 to 2 ml of water, which prevents the catheter from slipping during the procedure.

■ The patient then assumes the right posterior oblique position, with his right thigh drawn up to a 90-degree angle and the penis placed along its axis. The left thigh is extended.

■ The contrast medium is injected through the catheter. After three-fourths of the contrast medium has been injected, the first X-ray film is exposed while the remainder of the contrast medium is being injected. Left lateral oblique views may also be taken.

■ Fluoroscopic control may be helpful, especially for evaluating urethral injury.

For women and children

■ In women, this test may be used when urethral diverticula are suspected. A double-balloon catheter is used, which occludes the bladder neck from above and the external meatus from below.

■ In children, the procedure is the same as for adults except that a smaller catheter is used.

For all patients

■ Watch for chills and fever related to extravasation of contrast medium into the general circulation for 12 to 24 hours after retrograde urethrography. Also observe for signs of sepsis and allergic manifestations.

Precautions

■ Retrograde urethrography should be performed cautiously in patients with urinary tract infection.

■ Monitor for urinary tract infection. If urethral trauma is present, monitor for stricture, infection, and urinary extravasation. Prepare the patient for surgery if indicated.

Normal findings

The membranous, bulbar, and penile portions of the urethra — and occasionally the prostatic portion — appear normal in size, shape, and course.

Abnormal findings

Radiographs obtained during retrograde urethrography may show the following abnormalities: urethral diverticula, fistulas, strictures, false passages, calculi, and lacerations; congenital anomalies, such as urethral valves and perineal hypospadias; and rarely, tumors (in less than 1% of patients).

Interfering factors

- None significant

RETROGRADE CYSTOGRAPHY

Retrograde cystography involves the instillation of contrast medium into the bladder, followed by radiographic examination. This procedure is used to diagnose bladder rupture without urethral involvement because it can determine the location and extent of the rupture. Other indications for retrograde cystography include neurogenic bladder; recurrent urinary tract infections (UTIs), especially in children; suspected vesicoureteral reflux; and vesical fistulas, diverticula, and tumors. This test is also performed when cystoscopic examination is impractical, as in male infants, or when excretory urography has not adequately visualized the bladder. Voiding cystourethrography is commonly performed concomitantly.

Purpose

- To evaluate the structure and integrity of the bladder

Patient preparation

- Explain to the patient that this test permits radiographic examination of the bladder.
- Inform the patient that he need not restrict food or fluids.
- Tell the patient who will perform the test and where it will take place.
- Inform the patient that he may experience some discomfort when the catheter is inserted and when the contrast medium is instilled through the catheter.
- Tell the patient that he may hear loud, clacking sounds as the X-ray films are made.
- Make sure the patient or a responsible family member has signed an informed consent form.
- Check the patient's history for hypersensitivity to contrast media, iodine, or shellfish; mark it on the chart and inform the physician.

Equipment

Radiographic equipment, drip infusion set or syringes, standard contrast medium, urethral indwelling urinary catheters

Procedure and posttest care

- The patient is placed in a supine position on the X-ray table and a preliminary kidney-ureter-bladder radiograph is taken.
- The radiograph is developed immediately and scrutinized for renal shadows, calcifications, contours of the bone and psoas muscles, and gas patterns in the lumen of the GI tract.
- The bladder is catheterized and 200 to 300 ml of sterile contrast medium (50 to 100 ml for an infant) is instilled by gravity or gentle syringe injection. The catheter is then clamped.
- With the patient in a supine position, an anteroposterior film is taken. The patient is then tilted to one side, then the other, and two posterior oblique (and sometimes lateral) views are taken.

- If the patient's condition permits, he's placed in the jackknife position and a posteroanterior film is taken. A space-occupying vesical lesion may require additional exposures. Rarely, to enhance visualization, 100 to 300 ml of air may be insufflated into the bladder by syringe after removal of the contrast medium (double-contrast technique).
- The catheter is then unclamped, the bladder fluid is allowed to drain, and a radiograph is obtained to detect urethral diverticula, reflux into the ureters, fistulous tracts into the vagina, or intraperitoneal or extraperitoneal extravasation of the contrast medium.
- Monitor vital signs every 15 minutes for the first hour, every 30 minutes during the second hour, then every 2 hours for up to 24 hours.
- Record the time of the patient's voidings and the color and volume of the urine. Observe for hematuria that persists after the third voiding and notify the physician.
- Watch for signs of urinary sepsis from UTI (chills, fever, elevated pulse and respiration rates, and hypotension) or similar signs related to extravasation of contrast medium into the general circulation.
- Prepare for surgery and urinary diversion, if indicated. Strain urine if calculi are detected.
- Monitor for retention or distention if neurogenic bladder is diagnosed and administer medication as ordered (baclofen for spasms; bethanechol chloride for hypotonic bladder).
- Discuss the use of a percutaneous stimulator if one is being contemplated. Teach self-catheterization if indicated for neurogenic bladder.

Precautions

- Retrograde cystography is contraindicated during exacerbation of an acute UTI or in patients with an obstruction that prevents passage of a urinary catheter.
- This test shouldn't be performed in patients with urethral evulsion or transection, unless catheter passage and flow of contrast medium are monitored fluoroscopically.

Normal findings

Retrograde cystography shows a bladder with normal contours, capacity, integrity, and urethrovesical angle and with no evidence of tumor, diverticula, or rupture. Vesicoureteral reflux should be absent. The bladder shouldn't be displaced or externally compressed; the bladder wall should be smooth, not thick.

Abnormal findings

Retrograde cystography can identify vesical trabeculae or diverticula, space-occupying lesions (tumors), calculi or gravel, blood clots, high- or low-pressure vesicoureteral reflux, and a hypotonic or hypertonic bladder.

Interfering factors

- Gas, stool, or residual barium from recent diagnostic tests in the bowel (possible poor imaging)

RETROGRADE URETEROPYELOGRAPHY

Retrograde ureteropyelography allows radiographic examination of the renal collecting system after injection of a contrast medium through a ureteral catheter during cystoscopy. The contrast medium is usually iodine-based and, although some of it may be absorbed through the mucous membranes, this test is preferred for patients with hypersensitivity to iodine (in whom I.V. administration of an iodine-based contrast medium, as in excretory urography, is contraindicated). This test is also indicated when visualization of the renal collecting system by excretory urography is inadequate due to inferior films or marked renal insufficiency because retrograde ureteropyelography is not influenced by impaired renal function.

Purpose

- To assess the structure and integrity of the renal collecting system (calyces, renal pelvis, and ureter) (See *Sites and types of obstruction indicated by ureteropyelography.*)

Patient preparation

- Explain to the patient that this test permits visualization of the urinary collecting system.
- If a general anesthetic is to be used, instruct the patient to fast for 8 hours before the test. Generally, he should be well hydrated to ensure adequate urine flow.
- Tell the patient who will perform the test and where it will take place.
- Inform the patient that he'll be positioned on an examination table, with his legs in stirrups, and that the position may be tiring.
- If the patient will be awake throughout the procedure, tell him that he may feel pressure as the instrument is passed and a pressure sensation in the kidney area when the contrast medium is introduced. Also, he may feel an urgency to void.
- Make sure the patient or a responsible family member has signed an informed consent form.
- Just before the procedure, administer prescribed premedication.

Equipment

Cystoscopy setup, ureteral catheters, 10-ml syringes with ureteral adapters, contrast medium, radiographic equipment, tilt table with stirrups

Procedure and posttest care

- Place the patient in lithotomy position. Care must be taken to avoid pressure points or impairment to circulation while his legs are in the stirrups.
- After the patient is anesthetized, the urologist first performs a cystoscopic examination.
- After visual inspection of the bladder, one or both ureters are catheterized with opaque catheters, depending on the condition or abnormality suspected. Radiographic monitoring allows correct positioning of the catheter tip in the renal pelvis.
- The renal pelvis is emptied by gravity drainage or aspiration. About 5 ml of contrast medium is then slowly injected through the catheter using the syringe with the special adapter.
- When adequate filling and opacification have occurred, anteroposterior radiographic films are taken and immediately developed. Lateral and oblique films can be taken, as needed, after the injection of more contrast medium.
- After the radiographs of the renal pelvis are examined, a few more milliliters of contrast medium are injected to outline the ureters as the catheter is slowly withdrawn.
- Delayed films (10 to 15 minutes after complete catheter removal) are then taken to check for retention of the contrast medium, indicating urinary stasis.
- If ureteral obstruction is present, the ureteral catheter may be kept in place and, together with an indwelling urinary catheter, connected to a gravity drainage system until posttest urinary flow is corrected or returns to normal.

Sites and types of obstruction indicated by ureteropyelography

Ureteropyelography may detect a stricture, neoplasm, blood clot, or calculus that obstructs urine flow in the calyces, pelvis, or ureter. Small calculi may remain in the calyces and pelvis or pass down the ureter. A staghorn calculus (a cast of the calyceal and pelvic collecting system) may form from a calculus that stays in the kidney.

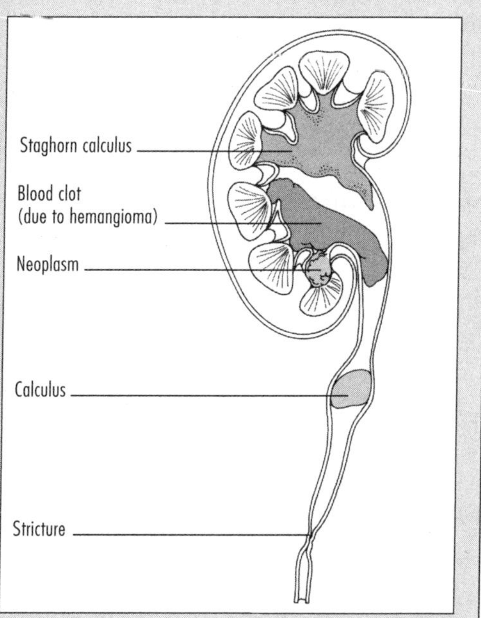

■ Check vital signs every 15 minutes for the first hour, then every 30 minutes for 1 hour, then every hour for the next 2 hours, and then every 4 hours for 24 hours.

■ Monitor fluid intake and urine output for 24 hours. Observe each specimen for hematuria. Gross hematuria or hematuria after the third voiding is abnormal and should be reported. If the patient doesn't void for 8 hours after the procedure, or immediately if the patient feels distress and his bladder is distended, urethral catheterization may be necessary.

Be especially attentive to catheter output if ureteral catheters have been left in place, because inadequate output may reflect catheter obstruction, requiring irrigation. Protect ureteral catheters from dislodgment. Note output amounts for each catheter (indwelling, urinary, urethral) separately; this helps determine the location of an obstruction that is causing reduced output.

■ Administer prescribed analgesics, tub baths, and increased fluid intake for dysuria, which commonly occurs after retrograde ureteropyelography.

■ Watch for and report severe pain in the area of the kidneys as well as any signs of sepsis (such as chills, fever, and hypotension).

■ If irrigation is ordered, never use more than 10 ml sterile saline solution.

Precautions

■ Retrograde ureteropyelography must be done carefully in patients with urinary stasis caused by ureteral obstruction to prevent further injury to the ureter.

■ This test is contraindicated in patients who are pregnant unless the benefits of the procedure outweigh the risks to the fetus.

Normal findings

Following a normal cystoscopic examination, ureteral catheterization, and injection of contrast medium through the catheters, opacification of the pelves and calyces should occur immediately. Normal structures should be outlined clearly and should appear symmetrical in bilateral testing. Ureters should fill uniformly and appear normal in size and course. Inspiratory and expiratory exposures, when superimposed, normally create two outlines of the renal pelvis ¾″ (2 cm) apart.

Abnormal findings

Incomplete or delayed drainage reflects an obstruction, most commonly at the ureteropelvic junction. Enlargement of the components of the collecting system or delayed emptying of contrast medium may indicate obstruction due to tumor, blood clot, stricture, or calculi.

Perinephric inflammation or suppuration often causes fixation of the kidney on the same side, resulting in a single sharp radiographic outline of the collecting system when inspiratory and expiratory exposures are superimposed. Upward, downward, or lateral renal displacement can result from renal abscess or tumor or from perinephric abscess. Neoplasms can cause displacement of either pole or of the entire kidney.

Interfering factors

■ Previous contrast studies or presence of stool or gas in the bowel (possible poor imaging)

ANTEGRADE PYELOGRAPHY

Antegrade pyelography allows examination of the upper collecting system when ureteral obstruction rules out retrograde ureteropyelography or when cystoscopy is contraindicated. It depends on percutaneous needle puncture for injection of contrast medium into the renal pelvis or calyces.

Renal pressure can be measured during this procedure. Also, urine can be collected for cultures and cytologic studies and for evaluation of renal functional reserve before surgery.

After completion of radiographic studies, a nephrostomy tube can be inserted to provide temporary drainage or access for other therapeutic or diagnostic procedures.

Purpose

■ To evaluate obstruction of the upper collecting system by stricture, calculus, clot, or tumor

■ To evaluate hydronephrosis revealed during excretory urography or ultrasonography and to enable placement of a percutaneous nephrostomy tube

■ To evaluate the function of the upper collecting system after ureteral surgery or urinary diversion

■ To assess renal functional reserve before surgery

Patient preparation

■ Explain to the patient that this test allows radiographic examination of the kidney.

- Tell the patient that he may be required to fast for 6 to 8 hours before the test.
- Tell the patient he may receive antimicrobial drugs before and after the procedure.
- Tell the patient who will perform the test and where it will take place.
- Explain to the patient that a needle will be inserted into the kidney after he's given a sedative and a local anesthetic. Explain that urine may be collected from the kidney for testing and that, if necessary, a tube will be left in the kidney for drainage.
- Tell the patient that he may feel mild discomfort during injection of the local anesthetic and contrast medium and that he may also feel transient burning and flushing from the contrast medium.
- Warn the patient that the X-ray machine makes loud, clacking sounds as films are taken.
- Check the patient's history for hypersensitivity reactions to contrast media, iodine, or shellfish. Mark any sensitivities clearly on the chart. Also check the history and recent coagulation studies for indications of bleeding disorders.
- Make sure the patient or a responsible family member has signed an informed consent form.
- Just before the procedure, administer a sedative, if needed, and check that pretest blood work, such as kidney function has been performed if ordered.

Equipment

Radiographic equipment, including a fluoroscope and, possibly, ultrasound equipment; percutaneous nephrostomy tray; manometer; preparatory tray; gloves and sterile containers for specimens; syringes and needles; contrast medium; local anesthetic; emergency resuscitation equipment

Procedure and posttest care

- The patient is placed in a prone position on the X-ray table. The skin over the kidney is cleaned with antiseptic solution, and a local anesthetic is injected.
- Previous urographic films or ultrasound recordings are studied for anatomic landmarks. (It's important to determine if the kidney to be studied is in normal position. If not, the angle of the needle entry must be adjusted during percutaneous puncture.)
- Under guidance of fluoroscopy or ultrasonography, the percutaneous needle is inserted below the 12th rib at the level of the transverse process of the 2nd lumbar vertebra. Aspiration of urine confirms that the needle has reached the dilated collecting system, which is usually 2¾″ to 3⅛″ (7 to 8 cm) below the skin surface in adults.
- Flexible tubing is connected to the needle to prevent displacement during the procedure. If intrarenal pressure is to be measured, the manometer is connected to the tubing as soon as it's in place. Urine specimens are then taken if needed.
- An amount of urine equal to the amount of contrast medium to be injected is withdrawn to prevent overdistention of the collecting system.
- The contrast medium is injected under fluoroscopic guidance. Posteroanterior, oblique, and anteroposterior radiographs are taken. Ureteral peristalsis is observed on the fluoroscope screen to evaluate obstruction.
- A percutaneous nephrostomy tube is inserted if drainage is needed because of increased renal pressure, dilation, or intrarenal reflux. If drainage isn't needed, the catheter is withdrawn and a sterile dressing is applied.
- Check vital signs every 15 minutes for the first hour, every 30 minutes for the second hour, and every 2 hours for the next 24 hours.

- Check dressings for bleeding, hematoma, or urine leakage at the puncture site at each check of vital signs. For bleeding, apply pressure. For a hematoma, apply warm soaks. Report urine leakage or the patient's failure to void within 8 hours.
- Monitor fluid intake and urine output for 24 hours. Observe each specimen for hematuria. Report hematuria if it persists after the third voiding.
- Watch for and report signs of sepsis or extravasation of contrast medium (chills, fever, rapid pulse or respirations, and hypotension).

CLINICAL ALERT *Also watch for and report signs that adjacent organs have been punctured, such as pain in the abdomen or flank, or pneumothorax (sudden onset of pleuritic chest pain, dyspnea, tachypnea, decreased breath sounds on the affected side, and tachycardia).*

- If a nephrostomy tube is inserted, check to make sure it's patent and draining well. Irrigate with 5 to 7 ml of sterile saline, as ordered, to maintain patency.
- Administer prescribed antibiotics for several days after the procedure and prescribed analgesics.
- If hydronephrosis is present, monitor intake and output, edema, hypertension, flank pain, acid-base status, and glucose level.

Precautions

- Antegrade pyelography is contraindicated in patients with bleeding disorders.
- Watch for signs of hypersensitivity to the contrast medium.
- This procedure is contraindicated in patients who are pregnant unless the benefits outweigh the risks to the fetus.

Normal findings

After injection of contrast medium, the upper collecting system should fill uniformly and appear normal in size and course. Normal structures should be outlined clearly.

Abnormal findings

Enlargements of the upper collecting system and parts of the ureteropelvic junction indicate obstruction. Antegrade pyelography shows the degree of dilation, clearly defines obstructions, and demonstrates intrarenal reflux. In hydronephrosis, the ureteropelvic junction shows marked distention. Results of recent surgery or urinary diversion will be obvious; for example, a ureteral stent or a dilated stenotic area will be clearly visualized.

Intrarenal pressure greater than 20 cm H_2O indicates obstruction. Cultures or cytologic studies of urine specimens taken during antegrade pyelography can confirm antegrade pyelonephrosis or malignancy.

Interfering factors

- Recent barium procedures, or stool or gas in the bowel (possible poor imaging)
- Obesity (possible difficulty in needle placement)

EXCRETORY UROGRAPHY

The cornerstone of a urologic workup, excretory urography (also called intravenous pyelography) requires I.V. administration of a contrast medium and allows visualization of the renal parenchyma, calyces, and pelvis, as well as the ureters, bladder and, in some cases, the urethra.

In some facilities, a nonenhanced computed tomography scan of the urinary tract is commonly performed instead of this test if urinary tract stones are suspected.

Purpose

- To evaluate the structure and excretory function of the kidneys, ureters, and bladder
- To support a differential diagnosis of renovascular hypertension

Patient preparation

- Explain to the patient that this test helps to evaluate the structure and function of the urinary tract.
- Make sure the patient is well hydrated; then instruct him to fast for 8 hours before the test. Tell him who will perform the test and where it will take place.
- Inform the patient that he may experience a transient burning sensation and metallic taste when the contrast medium is injected. Tell him to report other sensations he may experience.
- Warn the patient that the X-ray machine may make loud, clacking sounds during the test.
- Make sure the patient or a responsible family member has signed an informed consent form, if required.
- Check the patient's history for hypersensitivity to iodine, iodine-containing foods, or contrast media containing iodine. Mark sensitivities on the chart and notify the physician.
- Administer a laxative, if necessary, the night before the test, to minimize poor resolution of X-ray films due to stool and gas in the GI tract.

Equipment

Contrast medium (sodium diatrizoate or iothalamate, or meglumine diatrizoate or iothalamate); 50-ml syringe (or I.V. container and tubing); 19G to 21G needle, catheter, or butterfly needle; venipuncture equipment (tourniquet, antiseptic, adhesive bandage); X-ray table, X-ray and tomographic equipment, emergency resuscitation equipment

Procedure and posttest care

- The patient is placed in a supine position on the X-ray table.
- A kidney-ureter-bladder radiograph is exposed, developed, and studied for gross abnormalities of the urinary system. In the absence of any such abnormality, contrast medium is injected (dosage varies according to age), and the patient is observed for signs of hypersensitivity (flushing, nausea, vomiting, hives, or dyspnea).
- The first radiograph, visualizing the renal parenchyma, is obtained about 1 minute after the injection, possibly supplemented by tomography if small space-occupying masses, such as cysts or tumors, are suspected.
- Films are then exposed at regular intervals — usually 5, 10, and 15 or 20 minutes after the injection.
- Ureteral compression is performed after the 5-minute film is exposed. This can be accomplished through inflation of two small rubber bladders placed on the abdomen on both sides of the midline, secured by a fastener wrapped around the patient's torso. The inflated bladders occlude the ureters without causing the patient discomfort, and facilitate retention of the contrast medium by the upper urinary tract. (Ureteral compression is contraindicated by ureteral calculi, aortic aneurysm, pregnancy, or recent abdominal trauma or surgical procedure.)
- After the 10-minute film is exposed, ureteral compression is released. As the contrast flows into the lower urinary tract, another film is taken of the lower

halves of both ureters and then, finally, one is taken of the bladder.

- At the end of the procedure, the patient voids, and another film is made immediately to visualize residual bladder content or mucosal abnormalities of the bladder or urethra.
- If a hematoma develops at the injection site, ease the patient's discomfort by applying warm soaks.
- Observe for delayed reactions to the contrast medium.
- Continue I.V. fluids or provide oral fluid to increase hydration. Administer medications as ordered.

Precautions

- Premedication with corticosteroids may be indicated for patients with severe asthma or a history of sensitivity to the contrast medium.
- This test may be contraindicated in patients with abnormal renal function (as evidenced by increased creatinine and blood urea nitrogen levels) and in children or elderly patients with actual or potential dehydration.

Normal findings

The kidneys, ureters, and bladder show no gross evidence of soft- or hard-tissue lesions. Prompt visualization of the contrast medium in the kidneys demonstrates bilateral renal parenchyma and pelvicalyceal systems of normal conformity. The ureters and bladder should be outlined and the postvoiding radiograph should show no mucosal abnormalities and minimal residual urine.

Abnormal findings

Excretory urography can demonstrate many abnormalities of the urinary system, including renal or ureteral calculi; abnormal size, shape, or structure of kidneys, ureters, or bladder; supernumerary or absent kidney; polycystic kidney disease associated with renal hypertrophy; redundant pelvis or ureter; space-occupying lesion; pyelonephrosis; renal tuberculosis; hydronephrosis; and renovascular hypertension.

Interfering factors

- End-stage renal disease, stool or gas in the colon (possible poor imaging)
- Insufficient injection of contrast medium, a recent barium enema, GI or gallbladder series (possible poor imaging)

RENAL ANGIOGRAPHY

Renal angiography requires arterial injection of a contrast medium and permits radiographic examination of the renal vasculature and parenchyma. As the contrast pervades the renal vasculature, rapid-sequence radiographs show the vessels during three phases of filling: arterial, nephrographic, and venous.

This procedure usually follows standard bolus aortography, which shows individual variations in number, size, and condition of the main renal arteries, aberrant vessels, and the relationship of the renal arteries to the aorta.

Purpose

- To demonstrate the configuration of total renal vasculature before surgical procedures
- To determine the cause of renovascular hypertension, such as from stenosis, thrombotic occlusions, emboli, and aneurysms
- To evaluate chronic renal disease or renal failure
- To investigate renal masses and renal trauma
- To detect complications following renal transplantation, such as a nonfunctioning shunt or rejection of the donor organ

- To differentiate highly vascular tumors from avascular cysts

Patient preparation

- Explain to the patient that this test permits visualization of the kidneys, blood vessels, and functional units and aids in diagnosing renal disease or masses.
- Instruct the patient to fast for 8 hours before the test and to drink extra fluids the day before the test and the day after the test to maintain adequate hydration (or to start an I.V. line, if needed). Oral medication may be continued; a special order is needed for patients with diabetes.
- Tell the patient he may receive a laxative or an enema the evening before the test.
- Tell the patient who will perform the test and where it will take place.
- Describe the procedure to the patient and inform him that he may experience transient discomfort (flushing, burning sensation, and nausea) during injection of the contrast medium.
- Make sure the patient or a responsible family member has signed an informed consent form.
- Check the patient's history for hypersensitivity to iodine-based contrast media or iodine-containing foods such as shellfish. Mark sensitivities on the chart and inform the physician because the patient may require prophylactic antiallergenics (diphenhydramine or corticosteroids).
- Administer prescribed medications (usually a sedative and a narcotic analgesic) before the test.
- Instruct the patient to put on a gown and to remove all metallic objects that may interfere with test results.
- Ask the patient to void before leaving the unit.
- Record baseline vital signs. Ensure that recent laboratory test results (blood urea nitrogen and serum creatinine levels and bleeding studies) are documented on the patient's chart. Verification of adequate renal function and adequate clotting ability is vital. Evaluate peripheral pulse sites and mark them for easy access in postprocedure assessment.

Equipment

Image-intensified fluoroscope with television monitor, high-powered radiographic equipment, pressure-injection device, rapid cassette changer, polyethylene radiopaque vascular catheters, guide wire, contrast material (such as Hypaque or Renografin), preparation tray with 70% alcohol or povidone-iodine solution, emergency resuscitation equipment

Procedure and posttest care

- The patient is placed in a supine position, and a peripheral I.V. infusion is started. The skin over the arterial puncture site is cleaned with antiseptic solution and a local anesthetic is injected.
- The femoral artery is punctured and, under fluoroscopic visualization, cannulated. (If a femoral pulse is absent or the artery is convoluted or plaque-ridden, percutaneous transaxillary, transbrachial, or translumbar catheterization may be performed instead.)
- After passing the flexible guide wire through the artery, the cannula is withdrawn, leaving several inches of wire in the lumen.
- A polyethylene catheter is passed over the wire and advanced, under fluoroscopic guidance, up the femoroiliac vessels to the aorta. The guide wire is removed and the catheter is flushed with heparin flush solution.
- The contrast medium is injected and screening aortograms are taken before proceeding.

- On completion of the aortographic study, a renal catheter is exchanged for the vascular catheter.
- To determine the position of the renal arteries and ensure that the tip of the catheter is in the lumen, a test bolus (3 to 5 ml) of contrast medium is injected immediately.
- If the patient has no adverse reaction to the contrast medium, 20 to 25 ml of the substance is injected just below the origin of the renal arteries.
- A series of rapid-sequence X-ray films of the filling of the renal vascular tree is exposed.
- If additional selective studies are required, the catheter remains in place while the films are examined. If the films are satisfactory, the catheter is removed.
- Apply a sterile sponge firmly to the puncture site for 15 minutes.
- Before the patient is returned to his room, observe the puncture site for hematoma.
- Keep the patient flat in bed and instruct him to keep the punctured leg straight for at least 6 hours or as otherwise ordered.
- Check vital signs every 15 minutes for 1 hour, then every 30 minutes for 2 hours, and then every hour until they stabilize.
- Monitor popliteal and dorsalis pedis pulses for adequate perfusion at least every hour for 4 hours. Note the color and temperature of the involved extremity and compare with the uninvolved extremity. Watch for signs of pain or paresthesia in the involved limb.
- Watch for bleeding or hematomas at the injection site. Keep the pressure dressing in place and check for bleeding when you check all vital signs. If bleeding occurs, promptly notify the physician and apply direct pressure or a sandbag to the site.
- Apply cold compresses to the puncture site to reduce edema and lessen pain.
- Provide extra fluids (2,000 to 3,000 ml in the 24-hour period after the test) to prevent nephrotoxicity from the contrast medium.
- Monitor the patient for anaphylaxis from the contrast medium (signs include cardiorespiratory distress, renal failure, and shock).
- Monitor the patient for atrial arrhythmias and evaluate aspartate aminotransferase and lactate dehydrogenase activity if renal stenosis is observed.

Precautions

- Renal angiography is contraindicated during pregnancy and in patients with bleeding tendencies, allergy to contrast media, and renal failure caused by end-stage renal disease.

Normal findings

Renal arteriographs show normal arborization of the vascular tree and normal architecture of the renal parenchyma.

Abnormal findings

Renal tumors usually show hypervascularity; renal cysts typically appear as clearly delineated, radiolucent masses. Renal artery stenosis caused by arteriosclerosis produces a noticeable constriction in the blood vessels, usually within the proximal portion of its length; this is a crucial finding in confirming renovascular hypertension. Renal artery dysplasia, unlike renal artery stenosis, usually affects the middle and distal portions of the vessel. Alternating aneurysms and stenotic regions give this rare disorder a characteristic beads-on-a-string appearance.

In renal infarction, blood vessels may appear to be absent or cut off, with the normal tissue replaced by scar tissue. Another typical finding is the appearance of triangular areas of infarcted tissue near the periphery of the affected kidney. The kidney itself may appear shrunken due to tissue scarring.

Renal angiography may also detect renal artery aneurysms (saccular or fusiform) and renal arteriovenous fistula with abnormal widening of and direct passage between the renal artery and renal vein. Destruction, distortion, and fibrosis of renal tissue with areas of reduced and tortuous vascularity may be noted in severe or chronic pyelonephritis, and an increase in capsular vessels with abnormal intrarenal circulation may indicate renal abscesses or inflammatory masses.

When angiography is used to evaluate renal trauma, it may detect intrarenal hematoma, parenchymal laceration, shattered kidneys, and areas of infarction. Renal angiography may also be useful in distinguishing pseudotumors from tumors or cysts, in evaluating the volume of residual functioning renal tissue in hydronephrosis, and in evaluating donors and recipients before and after renal transplantation.

Interfering factors

- Patient movement
- Recent contrast studies, such as barium enema or an upper GI series (possible poor imaging)
- Presence of stool or gas in the GI tract (possible poor imaging)

RENAL VENOGRAPHY

Renal venography is a relatively simple procedure allowing radiographic examination of the main renal veins and their tributaries. In this test, contrast medium is injected by percutaneous catheter passed through the femoral vein and inferior vena cava into the renal vein. Indications for renal venography include renal vein thrombosis, tumor, and venous anomalies.

Purpose

- To detect renal vein thrombosis
- To evaluate renal vein compression due to extrinsic tumors or retroperitoneal fibrosis
- To assess renal tumors and detect invasion of the renal vein or inferior vena cava
- To detect venous anomalies and defects
- To differentiate renal agenesis from a small kidney
- To collect renal venous blood samples for evaluation of renovascular hypertension

Patient preparation

- Explain to the patient that this test permits radiographic study of the renal veins.
- If prescribed, instruct the patient to fast for 4 hours before the test.
- Tell the patient who will perform the test and where it will take place.
- Inform the patient that a catheter will be inserted into a vein in the groin area after he's given a sedative and a local anesthetic.
- Tell the patient that he may feel mild discomfort during injection of the local anesthetic and contrast medium and that he may also feel transient burning and flushing from the contrast medium.
- Warn the patient that the X-ray equipment may make loud, clacking noises as the films are taken.
- Check the patient's history for hypersensitivity to contrast media, iodine, or iodine-containing foods, such as shell-

fish. Mark sensitivities on the chart and report them to the physician.

■ Check the patient's history and any coagulation studies for indications of bleeding disorders.

■ If renin assays will be done, check the patient's diet and medications, and consult with the health care team. As ordered, restrict the patient's salt intake and discontinue antihypertensive drugs, diuretics, estrogen, and oral contraceptives.

■ Make sure the patient or a responsible family member has signed an informed consent form.

■ Just before the procedure, administer a sedative if necessary.

■ Record baseline vital signs. Make sure pretest blood urea nitrogen and urine creatinine levels are adequate because the kidneys clear contrast media.

Equipment

Radiographic equipment, renal venography tray with flexible guide wires, polyethylene radiopaque vascular catheters, needle and cannula or 18G needle, three-way stopcock, and flexible tubing; preparatory tray; syringes and needles; contrast medium; local anesthetic; emergency resuscitation equipment

Procedure and posttest care

■ The patient is placed in a supine position on the X-ray table, with his abdomen centered over the film. The skin over the right femoral vein near the groin is cleaned with antiseptic solution and draped. (The left femoral vein or jugular veins may be used.)

■ A local anesthetic is injected and the femoral vein is cannulated.

■ Under fluoroscopic guidance, a guide wire is threaded a short distance through the cannula, which is then removed. A catheter is passed over the wire into the inferior vena cava.

■ When catheterization of the femoral vein is contraindicated, the right antecubital vein is punctured, and the catheter is inserted and advanced through the right atrium of the heart into the inferior vena cava.

■ A test bolus of contrast medium is injected to determine that the vena cava is patent. If so, the catheter is advanced into the right renal vein and contrast medium (usually 20 to 40 ml) is injected.

■ When studies of the right renal vasculature are completed, the catheter is withdrawn into the vena cava, rotated, and guided into the left renal vein.

■ If visualization of the renal venous tributaries is indicated, epinephrine can be injected into the ipsilateral renal artery by catheter before contrast medium is injected into the renal vein. Epinephrine temporarily blocks arterial flow and allows filling of distal intrarenal veins. Obstructing the artery briefly with a balloon catheter produces the same effect.

■ After anteroposterior films are made, the patient lies prone for posteroanterior films.

■ For renin assays, blood samples are withdrawn under fluoroscopy within 15 minutes after venography. After catheter removal, apply pressure to the site for 15 minutes and put on a dressing.

■ Check vital signs and distal pulses every 15 minutes for the first hour, then every 30 minutes for the second hour, and then every 2 hours for 24 hours. Keep the patient on bed rest for 2 hours.

■ Observe the puncture site for bleeding or hematoma when checking vital signs; if bleeding occurs, apply pressure. Report bleeding as soon as possible.

■ Report signs of vein perforation, embolism, and extravasation of contrast medium. These include chills, fever, rapid pulse and respiration, hypotension, dyspnea, and chest, abdominal, or flank pain. Also report complaints of paresthesia or pain in the catheterized limb — symptoms of nerve irritation or vascular compromise.

- Administer prescribed sedatives and antimicrobials.
- Prepare for further arteriography or surgery as ordered.
- As ordered, instruct the patient to resume his normal diet and any discontinued medications.
- Instruct the patient to increase fluid intake (unless contraindicated) to help clear contrast media.

Precautions

- Renal venography is contraindicated in severe thrombosis of the inferior vena cava.
- The guide wire and catheter should be advanced carefully if severe renal vein thrombosis is suspected.
- Watch for signs of hypersensitivity to the contrast medium.

Normal findings

After injection of the contrast medium, opacification of the renal vein and tributaries should occur immediately.

Normal renin content of venous blood in an adult in a supine position is 1.5 to 1.6 ng/ml/hour.

Abnormal findings

Occlusion of the renal vein near the inferior vena cava or the kidney indicates renal vein thrombosis. If the clot is outlined by contrast medium, it may look like a filling defect. However, a clot can usually be identified because it's within the lumen and less sharply outlined than a filling defect. Collateral venous channels, which opacify with retrograde filling during contrast injection, often surround the occlusion. Complete occlusion prolongs transit of the contrast medium through the renal veins.

A filling defect of the renal vein may indicate obstruction or compression by extrinsic tumor or retroperitoneal fibrosis. A renal tumor that invades the renal vein or inferior vena cava usually produces a filling defect with a sharply defined border.

Venous anomalies are indicated by opacification of abnormally positioned or clustered vessels. Absence of a renal vein differentiates renal agenesis from a small kidney.

Elevated renin content in renal venous blood usually indicates essential renovascular hypertension when assay results correspond for both kidneys. Elevated renin levels in one kidney indicate a unilateral lesion and usually require further evaluation by arteriography.

Interfering factors

- Recent contrast studies or stool or gas in the bowel
- Failure to restrict salt, antihypertensive drugs, diuretics, estrogen, and oral contraceptives

VOIDING CYSTOURETHROGRAPHY

In voiding cystourethrography, a contrast medium is instilled by gentle syringe pressure or gravity into the bladder through a urethral catheter. Fluoroscopic films or overhead radiographs demonstrate bladder filling, and then show excretion of the contrast medium as the patient voids.

Purpose

- To detect abnormalities of the bladder and urethra, such as vesicoureteral reflux, neurogenic bladder, prostatic hyperplasia, urethral strictures, or diverticula

Patient preparation

- Explain to the patient that this test permits assessment of the bladder and the urethra.
- Inform the patient that he need not restrict food or fluids.
- Tell the patient who will perform the test and where it will take place.
- Inform the patient that a catheter will be inserted into his bladder and a contrast medium will be instilled through the catheter.
- Tell the patient he may experience a feeling of fullness and an urge to void when the contrast medium is instilled. Explain that X-rays will be taken of his bladder and urethra and that he'll be asked to assume various positions.
- Make sure the patient or a responsible family member has signed an informed consent form, if required.
- Check the patient's history for hypersensitivity to contrast media or iodine-containing foods such as shellfish; note sensitivities on the chart and notify the physician.
- Just before the procedure, administer a sedative, if prescribed.

Equipment

Radiographic equipment (fluoroscope and screen and accessories for spot-film radiography), indwelling urinary catheter, standard urographic contrast medium (up to 1,000 ml of 15% solution), 50-ml syringe (for infants) or gravity-feed apparatus

Procedure and posttest care

- The patient is placed in a supine position and an indwelling urinary catheter is inserted into the bladder.
- The contrast medium is instilled through the catheter until the bladder is full.
- The catheter is clamped and X-ray films are exposed with the patient in supine, oblique, and lateral positions.
- The catheter is removed and the patient assumes right oblique position (right leg flexed to 90 degrees, left leg extended, penis parallel to right leg) and begins to void.
- Four high-speed exposures of the bladder and urethra, coned down to reduce radiation exposure, are usually made on one film during voiding.
- If the right oblique view doesn't delineate both ureters, the patient is asked to stop urinating and to begin again in the left oblique position.
- The most reliable voiding cystourethrograms are obtained with the patient recumbent. Patients who can't void recumbent may do so standing (not sitting).
- Expression cystourethrography may have to be performed, under a general anesthetic, for young children who cannot void on command.
- Observe and record the time, color, and volume of the patient's voidings. Report hematuria if present after the third voiding.
- Encourage the patient to drink large quantities of fluids to reduce burning on urination and to flush out residual contrast medium.
- Monitor for chills and fever related to extravasation of contrast material or urinary sepsis.
- If stricture is present, prepare for surgery as indicated.
- Monitor for symptoms of urinary tract infection.

Precautions

■ Voiding cystourethrography is contraindicated in patients with an acute or exacerbated urethral or bladder infection, or an acute urethral injury.
■ Hypersensitivity to the contrast medium may also contraindicate this test.

Normal findings

Delineation of the bladder and urethra shows normal structure and function, with no regurgitation of contrast medium into the ureters.

Abnormal findings

Voiding cystourethrography may show urethral stricture, vesical or urethral diverticula, ureterocele, cystocele, prostate enlargement, vesicoureteral reflux, or neurogenic bladder. The severity and location of such abnormalities are then evaluated to determine whether surgical intervention is necessary.

Interfering factors

■ Embarrassment (inhibits patient from voiding on command)
■ Interrupted or less vigorous voiding, muscle spasm or incomplete sphincter relaxation (due to urethral trauma during catheterization)
■ Presence of contrast media from recent tests, stool, or gas in the bowel (possible poor imaging)

WHITAKER TEST

Also called a pressure or flow study, the Whitaker test correlates radiographic findings with measurements of pressure and flow in the kidneys and ureters, and facilitates assessment of the upper urinary tract's efficiency in emptying.

In this procedure, radiographs are taken after urethral catheterization, I.V. administration of a contrast medium, percutaneous cannulation of the kidney, and renal perfusion of the contrast medium. Intrarenal and bladder pressures are then measured.

Purpose

■ To identify and evaluate renal obstruction

Patient preparation

■ Explain to the patient that this test helps to evaluate kidney function.
■ Instruct the patient to avoid food and fluids for at least 4 hours before the test.
■ Tell the patient who will perform the test, where it will take place, and that it will take about 1 hour.
■ Describe the procedure to the patient. Inform him that he'll be given a mild sedative before the test, that he may feel some discomfort during insertion of the urethral catheter and injection of the local anesthetic, and that he may also feel transient burning and flushing after injection of the contrast medium.
■ Warn the patient that the X-ray machine makes loud clacking sounds as films are exposed.
■ Make sure the patient or a responsible family member has signed an informed consent form.
■ Check the patient's history and recent coagulation studies for bleeding disorders. Also check for hypersensitivity reactions to iodine, iodine-containing foods, such as shellfish, and contrast media. Mark sensitivities on the chart and inform the physician.
■ Just before the procedure, instruct the patient to void, and administer prescribed sedatives. Check that pretest blood work (such as kidney function) was done if ordered.

■ Administer prophylactic antimicrobials, as prescribed, to prevent infection from instrumentation.

Equipment

Radiographic equipment, perfusion pump with 50-ml luer-lock syringe, transducer and recorder, manometer, three-way and four-way stopcocks, I.V. extension set, manometer lines, one double-male connector to connect urethral catheter and stopcock, sterile water and normal saline solution, contrast medium, local anesthetic, percutaneous puncture tray with 4″ to 6″ 18G Longdwel cannula, gloves, preparatory tray, emergency resuscitation equipment

Procedure and posttest care

■ Place the patient in a supine position on the X-ray table. The table must be horizontal and must remain at the same height throughout the test.

■ To prepare for measurement of bladder pressure, a urethral catheter is placed in the bladder. The patient's bladder may be emptied, depending on his suspected condition. (If an obstruction is suspected, the patient will be asked to void before the test. If a condition, such as a bladder hypertonia, is the suspected cause of insufficient emptying, he shouldn't void.)

■ A plain film of the urinary tract is taken to obtain anatomic landmarks.

■ The catheter is then connected to a three-way stopcock on a manometer line linked to the transducer and recorder. The line is then filled with sterile water.

■ Contrast medium is injected I.V.

■ The patient is placed prone and made comfortable with pillows. When urography demonstrates contrast medium in the kidney, the skin is cleaned with antiseptic solution and draped.

■ Pressure recording equipment is calibrated. The renal perfusion tubing is filled with sterile water or normal saline solution and held at the level of the kidney.

■ Local anesthetic is injected and an incision is made through the flank for cannulation of the kidney.

■ The patient is asked to hold his breath while the needle is inserted into the renal pelvis. Aspiration of urine confirms that the needle is in position.

■ The cannula is then connected by a four-way stopcock to the perfusion tubing and the manometer line.

■ Perfusion of the contrast medium is begun, serial X-rays are taken, and intrarenal pressure is measured. Bladder pressure is then measured.

■ Perfusion continues at a steady rate of 10 ml/minute until bladder pressure is constant. When pressure holds steady for a few minutes and adequate films have been taken, perfusion is discontinued. Residual fluid is aspirated from the kidney, the cannula is removed, and the wound is dressed.

■ Keep the patient in a supine position for 12 hours after the test.

■ Check vital signs every 15 minutes for the first hour, every 30 minutes for the next hour, and then every 2 hours for 24 hours.

■ Check the puncture site for bleeding, hematoma, or urine leakage each time vital signs are checked. If bleeding occurs, apply pressure. If a hematoma develops, apply warm soaks. Report urine leakage.

■ Monitor fluid intake and urine output for 24 hours. Report hematuria that persists after the third voiding.

■ Watch for signs of sepsis (chills, fever, tachycardia, tachypnea, or hypotension) or similar signs of extravasation of the contrast medium.

■ Inform the patient that colicky pains are transient.

■ Administer prescribed analgesics.

■ Administer antimicrobials for several days after the test as ordered to prevent infection.
■ If an obstruction is present, prepare the patient for surgery.

Precautions

■ Contraindications include bleeding disorders and severe infection.

Normal findings

Visualization of the kidney after gradual perfusion of the contrast medium shows normal outlines of the renal pelvis and calyces. The ureter should fill uniformly and appear normal in size and course.

The normal value for intrarenal pressure is 15 cm H_2O. The normal value for bladder pressure may range from 5 to 10 cm H_2O.

Abnormal findings

Enlargement of the renal pelvis, calyces, or ureteropelvic junction may indicate obstruction. Subtraction of bladder pressure from intrarenal pressure results in a differential that aids diagnosis. A differential of 12 to 15 cm H_2O indicates obstruction. A differential of less than 10 cm H_2O indicates a bladder abnormality, such as hypertonia or neurogenic bladder.

Interfering factors

■ Recent barium studies or stool or gas in the bowel (hinders accurate needle placement and visualization of the upper urinary tract)
■ Patient movement

REPRODUCTIVE SYSTEM

MAMMOGRAPHY

Mammography is used as a screening test for breast cancer. It helps to detect breast cysts or tumors, especially those not palpable on physical examination. Biopsy of suspicious areas may be required to confirm malignancy. Mammography may follow screening procedures such as ultrasonography or thermography. (See *Using ultrasonography to detect breast cancer,* page 622.) Although mammography can detect 90% to 95% of breast cancers, this test produces many false-positive results.

The American College of Radiologists and the American Cancer Society have established separate guidelines for the use and potential risks of mammography. Both groups agree that despite low radiation levels, the test is contraindicated during pregnancy. Magnetic resonance imaging, which is highly sensitive, is becoming a more popular method of breast imaging; however, it isn't very specific and leads to biopsies of many benign lesions.

For patients at high risk for breast cancer, a newer test, ductal lavage, may identify abnormal cells before they are large enough to form a tumor. (See *Ductal lavage,* page 623.)

Purpose

■ To screen for malignant breast tumors
■ To investigate palpable and unpalpable breast masses, breast pain, or nipple discharge
■ To help differentiate between benign breast disease and breast cancer

Using ultrasonography to detect breast cancer

Ultrasonography is especially useful for diagnosing tumors less than ¼" (0.6 cm) in diameter and in distinguishing cysts from solid tumors in dense breast tissue. As in other ultrasound techniques, a transducer sends a beam of high-frequency sound waves through the patient's skin and into the breast. The sound waves are then processed and displayed for interpretation.

A benefit to ultrasonography is that it can show all areas of the breast, including the area close to the chest wall, which is hard to study with X-rays. When used as an adjunct to mammography, ultrasound increases diagnostic accuracy; when used alone, it's more accurate than mammography in examining the denser breast tissue of young patients.

■ To monitor patients with breast cancer who have been treated with breast-conserving surgery and radiation

Patient preparation

■ Assess the patient's understanding of the test, answer her questions, and correct any misconceptions.
■ Tell the patient who will perform the test and where it will take place.
■ Tell the patient not to use underarm deodorant or powder on the day of the examination.
■ If the patient has breast implants, tell her to inform the staff when she schedules the mammogram so that a technologist familiar with imaging implants is on duty.
■ Inform the patient that although the test takes only about 15 minutes to perform, she may be asked to wait while the films are checked to make sure they're readable. Advise her that there's a high rate of false-positive results.
■ Just before the test, give the patient a gown to wear that opens in the front, and ask her to remove all jewelry and clothing above the waist.

Procedure and posttest care

■ The patient stands and is asked to rest one of her breasts on a table above an X-ray cassette.
■ The compression plate is placed on the breast and the patient is told to hold her breath. A radiograph is taken of the craniocaudal view. The machine is rotated, the breast is compressed again, and a radiograph of the lateral view is taken.
■ The procedure is repeated on the other breast.
■ After the films are developed, they're checked to make sure they're readable.

Normal findings

A normal mammogram reveals normal duct, glandular tissue, and fat architecture. No abnormal masses or calcifications should be seen.

Abnormal findings

Well-outlined, regular, and clear spots suggest benign cysts; irregular, poorly outlined, and opaque areas suggest a malignant tumor. Malignant tumors are generally solitary and unilateral; benign cysts tend to occur bilaterally. Findings that suggest cancer require further tests, such as biopsy, for confirmation.

Interfering factors

■ Powders or salves on the breasts (possible false-positive results)
■ Failure to remove jewelry and clothing (possible false-positive results or poor imaging)
■ Glandular breasts (common under age 30), active lactation, and previous breast surgery (possible poor imaging)
■ Breast implants (may hinder detection of masses)

Ductal lavage

Ductal lavage is a minimally invasive procedure that's used to determine the existence of abnormal cells inside the milk ducts, where most breast cancer originates. Without the procedure, 8 to 10 years may pass before the abnormal cells, which indicate a significantly increased risk for breast cancer, grow into a tumor large enough to be detected by either mammogram or physical exam.

The procedure may be performed on an outpatient basis or in the physician's office. An anesthetic cream is applied to the patient's nipple area and gentle suction is used to draw tiny amounts of fluid from the milk ducts to the nipple surface, which helps the physician locate the milk duct's natural openings. A thin catheter is then inserted into a milk duct opening and a small amount of anesthetic is infused into it. Saline is introduced into the catheter to gently rinse the duct and collect cells. The ductal cell fluid is then withdrawn through the catheter, deposited into a collection vial, and sent to a cytology laboratory for analysis.

High-risk women can undergo repeated testing or may opt for early intervention, such as tamoxifen chemotherapy or surgical intervention.

HYSTEROSALPINGOGRAPHY

Hysterosalpingography is a radiologic examination for visualizing the uterine cavity, the fallopian tubes, and the peritubal area. In this procedure, fluoroscopic X-ray films are taken as a contrast medium flows through the uterus and the fallopian tubes.

This test is generally performed as part of an infertility study. Although ultrasonography has virtually replaced hysterosalpingography in the detection of foreign bodies, such as a dislodged intrauterine device, it can't evaluate tubal patency, which is the main purpose of hysterosalpingography. Risks of this test include uterine perforation, intravascular injection of the contrast medium, and exposure to potentially harmful radiation.

Purpose

- To confirm tubal abnormalities, such as adhesions and occlusion
- To confirm uterine abnormalities, such as the presence of foreign bodies, congenital malformations, and traumatic injuries
- To confirm the presence of fistulas or peritubal adhesions

Patient preparation

- Explain to the patient that this test confirms uterine and fallopian tube abnormalities.
- Tell the patient who will perform the test and where it will take place. The test should be performed 2 to 5 days after menstruation ends.
- Advise the patient that she may experience moderate cramping from the procedure; however, she may receive a mild sedative, such as diazepam, or a nonprescription prostaglandin inhibitor, if ordered, 30 minutes before the procedure.

Equipment

Antiseptic cleaning solution, sterile needle, contrast medium, vaginal speculum, tenaculum, cannula with acorn tip on one end and luer-lock on the other, radiograph machine with fluoroscopic capabilities

Procedure and posttest care

■ With the patient in lithotomy position, a scout film is taken.
■ A speculum is inserted in the vagina, the tenaculum is placed on the cervix, and the cervix is cleaned.
■ The cannula is inserted into the cervix and anchored to the tenaculum. After the contrast medium is injected through the cannula, the uterus and the fallopian tubes are viewed fluoroscopically, and radiographs are taken. To take oblique views, the X-ray table may be tilted or the patient asked to change position. Films may also be taken later to evaluate spillage of contrast medium into the peritoneal cavity.
■ Watch for signs of infection, such as fever, pain, increased pulse rate, malaise, and muscle ache.
■ Assure the patient that cramps and vagal reaction (slow pulse rate, nausea, and dizziness) are transient.

Precautions

■ Hysterosalpingography is contraindicated in patients with menses, undiagnosed vaginal bleeding, or pelvic inflammatory disease.
■ Watch for an allergic reaction to the contrast medium, such as urticaria, itching, or hypotension.

Normal findings

Normally, radiographs reveal a symmetrical uterine cavity; the contrast medium courses through fallopian tubes of normal caliber, spills freely into the peritoneal cavity, and doesn't leak from the uterus.

Abnormal findings

An asymmetrical uterus suggests intrauterine adhesions or masses, such as fibroids or foreign bodies; impaired contrast flow through the fallopian tubes suggests partial or complete blockage, resulting from intraluminal agglutination, extrinsic compression by adhesions, or perifimbrial adhesions; leakage of the contrast medium through the uterine wall suggests fistulas. Laparoscopy with contrast medium confirms positive or equivocal findings.

Interfering factors

■ Tubal spasm or excessive traction (may show as a stricture in normal fallopian tubes)
■ Excessive traction (may displace adhesions, making the fallopian tubes appear normal)

SKELETAL SYSTEM

VERTEBRAL RADIOGRAPHY

Vertebral radiography visualizes all or part of the vertebral column. A commonly performed test, it's used to evaluate the vertebrae for deformities, fractures, dislocations, tumors, and other abnormalities. Bone films determine bone density, texture, erosion, and changes in bone relationships. X-rays of the cortex of the bone reveal the presence of any widening, narrowing, and signs of irregularity. Joint X-rays can reveal the presence of fluid, spur formation, narrowing, and changes in the joint structure.

Anatomically, the vertebral column is divided in descending order into five segments: cervical, thoracic, lumbar, sacral, and coccygeal. All vertebrae are similar in structure, but vary in size, shape, and articular surface, according to location. The type and extent of vertebral radiography depends on the patient's clinical condition. For example, a patient with lower back pain requires only study of the lumbar and sacral segments.

Purpose

- To detect vertebral fractures, dislocations, subluxations, and deformities
- To detect vertebral degeneration, infection, and congenital disorders
- To detect disorders of the intervertebral disks
- To determine the vertebral effects of arthritic and metabolic disorders

Patient preparation

- Explain to the patient that this test permits examination of the spine.
- Inform the patient that he need not restrict food or fluids.
- Tell the patient the test requires X-ray films. Also tell him who will perform the test and where it will take place.
- Advise the patient that he'll be placed in various positions for the X-ray films.
- Tell the patient that although some positions may cause slight discomfort, his cooperation is needed to ensure accurate results.
- Stress to the patient that he must keep still and hold his breath during the procedure.

Procedure and posttest care

The procedure varies considerably depending on the vertebral segment being examined.

- Initially, the patient is placed in a supine position on the X-ray table for an anteroposterior view.
- The patient may be repositioned for lateral or right and left oblique views; specific positioning depends on the vertebral segment or adjacent structure of interest.
- Analgesics or local heat applications may relieve pain.

Precautions

- Vertebral radiography is contraindicated during the first trimester of pregnancy, unless the benefits outweigh the risk of fetal radiation exposure.
- Exercise extreme caution when handling trauma patients with suspected spinal injuries, particularly of the cervical area. Such patients should be filmed while on the stretcher to avoid further injury during transfer to the radiographic table.

Normal findings

Normal vertebrae show no fractures, subluxations, dislocations, curvatures, or other abnormalities. Specific positions and spacing of the vertebrae vary with the patient's age.

In the lateral view, adult vertebrae are aligned to form four alternately concave and convex curves. The cervical and lumbar curves are convex anteriorly; the thoracic and sacral curves are concave anteriorly. Although the structure of the coccyx varies, it usually points forward and downward.

Neonatal vertebrae form only one curve, which is concave anteriorly.

Abnormal findings

The vertebral radiograph readily shows spondylolisthesis, fractures, subluxations, dislocations, wedging, and such deformities as kyphosis, scoliosis, and lordosis.

To confirm other disorders, spinal structures and their spatial relationships on the radiograph must be examined, and the patient's history and clinical status must be considered. These disorders include congenital abnormalities, such as torticollis (wryneck), absence of sacral or lumbar vertebrae, hemivertebrae, and Klippel-Feil syndrome; degenerative processes, such as hypertrophic spurs, osteoarthritis, and narrowed disk spaces; tuberculosis (Pott's disease); benign or malignant intraspinal tumors; ruptured disk and cervical disk syndrome; and systemic disorders, such as rheumatoid arthritis, Charcot's disease, ankylosing spondylitis, osteoporosis, and Paget's disease.

Depending on radiographic results, definitive diagnosis may also require additional tests, such as myelography or computed tomography scanning.

Interfering factors

- Improper positioning of the patient or patient movement (possible poor imaging)

BONE DENSITOMETRY

Bone densitometry assesses bone mass quantitatively. This noninvasive technique, also known as dual energy X-ray absorptiometry (DEXA), uses an X-ray tube to measure bone mineral density, but exposes the patient to only minimal radiation. The images detected are computer-analyzed to determine bone mineral status. The computer calculates the size and thickness of the bone as well as its volumetric density to determine its potential resistance to mechanical stress. It may be performed in the radiology department of a hospital, a physician's office, or a clinic.

Purpose

- To determine bone mineral density
- To identify risk for osteoporosis
- To evaluate clinical response to therapy for reducing the rate of bone loss

Patient preparation

- Reassure the patient that the test is painless and that the exposure to radiation is minimal.
- Tell the patient that the test will take from 10 minutes to 1 hour, depending on the areas to be scanned.
- Tell the patient who will perform the test and where it will take place.

Procedure and posttest care

- Instruct the patient to remove all metallic objects from the area to be scanned.
- The patient is positioned on a table under the scanning device, with the radiation source below and the detector above. The detector measures the bone's radiation absorption and produces a digital readout.

Precautions

- Bone densitometry is contraindicated during pregnancy.

Normal findings

Computer-analyzed results of the bone densitometry scan are within normal limits for the patient's age, sex, and height.

The patient's rate of bone loss can be treated over time.

Abnormal findings

The value and reliability of bone densitometry as a predictor of fractures are under investigation. Controversy exists regarding the scanning site and whether bone loss occurs as a general phenomenon or occurs first in the spine. Also, large-scale studies are being conducted to establish an "at-risk" level of bone density to help predict fractures.

Interfering factors

- Osteoarthritis (possible decrease)
- Fat tissue (poor visualization)
- Fractures

■ Size of region to be scanned

ARTHROGRAPHY

Arthrography allows radiographic examination of a joint after injection of a radiopaque dye, air, or both (double-contrast arthrogram) to outline soft-tissue structures and the contour of the joint. The joint is put through its range of motion while a series of radiographs are taken.

Indications for arthrography include persistent unexplained joint discomfort or pain. Complications may include persistent joint crepitus and allergic reactions to the contrast dye. Magnetic resonance imaging of the joint may be used in place of this test.

Purpose

■ To identify acute or chronic tears or other abnormalities of the joint capsule or supporting ligaments of the knee, shoulder, ankle, hips, or wrist
■ To detect internal joint derangements
■ To locate synovial cysts

Patient preparation

■ Describe the procedure to the patient and answer any questions he may have. Explain that this test permits examination of a joint.
■ Inform the patient he need not restrict food or fluids.
■ Tell the patient who will perform the procedure and where it will take place.
■ Explain that the fluoroscope allows the physician to track the contrast medium as it fills the joint space.
■ Inform the patient that standard X-ray films will also be taken after diffusion of the contrast medium.
■ Tell the patient that, although the joint area will be anesthetized, he may experience a tingling sensation or pressure in the joint when the contrast medium is injected.
■ Instruct the patient to remain as still as possible during the procedure, except when following instructions to change position.
■ Stress to the patient the importance of his cooperation in assuming various positions because films must be taken as quickly as possible to ensure optimum quality.
■ Check the patient's history to determine if he's hypersensitive to local anesthetics, iodine, seafood, or dyes used for other diagnostic tests.

Equipment

Fluoroscope, skin-cleansing solution, local anesthetic, two 2″ 20G needles, two 24G needles, three 3-ml syringes, short lumbar puncture needle (3″ 22G needle for arthrography of the shoulder), water-soluble radiopaque dye (5 to 15 ml), four sterile sponges, elastic knee bandage, sterile towels, sterile specimen container for fluid, culture tube, sterile adhesive bandage, collodion (optional), shave preparation kit

Procedure and posttest care

Knee arthrography

■ The knee is cleaned with an antiseptic solution and the area around the puncture site is anesthetized. (It isn't usually necessary to anesthetize the joint space itself.)
■ A 2″ needle is then inserted into the joint space between the patella and femoral condyle, and fluid is aspirated. The aspirated fluid is usually sent to the laboratory for analysis.
■ While the needle is still in place, the aspirating syringe is removed and replaced with a syringe containing dye.
■ If fluoroscopic examination demonstrates correct placement of the needle, the dye is injected into the joint space.

- After the needle is removed, the site is rubbed with a sterile sponge and the wound may be sealed with collodion.
- The patient is asked to walk a few steps or to move his knee through a range of motion to distribute the dye in the joint space. A film series is quickly taken with the knee held in various positions.
- If the films are clean and demonstrate proper dye placement, the knee is bandaged, possibly with an elastic bandage.
- Tell the patient to keep the bandage in place for several days and teach him how to rewrap it.

Shoulder arthrography

- The skin is prepared and a local anesthetic is injected subcutaneously just in front of the acromioclavicular joint.
- Additional anesthetic is injected directly onto the head of the humerus.
- The short lumbar puncture needle is inserted until the point is embedded in the joint cartilage.
- The stylet is removed, a syringe of contrast medium is attached and, using fluoroscopic guidance, about 1 ml of dye is injected into the joint space, as the needle is withdrawn slightly.
- If fluoroscopic examination demonstrates correct needle placement, the remainder of the dye is injected while the needle is slowly withdrawn and the site is wiped with a sterile sponge.
- A film series is taken quickly to achieve maximum contrast.

Both types

- Tell the patient to rest the joint for at least 12 hours.
- Inform the patient that he may experience some swelling or discomfort, or may hear crepitant noises in the joint after the test, but that these symptoms usually disappear after 1 or 2 days; tell him to report persistent symptoms.
- Advise the patient to apply ice to the joint if swelling occurs and to take a mild analgesic for pain.
- Instruct the patient to report any signs of infection at the needle insertion site, such as warmth, redness, swelling, or foul-smelling drainage.

Precautions

- Arthrography is contraindicated during pregnancy and in patients with active arthritis, joint infection, or previous sensitivity to radiopaque media.

Normal findings

A normal knee arthrogram shows a characteristic wedge-shaped shadow, pointed toward the interior of the joint, which indicates a normal medial meniscus. A normal shoulder arthrogram shows the bicipital tendon sheath, redundant inferior joint capsule, and subscapular bursa intact.

Abnormal findings

Arthrography accurately detects medial meniscal tears and lacerations in 90% to 95% of cases. Because the entire joint lining is opacified, arthrography can demonstrate extrameniscal lesions, such as osteochondritis dissecans, chondromalacia patellae, osteochondral fractures, cartilaginous abnormalities, synovial abnormalities, tears of the cruciate ligaments, and disruption of the joint capsule and collateral ligaments.

Arthrography can reveal shoulder abnormalities, such as adhesive capsulitis, bicipital tenosynovitis or rupture, and rotator cuff tears. It can also evaluate damage from recurrent dislocations.

Interfering factors

- Dilution of the contrast medium due to incomplete aspiration of joint effusion (possible poor imaging)
- Improper injection technique (possible displacement of contrast medium)

Miscellaneous Tests

Lymphangiography

Lymphangiography (or lymphography) is the radiographic examination of the lymphatic system after the injection of an oil-based contrast medium into a lymphatic vessel in each foot or, less commonly, in each hand. This test is no longer used widely.

Injection into the foot allows visualization of the lymphatics of the leg, inguinal and iliac regions, and the retroperitoneum up to the thoracic duct.

Injection into the hand allows visualization of the axillary and supraclavicular nodes. This procedure may also be used to study the cervical region (retroauricular area), but this is less useful and less common.

X-ray films are taken immediately after injection to demonstrate the filling of the lymphatic system and then again 24 hours later to visualize the lymph nodes. Because the contrast medium remains in the nodes for up to 2 years, subsequent X-ray films can assess progression of disease and monitor effectiveness of treatment.

Purpose

- To detect and stage lymphomas and to identify metastatic involvement of the lymph nodes (computed tomography is used more commonly for staging)
- To distinguish primary from secondary lymphedema
- To suggest surgical treatment or evaluate the effectiveness of chemotherapy and radiation therapy in controlling malignancy
- To investigate enlarged lymph nodes detected by computed tomography or ultrasonography

Patient preparation

- Explain to the patient that this test permits examination of the lymphatic system through X-ray films taken after the injection of a contrast medium.
- Inform the patient that he need not restrict food or fluids.
- Tell the patient who will perform this procedure and where it will take place.
- Mention that additional X-ray films are also taken the following day but that these take less than 30 minutes.
- Inform the patient that blue contrast medium will be injected into each foot to outline the lymphatic vessels; that the injection causes transient discomfort; and that the contrast medium discolors urine and stool for 48 hours, and may give his skin and vision a bluish tinge for 48 hours.
- Tell the patient that a local anesthetic will be injected before a small incision is made in each foot.
- Inform the patient that the contrast medium is then injected for the next 1½ hours using a catheter inserted into a lymphatic vessel.
- Advise the patient that he must remain as still as possible during injection of the contrast medium, and that he may experience some discomfort in the popliteal or inguinal areas at the beginning of the injection of the contrast medium.
- If this test is performed on an outpatient basis, advise the patient to have a friend or relative accompany him.
- Warn the patient that the incision site may be sore for several days after lymphangiography.
- Make sure the patient or a responsible family member has signed an informed consent form.

■ Check the patient's history to determine if he's hypersensitive to iodine, seafood, or the contrast media used in other diagnostic tests such as excretory urography. Alert the physician to any sensitivities.
■ Just before the procedure, instruct the patient to void and check his vital signs for a baseline. If prescribed, administer a sedative and an oral antihistamine (if hypersensitivity to the contrast medium is suspected).

Procedure and posttest care

■ A preliminary X-ray of the chest is taken with the patient in an erect or a supine position.
■ The skin over the dorsum of each foot is cleaned with antiseptics.
■ Blue contrast dye is injected intradermally into the area between the toes, usually the first and fourth toe webs.
■ The contrast medium infiltrates the lymphatic system and within 15 to 30 minutes the lymphatic vessels appear as small blue lines on the upper surface of the instep of each foot.
■ A local anesthetic is then injected into the dorsum of each foot and a transverse incision is made to expose the lymphatic vessel.
■ Each vessel is cannulated with a 30G needle attached to polyethylene tubing and a syringe filled with ethiodized oil.
■ Once the needles are positioned, the patient is instructed to remain still throughout the injection period to avoid dislodging the needles.
■ The syringe is then placed within an infusion pump that injects the contrast medium at a constant rate of 0.1 to 0.2 ml/minute for about 1½ hours to avoid injury to delicate lymphatic vessels.
■ Fluoroscopy may be used to monitor filling of the lymphatic system.
■ The needles are removed, the incisions are sutured, and sterile dressings are applied.
■ X-ray films of the legs, pelvis, abdomen, and chest are taken.
■ The patient is then taken to his room but must return 24 hours later for additional films.
■ Check the patient's vital signs every 4 hours for 48 hours.
■ Watch for pulmonary complications, such as shortness of breath, pleuritic pain, hypotension, low-grade fever, and cyanosis caused by embolization of the contrast medium.
■ Enforce bed rest for 24 hours, with the patient's feet elevated to help reduce swelling.
■ Apply ice packs to the incision sites to help reduce swelling, and administer prescribed analgesics.
■ Check the incision sites for infection and leave the dressings in place for 2 days, making sure the wounds remain dry. Tell the patient the sutures will be removed in 7 to 10 days.
■ Prepare the patient for follow-up X-rays, as needed.

Precautions

■ Lymphangiography is contraindicated in patients with hypersensitivity to iodine, pulmonary insufficiencies, cardiac diseases, and severe renal or hepatic diseases.

Normal findings

The lymphatic system normally demonstrates homogeneous and complete filling with contrast medium on the initial films. On the 24-hour films, the lymph nodes are fully opacified and well circumscribed; the lymphatic channels are emptied a few hours after injection of the contrast medium.

Abnormal findings

Enlarged, foamy-looking nodes indicate Hodgkin's disease or malignant lymphoma. Filling defects or lack of opacification indicates metastatic involve-

Staging malignant lymphoma

Malignant lymphoma may be staged according to the following levels:

- Stage I: Involvement of a single lymph node region or of a single extralymphatic organ or site
- Stage II: Involvement of two or more lymph node regions on the same side of the diaphragm or localized involvement of an extralymphatic organ or the site of one or more lymph node regions on the same side of the diaphragm
- Stage III: Involvement of lymph node regions on both sides of the diaphragm, which may also be accompanied by localized involvement of an extralymphatic organ or site or of the spleen (or both)
- Stage IV: Diffuse or disseminated involvement of one or more extralymphatic organs or tissue with or without associated lymph node enlargement

ment of the lymph nodes. The number of nodes affected, unilateral or bilateral involvement, and the extent of extranodal involvement help determine staging of lymphoma. However, definitive staging may require additional diagnostic tests such as computed tomography, ultrasonography, selective biopsy, and laparotomy. (See *Staging malignant lymphoma.*)

In differential diagnosis of primary and secondary lymphedema, shortened lymphatic vessels and a deficient number of vessels indicate primary lymphedema. Abruptly terminating lymphatic vessels, caused by retroperitoneal tumors impinging on the vessels, inflammation, filariasis, and trauma resulting from surgery or radiation, indicate secondary lymphedema.

Interfering factors

- Inability to cannulate the lymphatic vessels (precludes use of this test)

13

Computed tomography and magnetic resonance imaging

NEUROLOGIC SYSTEM

INTRACRANIAL COMPUTED TOMOGRAPHY

Intracranial computed tomography (CT) provides a series of tomograms, translated by a computer and displayed on a monitor, representing cross-sectional images of various layers of the brain. This technique can reconstruct cross-sectional, horizontal, sagittal, and coronal plane images. Hundreds of thousands of readings of radiation levels absorbed by brain tissues may be combined to depict anatomic slices of varying thickness. Specificity and accuracy are enhanced by the degree of resolution, which depends on the number of radiation density calculations made by the computer. Although magnetic resonance imaging (MRI) has surpassed CT scanning in diagnosing neurologic anatomy and pathology, the CT scan is more widely available and cost-effective and can be performed more easily in acute situations.

Purpose

- To diagnose intracranial lesions and abnormalities
- To monitor the effects of surgery, radiation therapy, or chemotherapy on intracranial tumors
- To serve as a guide for cranial surgery

Patient preparation

- Explain to the patient that this test permits assessment of the brain.
- Unless contrast enhancement is scheduled, inform the patient that there are no food or fluid restrictions. If contrast enhancement is scheduled, instruct him to fast for 4 hours before the test.
- Tell the patient that a series of X-ray films will be taken of his brain. Describe who will perform the test and where it will take place. Explain that the test will cause minimal discomfort.
- Tell the patient that he'll be positioned on a moving CT bed, with his head immobilized and his face uncovered. The head of the table will then be moved into the scanner, which rotates around his head and makes loud clacking sounds.
- If a contrast medium is used, tell the patient that he may feel flushed and warm and may experience a transient head-ache, a salty or metallic taste, or nausea and vomiting after the contrast medium is injected.
- Instruct the patient to wear a gown (outpatients may wear any comfortable clothing) and to remove all metal objects from the CT scan field.
- If the patient is restless or apprehensive, a sedative may be prescribed.
- Check the patient's history for hypersensitivity to shellfish, iodine, or contrast media, and mark your findings in his chart. Inform the physician of any sensitivities because he may order prophylactic medications or may choose not to use contrast enhancement.

Equipment

CT scanner, oscilloscope, contrast medium (iothalamate meglumine or diatrizoate sodium), 60-ml syringe, 19G to 21G needle, I.V. tubing, and I.V. insertion equipment, if needed

Procedure and posttest care

- Place the patient in a supine position on an X-ray table, with his head immobilized by straps, if required, and ask him to lie still.

- The head of the table is moved into the scanner, which rotates around the patient's head, taking radiographs at 1-degree intervals in a 180-degree arc.
- When this series of radiographs is completed, a contrast enhancement is performed. Usually 50 to 100 ml of contrast medium is administered by I.V. injection or I.V. drip over 1 to 2 minutes. Monitor for hypersensitivity reactions, such as urticaria, respiratory difficulty, or rash. Reactions usually develop within 30 minutes.
- After injection of the contrast medium, another series of scans is taken. Information from the scans is stored on magnetic tapes, fed into a computer, and converted into images on an oscilloscope. Photographs of selected views are taken for further study.
- If a contrast medium was used, watch for residual adverse reactions (headache, nausea, and vomiting) and inform the patient that he may resume his usual diet.

Precautions

- Intracranial CT scanning with contrast enhancement is contraindicated in persons who are hypersensitive to iodine or contrast medium.
- Iodine or contrast medium may be harmful or fatal to a fetus, especially during the first trimester.

Normal findings

The density of tissue determines the amount of radiation that passes through it. Tissue densities appear as white, black, or shades of gray on the computed image obtained by intracranial CT scanning. Bone, the densest tissue, appears white; ventricular and subarachnoid cerebrospinal fluid, the least dense, appears black. Brain matter appears in shades of gray. Structures are evaluated according to their density, size, shape, and position.

Abnormal findings

Areas of altered density (they may be lighter or darker) or displaced vasculature or other structures may indicate intracranial tumor, hematoma, cerebral atrophy, infarction, edema, or congenital anomalies such as hydrocephalus.

Intracranial tumors vary significantly in appearance and characteristics. Metastatic tumors generally cause extensive edema in early stages and can usually be defined by contrast enhancement. Primary tumors vary in density and in their capacity to cause edema, displace ventricles, and absorb contrast medium in contrast enhancement. Astrocytomas, for example, usually have low densities; meningiomas have higher densities and can generally be defined with contrast enhancement; glioblastomas, usually ill-defined, are also enhanced after injection of a contrast medium.

Because the high density of blood contrasts markedly with low-density brain tissue, it's normally easy to detect subdural and epidural hematomas and other acute hemorrhages. Contrast enhancement helps locate subdural hematomas.

Cerebral atrophy customarily appears as enlarged ventricles with large sulci. Cerebral infarction may appear as low-density areas at the obstruction site or may not be apparent, especially within the first 24 hours or if the infarction is small or doesn't cause edema. With contrast enhancement, the infarcted area may not show in the acute phase but will show clearly after resolution of the lesion. Cerebral edema usually appears as an area of marked generalized decreased density. In children, enlargement of the fourth ventricle generally indicates hydrocephalus.

Normally, the cerebral vessels don't appear on CT images. However, in patients with arteriovenous malformation,

Understanding PET and SPECT

Like computed tomography (CT) scanning and magnetic resonance imaging (MRI), positron emission tomography (PET) and single-photon emission computed tomography (SPECT) provide images of the brain through sophisticated computer reconstruction algorithms. However, PET and SPECT images detail brain function as well as structure and thus differ significantly from the images provided by these other advanced techniques. PET and SPECT combine elements of both CT scanning and conventional radionuclide imaging. For example, they measure the emissions of injected radioisotopes and convert them to a tomographic image of the brain. SPECT scanning uses gamma radiation with radionucleotides within the brain, and PET uses radioisotopes of biologically important elements — oxygen, nitrogen, carbon, and fluorine — that emit particles called positrons.

HOW IT WORKS

During PET and SPECT, pairs of gamma rays are emitted; the scanner detects them and relays the information to a computer for reconstruction as an image. SPECT scanners use radionucleotides labeled with iodine or hexamethylpropyline amineoxime to detect blood flow. PET scanners omit positrons that can be chemically "tagged" to biologically active molecules such as carbon monoxide, neurotransmitters, hormones, and metabolites (especially glucose), enabling study of their uptake and distribution in brain tissue. For example, blood tagged with ^{11}C-carbon monoxide allows study of hemodynamic patterns in brain tissue; tagged neurotransmitters, hormones, and drugs allow mapping of receptor distribution.

Isotope-tagged glucose (which penetrates the blood-brain barrier rapidly) allows dynamic study of brain function because PET scans can pinpoint the sites of glucose metabolism in the brain under various conditions. Researchers expect SPECT and PET scanning to prove useful in the diagnosis of psychiatric disorders, transient ischemic attacks, amyotrophic lateral sclerosis, Parkinson's disease, Wilson's disease, multiple sclerosis, seizure disorders, cerebrovascular disease, and Alzheimer's disease. The reason is that all of these disorders may alter the location and patterns of cerebral glucose metabolism.

COST FACTORS

PET scanning is a costly test because the radioisotopes used have very short half-lives and must be produced at an on-site cyclotron and attached quickly to the desired tracer molecules.

cerebral vessels may appear with slightly increased density. Contrast enhancement allows a better view of the abnormal area, but MRI is now the preferred procedure for imaging cerebral vessels.

Another technology for obtaining images of the brain is positron emission tomography. (See *Understanding PET and SPECT.*)

Interfering factors

- Patient's head movement (possible poor imaging)
- Failure to remove metal objects from the scanning field (possible poor imaging)
- Hemorrhage (possible false-negative imaging due to change in hematoma)

INTRACRANIAL MAGNETIC RESONANCE IMAGING

Intracranial magnetic resonance imaging (MRI) produces highly detailed, cross-sectional images of the brain and spine in multiple planes. The primary advantage of MRI is its ability to "see through" bone and to delineate fluid-filled soft tissue. It has proved useful in the diagnosis of cerebral infarction, tumors, abscesses, edema, hemorrhage, nerve fiber demyelination (as in multiple sclerosis), and other disorders that increase the fluid content of affected tissues. It can also show irregularities of the spinal cord with a resolution and detail previously unobtainable. It can also produce images of organs and vessels in motion.

MRI technology makes use of magnetic fields and radio frequency waves, which are imperceptible by the patient; no harmful effects have been documented. Research continues on the optimal magnetic fields and radio frequency waves for each type of tissue. (See *New methods of monitoring cerebral function* and *Applications for MRI.*)

New methods of monitoring cerebral function

OPTICAL IMAGING

Optical imaging uses fiber-optic light and a camera to produce visual images of the brain as it responds to stimulation. This technique produces higher-resolution pictures of the brain than either MRI or PET scans. Researchers believe it may be valuable during neurosurgery to minimize damage to crucial areas of the brain that control speech, movement, and other activities. Because the procedure scans only the brain's surface, it is meant to be used in combination with other diagnostic techniques.

FAST MRI

Fast MRI produces pictures less than a second apart. These images display blood flow through the brain and the changes that occur in blood flow when the patient performs different tasks. Neuroscientists believe that active areas of the brain must consume more oxygen and that areas of the brain that are currently working become laden with oxygen. Fast MRI can distinguish between oxygen-laden blood and oxygen-depleted blood. Thus, this test may be used to help identify which areas of the normal brain are involved in certain activities and emotions. Possible applications for fast MRI include guiding neurosurgeons during surgery and helping researchers better understand epilepsy, brain tumors, and even psychiatric illnesses.

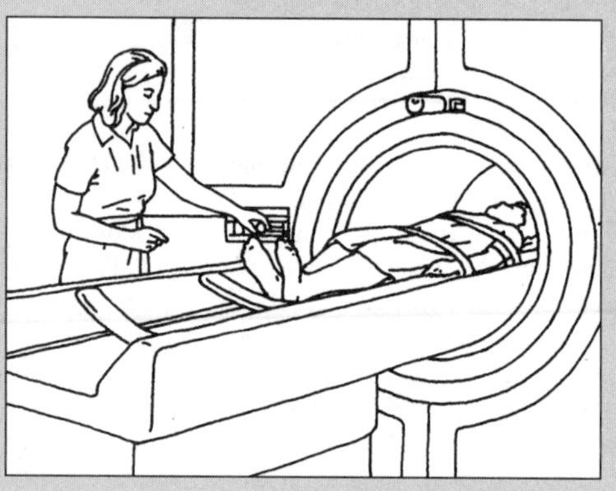

Applications for MRI

Magnetic resonance imaging (MRI) is used to provide clear images of parts of the brain, such as the brain stem and cerebellum, that are difficult to image by other methods. Four MRI techniques are now available to examine other aspects of the brain.

MAGNETIC RESONANCE ANGIOGRAPHY
Magnetic resonance angiography allows the visualization of blood flowing through the cerebral vessels.

MAGNETIC RESONANCE SPECTROSCOPY
Magnetic resonance spectroscopy creates images over time that show the metabolism of certain chemical markers in a specific area of the brain. Some researchers have dubbed this test a "metabolic biopsy" because it reveals pathologic neurochemistry over time.

DIFFUSION-PERFUSION IMAGING
Diffusion-perfusion imaging uses a stronger-than-normal magnetic gradient to reveal areas of focal cerebral ischemia within minutes. Currently used in stroke research, this MRI technique may be used by diagnosticians to distinguish permanent from reversible ischemia.

NEUROGRAPHY
Neurograms provide a three-dimensional image of nerves. They may be used in the future to find the exact location of nerves that are damaged, crimped, or in disarray.

Purpose

- To aid diagnosis of intracranial and spinal lesions and soft-tissue abnormalities

Patient preparation

- Explain to the patient that this test assesses bone and soft tissue. Tell him who will perform the test and where it will take place.
- Explain to the patient that MRI is painless and involves no exposure to radiation from the scanner. A radioactive contrast dye may be used, depending on the type of tissue being studied.
- Advise the patient that he'll have to remain still for the entire procedure.
- Inform the patient that the opening for the head and body is quite small and deep. Tell him that he'll hear the scanner clicking, whirring, and thumping as it moves inside its housing.
- Explain to the patient that sedation may be administered if he suffers from claustrophobia or if extensive time is required for scanning.
- Reassure the patient that he'll be able to communicate with the technician at all times.
- Instruct the patient to remove all metallic objects, including jewelry, hair pins, and a watch, and ask if he has any surgically implanted joints, pins, clips, valves, pumps, or pacemakers containing metal that could be attracted to the strong MRI magnet. If he does, he won't be able to undergo the test.
- Ensure that the patient or a responsible family member has signed an informed consent form, if required.

Procedure and posttest care

- The patient is placed in a supine position on a narrow bed, which then slides him to the desired position inside the scanner where radio frequency energy is directed at his head or spine.

- The resulting images are displayed on a monitor and recorded on film or magnetic tape for permanent storage.
- The radiologist may vary radio frequency waves and use the computer to manipulate and enhance the images.
- During the procedure the patient must remain still.
- Tell the patient that he may resume normal activity after the test.
- If the patient was sedated, ensure that a responsible person drives him home.
- If the test took a long time and the patient was lying flat for an extended period, observe him for orthostatic hypotension.

Precautions

- Because MRI works through a powerful magnetic field, it can't be performed on patients with pacemakers, intracranial aneurysm clips, or other ferrous metal implants or on a patient with gunshot wounds to the head.
- Because of the strong magnetic field, metallic or computer-based equipment (for example, ventilators and I.V. pumps) can't enter the MRI area.

Normal findings

MRI can show normal anatomic details of the central nervous system in any plane, without bone interference. Brain and spinal cord structures should appear distinct and sharply defined. Tissue color and shading will vary, depending on the radio frequency energy, magnetic strength, and degree of computer enhancement.

Abnormal findings

Because MRI depicts the density (water content) of tissue, it clearly shows structural changes resulting from disorders that increase tissue water content, such as cerebral edema, demyelinating disease, and pontine and cerebellar tumors. Edematous fluid, for example, generally appears cloudy or gray, whereas blood generally appears dark. Lesions of multiple sclerosis appear as areas of demyelination (curdlike, gray or gray-white areas) around the edges of ventricles. Tumors appear as changes in normal anatomy, which computer enhancement may further delineate.

Interfering factors

- Excessive patient movement (possible poor imaging)

GASTROINTESTINAL SYSTEM

LIVER AND BILIARY TRACT COMPUTED TOMOGRAPHY

In computed tomography (CT) of the biliary tract and liver, multiple X-rays pass through the upper abdomen and are measured while detectors record differences in tissue attenuation. A computer reconstructs this data as a two-dimensional image on a monitor. CT scanning accurately distinguishes the biliary tract and the liver if the ducts are large. Use of I.V. contrast media during CT scanning can accentuate different densities.

Although CT scanning and ultrasonography detect biliary tract and liver disease equally well, the latter technique is performed more commonly. CT scanning is more expensive than ultrasonography and requires exposure to moderate amounts of radiation. However, it's the test of choice in patients who are obese and in those with livers positioned high under the rib cage because bone and excessive fat hinder ultrasound transmission.

Purpose

- To distinguish between obstructive and nonobstructive jaundice
- To detect intrahepatic tumors and abscesses, subphrenic and subhepatic abscesses, cysts, and hematomas

Patient preparation

- Explain to the patient that this test helps detect biliary tract and liver disease.
- Tell the patient he'll be given a contrast medium to drink and then he should fast until after the examination. If contrast isn't ordered, fasting isn't necessary.
- Explain to the patient who will perform the test and where it will take place.
- Inform the patient that he'll be placed on an adjustable table, which is positioned inside a scanning gantry. Assure him that the test will be painless.
- Tell the patient he'll be asked to remain still during the test and to hold his breath when instructed. Stress the importance of remaining still during the test because movement can cause artifacts, thereby prolonging the test and limiting its accuracy.
- If I.V. contrast medium is being used, inform the patient that he may experience transient discomfort from the needle puncture and a localized feeling of warmth on injection as well as a salty or metallic taste. Tell him to immediately report nausea, vomiting, dizziness, headache, and hives.
- Check the patient's history for hypersensitivity to iodine, seafood, or the contrast media used in other diagnostic tests.
- If a contrast medium has been ordered, give the patient the oral contrast medium supplied by the radiology department.
- Ensure that the patient or a responsible family member has signed an informed consent form, if required.

Procedure and posttest care

- The patient is placed in a supine position on an X-ray table, and the table is positioned within the opening in the scanning gantry.
- A series of transverse X-ray films is taken and recorded on magnetic tape. This information is reconstructed by a computer and appears as images on a television screen.
- These images are studied, and selected ones are photographed. When the first series of films is completed, the images are reviewed.
- Contrast enhancement may be performed. After the contrast medium is injected, a second series of films is taken, and the patient is carefully observed for an allergic reaction.
- After the procedure, tell the patient that he may resume his usual diet.

Precautions

- CT scanning of the biliary tract and liver is usually contraindicated during pregnancy.
- Use of an I.V. contrast medium is contraindicated in patients with hypersensitivity to iodine or with severe renal or hepatic disease.

Normal findings

Normally, the liver has a uniform density that's slightly greater than that of the pancreas, kidneys, and spleen. Linear and circular areas of slightly lower density, representing hepatic vascular structures, may interrupt this uniform appearance. The portal vein is usually visible; the hepatic artery usually isn't. I.V. contrast medium enhances the isodensity of vascular structures and liver parenchyma.

Typically, intrahepatic biliary radicles aren't visible, but the common hepatic and bile ducts may be visible as low-density structures. Because bile has the same density as water, use of an I.V. contrast medium improves demarcation of the biliary tract by enhancing surrounding parenchyma and vascular structures.

Like the biliary ducts, the gallbladder is visible as a round or elliptic low-density structure. A contracted gallbladder may be impossible to visualize.

Abnormal findings

Most focal hepatic defects appear less dense than the normal parenchyma, and CT scans can detect small lesions. Use of rapid-sequence scanning with an I.V. contrast medium helps distinguish between the two because the normal parenchyma shows greater enhancement than focal defects.

Primary and metastatic neoplasms may appear as well-circumscribed or poorly defined areas of slightly lower density than the normal parenchyma. However, some lesions have the same density as the liver parenchyma and may be undetectable. Neoplasms that are especially large may distort the liver's contour. Hepatic abscesses appear as relatively low-density, homogeneous areas, usually with well-defined borders. Hepatic cysts appear as sharply defined round or oval structures and have a density lower than abscesses and neoplasms.

The density of a hepatic hematoma varies with its age. A recent clot is as dense as or slightly more dense than the normal parenchyma; a resolving clot is somewhat less dense than the normal parenchyma. Intrahepatic hematomas vary in shape; subcapsular hematomas are usually crescent-shaped and compress the liver away from the capsule.

When distinguishing between obstructive and nonobstructive jaundice, biliary duct dilation indicates the former and an absence of dilation indicates the latter. Dilated intrahepatic bile ducts appear as low-density linear and circular branching structures. Dilation of the common hepatic duct, common bile duct, and gallbladder may also be apparent, depending on the site and severity of obstruction. Use of an I.V. contrast medium helps detect biliary dilation, especially when the ducts are only slightly dilated.

Usually, CT scanning can identify the cause of obstruction — for example, calculi or pancreatic carcinoma. However, if the site of obstruction must be located before surgery, percutaneous transhepatic cholangiography or endoscopic retrograde cholangiopancreatography (less common) may be performed as well.

Interfering factors

- Presence of oral or I.V. contrast media, including barium, in the bile from earlier tests (possible poor imaging)

PANCREATIC COMPUTED TOMOGRAPHY

In computed tomography (CT) of the pancreas, multiple X-rays penetrate the upper abdomen while a detector records the differences in tissue attenuation, which is then displayed as an image on a television screen. A series of cross-sectional views can provide a detailed look at the pancreas. CT scanning accurately distinguishes the pancreas and surrounding organs and vessels if enough fat is present between the structures. Use of an I.V. or oral contrast medium can further accentuate differences in tissue density.

CT scanning is replacing ultrasonography as the test of choice for examining the pancreas. Although ultrasonography costs less and involves less risk for the patient, it's also less accurate. In retroperitoneal disorders, specifically when pancreatitis is suspected, CT scanning goes beyond ultrasonography by showing the general swelling that accompanies acute inflammation of the gland. In chronic cases, CT scanning easily detects calcium deposits commonly missed by simple radiography, particularly in patients who are obese.

Purpose

- To detect pancreatic carcinoma or pseudocysts
- To detect or evaluate pancreatitis
- To distinguish between pancreatic disorders and disorders of the retroperitoneum

Patient preparation

- Explain to the patient that this test helps detect disorders of the pancreas.
- Instruct the patient to fast after administration of the oral contrast medium.
- Describe the test, including who will perform it and where it will take place.
- Tell the patient that he'll be placed on an adjustable table that is positioned inside a scanning gantry. Assure him that the procedure is painless.
- Explain to the patient that he'll need to remain still during the test and periodically hold his breath.
- Inform the patient that he may be given an I.V. contrast medium, an oral contrast medium, or both to enhance visualization of the pancreas. Describe possible adverse reactions to the medium, such as nausea, flushing, dizziness, and sweating, and tell him to report these symptoms.
- Check the patient's history for recent barium studies and for hypersensitivity to iodine, seafood, or contrast media used in prior tests.
- Ensure that the patient or a responsible family member has signed an informed consent form, if required.
- Administer the oral contrast medium.

Procedure and posttest care

- Help the patient into the supine position on the X-ray table and position the table within the opening in the scanning gantry.
- A series of transverse X-rays is taken and recorded on magnetic tape. The varying tissue absorption is calculated by a computer, and the information is reconstructed as images on a television screen. These images are studied, and selected ones are photographed.
- After the first series of films is completed, the images are reviewed. Then contrast enhancement may be ordered. After the contrast medium is administered, another series of films is taken, and the patient is observed for an allergic reaction, such as itching, hypotension, hypertension, diaphoresis, or dyspnea.
- After the procedure, tell the patient he may resume his usual diet.
- Observe for a delayed allergic reaction to the contrast dye, such as urticaria, headache, and vomiting.

Precautions

- CT scanning of the pancreas is contraindicated during pregnancy.
- If a contrast medium is used, the test is contraindicated in patients with a history of hypersensitivity to iodine or severe renal or hepatic disease.

Normal findings

Usually, the pancreatic parenchyma displays a uniform density, especially when an I.V. contrast medium is used. The

Normal CT scan of the pancreas

This normal pancreatic computed tomography (CT) scan shows the pancreas opacified by contrast medium.

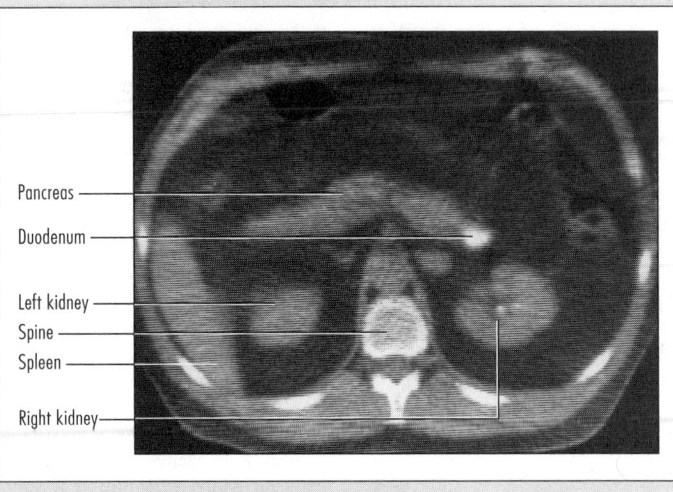

gland normally thickens from tail to head and has a smooth surface. A contrast medium administered orally opacifies the adjacent stomach and duodenum and helps outline the pancreas, particularly in patients with little peripancreatic fat, such as children and thin adults. (See *Normal CT scan of the pancreas.*)

Abnormal findings

Because the tissue density of pancreatic carcinoma resembles that of the normal parenchyma, changes in pancreatic size and shape help demonstrate carcinoma and pseudocysts. Usually, carcinoma first appears as a localized swelling of the head, body, or tail of the pancreas and may spread to obliterate the fat plane, dilate the main pancreatic duct and common bile duct by obstructing them, and produce low-density focal lesions in the liver from metastasis. Use of an I.V. contrast medium helps detect metastases by opacifying the pancreatic and hepatic parenchyma.

Adenocarcinoma and islet cell tumor are the most common carcinomas of the pancreas. Cystadenomas and cystadenocarcinomas, usually multilocular, occur most frequently in the body and tail of the pancreas and appear as low-density focal lesions marked by internal septa. Contrast medium administered by mouth helps distinguish between bowel loops and tumors in the tail of the pancreas.

Acute pancreatitis, either edematous (interstitial) or necrotizing (hemorrhagic), produces diffuse enlargement of the pancreas. In acute edematous pancreatitis, the density of the parenchyma is uniformly decreased. In acute necrotizing pancreatitis, the density is nonuniform because of the presence of both necrosis and hemorrhage. The areas of tissue necrosis have diminished density. In acute pancreatitis, inflammation often spreads into the peripancreatic fat, causes stranding in the mesenteric fat, and blurs the margin of the gland.

Abscesses, phlegmons, and pseudocysts may occur as complications of acute pancreatitis. Abscesses, either within or outside the pancreas, appear as low-density areas and are most readily detected when they contain gas. Pseudocysts, which may be unilocular or multilocular, appear as sharply circumscribed, low-density areas that may contain debris. Ascites and pleural effusion may also be apparent in acute pancreatitis.

In chronic pancreatitis, the pancreas may appear normal, enlarged (localized or generalized), or atrophic, depending on the severity of the disease. Calcification of the ducts and dilation of the main pancreatic duct are characteristic. Pseudocysts, obliteration of the fat plane, and secondary complications (such as biliary obstruction) may occur.

Interfering factors

- Barium or other contrast media in the GI tract from earlier tests (possible poor imaging)
- Excessive peristalsis or excessive patient movement

GIVEN DIAGNOSTIC IMAGING SYSTEM

The given diagnostic imaging system (also called the *camera pill*) is a tiny video camera with a light source and transmitter inside a capsule, allowing recording of images along its path. The "capsule endoscope" measures 11 × 30 mm and is propelled along the digestive tract by peristalsis. The clear end records images of the walls of the stomach and, particularly, the small intestine, where many other diagnostic techniques may not reach or otherwise visualize. (See *Looking inside,* page 644.) The images are transmitted to a data recorder on a belt placed around the patient's waist. After swallowing the pill, the patient doesn't need to stay at the hospital and is able to return to work or other activities of daily living.

Purpose

- To detect polyps or cancer
- To detect causes of bleeding and anemia

Patient preparation

- Explain to the patient that this test helps visualize the stomach and small intestine, helping to detect disorders there.
- Tell the patient who will perform the test and where it will take place.
- Inform the patient he may need to fast for 12 hours before the test but may have fluids for up to 2 hours before the test, unless ordered otherwise (usually no preparation is involved, but some patients may benefit from it).
- Explain to the patient that he'll need to swallow the camera pill and that it will send information to a receiver he'll need to wear on his belt.
- Tell the patient that the procedure is painless and after swallowing the pill he can go home or go to work.
- Explain to the patient that walking helps facilitate movement of the pill.
- Tell the patient he'll need to return to the facility in 24 hours (or as directed) so the recorder can be removed from his belt.

Looking inside

After the patient swallows the capsule, it travels through the body by the natural movement of the digestive tract. A receiver worn outside the body records the images. The strength of the signal indicates the capsule's location.

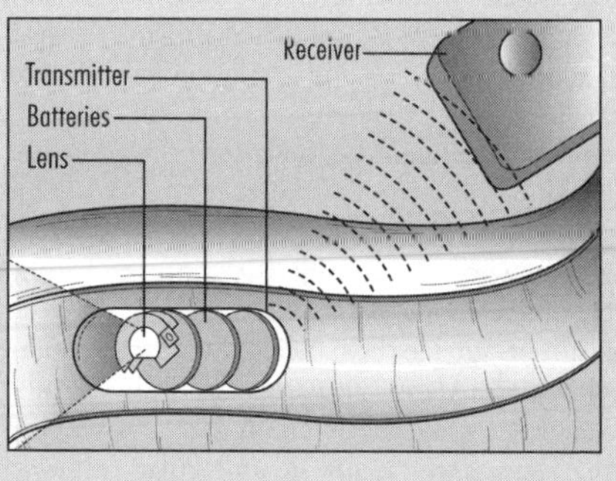

■ Tell the patient the pill will be excreted normally in the feces in 8 to 72 hours.

Procedure and posttest care

■ The patient ingests the camera pill as ordered, and a receiver is attached to his belt.

■ The pill records images for up to 6 hours along its path of the stomach, small intestine, and mouth of the large intestine, transmitting the information to the receiver.

■ The patient returns to the facility as ordered so the images can be transmitted into the computer, where they're displayed on the screen.

■ The patient may resume normal diet after the images are obtained.

■ The pill is excreted in the feces normally.

Precautions

■ The procedure is contraindicated in cases of suspected obstruction, fistulas or strictures, and in those who can't swallow (infants, young children, those who have swallowing impairment).

Normal findings

Normally, the camera illustrates normal anatomy of the stomach and small intestine.

Abnormal findings

The camera may detect sites of bleeding.

Interfering factors

■ Narrowing or obstruction of the intestine may cause the pill to become lodged.

■ The battery is short-lived, so images of the large intestine are unobtainable.

■ The pill can't be used to stop bleeding, take tissue samples, remove growths, or repair any problems detected. Other invasive studies may be needed.

MUSCULOSKELETAL SYSTEM

SPINAL COMPUTED TOMOGRAPHY

Much more versatile than conventional radiography, computed tomography (CT) of the spine provides detailed high-resolution images in the cross-sectional, longitudinal, sagittal, and lateral planes. Multiple X-ray beams from a computerized body scanner are directed at the spine from different angles; these pass through the body and strike radiation detectors, producing electrical impulses. A computer then converts these impulses into digital information, which is displayed as a three-dimensional image on a monitor. Storage of the digital information allows electronic recreation and manipulation of the image, creating a permanent record of the images to enable reexamination without repeating the procedure.

CT scans are helpful in defining the lesions causing spinal cord compression. Metastatic disease and discogenic disease with osteophyte formation and calcification are examples of pathologic processes diagnosed by CT scans. Since the advent of magnetic resonance imaging, CT scans are used less frequently to diagnose infection, abscesses, hematomas, and some disk herniations.

Purpose

- To diagnose spinal lesions and abnormalities
- To monitor the effects of spinal surgery or therapy

Patient preparation

- Explain to the patient that this procedure allows visualization of his spine.
- If contrast medium isn't ordered, tell the patient that he need not restrict food or fluids. If contrast medium is ordered, instruct him to fast for 4 hours before the test.
- Tell the patient that a series of scans will be taken of his spine. Explain who will perform the procedure and where it will take place.
- Reassure the patient that the procedure is painless, but that he may find having to remain still for a prolonged period uncomfortable.
- Explain to the patient that he'll be positioned on an X-ray table inside a CT body scanning unit and he'll be told to lie still because movement during the procedure may cause distorted images. The computer-controlled scanner will revolve around him taking multiple scans.
- If a contrast medium is used, tell the patient that he may feel flushed and warm and may experience a transient headache, a salty taste, and nausea or vomiting after injection of the contrast medium. Reassure him that these reactions are normal.
- Instruct the patient to wear a radiologic examining gown and to remove all metal objects and jewelry.
- Check the patient's history for hypersensitivity reactions to iodine, shellfish, or contrast media. If such reactions have occurred, note them in the patient's chart and notify the physician who may order prophylactic medications or choose not to use contrast enhancement.
- If the patient appears restless or apprehensive about the procedure, a mild sedative may be prescribed.
- Ensure that the patient or a responsible family member has signed an informed consent form, if required.

Equipment

CT body scanner, oscilloscope, recording equipment, contrast medium (iothalamate meglumine or diatrizoate sodium), 60-ml syringe, 19G to 20G needle

Procedure and posttest care

- Place the patient in a supine position on an X-ray table, and tell him to lie as still as possible.
- The table slides into the circular opening of the CT scanner and the scanner revolves around the patient, taking radiographs at preselected intervals.
- After the first set of scans is taken, the patient is removed from the scan-

ner. Contrast medium may be administered.

- Observe the patient for signs and symptoms of a hypersensitivity reaction, including pruritus, rash, and respiratory difficulty, for 30 minutes after the contrast medium has been injected.
- After contrast medium injection, the patient is moved back into the scanner, and another series of scans is taken. The images obtained from the scan are displayed on a monitor during the procedure and stored on magnetic tape.
- After testing with contrast enhancement, observe the patient for residual effects, such as headache, nausea, and vomiting.
- Inform the patient that he may resume his usual diet, as ordered.

Precautions

- Body CT scanning with contrast enhancement is contraindicated in patients who are hypersensitive to iodine, shellfish, or contrast media used in radiographic studies.
- Some patients may experience strong feelings of claustrophobia or anxiety when inside the CT body scanner. For such patients, a mild sedative to help reduce anxiety may be ordered.
- For patients with significant back pain, administer prescribed analgesics before the scan.

Normal findings

In the CT image, spinal tissue appears white, black, or gray, depending on its density. Vertebrae, the densest tissues, are white; cerebrospinal fluid is black; soft tissues appear in shades of gray.

Abnormal findings

By highlighting areas of altered density and depicting structural malformation, CT scanning can reveal all types of spinal lesions and abnormalities. It's particularly useful in detecting and localizing tumors, which appear as masses varying in density. Measuring this density and noting the configuration and location relative to the spinal cord can usually identify the type of tumor. For example, a neurinoma (schwannoma) appears as a spherical mass dorsal to the cord. A darker, wider mass lying more laterally or ventrally to the cord may be a meningioma.

CT scans also reveal degenerative processes and structural changes in detail. Herniated nucleus pulposus shows as an obvious herniation of disk material with unilateral or bilateral nerve root compression; if the herniation is midline, spinal cord compression will be evident. Cervical spondylosis shows as cervical cord compression due to bony hypertrophy of the cervical spine; lumbar stenosis as hypertrophy of the lumbar vertebrae, causing cord compression by decreasing space within the spinal column. Facet disorders show as soft-tissue changes, bony overgrowth, and spurring of the vertebrae, which result in nerve root compression. Fluid-filled arachnoidal and other paraspinal cysts show as dark masses displacing the spinal cord. Vascular malformations, evident after contrast enhancement, show as masses or clusters, usually on the dorsal aspect of the spinal cord.

Congenital spinal malformations, such as meningocele, myelocele, and spina bifida, show as abnormally large, dark gaps between the white vertebrae.

Interfering factors

- Excessive patient movement
- Failure to remove metallic objects from the scan area (possible poor imaging)

SKELETAL COMPUTED TOMOGRAPHY

Skeletal computed tomography (CT) provides a series of tomograms, translated by a computer and displayed on a monitor, representing cross-sectional images of various layers (or slices) of bone. This technique can reconstruct cross-sectional, horizontal, sagittal, and coronal plane images.

Taking collimated (parallel) radiographs increases the number of radiation density calculations the computer makes, thereby improving the degree of resolution and thus specificity and accuracy. Hundreds of thousands of readings of radiation levels absorbed by tissues may be combined to depict anatomic slices of varying thickness.

Purpose

- To determine the existence and extent of primary bone tumors, skeletal metastases, soft-tissue tumors, injuries to ligaments or tendons, and fractures
- To diagnose joint abnormalities difficult to detect by other methods

Patient preparation

- Explain to the patient that this procedure allows visualization of bones and joints. If contrast medium isn't ordered, tell him that he need not restrict food or fluids. If contrast medium is ordered, instruct him to fast for 4 hours before the test.
- Explain to the patient who will perform the procedure and where it will take place. Reassure him that the procedure is painless.
- Explain to the patient that he'll be positioned on an X-ray table inside a CT scanner and asked to lie still; the computer-controlled scanner will revolve around him taking multiple scans. Stress that he should lie as still as possible because movement may cause distorted images.
- If a contrast medium is used, tell the patient that he may feel flushed and warm and may experience a transient headache, a salty or metallic taste, and nausea or vomiting after its injection. Reassure him that these reactions are normal.
- Instruct the patient to wear a radiologic examining gown and to remove all metal objects and jewelry in the X-ray field.
- Check the patient's history for hypersensitivity reactions to iodine, shellfish, or contrast media. Mark any such reactions in the chart and notify the physician who may order prophylactic medications or choose not to use a contrast medium.
- If the patient appears restless or apprehensive about the procedure, a mild sedative may be prescribed.
- Ensure that the patient or a responsible family member has signed an informed consent form, if required.

Equipment

CT scanner; contrast medium; I.V. insertion equipment, if needed

Procedure and posttest care

- Place the patient in a supine position on an X-ray table, and tell him to lie as still as possible.
- The table is slid into the circular opening of the CT scanner. The scanner revolves around the patient, taking radiographs at preselected intervals.
- After the first set of scans is taken, the patient is removed from the scanner and a contrast medium is administered if necessary.
- Observe the patient for signs and symptoms of a hypersensitivity reaction, including pruritus, rash, and respiratory difficulty, for 30 minutes after the contrast medium has been injected.

■ After contrast medium I.V. injection, the patient is moved back into the scanner, and another series of scans is taken. The images obtained from the scan are displayed on a monitor during the procedure and stored on magnetic tape to create a permanent record for subsequent study.
■ If contrast media is used, observe for a delayed allergic reaction and treat as necessary. (Diphenhydramine is the drug of choice.)
■ Encourage fluids to assist in elimination of the contrast medium.
■ Tell the patient that he may resume his usual activity level and diet, if appropriate.
■ Provide comfort measures and pain medication as ordered because of prolonged positioning on table.

Precautions

■ This procedure is contraindicated during pregnancy and in patients who are hypersensitive to iodine, shellfish, or contrast media, or in those who have renal insufficiency (if they aren't on dialysis).
■ Some patients may experience strong feelings of claustrophobia or anxiety when inside the CT body scanner. For such patients, a mild sedative may be ordered to help reduce anxiety.
■ For patients with significant bone or joint pain, administer analgesics so that the patient can lie still comfortably during the scan.

Normal findings

The scan should reveal no pathology in the bones or joints. It produces crisp images of the structure while blurring or eliminating details of surrounding structures.

Abnormal findings

Because of its ability to display cross-sectional anatomy, CT scanning is useful for detecting the shoulder, spine, hip, and pelvis. This cross-sectional view eliminates the confusing shadows of superimposed structures that occur with conventional radiographs. The scan can reveal primary bone tumors and soft-tissue tumors as well as skeletal metastasis. It can also reveal joint abnormalities difficult to detect by other methods.

Interfering factors

■ Claustrophobia (possible interference with patient's ability to lie in scanner for long periods)
■ Excessive patient movement
■ Failure to remove metallic objects from examination field (possible poor imaging)

SKELETAL MAGNETIC RESONANCE IMAGING

A noninvasive technique, skeletal magnetic resonance imaging (MRI) produces clear and sensitive tomographic images of bone and soft tissue. The scan provides superior contrast of body tissues and allows imaging of multiple planes, including direct sagittal and coronal views in regions that can't be easily visualized with X-rays or computed tomography (CT) scans. MRI eliminates any risks associated with exposure to X-ray beams and causes no known harm to cells.

MRIs are most easily generated from the proton of the hydrogen atom. Each water molecule has two hydrogen atoms, but the distribution of water molecules varies according to specific body tissue. For example, bone is considered "dry" because it doesn't contain much hydrogen. Consequently, bone produces a weak signal and can't be visualized. However, normal bone marrow has the brightest signal and can be seen well.

Purpose

- To evaluate bony and soft-tissue tumors
- To identify changes in bone marrow composition
- To identify spinal disorders

Patient preparation

- Make sure the scanner can accommodate the patient's weight and abdominal girth.
- Explain to the patient that this test assesses bone and soft tissue. Tell him who will perform the test and where it will take place.
- Explain to the patient that although MRI is painless and involves no exposure to radiation from the scanner, a contrast medium may be used, depending on the type of tissue being studied.
- Explain to the patient that if he's claustrophobic or if extensive time is required for scanning, a mild sedative may be administered to reduce anxiety. Open scanners have been developed for use on patients with extreme claustrophobia or morbid obesity, but tests using such machines take longer.
- Explain to the patient the need to lie flat, and describe the test procedure.
- Explain to the patient that he'll hear the scanner clicking, whirring, and thumping as it moves inside its housing.
- Reassure the patient that he'll be able to communicate with the technician at all times.
- Instruct the patient to remove all metallic objects, including jewelry, hair pins, or watches.
- Ask whether the patient has any surgically implanted joints, pins, clips, valves, pumps, or pacemakers containing metal that could be attracted to the strong MRI magnet. If he does, he won't be able to have the test.
- Ensure that the patient or a responsible family member has signed an informed consent form, if required.

Procedure and posttest care

- At the scanner room door, check the patient one last time for metal objects.
- The patient is placed on a narrow, padded, nonmetallic table that moves into the scanner tunnel. Fans continuously circulate air in the tunnel, and a call bell or intercom is used to maintain verbal contact.
- Remind the patient to remain still throughout the procedure.
- While the patient lies within the strong magnetic field, the area to be studied is stimulated with radio frequency waves.
- If the test is prolonged with the patient lying flat, monitor him for orthostatic hypotension.
- Provide comfort measures and pain medication as needed and ordered because of prolonged positioning in the scanner.
- After the test, tell the patient that he may resume normal activity.
- Provide emotional support to the patient with claustrophobia or anxiety over his diagnosis.

Precautions

- MRI can't be performed on patients with pacemakers, intracranial aneurysm clips, or other ferrous metal implants. Ventilators, I.V. infusion pumps, oxygen tanks, and other metallic or computer-based equipment must be kept out of the MRI area.
- If the patient is unstable, make sure an I.V. line without metal components is in place and that all equipment is compatible with MRI imaging. If necessary, monitor oxygen saturation, cardiac rhythm, and respiratory status dur-

ing the test. An anesthesiologist may be needed to monitor a heavily sedated patient.

■ A technician should maintain verbal contact with the conscious patient.

Normal findings

MRI should reveal no pathology in bone, muscles, and joints.

Abnormal findings

MRI is excellent for visualizing diseases of the spinal canal and cord and for identifying primary and metastatic bone tumors. It's beneficial in anatomic delineation of muscles, ligaments, and bones. The images show superior contrast of body tissues and sharply define healthy, benign, and malignant tissues.

Interfering factors

■ Excessive patient movement
■ Patient unable to fit into scanner

Miscellaneous Tests

Orbital Computed Tomography

Orbital computed tomography (CT) allows visualization of abnormalities not readily seen on standard radiographs, delineating their size, position, and relationship to adjoining structures. A series of tomograms reconstructed by a computer and displayed as anatomic slices on a monitor, the orbital CT scan identifies space-occupying lesions earlier and more accurately than other radiographic techniques and provides three-dimensional images of orbital structures, especially the ocular muscles and the optic nerve.

Purpose

■ To evaluate pathologies of the orbit and eye — especially expanding lesions and bone destruction
■ To evaluate fractures of the orbit and adjoining structures
■ To determine the cause of unilateral exophthalmos

Patient preparation

■ Describe the procedure to the patient, and explain that this test visualizes the anatomy of the eye and its surrounding structures.

■ If contrast enhancement isn't scheduled, inform the patient that he need not restrict food or fluids. If contrast enhancement is scheduled, withhold food and fluids from the patient for 4 hours before the test.

■ Tell the patient that a series of X-ray films will be taken of his eye and explain who will perform the test and where it will take place.

■ Reassure the patient that the test will cause him no discomfort.

■ Tell the patient that he'll be positioned on an X-ray table and that the head of the table will be moved into the scanner, which will rotate around his head and make loud clacking sounds.

■ If a contrast medium will be used for the procedure, tell the patient that he may feel flushed and warm and may experience a transient headache, a salty or metallic taste, and nausea or vomiting after the contrast medium is injected. Reassure him that these reactions are normal.

■ Ensure that the patient or a responsible family member has signed an informed consent form, if required.

■ Check the patient's history for hypersensitivity reactions to iodine, shellfish, or contrast media, and notify the physician of the sensitivities.

■ Instruct the patient to remove jewelry, hairpins, or other metal objects in the X-ray field to allow for precise imaging of the orbital structures.

Equipment

CT scanner; contrast medium; I.V. insertion equipment, if needed

Procedure and posttest care

■ The patient is placed in a supine position on the X-ray table, with his head immobilized by straps, if required. Ask him to lie still.

■ The head of the table is moved into the scanner, which rotates around the patient's head taking radiographs.

■ Information obtained is stored on magnetic tapes, and the images are displayed on a monitor. Photographs may be made if a permanent record is desired.

■ When this series of radiographs has been taken, contrast enhancement is performed. The contrast medium is injected I.V. and a second series of scans is recorded.

■ If a contrast medium was used, watch for its residual adverse effects, including headache, nausea, or vomiting. After the procedure, advise the patient that he may resume his usual diet.

Precautions

■ Use of contrast enhancement is contraindicated in patients with known hypersensitivity reactions to iodine, shellfish, or contrast media used in other tests.

Normal findings

Orbital structures are evaluated for size, shape, and position. Dense orbital bone provides a marked contrast to less dense periocular fat. The optic nerve and the medial and lateral rectus muscles are clearly defined. The rectus muscles appear as thin dense bands on each side, behind the eye. The optic canals should be equal in size.

Abnormal findings

Orbital CT scans can identify intraorbital and extraorbital space-occupying lesions that obscure the normal structures or cause orbital enlargement, indentation of the orbital walls, or bone destruction. This test can also help determine the type of lesion. For example, infiltrative lesions, such as lymphomas and metastatic carcinomas, appear as irregular areas of density. However, encapsulated tumors, such as benign hemangiomas and meningiomas, appear as clearly defined masses of consistent density. CT scans can also visualize intracranial tumors that invade the orbit, thickening of the optic nerve that may occur with gliomas, meningiomas, and secondary tumors that may cause enlargement of the optic canal.

In evaluating fractures, CT scans allow a complete three-dimensional view of the affected structures. In determining the cause of unilateral exophthalmos, CT scans can show early erosion or expansion of the medial orbital wall that may arise from lesions in the ethmoidal cells. It can also detect space-occupying lesions in the orbit or paranasal sinuses that cause exophthalmos. CT scans can also show thickening of the medial and lateral rectus muscles in proptosis resulting from Graves' disease.

Enhancement with a contrast medium may provide information about the circulation through abnormal ocular tissues.

Interfering factors

■ Head movement

■ Failure to remove metallic objects from examination field (possible poor imaging)

THORACIC COMPUTED TOMOGRAPHY

Thoracic computed tomography (CT) provides cross-sectional views of the chest by passing an X-ray beam from a computerized scanner through the body at different angles. CT scanning may be done with or without an injected contrast medium, which is primarily used to highlight blood vessels and to allow greater visual discrimination.

This test provides a three-dimensional image and is especially useful in detecting small differences in tissue density. The thoracic CT scan may replace mediastinoscopy in diagnosis of mediastinal masses and Hodgkin's disease; its value in the evaluation of pulmonary pathology is proven.

Purpose

- To locate suspected neoplasms (such as in Hodgkin's disease), especially with mediastinal involvement
- To differentiate coin-size calcified lesions (indicating tuberculosis) from tumors
- To differentiate emphysema or bronchopleural fistula from lung abscess
- To distinguish tumors adjacent to the aorta from aortic aneurysms
- To detect the invasion of a neck mass in the thorax
- To evaluate primary malignancy that may metastasize to the lungs, especially in patients with primary bone tumors, soft-tissue sarcomas, and melanomas
- To evaluate the mediastinal lymph nodes
- To evaluate the severity of lung disease, such as emphysema
- To detect a dissection or leak of an aortic aneurysm or aortic arch aneurysm
- To plan radiation treatment

Patient preparation

- Explain to the patient that this test provides cross-sectional views of the chest and distinguishes small differences in tissue density.
- If a contrast medium won't be used, inform the patient that he need not restrict food or fluids. If the test is to be performed with contrast enhancement, instruct him to fast for 4 hours before the test.
- Tell the patient who will perform the test and where it will take place.
- Inform the patient that he'll be positioned on an X-ray table that moves into the center of a large ring-shaped piece of X-ray equipment and that the equipment may be noisy.
- Inform the patient that a contrast medium may be injected into a vein in his arm. If so, he may experience nausea, warmth, flushing of the face, and a salty or metallic taste. Reassure him that these symptoms are normal and that radiation exposure is minimal.
- Tell the patient not to move during the test, but to breathe normally until told to follow specific breathing instructions. Instruct him to remove all jewelry and metallic objects in the X-ray field.
- Check the patient's history for hypersensitivity to iodine, shellfish, or contrast media.
- Ensure that the patient or a responsible family member has signed an informed consent form, if required.

Equipment

CT scanner; contrast medium, if ordered; I.V. insertion equipment, if necessary

Procedure and posttest care

- After the patient is placed in a supine position on the X-ray table and the contrast medium has been injected, the machine scans the patient at different angles while the computer calculates small differences in the densities of various tissues, water, fat, bone, and air.

■ This information is displayed as a printout of numerical values and as a projection on a monitor. Images may be recorded for further study.

■ Watch for signs of delayed hypersensitivity to the contrast medium (itching, hypotension or hypertension, or respiratory distress).

■ After the test, encourage the patient to drink lots of fluids.

Precautions

■ Thoracic CT scanning is contraindicated during pregnancy and, if a contrast medium is used, in persons who have a history of hypersensitivity reactions to iodine, shellfish, or contrast media.

Normal findings

Black and white areas on a thoracic CT scan refer, respectively, to air and bone densities. Shades of gray correspond to water, fat, and soft-tissue densities.

Abnormal findings

Abnormal thoracic CT findings include tumors, nodules, cysts, aortic aneurysms, enlarged lymph nodes, pleural effusion, and accumulations of blood, fluid, or fat.

Interfering factors

■ Failure to remove all metallic objects from the scanning field (possible poor imaging)

■ Patient's inability to remain still during the procedure

■ Obese patient (may be too heavy for scanning table)

CARDIAC MAGNETIC RESONANCE IMAGING

A great asset in the diagnosis of cardiac disorders, cardiac magnetic resonance imaging (MRI) has the ability to "see through" bone and to delineate fluid-filled soft tissue in great detail as well as produce images of organs and vessels in motion.

In this noninvasive procedure, the patient is placed in a magnetic field, into which a radio frequency beam is introduced. Resulting energy changes are measured and used by the MRI computer to generate images on a monitor. Cross-sectional images of the anatomy are viewed in multiple planes and recorded for permanent record.

Another technology for evaluating cardiac pathology is positron emission tomography. (See *Cardiac PET scan,* page 654.)

Purpose

■ To identify anatomic sequelae related to myocardial infarction, such as formation of ventricular aneurysm, ventricular wall thinning, and mural thrombus

■ To detect and evaluate cardiomyopathy

■ To detect and evaluate pericardial disease

■ To identify paracardiac or intracardiac masses

■ To detect congenital heart disease, such as atrial or ventricular septal defects, and the degree of malposition of the great vessel

■ To identify vascular disease, such as thoracic aneurysm and thoracic dissection

■ To assess the structure of the pulmonary vasculature

Cardiac PET scan

Positron emission tomography (PET) scanning combines elements of computed tomography (CT) scanning and conventional radionuclide imaging. The cardiac PET scan is used to detect coronary artery disease, to evaluate myocardial metabolism and contractility, and to distinguish viable from infarcted cardiac tissue, especially during early stages of myocardial infarction.

HOW IT WORKS

Like radionuclide imaging, cardiac PET scans measure emissions of injected radioisotopes and convert these values to tomographic images. PET uses radioisotopes of biologically important elements — oxygen, nitrogen, carbon, and fluorine — which emit particles called positrons. During positron emissions, gamma rays are detected by the PET scanner and reconstructed to form an image. One distinct advantage of PET scans is that positron emitters can be chemically "tagged" to biologically active molecules such as carbon monoxide, neurotransmitters, hormones, and metabolites (particularly glucose), enabling study of their uptake and distribution in tissue.

PATIENT PREPARATION

When preparing a patient for a cardiac PET scan, explain the following key points:

◆ If the test is ordered to assess myocardial contractility, explain to the patient that the test distinguishes viable tissue from tissue injured by infarction and may also help the physician assess mitochondrial impairment associated with ischemia or evaluate coronary artery obstruction.

◆ Explain to the patient that he'll be given a radioactive substance, either by injection, inhalation, or I.V. infusion, and that a highly specialized camera will detect the radioactive decay of this substance and send this data to a computer, which converts it to an image.

◆ Describe the test to the patient, including who will perform it and where it will take place. Take time to describe the equipment.

◆ Tell the patient that the test is painless, unless an I.V. infusion is planned, in which case he may experience some discomfort from the needle puncture and the tourniquet. If the radioisotope will be inhaled, explain this painless procedure.

◆ If fasting is ordered, describe to the patient food and fluid restrictions.

◆ Tell the patient that he'll undergo an attenuation scan for about 30 minutes. Then he'll receive the appropriate positron emitter and undergo PET scanning.

Because the radioisotope may be harmful to a fetus, female patients of childbearing age should be screened carefully before undergoing this procedure.

Patient preparation

■ Explain to the patient that this test assesses the heart's function and structure.

■ Tell the patient who will perform the test and where it will be done.

■ Inform the patient that he'll be positioned on a narrow bed, which slides into a large cylinder that houses the MRI magnets. Tell him that the scanner will make clicking, whirring, and thumping noises as it moves inside its housing and that he may receive earplugs.

■ Explain to the patient who's claustrophobic or anxious about the test's duration that he'll receive a mild sedative to reduce his anxiety.

■ Explain to the patient the need to lie flat.

■ Reassure the patient that he'll be able to communicate with the technician at all times and that the procedure will be stopped if he feels claustrophobic.

- Immediately before the test, have the patient remove all metal objects. Double-check to make sure he doesn't have a pacemaker or any surgically implanted joints, pins, clips, valves, or pumps containing metal that could be attracted to the strong MRI magnet. If he does, he won't be able to undergo the test.
- Ensure that the patient or a responsible family member has signed an informed consent form, if required.
- Administer the prescribed sedative.

Procedure and posttest care

- At the scanner room door, check the patient one last time for metal objects.
- The patient is placed supine on a narrow, padded, nonmetallic bed that slides to the desired position inside the scanner. Radio frequency waves are directed at his chest. The resulting images are displayed on a monitor and recorded on film or magnetic tape for permanent storage.
- The radiologist may vary the waves and use the computer to manipulate and enhance the images.
- Remind the patient to remain still throughout the procedure.
- Assess how the patient responds to the enclosed environment. Provide reassurance, if necessary.
- Monitor the sedated patient's hemodynamic, cardiac, respiratory, and mental status until the effects of the sedative have worn off.

Precautions

- Claustrophobic patients may experience anxiety. Monitor cardiac patients for signs of ischemia (chest pressure, shortness of breath, or changes in hemodynamic status).
- MRI can't be performed on patients with pacemakers or intracranial aneurysm clips.
- If the patient is unstable, make sure an I.V. line with no metal components is in place and that all equipment is compatible with MRI imaging. If necessary, monitor the patient's oxygen saturation, cardiac rhythm, and respiratory status during the test.
- An anesthesiologist may be needed to monitor a heavily sedated patient.
- A nurse or radiology technician should maintain verbal contact with the conscious patient.

Normal findings

MRI should reveal no anatomic or structural dysfunctions in cardiovascular tissue.

Abnormal findings

MRI can detect cardiomyopathy and pericardial disease. It can also detect atrial or ventricular septal defects or other congenital defects. MRI is useful for identifying paracardiac or intracardiac masses. In addition, it can evaluate the extent of pericardial or vascular disease.

Interfering factors

- Patient's inability to remain still during the procedure

RENAL COMPUTED TOMOGRAPHY

Renal computed tomography (CT) provides a useful image of the kidneys made from a series of tomograms or cross-sectional slices, which are then translated by a computer and displayed on a monitor. The image density reflects the amount of radiation absorbed by renal tissue and permits identification of masses and other lesions. An I.V. contrast medium may be injected to accentuate the renal parenchyma's density and help differentiate renal masses. This highly accurate test is usually performed to investigate diseases found by other diagnostic procedures such as excretory urography.

Purpose

- To detect and evaluate renal abnormalities, such as tumor, obstruction, calculi, polycystic kidney disease, congenital anomalies, and abnormal fluid accumulation around the kidneys
- To evaluate the retroperitoneum

Patient preparation

- Explain to the patient that this test permits examination of the kidneys.
- If contrast enhancement isn't scheduled, inform the patient that he need not restrict food or fluids. If contrast enhancement is scheduled, instruct him to fast for 4 hours before the test.
- Tell the patient who will perform the test and where it will take place.
- Inform the patient that he'll be positioned on an X-ray table, and that a scanner will take films of his kidneys.
- Warn the patient that the scanner may make loud, clacking sounds as it rotates around his body.
- Tell the patient that he may experience transient adverse effects, such as flushing, metallic taste, and headache, after injection of the contrast medium.
- Make sure that the patient or a responsible family member has signed a consent form, if required.
- Check the patient's history for hypersensitivity to shellfish, iodine, or contrast media. Mark any sensitivities in the patient's chart.
- Just before the procedure, instruct the patient to put on a gown and to remove any metallic objects that could interfere with the scan.
- Administer prescribed sedatives.

Equipment

CT scanner; contrast medium, if ordered; I.V. insertion equipment, if necessary

Procedure and posttest care

- The patient is placed in a supine position on the X-ray table and secured with straps.
- The table is moved into the scanner.
- Instruct the patient to lie still.
- The scanner then rotates around the patient, taking multiple images at different angles within each cross-sectional slice.
- When one series of tomograms is complete, I.V. contrast enhancement may be performed. Another series of tomograms is then taken.
- After the I.V. contrast medium is administered, monitor for allergic reactions, such as respiratory difficulty, urticaria, or other skin eruptions.
- Information from the scan is stored on a disk or on a magnetic tape, fed into a computer, and converted into an image for display on a monitor. Radiographs and photographs are taken of selected views.
- If the procedure was performed with contrast enhancement, observe the patient for hypersensitivity to the contrast medium.
- After the test, tell the patient that he may resume his usual diet.
- If calculi are present, strain urine, hydrate the patient, and discuss nutritional adaptations as indicated.
- Support the patient and his family if surgery is indicated for a neoplasm.
- Monitor the patient's vital signs if a sedative was administered.

Precautions

- Watch for signs of hypersensitivity to the contrast medium if contrast enhancement is required.

Normal findings

Normally, the density of the renal parenchyma is slightly higher than that of the liver, but is much less dense than bone, which appears white on a CT scan. The density of the collecting system is generally low (black), unless a contrast medium is used to enhance it to a higher (whiter) density. The position of the kidneys is evaluated according to the surrounding structures; the size and shape of the kidneys are determined by counting cuts between the superior and inferior poles and following the contour of the renal outline.

Abnormal findings

Renal masses appear as areas of different density than normal parenchyma, possibly altering the kidneys' shape or projecting beyond their margins. Renal cysts, for example, appear as smooth, sharply defined masses, with thin walls and a lower density than normal parenchyma. Tumors such as renal cell carcinoma, however, are usually not as well delineated; they tend to have thick walls and nonuniform density. With contrast enhancement, solid tumors show a higher density than renal cysts but lower density than normal parenchyma. Tumors with hemorrhage, calcification, or necrosis show higher densities. Vascular tumors are more clearly defined with contrast enhancement. Adrenal tumors are confined masses, usually detached from the kidneys and from other retroperitoneal organs.

Renal CT scanning may also identify other abnormalities, including obstructions, calculi, polycystic kidney disease, congenital anomalies, and abnormal accumulations of fluid around the kidneys, such as hematomas, lymphoceles, and abscesses. After nephrectomy, CT scanning can detect abnormal masses, such as recurrent tumors, in a renal fossa that should be empty.

Interfering factors

- Patient's inability to remain still during the procedure
- Presence of contrast media from other recent tests or of foreign bodies such as catheters or surgical clips (possible poor imaging)

14

Nuclear medicine scans

Thyroid

RADIOACTIVE IODINE UPTAKE TEST

The radioactive iodine uptake (RAIU) test evaluates thyroid function by measuring the amount of orally ingested iodine 123 (^{123}I) or iodine 131 (^{131}I) that accumulates in the thyroid gland after 2, 6, and 24 hours. An external single counting probe measures the radioactivity in the thyroid as a percentage of the original dose, thus indicating its ability to trap and retain iodine. The RAIU test accurately diagnoses hyperthyroidism but is less accurate for hypothyroidism. Indications for this test include abnormal results of chemical tests used to evaluate thyroid function.

Purpose

- To evaluate thyroid function
- To help diagnose hyperthyroidism or hypothyroidism
- To help distinguish between primary and secondary thyroid disorders (in combination with other tests)

Patient preparation

- Tell the patient that RAIU testing assesses thyroid function.
- Instruct the patient to begin fasting at midnight the night before the test.
- Explain to the patient that he'll receive radioactive iodine (capsule or liquid) and that he'll then be scanned after 2 hours, 6 hours, and 24 hours.
- Assure the patient that the test is painless and that the small amount of radioactivity used is harmless.
- Check the patient's history for iodine exposure, which may interfere with test results. Note any prior radiologic tests using contrast media, nuclear medicine procedures, or current use of iodine preparations or thyroid medications on the film request slip. Iodine hypersensitivity isn't considered a contraindication because the amount of iodine used is similar to the amount consumed in a normal diet.
- Ensure that the patient or a responsible family member has signed an informed consent form, if required.

Equipment

Oral dose of ^{123}I or ^{131}I (the radiologist determines the exact dosage), external single counting probe

Procedure and posttest care

- After ingesting an oral dose of radioactive iodine, the patient's thyroid is scanned at 2 hours, 6 hours, and 24 hours by placing the anterior portion of his neck in front of an external single counting probe.
- The amount of radioactivity detected by the probe is compared with the amount of radioactivity contained in the original dose to determine the percentage of radioactive iodine retained by the thyroid.
- Instruct the patient to resume a light diet 2 hours after taking the oral dose of radioactive iodine. When the study is complete, the patient may resume a normal diet.

Precautions

- Radioactive iodine uptake testing is contraindicated during pregnancy and lactation because of possible teratogenic effects. It's also contraindicated in patients who are allergic to iodine and shellfish.

Normal findings

After 2 hours, 4% to 12% of the radioactive iodine should have accumulated in the thyroid; after 6 hours,

5% to 20%; at 24 hours, accumulation should be 8% to 29%. The remaining radioactive iodine is excreted in the urine. Local variations in the normal range of iodine uptake may occur due to regional differences in dietary iodine intake and procedural differences among laboratories.

Abnormal findings

Below-normal iodine uptake may indicate hypothyroidism, subacute thyroiditis, or iodine overload. Above-normal uptake may indicate hyperthyroidism, early Hashimoto's thyroiditis, hypoalbuminemia, lithium ingestion, or iodine-deficient goiter. However, in hyperthyroidism, the rate of turnover may be so rapid that a false normal measurement occurs at 24 hours.

Interfering factors

- Renal failure; diuresis; severe diarrhea; X-ray contrast media studies; ingestion of iodine preparations including iodized salt, cough syrups, and some multivitamins (decrease)
- Thyroid hormones, thyroid hormone antagonists, salicylates, penicillins, antihistamines, anticoagulants, corticosteroids, and phenylbutazone (decrease)
- Phenothiazines or iodine-deficient diet (increase)

RADIONUCLIDE THYROID IMAGING

In radionuclide thyroid imaging, the thyroid is studied by gamma camera after the patient receives a radioisotope (iodine 123 [^{123}I], technetium [^{99m}Tc] pertechnetate, or iodine 131 [^{131}I]). Thyroid imaging typically follows discovery of a palpable mass, an enlarged gland, or an asymmetrical goiter and is performed concurrently with thyroid uptake tests and measurements of serum triiodothyronine (T_3) and serum thyroxine levels. Later, thyroid ultrasonography may be performed.

Purpose

- To assess the size, structure, and position of the thyroid gland
- To evaluate thyroid function (in conjunction with other thyroid tests)

Patient preparation

- Tell the patient that this test helps determine the cause of thyroid dysfunction.
- If ^{123}I or ^{131}I will be used, tell the patient to fast after midnight the night before the test. Fasting isn't required if an I.V. injection of ^{99m}Tc pertechnetate is used.
- Explain to the patient that after he receives the radiopharmaceutical, a gamma camera will be used to produce an image of his thyroid. Tell him that the imaging procedure will take about 30 minutes and assure him that his exposure to radiation is minimal.
- Ask the patient if he has undergone tests that used radiographic contrast media within the past 60 days. Note previous radiographic contrast media exposure on the X-ray request.
- Check the patient's diet and medication history. Medications, such as thyroid hormones, thyroid hormone antagonists, and iodine preparations (Lugol's solution, some multivitamins, and cough syrups) should be discontinued 2 to 3 weeks before the test as ordered. Phenothiazines, corticosteroids, salicylates, anticoagulants, and antihistamines should be discontinued 1 week before the test as ordered. Instruct the patient to stop consuming iodized salt, iodinated salt substitutes, and seafood for 14 to 21 days as ordered. Liothyro-

nine, propylthiouracil, and methimazole should be discontinued 3 days before the test, and thyroxine should be discontinued 10 days before the test as ordered.

- The patient receives ^{123}I or ^{131}I (oral) or ^{99m}Tc pertechnetate (I.V.). Record the date and the time of administration.
- The patient receiving an oral radioisotope should fast for another 2 hours after administration.
- Just before the test, tell the patient to remove dentures, jewelry, and other materials that may interfere with the imaging process.
- Ensure that the patient or a responsible family member has signed an informed consent form, if required.

Procedure and posttest care

- The test is performed 24 hours after oral administration of ^{123}I or ^{131}I or 20 to 30 minutes after I.V. injection of ^{99m}Tc pertechnetate. Just before the test, tell the patient to remove his dentures and any jewelry that could interfere with visualization of the thyroid.
- The patient is placed in a supine position with his neck extended; the thyroid gland is palpated. The gamma camera is positioned above the anterior portion of his neck.
- Images of the patient's thyroid gland are projected on a monitor and are recorded on X-ray film. Three views of the thyroid are obtained: a straight-on anterior view and two bilateral oblique views.
- Following the procedure, tell the patient he may resume medications suspended for the test as ordered. Instruct him to resume his normal diet.

Precautions

- Radionuclide thyroid imaging is contraindicated during pregnancy and lactation and in patients with a previous allergy to iodine, shellfish, or radioactive tracers.

Normal findings

Normally, radionuclide thyroid imaging reveals a thyroid gland that's about 2″ (5 cm) long and 1″ (2.5 cm) wide, with a uniform uptake of the radioisotope and without tumors. The gland is butterfly-shaped, with the isthmus located at the midline. Occasionally, a third lobe called the *pyramidal lobe* may be present; this is a normal variant.

Abnormal findings

During radionuclide thyroid imaging, hyperfunctioning nodules (areas of excessive iodine uptake) appear as black regions called *hot spots.* The presence of hot spots requires a follow-up T_3 thyroid suppression test to determine if the hyperfunctioning areas are autonomous. Hypofunctioning nodules (areas of little or no iodine uptake) appear as white or light gray regions called *cold spots.* If a cold spot appears, subsequent thyroid ultrasonography may be performed to rule out cysts; in addition, fine needle aspiration and biopsy of such nodules may be performed to rule out malignancy. (See *Results of thyroid imaging in thyroid disorders,* page 662.)

Interfering factors

- Iodine-deficient diet, phenothiazines (increase)
- Decrease uptake of radioactive iodine due to renal disease; ingestion of iodized salt, iodine preparations, iodinated salt substitutes, or seafood; and use of thyroid hormones, thyroid hormone antagonists, aminosalicylic acid, corticosteroids, multivitamins or cough syrups containing inorganic iodine (decrease)
- Severe diarrhea and vomiting, impairing GI absorption of radioiodine (decrease)

Results of thyroid imaging in thyroid disorders

The chart below shows the characteristic findings in radionuclide imaging tests that are associated with various thyroid disorders as well as the possible causes of those disorders.

CONDITION	FINDINGS	CAUSES
Hypothyroidism	◆ Glandular damage or absent gland	◆ Surgical removal of gland ◆ Inflammation ◆ Radiation ◆ Neoplasm (rare)
Hypothyroid goiter	◆ Enlarged gland ◆ Decreased uptake (of radioactive iodine) if glandular destruction is present ◆ Increased uptake possible from congenital error in thyroxine synthesis	◆ Insufficient iodine intake ◆ Hypersecretion of thyroid-stimulating hormone (TSH) caused by thyroid hormone deficiency
Myxedema (cretinism in children)	◆ Normal or slightly reduced gland size ◆ Uniform pattern ◆ Decreased uptake	◆ Defective embryonic development, resulting in congenital absence or underdevelopment of thyroid gland ◆ Maternal iodine deficiency
Hyperthyroidism (Graves' disease)	◆ Enlarged gland ◆ Uniform pattern ◆ Increased uptake	◆ Unknown, but may be hereditary ◆ Production of thyroid-stimulating immunoglobulins
Toxic nodular goiter	◆ Multiple hot spots	◆ Long-standing simple goiter
Hyperfunctioning adenomas	◆ Solitary hot spot	◆ Adenomatous production of triiodothyronine and thyroxine, suppressing TSH secretion and producing atrophy of other thyroid tissue
Hypofunctioning adenomas	◆ Solitary cold spot	◆ Cyst or nonfunctioning nodule
Benign multinodular goiter	◆ Multiple nodules with variable or no function	◆ Local inflammation ◆ Degeneration
Thyroid carcinoma	◆ Usually a solitary cold spot with occasional or no function	◆ Neoplasm

RESPIRATORY SYSTEM

LUNG PERFUSION SCAN

A lung perfusion scan produces an image of pulmonary blood flow after I.V. injection of a radiopharmaceutical, either human serum albumin microspheres or macroaggregated albumin bonded to technetium.

Purpose

- To assess arterial perfusion of the lungs
- To detect pulmonary emboli
- To evaluate pulmonary function before lung resection

Patient preparation

- Tell the patient that this test helps evaluate respiratory function.
- Explain to the patient that he need not restrict food or fluids before the test.
- Describe to the patient the test, including who will perform it and where it will take place.
- Tell the patient that a radiopharmaceutical will be injected into a vein in his arm and that he'll then sit in front of a camera or lie under it. Explain that neither the camera nor the uptake probe emits radiation and that the amount of radioactivity in the radiopharmaceutical is minimal.
- Assure the patient that he'll be comfortable during the test and that he doesn't have to remain perfectly still.
- On the test request, note if the patient has conditions such as chronic obstructive pulmonary disease (COPD), vasculitis, pulmonary edema, tumor, sickle cell disease, or parasitic disease.
- Ensure that the patient or a responsible family member has signed an informed consent form, if required.

Equipment

Scanner; radiopharmaceutical agent for I.V. use; I.V. insertion equipment, if needed

Procedure and posttest care

- With the patient supine and taking moderately deep breaths, the radiopharmaceutical is injected I.V. slowly over 5 to 10 seconds to allow more even distribution of pulmonary blood flow.
- After the injection, the gamma camera takes a series of single stationary images in the anterior, posterior, oblique, and both lateral chest views.
- Images, which are projected on an oscilloscope screen, show the distribution of radioactive particles.
- If a hematoma develops at the injection site after the test, apply warm soaks.

Precautions

- A lung scan is contraindicated in patients hypersensitive to the radiopharmaceutical.

Normal findings

Areas with normal blood perfusion called hot spots show a high uptake of the radioactive substance; a normal lung shows a uniform uptake pattern.

Abnormal findings

Areas of low radioactive uptake called cold spots indicate poor perfusion, suggesting an embolism; however, a ventilation scan is necessary to confirm diagnosis. Decreased regional blood flow that occurs without vessel obstruction may indicate pneumonitis.

Interfering factors

- Scheduling more than one radionuclide test per day, especially if using different tracing substances (may hinder diffusion of tracer isotope in second test)
- Administering all the radiopharmaceutical while the patient is in sitting position (possible poor imaging due to settling of tracer isotope in lung bases)
- Conditions such as COPD, vasculitis, pulmonary edema, tumor, sickle cell disease, and parasitic disease (possible poor imaging)

LUNG VENTILATION SCAN

The lung ventilation scan is performed after the patient inhales a mixture of air and radioactive gas that delineates areas of the lung ventilated during respiration. The scan records the distribution of the gas during three phases: the buildup of radioactive gas (wash-in phase), the time after rebreathing when radioactivity reaches a steady level (equilibrium phase), and after removal of the radioactive gas from the lungs (wash-out phase).

Purpose

- To help diagnose pulmonary emboli
- To identify areas of the lung capable of ventilation
- To help evaluate regional respiratory function
- To locate regional hypoventilation which may indicate atelectasis, obstructing tumors, or chronic obstructive pulmonary disease

Patient preparation

- Describe the procedure to the patient, and explain that this test helps evaluate respiratory function.
- Tell the patient that he need not restrict food or fluids.
- Tell the patient who will perform the test and where it will take place.
- Ask the patient to remove all jewelry and metal objects from the scanning field.
- Explain to the patient that he'll be asked to hold his breath for a short time after inhaling a gas and to remain still while a machine scans his chest.
- Reassure the patient that a minimal amount of radioactive gas is used.
- Ensure that the patient or a responsible family member has signed an informed consent form, if required.

Equipment

Nuclear scanner, radioactive gas, mask

Procedure and posttest care

- After the patient inhales air mixed with a small amount of radioactive gas through a mask, its distribution in the lungs is monitored on a nuclear scanner.
- The patient's chest is scanned as he exhales.

Precautions

- Watch for leaks in the closed system of radioactive gas, such as through the mask, which can contaminate the surrounding atmosphere.

Normal findings

Normal findings include an equal distribution of gas in both lungs and normal wash-in and wash-out phases.

Abnormal findings

Unequal gas distribution in both lungs indicates poor ventilation or airway obstruction in areas with low radioactivity.

When compared with a lung scan (perfusion scan), in vascular obstructions, such as pulmonary embolism, the perfusion to the embolized area is decreased, but the ventilation to this area is maintained; in parenchymal disease such as pneumonia, ventilation is abnormal within the areas of consolidation.

Interfering factors

- Failure to remove jewelry and other metal objects from the scanning field (possible poor imaging)

CARDIOVASCULAR SYSTEM

TECHNETIUM PYROPHOSPHATE SCAN

Technetium pyrophosphate scanning (also called *hot spot myocardial imaging* or *infarct avid imaging*) is used to detect a recent myocardial infarction (MI) and to determine its extent. This test uses an I.V. tracer isotope (technetium Tc 99m [^{99m}Tc] pyrophosphate). This isotope accumulates in damaged myocardial tissue (possibly by combining with calcium in the damaged myocardial cells), where it forms a "hot spot" on a scan made with a scintillation camera. Such hot spots first appear within 12 hours of infarction, are most apparent after 48 to 72 hours, and usually disappear after 1 week. Hot spots that persist longer than 1 week usually suggest ongoing myocardial damage.

Purpose

- To confirm recent MI
- To help define the size and location of an MI
- To assess the prognosis after acute MI

Patient preparation

- Explain to the patient that this test helps assess if the heart muscle is injured.
- Inform the patient that he need not restrict food or fluids. Tell him who will perform the test and where it will take place.
- Inform the patient that he'll receive a tracer isotope I.V. 2 or 3 hours before the procedure and that multiple images of his heart will be made.
- Reassure the patient that the injection causes only transient discomfort, that the scan itself is painless, and that the test involves less exposure to radiation than a chest X-ray.
- Instruct the patient to remain quiet and motionless while he's being scanned.
- Make sure the patient or a responsible family member has signed an informed consent form, if required.

Equipment

Scanner; ^{99m}Tc pyrophosphate; I.V. equipment, if needed

Procedure and posttest care

- Usually, 20 millicuries of ^{99m}Tc pyrophosphate are injected I.V. into the antecubital vein.
- After 2 or 3 hours, the patient is placed in a supine position and electrocardiography electrodes are attached for continuous monitoring during the test.
- Generally, scans are taken with the patient in several positions, including anterior, left anterior oblique, right anterior oblique, and left lateral. Each scan takes 10 minutes.

Precautions

- Monitor the patient for adverse reactions to the injected media.

Normal findings

A normal technetium pyrophosphate scan shows no isotope in the myocardium.

Abnormal findings

The isotope is taken up by the sternum and ribs, and their activity is compared with the heart's; 2+, 3+, and 4+ activity (equal to or greater than bone) indicates a positive myocardial scan. The technetium pyrophosphate scan can reveal areas of isotope accumulation, or hot spots, in damaged myocardium, particularly 48 to 72 hours after onset of acute MI; however, hot spots are apparent as early as 12 hours after acute MI. In most patients with MI, hot spots disappear after 1 week; in some, they persist for several months if necrosis continues in the area of infarction.

Knowing where the infarct is makes it possible to anticipate complications and to plan patient care. About one-fourth of patients with unstable angina pectoris show hot spots due to subclinical myocardial necrosis and may require coronary arteriography and bypass grafting.

Interfering factors

- Isotope accumulation (in about 10% of patients, may result from ventricular aneurysm associated with dystrophic calcification, pulmonary neoplasm, recent cardioversion, or valvular heart disease due to severe calcification)

THALLIUM IMAGING

Also called *cold spot myocardial imaging* or *thallium scintigraphy,* thallium imaging evaluates myocardial blood flow after I.V. injection of the radioisotope thallium 201 or Cardiolite. The main difference between these two tracers is that Cardiolite has a better energy spectrum for imaging. Cardiolite requires living myocardial cells for uptake and allows for imaging the myocardial blood flow before and after reperfusion. This allows for better estimation of myocardial salvage. Because thallium, the physiologic analogue of potassium, concentrates in healthy myocardial tissue but not in necrotic or ischemic tissue, areas of the heart with a normal blood supply and intact cells rapidly take it up. Areas with poor blood flow and ischemic cells fail to take up the isotope and appear as "cold spots" on a scan.

This test is performed in a resting state or after stress. Resting imaging can detect acute myocardial infarction (MI) within the first few hours of symptoms but doesn't distinguish an old from a new infarct. Stress imaging, performed after the patient exercises on a treadmill until he experiences angina or rate-limiting fatigue, can assess known or suspected coronary artery disease (CAD) and can evaluate the effectiveness of antianginal therapy or balloon angioplasty and the patency of grafts after coronary artery bypass surgery. Possible complications of stress testing include arrhythmias, angina pectoris, and MI.

Purpose

- To assess myocardial scarring and perfusion
- To demonstrate the location and extent of acute or chronic MI, including

transmural and postoperative infarction (resting imaging)

- To diagnose CAD (stress imaging)
- To evaluate the patency of grafts after coronary artery bypass surgery
- To evaluate the effectiveness of antianginal therapy or balloon angioplasty (stress imaging)

Patient preparation

- Explain to the patient that these tests help determine if any areas of the heart muscle aren't receiving an adequate supply of blood.
- If the patient will be undergoing stress imaging, instruct him to restrict alcohol, tobacco, and nonprescribed medications for 24 hours before the test and to have nothing by mouth for 3 hours before the test.
- Describe the test, including who will perform it and where it will take place. Explain that additional scans may be required.
- Tell the patient that he'll receive a radioactive tracer I.V. and that multiple images of his heart will be scanned.
- Explain to the patient that it's important to lie still when images are taken.
- Warn the patient that he may experience discomfort from skin abrasion during preparation for electrode placement. Assure him that the test involves minimal radiation exposure.
- Make sure the patient or a responsible family member has signed an informed consent form, if required.
- Tell the patient undergoing stress imaging to wear walking shoes during the treadmill exercise and to report fatigue, pain, or shortness of breath immediately.

Equipment

Scanner; I.V. insertion equipment, if needed; radioactive tracer

Procedure and posttest care

Resting imaging

- Optimally, within the first few hours of symptoms of MI, the patient receives an injection of thallium I.V. or Cardiolite and scanning begins after 10 minutes.
- If further scanning is required, have the patient rest and restrict food and beverages other than water.

Stress imaging

- The patient, wired with electrodes, walks on a treadmill at a regulated pace that's gradually increased, while the electrocardiogram (ECG), blood pressure, and heart rate are monitored.
- When the patient reaches peak stress, the examiner injects 1.5 to 3 millicuries of thallium into the antecubital vein and then flushes it with 10 to 15 ml of normal saline solution or an infusion of Cardiolite.
- The patient exercises an additional 45 to 60 seconds to permit circulation and uptake of the isotope, and then lies on his back under the scintillation camera.
- If the patient is asymptomatic, the precordial leads are removed. Scanning begins after 10 minutes with the patient in anterior, left anterior oblique, and left lateral positions.
- Additional scans may be taken after the patient rests and occasionally after 24 hours. Taking a scan after the patient rests is helpful in differentiating between an ischemic area and an infarcted or scarred area of the myocardium.

Precautions

- Contraindications include impaired neuromuscular function, pregnancy, locomotor disturbances, acute MI or myocarditis, aortic stenosis, acute infection, unstable metabolic conditions (such as diabetes), digoxin toxicity, and recent pulmonary infarction.

■ Stop stress imaging at once if the patient develops chest pain, dyspnea, fatigue, syncope, hypotension, ischemic ECG changes, significant arrhythmias, or critical signs (pale, clammy skin, confusion, or staggering).
■ Emergency medical equipment should be readily available, if needed.

Normal findings

Imaging should show normal distribution of the isotope throughout the left ventricle and no defects (cold spots). The results may be normal if the patient has narrowed coronary arteries but adequate collateral circulation.

Abnormal findings

Persistent defects indicate MI; transient defects (those that disappear after 3 to 6 hours of rest) indicate ischemia from CAD. After coronary artery bypass surgery, improved regional perfusion suggests patency of the graft. Increased perfusion after ingestion of antianginal drugs can show that they relieve ischemia. Improved perfusion after balloon angioplasty suggests increased coronary flow.

Interfering factors

■ Cold spots (possible result of sarcoidosis, myocardial fibrosis, cardiac contusion, attenuation due to soft tissue, apical cleft, coronary spasm and artifacts such as implants and electrodes)
■ Absence of cold spots in the presence of CAD (possibly due to insignificant obstruction, inadequate stress, delayed imaging, collateral circulation, or single-vessel disease, particularly of the right or left circumflex coronary arteries)

PERSANTINE-THALLIUM IMAGING

Persantine-thallium imaging is an alternative method of assessing coronary vessel function for patients who can't tolerate exercise or stress electrocardiography (ECG). Dipyridamole (Persantine) infusion simulates the effects of exercise by increasing blood flow to the collateral circulation and away from the coronary arteries, thereby inducing ischemia. Thallium infusion allows the examiner to evaluate the cardiac vessels' response. The heart is scanned immediately after the thallium infusion and again 2 to 4 hours later. Diseased vessels can't deliver thallium to the heart, and thallium lingers in diseased areas of the myocardium.

Purpose

■ To identify exercise- or stress-induced arrhythmias
■ To assess the presence and degree of cardiac ischemia

Patient preparation

■ Tell the patient that a painless, 5- to 10-minute baseline ECG will precede the test.
■ Explain to the patient that he'll need to restrict food and fluids before the test. Tell him to avoid caffeine and other stimulants (which may cause arrhythmias).
■ Instruct the patient to continue to take all his regular medications, with the possible exception of beta-adrenergic blockers, as prescribed.
■ Explain to the patient that an I.V. line infuses the medications for the study. Tell him who will start the I.V. and when, and that the needle insertion and the tourniquet may cause some discomfort.

■ Inform the patient that he may experience mild nausea, headache, dizziness, or flushing after Persantine administration. Reassure him that these adverse reactions are usually temporary and rarely need treatment.

■ Make sure the patient or a responsible family member has signed an informed consent form, if required.

Procedure and posttest care

■ The patient reclines or sits while a resting ECG is performed. Then Persantine is given either orally or I.V. over 4 minutes. Blood pressure, pulse rate, and cardiac rhythm are monitored continuously.

■ After administration of Persantine, the patient is asked to get up and walk. After Persantine takes effect, thallium is injected.

■ The patient is placed in a supine position for about 40 minutes while the scan is performed. Then the scan is reviewed. If necessary, a second scan is performed.

■ If the patient must return for further scanning, tell him to rest and to restrict food and fluids in the interim.

Precautions

■ The patient may experience arrhythmias, angina, ST-segment depression, or bronchospasm. Make sure resuscitation equipment is readily available.

■ More common adverse reactions are nausea, headache, flushing, dizziness, and epigastric pain.

Normal findings

Imaging should reveal characteristic distribution of the isotope throughout the left ventricle and no visible defects.

Abnormal findings

The presence of ST-segment depression, angina, and arrhythmias strongly suggests coronary artery disease (CAD). Persistent ST-segment depression generally indicates myocardial infarction. In contrast, transient ST-segment depression indicates ischemia from CAD.

"Cold spots" usually indicate CAD but may result from sarcoidosis, myocardial fibrosis, cardiac contusion, attenuation due to soft tissue (for example, breast and diaphragm), apical cleft, and coronary spasm. The absence of cold spots in the presence of CAD may result from insignificant obstruction, single-vessel disease, or collateral circulation.

Interfering factors

■ Failure to observe pretest restrictions

■ Artifacts such as implants and electrodes (possible false-positive)

■ Absence of cold spots with CAD (possible delay in imaging)

CARDIAC BLOOD POOL IMAGING

Cardiac blood pool imaging evaluates regional and global ventricular performance after I.V. injection of human serum albumin or red blood cells (RBCs) tagged with the isotope technetium 99m (^{99m}Tc) pertechnetate. In first-pass imaging, a scintillation camera records the radioactivity emitted by the isotope in its initial pass through the left ventricle. Higher counts of radioactivity occur during diastole because there's more blood in the ventricle; lower counts occur during systole as the blood is ejected. The portion of isotope ejected during each heartbeat can then be calculated to determine the ejection fraction; the presence and size of intracardiac shunts can also be determined.

Gated cardiac blood pool imaging, performed after first-pass imaging or as a separate test, has several forms; however, most forms use signals from an electrocardiogram (ECG) to trigger the scintillation camera. In two-frame gated imaging, the camera records left ventricular end-systole and end-diastole for 500 to 1,000 cardiac cycles; superimposition of these gated images allows assessment of left ventricular contraction to find areas of hypokinesia or akinesia.

In multiple-gated acquisition (MUGA) scanning, the camera records 14 to 64 points of a single cardiac cycle, yielding sequential images that can be studied like motion picture films to evaluate regional wall motion and determine the ejection fraction and other indices of cardiac function. In the stress MUGA test, the same test is performed at rest and after exercise to detect changes in ejection fraction and cardiac output. In the nitroglycerine MUGA test, the scintillation camera records points in the cardiac cycle after the sublingual administration of nitroglycerin to assess its effect on ventricular function.

Blood pool imaging is more accurate and involves less risk to the patient than left ventriculography in assessing cardiac function.

Purpose

- To evaluate left ventricular function
- To detect aneurysms of the left ventricle and other motion abnormalities of the myocardial wall (areas of akinesia or dyskinesia)
- To detect intracardiac shunting

Patient preparation

- Explain to the patient that this test permits assessment of the heart's left ventricle.
- Describe the test, including who will perform it, where it will take place, and its expected duration.
- Tell the patient that he need not restrict food or fluids before the test.
- Explain to the patient that he'll receive an I.V. injection of a radioactive tracer and that a detector positioned above his chest will record the circulation of this tracer through the heart.
- Reassure the patient that the tracer poses no radiation hazard and rarely produces adverse effects.
- Inform the patient that he may experience transient discomfort from the needle puncture, but that the imaging itself is painless.
- Instruct the patient to remain silent and motionless during imaging, unless otherwise instructed.
- Make sure the patient or a responsible family member has signed an informed consent form, if required.

Equipment

Scanner; ECG recorder; nitroglycerine; I.V. insertion equipment, if necessary

Procedure and posttest care

- The patient is placed in a supine position beneath the detector of a scintillation camera, and 15 to 20 millicuries of albumin or RBCs tagged with ^{99m}Tc pertechnetate are injected I.V.
- For the next minute, the scintillation camera records the first pass of the isotope through the heart so that the aortic and mitral valves can be located.
- Then, using an ECG, the camera is gated for selected 60-millisecond intervals, representing end-systole and end-diastole, and 500 to 1,000 cardiac cycles are recorded on X-ray or Polaroid film.
- To observe septal and posterior wall motion, the patient may be assisted to modified left anterior oblique position; or he may be assisted to right anterior oblique position and given 0.4 mg of nitroglycerin sublingually. The scintillation camera then records additional gated images to evaluate abnormal contraction in the left ventricle.

- The patient may be asked to exercise as the scintillation camera records gated images.
- If the patient is elderly or physically compromised, assist him to a sitting position and make sure he isn't dizzy. Then provide assistance in getting off the examination table.

Precautions

- Cardiac blood pool imaging is contraindicated during pregnancy.

Normal findings

Normally, the left ventricle contracts symmetrically, and the isotope appears evenly distributed in the scans. Normal ejection fraction is 55% to 65%.

Abnormal findings

Patients with coronary artery disease usually have asymmetrical blood distribution to the myocardium, which produces segmental abnormalities of ventricular wall motion; such abnormalities may also result from preexisting conditions, such as myocarditis. In contrast, patients with cardiomyopathies show globally reduced ejection fractions. In patients with left-to-right shunts, the recirculating radioisotope prolongs the downslope of the curve of scintigraphic data; early arrival of activity in the left ventricle or aorta signifies a right-to-left shunt.

Interfering factors

- None significant

MISCELLANEOUS TESTS

BONE SCAN

A bone scan involves imaging the skeleton by a scanning camera after I.V. injection of a radioactive tracer compound. The tracer of choice, radioactive technetium diphosphonate, collects in bone tissue in increased concentrations at sites of abnormal metabolism. When scanned, these sites appear as hot spots that are often detectable months before an X-ray can reveal any lesion. To promote early detection of lesions, this test may be performed with a gallium scan.

Purpose

- To detect or to rule out malignant bone lesions when radiographic findings are normal but cancer is confirmed or suspected
- To detect occult bone trauma due to pathologic fractures
- To monitor degenerative bone disorders
- To detect infection
- To evaluate unexplained bone pain
- To stage cancer

Patient preparation

- Describe the procedure to the patient. Explain that this test may detect skeletal abnormalities sooner than is possible with ordinary X-rays.
- Tell the patient who will perform the test, where it will take place, and that he may have to assume various positions on a scanner table. Emphasize that he must keep still for the scan.
- Assure the patient that the scan itself is painless and that the isotope, al-

though radioactive, emits less radiation than a standard X-ray machine.

- Make sure the patient or a responsible family member has signed an informed consent form, if required.
- If a bone scan is ordered to diagnose cancer, evaluate the patient's emotional state and offer support.
- Administer prescribed analgesics.
- After the patient receives an I.V. injection of the tracer and imaging agent, encourage him to increase his intake of fluids for the next 1 to 3 hours to facilitate renal clearance of the circulating free tracer.

Equipment

Bone mineral tracer; 3-ml syringe; 21G needle; I.V. insertion equipment, if needed; scanning camera

Procedure and posttest care

- The patient receives an I.V. injection of tracer and imaging agent. Encourage increased fluids for the next 1 to 3 hours to facilitate renal clearance.
- Instruct the patient to void immediately before the procedure (otherwise, a urinary catheter may be inserted to empty the bladder), then position him on the scanner table.
- As the scanner head moves back and forth over the patient's body, it detects low-level radiation emitted by the skeleton and translates this into a film or paper chart, or both, to produce two-dimensional pictures of the area scanned.
- The scanner takes as many views as needed to cover the specified area. The patient may have to be repositioned several times during the test to obtain adequate views. Children who can't hold still for the scan may need to be sedated.
- Check the injection site for redness or swelling. If a hematoma develops, apply warm soaks.
- Don't schedule any other radionuclide tests for 24 to 48 hours.
- Instruct the patient to drink lots of fluids and to empty his bladder frequently for the next 24 to 48 hours.
- Provide analgesics for pain resulting from positioning on the scanning table as needed.

Precautions

- To avoid exposing the fetus or infant to radiation, a bone scan is contraindicated during pregnancy or lactation.
- Allergic reactions to radionuclides may occur.

Normal findings

The tracer concentrates in bone tissue at sites of new bone formation or increased metabolism. The epiphyses of growing bone are normal sites of high concentration, or hot spots.

Abnormal findings

Although a bone scan demonstrates hot spots that identify sites of bone formation, it doesn't distinguish between normal and abnormal bone formation. But scan results can identify all types of bone malignancy, infection, fracture, and other disorders, if viewed in light of the patient's medical and surgical history, X-rays, and other laboratory tests.

Interfering factors

- Distended bladder (possible obscuring of pelvic detail)
- Improper injection technique (possible seepage of tracer into muscle tissue, creating false hot spots)
- Antihypertensives (invalidate test results)

LIVER-SPLEEN SCAN

In liver-spleen scanning, a gamma camera records the distribution of radioactivity within the liver and spleen after I.V. injection of a radioactive colloid. The colloid most commonly used, technetium 99m (^{99m}Tc) sulfide, concentrates in the reticuloendothelial cells through phagocytosis. About 80% to 90% of the injected colloid is taken up by Kupffer's cells in the liver, 5% to 10% by the spleen, and 3% to 5% by bone marrow. The gamma camera images either organ instantaneously without moving.

Although the indications for this test include the detection of focal disease, such as tumors, cysts, and abscesses, liver-spleen scanning demonstrates focal disease nonspecifically as a "cold spot" (a defect that fails to take up the colloid) and may fail to detect focal lesions smaller than ¾" (2 cm) in diameter. Although clinical signs and symptoms may aid diagnosis, liver-spleen scanning frequently requires confirmation by ultrasonography, computed tomography (CT), gallium scanning, or biopsy. CT scan is the fastest method of evaluating liver or splenic injury in abdominal trauma and is preferred to other scans.

Purpose

- To screen for hepatic metastases and hepatocellular disease, such as cirrhosis and hepatitis
- To detect focal disease, such as tumors, cysts, and abscesses, in the liver and spleen
- To demonstrate hepatomegaly or splenomegaly (in patients with palpable abdominal masses)
- To assess the condition of the liver and spleen after abdominal trauma

Patient preparation

- Explain to the patient that this procedure permits examination of the liver and spleen through scintigrams or scans taken after I.V. injection of a radioactive substance.
- Inform the patient that he need not restrict food or fluids before the test.
- Tell the patient who will perform the test and where it will take place.
- Explain to the patient that he may experience transient discomfort from the needle puncture.
- Make sure the patient isn't scheduled for more than one radionuclide scan on the same day.
- Assure the patient that the injection isn't dangerous because the test substance contains only trace amounts of radioactivity and allergic reactions to it are rare.
- Explain to the patient that the detector head of the gamma camera may touch his abdomen (if appropriate), and reassure him that this isn't dangerous.
- Advise the patient that he'll be asked to lie still and to breathe quietly during the procedure to ensure images of good quality; he may also be asked to hold his breath briefly. Explain that this technique helps to evaluate liver mobility and pliability.
- Make sure the patient or a responsible family member has signed an informed consent form, if required.

Equipment

Scanner; ^{99m}Tc sulfide; I.V. insertion equipment, if needed

Procedure and posttest care

- The ^{99m}Tc sulfide is injected I.V.; after 10 to 15 minutes, the patient's abdomen is scanned with the patient placed in supine, left and right lateral, left and right anterior oblique, and prone positions to ensure optimal visualization of the liver and spleen.

- The left anterior oblique position provides the best view of the spleen separate from the left lobe of the liver. With the patient supine, liver mobility and pliability may be evaluated by marking the costal margin and scanning as the patient breathes deeply (fixation suggests pathology).
- The scintigrams are reviewed for clarity before the patient is allowed to leave. If necessary, additional views are obtained.
- Watch for anaphylactoid reactions (shortness of breath, chest tightness, itching, headache) or pyrogenic (fever-producing) reactions, which may result from a stabilizer, such as dextran or gelatin, added to ^{99m}Tc sulfide.
- Inform the patient that the radioactive substance is eliminated from the body within 6 to 24 hours. Urge him to increase his fluid intake (unless contraindicated) to encourage this process.
- Instruct the patient to flush the toilet immediately after urinating to reduce exposure to radiation in the urine.

Precautions

- Liver-spleen scanning is usually contraindicated in children and during pregnancy and lactation.

Normal findings

Because the liver and spleen contain equal numbers of reticuloendothelial cells, both organs normally appear equally bright on the image. However, distribution of radioactive colloid is generally more uniform and homogeneous in the spleen than in the liver. The liver has various normal indentations and impressions, such as the gallbladder fossa and falciform ligament, that may mimic focal disease. (See *Identifying liver indentations in nuclear imaging.*)

Abnormal findings

Although liver-spleen scanning may fail to detect early hepatocellular disease, it shows characteristic, distinct patterns as such disease progresses. The most prominent sign of hepatocellular disease is a shift of the radioactive colloid that's caused by reduced hepatic blood flow and impaired function of Kupffer's cells. This inhibits distribution of the colloid in the liver, causing the liver to appear uniformly decreased or patchy. The spleen and bone marrow then take up the abnormally large amounts of the colloid unabsorbed by the liver, thus concentrating more radioactivity than the liver, and appear brighter on the scan. This same distribution pattern (colloid shift) also accompanies portal hypertension due to extrahepatic causes.

Hepatitis and cirrhosis are both associated with hepatomegaly and a colloid shift, but certain characteristics help distinguish them. In hepatitis, distribution of the colloid is usually uniformly decreased; in cirrhosis, it's patchy. Splenomegaly is typical in cirrhosis but not in hepatitis.

Metastasis to the liver or spleen may appear on the scan as a focal defect and requires biopsy to confirm the diagnosis. Liver metastasis usually originates in the GI or genitourinary tract, the breasts, or the lungs and is more common than metastasis to the spleen. After metastasis is confirmed, serial liver-spleen studies are useful in evaluating effectiveness of therapy.

Because cysts, abscesses, and tumors fail to take up the radioactive colloid, they appear on the scan as solitary or multiple focal defects. Hepatic cysts may appear as solitary defects; polycystic hepatic disease, as multiple defects. Splenic cysts are less common than he-

Identifying liver indentations in nuclear imaging

In nuclear imaging, normal indentations and impressions may be mistaken for focal lesions. These drawings of the liver — anterior view and posterior view — identify the contours and impressions that may be misread.

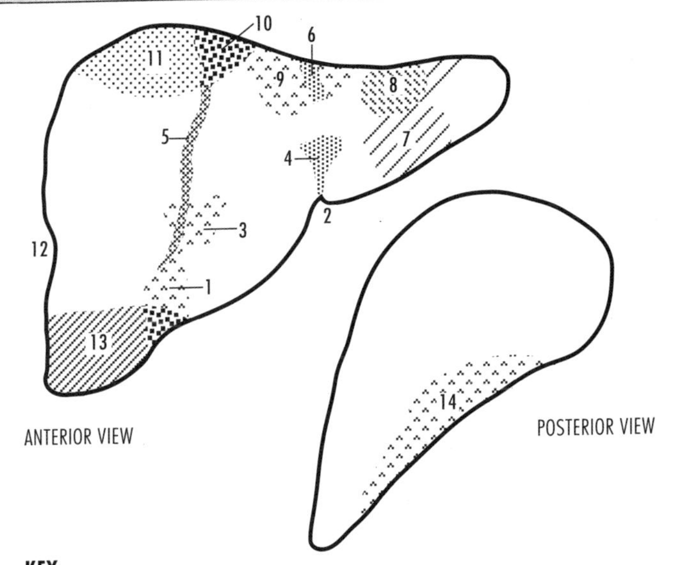

KEY:

1. Gallbladder fossa
2. Ligamentum teres and falciform ligament
3. Hilum, main branching of the portal vein
4. Pars umbilicalis portion, left portal vein
5. Variable stripe of lobar fissure between right and left lobes
6. Variable stripe of segmental fissure, left lobe
7. Thinning of left lobe
8. Impression of pectus excavatum
9. Cardiac impression
10. Hepatic veins and inferior vena cava
11. Shielding from right female breast
12. Harrison's groove or costal impression
13. Impression of hepatic flexure of colon
14. Right renal impression

patic cysts and may have a parasitic or nonparasitic origin. Ultrasonography can confirm hepatic or splenic cysts.

Intrahepatic abscesses are usually pyogenic or amebic. Subphrenic abscesses, located beneath the diaphragm, may distort the dome of the right lobe. Splenic abscesses are characteristic in bacterial endocarditis. All abscesses require gallium scanning or ultrasonography to confirm diagnosis.

Benign hepatic tumors — such as hemangiomas, adenomas, and hamartomas — require confirming biopsy or flow studies. Primary malignant tumors, such as hepatomas, also require biopsy. Benign splenic tumors are rare and include hemangiomas, fibromas, myomas, and hamartomas. Primary malignant splenic tumors are also rare, except in lymphoreticular malignancies such as Hodgkin's disease. Splenic tumors also require biopsy to confirm diagnosis. Although focal disease usually inhibits uptake of radioactive colloid, both obstruction of the superior vena cava and Budd-Chiari syndrome cause markedly increased uptake.

Liver-spleen scanning can verify palpable abdominal masses and differentiate between splenomegaly and hepatomegaly. A left upper quadrant mass may result from splenomegaly or, if the liver is grossly extended across the abdomen, from hepatomegaly. A right upper quadrant mass may result from hepatomegaly; a right lower quadrant mass may be a Riedel's lobe or a large dependent gallbladder. Splenic infarcts, often associated with bacterial endocarditis and massive splenomegaly, appear as peripheral defects, with decreased and irregular colloid distribution.

Scanning can assess hepatic injury after abdominal trauma. Intrahepatic hematoma appears as a focal defect; subcapsular hematoma, as a lentiform defect on the periphery of the liver; hepatic laceration, as a linear defect.

Scanning can also detect splenic injury after abdominal trauma. Intrahepatic hematoma appears as a focal defect; hepatic laceration appears as a linear defect. Splenic hematoma appears as a focal defect in or next to the spleen and may transect it. Subcapsular hematoma appears as a lentiform defect on the periphery of the spleen.

Interfering factors

- Radionuclides administered in other studies on the same day (possible poor imaging)
- Patient's inability to remain still during the procedure

GALLIUM SCAN

A gallium scan is a total body scan used to assess certain neoplasms and inflammatory lesions that attract gallium. It's usually performed 24 to 48 hours after the I.V. injection of radioactive gallium Ga (^{67}Ga) citrate; occasionally, it's performed 72 hours after the injection or, in acute inflammatory disease, 4 to 6 hours after the injection.

Because gallium has an affinity for benign and malignant neoplasms and inflammatory lesions, exact diagnosis requires additional confirming tests, such as ultrasonography and computed tomography scanning. Also, be aware that many neoplasms and a few inflammatory lesions may fail to demonstrate abnormal gallium activity.

Purpose

- To detect primary or metastatic neoplasms and inflammatory lesions when the site of the disease hasn't been clearly defined
- To evaluate malignant lymphoma and identify recurrent tumors following chemotherapy or radiation therapy
- To clarify focal defects in the liver when liver-spleen scanning and ultrasonography prove inconclusive
- To evaluate bronchogenic carcinoma

Patient preparation

- Explain to the patient that this test helps detect abnormal or inflammatory tissue.
- Tell the patient he need not restrict food or fluids before the test.
- Explain to the patient hat the test requires a total body scan (usually per-

formed 24 to 48 hours after the I.V. injection of radioactive gallium).

- Tell the patient who will perform the test and where it will take place.
- Warn the patient that he may experience transient discomfort from the needle puncture during injection of the radioactive gallium. Reassure him, however, that the dosage is only slightly radioactive and isn't harmful.
- If a gamma scintillation camera is to be used, assure the patient that although the uptake probe and detector head may touch his skin, he'll experience no discomfort.
- If a rectilinear scanner is to be used, mention that it makes a soft, irregular clicking noise as it registers the radiation emissions.
- Make sure the patient or a responsible family member has signed an informed consent form, if required.
- Administer a laxative, an enema, or both, as ordered.

Equipment

Scanner; I.V. insertion equipment, if needed; radioactive gallium

Procedure and posttest care

- The patient may be positioned erect or recumbent or in an appropriate combination of these positions, depending on his physical condition.
- Scans or scintigrams of the patient are taken 24 to 48 hours after ^{67}Ga citrate injection, from anterior and posterior views and, occasionally, lateral views.
- If the initial gallium scan suggests bowel disease and additional scans are necessary, give the patient a cleansing enema before continuing the test.

Precautions

- This test should precede barium studies because barium retention may hinder visualization of gallium activity in the bowel.
- Gallium scanning is usually contraindicated in children and during pregnancy or lactation; however, it may be performed if the potential diagnostic benefit outweighs the risks of exposure to radiation.

Normal findings

Gallium activity is normally demonstrated in the liver, spleen, bones, and large bowel. Activity in the bowel results from mucosal uptake of gallium and fecal excretion of gallium.

Abnormal findings

Gallium scanning may reveal inflammatory lesions — discrete abscesses or diffuse infiltration. In pancreatic or perinephric abscess, gallium activity is relatively localized; in bacterial peritonitis, gallium activity is spread diffusely within the abdomen.

Abnormally high gallium accumulation is characteristic in inflammatory bowel diseases, such as ulcerative colitis and regional ileitis (Crohn's disease), and in carcinoma of the colon. However, because gallium normally accumulates in the colon, the detection of inflammatory and neoplastic diseases is sometimes difficult.

Abnormal gallium activity may be present in various sarcomas, Wilms' tumor, and neuroblastomas; carcinoma of the kidney, uterus, vagina, and stomach; and testicular tumors, such as seminoma, embryonal carcinoma, choriocarcinoma, and teratocarcinoma, which often metastasize via the lymphatic system. In Hodgkin's disease and malignant lymphoma, gallium scanning can demonstrate abnormal activity in one or more lymph nodes or in extranodal locations. However, gallium scanning supported by results of lymphangiography can gauge the extent of metastases more accurately than either test alone because neither test consistently identifies all neoplastic nodes.

After chemotherapy or radiation therapy, gallium scanning may be used to detect new or recurrent tumors. However, these forms of therapy tend to diminish tumor affinity for gallium without necessarily eliminating the tumor.

In the differential diagnosis of focal hepatic defects, abnormal gallium activity may help narrow the diagnostic possibilities. Gallium localizes in hepatomas, but not in pseudotumors; in abscesses, but not in pleural effusions; and in tumors, but not in cysts or hematomas.

In examining patients with suspected bronchogenic carcinoma, abnormal activity confirms the presence of tumor. However, because gallium also localizes in inflammatory pulmonary diseases, such as pneumonia and sarcoidosis, a chest X-ray should be performed to distinguish a tumor from an inflammatory lesion.

Interfering factors

- Hepatic and splenic intake (possible false-negative scans due to possible obscuring of abnormal para-aortic nodes in Hodgkin's disease)
- Fecal accumulation in bowel (poor imaging of retroperitoneal space)
- Residual barium from other tests done 1 week before the scan (possible poor imaging)

RED BLOOD CELL SURVIVAL TIME

Normally, red blood cells (RBCs) are destroyed only when they reach senility. However, in hemolytic diseases, RBCs of all ages are randomly destroyed, resulting in anemia. The RBC survival time test measures the survival time of circulating RBCs and detects sites of abnormal RBC sequestration and destruction.

Survival time is measured by labeling a random sample of RBCs with radioactive chromium-51 sodium chromate (^{51}Cr). This labeled group of RBCs is then injected back into the patient. Serial blood samples measure the percent of labeled cells per unit volume over 3 to 4 weeks until 50% of the cells disappear (disappearance rate corresponds to destruction of a random cell population).

A normal RBC survives about 120 days (half-life of 60 days); the ^{51}Cr-labeled RBCs have a shorter half-life (25 to 30 days) because about 1% of senescent RBCs are removed from the circulation each day and about 1% of ^{51}Cr is spontaneously eluted from the labeled RBCs each day.

During the test period, a gamma camera scans the body for sites of abnormally high radioactivity, which indicate sites of excessive RBC sequestration and destruction. Other tests performed with the RBC survival time test may include spot-checks of the stool to detect GI blood loss; hematocrit; blood volume studies; and radionuclide iron uptake and clearance tests to aid differential diagnosis of anemia.

Purpose

- To help evaluate unexplained anemia, particularly hemolytic anemia
- To identify sites of abnormal RBC sequestration and destruction

Patient preparation

- Explain to the patient that this test helps identify the cause of his anemia.
- Advise the patient that he need not restrict food or fluids.
- Explain to the patient that the test involves labeling a blood sample with a radioactive substance and requires regular blood samples at 3-day intervals for 3 to 4 weeks. Tell him who will perform the testing and where it will take place.
- Tell the patient that he may experience discomfort from the needle punctures and the tourniquet. Reassure him that collecting each sample takes less than 3 minutes and that the small amount of radioactive substance used is harmless.
- If stool collection is required to test for GI bleeding, teach the patient the proper collection technique.
- Make sure the patient or a responsible family member has signed an informed consent form, if required.

Equipment

18G to 20G needle; I.V. insertion equipment, if needed; injectant, as ordered; heparinized blood collection tube

Procedure and posttest care

- A 30-ml blood sample is drawn and mixed with 100 microcuries of ^{51}Cr for an adult (less for a child).
- After an incubation period, the mixture is injected I.V. into the patient. A blood sample is drawn 30 minutes after injection to determine blood and RBC volumes.
- A 6-ml sample is collected in a heparinized tube after 24 hours; follow-up samples are collected at 3-day intervals for 3 to 4 weeks. (Intervals between samples may vary, depending on the laboratory.)
- To avoid error from physical decay of the ^{51}Cr, each sample is measured with a scintillation well counter on the day it's drawn.
- Radioactivity per milliliter of RBCs is calculated and the values are plotted to determine mean RBC survival time. Simultaneous gamma camera scans of the precordium, sacrum, liver, and spleen detect radioactivity at sites of excess RBC sequestration. A hematocrit test is done on a small portion of each blood sample to check for blood loss.
- At the end of the study, a sample is drawn to compare ending blood and RBC volumes with beginning volumes.
- If a hematoma develops at the venipuncture site, apply warm soaks.

Precautions

- This test is contraindicated during pregnancy because it exposes the fetus to radiation.
- Because excess blood loss can invalidate test results, this test is usually contraindicated for a patient with active bleeding or poor clotting function. However, if the test is necessary for a patient with poor clotting function, observe the venipuncture sites carefully for signs of hemorrhage.
- The patient shouldn't receive blood transfusions during the test period and should not have blood samples drawn for other tests.

Normal findings

Normal half-life for RBCs labeled with ^{51}Cr is 25 to 30 days. Normal gamma camera scans reveal slight radioactivity in the spleen, liver, and sometimes the bone marrow.

Abnormal findings

Decreased RBC survival time indicates a hemolytic disease, such as chronic lymphocytic leukemia, congenital nonspherocytic hemolytic anemia, hemoglobin C disease, hereditary spherocytosis, idiopathic acquired hemolytic anemia, paroxysmal nocturnal hemoglobinuria, elliptocytosis, pernicious anemia, sickle cell anemia, sickle cell hemoglobin C disease, or hemolytic-uremic syndrome. If hemolytic anemia is diagnosed, additional tests using cross-transfusion of labeled RBCs can determine whether anemia results from an intrinsic RBC defect or an extrinsic factor.

A gamma camera scan that detects a site of excess RBC sequestration provides direction for treatment. For example, abnormally high RBC sequestration in the spleen may require a splenectomy.

Interfering factors

- Dehydration, overhydration, or blood loss (possible invalidation of results due to changed circulating RBC volume)
- Blood transfusions during the test period (alters proportion of labeled RBCs to total RBCs)

RADIONUCLIDE RENAL IMAGING

Radionuclide renal imaging, which involves I.V. injection of a radionuclide followed by scintigram, provides a wealth of information for evaluating the kidneys. Observing the uptake concentration and transit of the radionuclide during this test allows assessment of renal blood flow, renal structure, and nephron and collecting system function. Depending on the patient's clinical presentation, this procedure may include dynamic scans to assess renal perfusion and function or static scans to assess structure.

The radioisotope injected depends on the specific information required and the examiner's preference. However, this procedure often includes double isotope technique to obtain a sequence of perfusion and function studies, followed by static images. This test may also be substituted for excretory urography in patients with hypersensitivity to contrast agents.

Purpose

- To detect and assess functional and structural renal abnormalities (such as lesions, renovascular hypertension) and acute or chronic disease (such as pyelonephritis or glomerulonephritis)
- To assess renal transplantation or renal injury due to trauma and obstruction of the urinary tract

Patient preparation

- Explain to the patient that this test permits evaluation of the structure, blood flow, and function of the kidneys.
- Tell the patient who will perform the test and where. (If static scans are ordered, there will be a delay of several hours before the images are taken.)
- Inform the patient that he'll receive an injection of a radionuclide and that he may experience transient flushing and nausea.
- Emphasize that only a small amount of radionuclide is administered and that it's usually excreted within 24 hours.
- Tell the patient several series of films will be taken of his bladder.
- Make sure the patient or a responsible family member has signed an informed consent form, if required.

■ Make sure the patient isn't scheduled for other radionuclide scans on the same day as this test.
■ If the patient receives antihypertensive medication, ask the physician if it should be withheld before the test.
■ Women who are pregnant and young children may receive supersaturated solution of potassium iodide 1 to 3 hours before the test to block thyroid uptake of iodine.

Equipment

Computerized gamma scintillation camera, technetium 99m (^{99m}Tc) for perfusion study, iodohippurate sodium I 131 (Hippuran) for function study, oscilloscope, magnetic tape, I.V. equipment

Procedure and posttest care

■ The patient is commonly placed in a prone position so that posterior views may be obtained. If the test is being performed to evaluate transplantation, the patient is positioned supine for anterior views.
■ Instruct the patient not to change his position.
■ A perfusion study (radionuclide angiography) is performed first to evaluate renal blood flow. The ^{99m}Tc is administered I.V., and rapid-sequence photographs (one per second) are taken for 1 minute.
■ Next, a function study is performed to measure the transit time of the radionuclide through the kidneys' functional units. After Hippuran is administered I.V., images are obtained at a rate of one per minute for 20 minutes. Alternatively, this entire procedure can be recorded on computer-compatible magnetic tape and concurrent renogram curves plotted.
■ Finally, static images are obtained 4 or more hours later, after the radionuclide has drained through the pelvicaliceal system.
■ Instruct the patient to flush the toilet immediately after each voiding for 24 hours as a radiation precaution.
■ If the patient is incontinent, change bed linens promptly and wear gloves to maintain standard precautions and prevent unnecessary skin contact.
■ Monitor the infection site for signs of hematoma, infection, and discomfort. Apply warm compresses for comfort.
■ Monitor intake and output and electrolyte, acid-base, BUN, and creatinine levels as indicated.

Precautions

■ This test is contraindicated in pregnant women unless the benefits to the mother outweigh the risk to the fetus.

Normal findings

Because 25% of cardiac output goes directly to the kidneys, renal perfusion should be evident immediately following uptake of the ^{99m}Tc in the abdominal aorta. Within 1 to 2 minutes, a normal pattern of renal circulation should appear. The radionuclide should delineate the kidneys simultaneously, symmetrically, and with equal intensity.

Hippuran administered for the function study rapidly outlines the kidneys — which should be normal in size, shape, and position — and also defines the collecting system and bladder. Maximum counts of the radionuclide in the kidneys occur within 5 minutes after injection (and within 1 minute of each other) and should fall to approximately one-third or less of the maximum counts in the same kidney within 25 minutes. Within this time, the function of both kidneys can be compared as the concentration of radionuclide shifts from the cortex to the pelvis and, finally, to the bladder.

Renal function is best evaluated by comparing these images with the renogram curves. Total function is considered normal when the effective renal plasma flow is 420 ml/minute or greater and the percentage of the dose excreted in the urine at 30 to 35 minutes is greater than 66%.

Abnormal findings

Images from the perfusion study can identify impeded renal circulation, such as that caused by trauma and renal artery stenosis or renal infarction. These conditions may occur in patients with renovascular hypertension and abdominal aortic disease. Because malignant renal tumors are usually vascular, these images can help differentiate tumors from cysts.

In evaluating a kidney transplant, abnormal perfusion may indicate obstruction of the vascular grafts. The function study can detect abnormalities of the collecting system and extravasation of the urine. Markedly decreased tubular function causes reduced radionuclide activity in the collecting system; outflow obstruction causes decreased radionuclide activity in the tubules, with increased activity in the collecting system. This test can also define the level of ureteral obstruction.

Static images can demonstrate lesions, congenital abnormalities, and traumatic injury. These images also detect space-occupying lesions within or surrounding the kidney, such as tumors, infarcts, and inflammatory masses (abscesses, for example); they can also identify congenital disorders, such as horseshoe kidney and polycystic kidney disease. They can define regions of infarction, rupture, or hemorrhage after trauma.

A lower-than-normal total concentration of the radionuclide, as opposed to focal defects, suggests a diffuse renal disorder, such as acute tubular necrosis, severe infection, or ischemia. In a patient who has had a kidney transplant, decreased radionuclide uptake generally indicates organ rejection. Failure of visualization may indicate congenital ectopia or aplasia.

Definitive diagnosis usually requires the combined analysis of static images, perfusion studies, and function studies.

Interfering factors

- Antihypertensives (possible masking of abnormalities)
- Scans of different organs performed on the same day (possible poor imaging)

HIDA SCAN

Also known as *hepatobiliary imaging, cholescintigraphy,* or *gallbladder nuclear scanning,* the hepatobiliary iminodiacetic acid (HIDA) scan obtains images of the hepatobiliary system to determine the patency of the cystic and common bile ducts through noninvasive scanning. The scanning is accomplished through injection of iminodiacetic acid (IDAs) analogues labeled with technetium 99m (^{99m}Tc). This test also evaluates gallbladder emptying.

Purpose

- To diagnose gallbladder disorders and determine degree of patency
- To diagnose acute and chronic cholecystitis
- To evaluate the patency of the biliary enteric bypass
- To assess obstructive jaundice in combination with radiography or ultrasonography

Patient preparation

- Explain to the patient that this test detects inflammation or obstruction of the gallbladder and its ducts.
- Tell the patient who will perform the test and where.
- Inform the patient that he'll receive an I.V. injection of a radionuclide. Tell him the needle insertion and the tourniquet may cause some discomfort.
- Explain to the patient that the radionuclide will be eliminated from the body within 6 to 24 hours.
- Inform the patient that repeat pictures may be taken up to 24 hours after the injection.
- Ensure that the patient has no allergies to the media used, that he has fasted for 2 to 6 hours before the scan, and that he can comply with activity restriction during the scan.
- Ask the patient to remove all jewelry and metallic objects and to put on a gown and void before the test.
- Explain to the patient that sincalide may be given before the test to promote gallbladder contraction and emptying.
- Make sure the patient or a responsible family member has signed an informed consent form, if required.

Equipment

Scanner; I.V. insertion equipment, if needed; radionuclide injectant, as ordered

Procedure and posttest care

- Immediately after the radionuclide is injected I.V., the right quadrant of the abdomen is scanned while the patient is in a supine position; images are taken every 5 minutes for the first 30 minutes, then every 10 minutes for the next 30 minutes.
- Delayed views may be taken after 2, 4, and 24 hours if the gallbladder can't be visualized.
- If the gallbladder can't be visualized, morphine may also be given I.V. during the study to initiate spasms of Oddi's sphincter in an effort to move the radionuclide into the gallbladder.
- Monitor vital signs at baseline and every 15 to 30 minutes.
- Observe the patient carefully for up to 60 minutes after the study for a possible hypersensitivity reaction.
- Advise the patient to drink plenty of fluids, unless contraindicated, for 24 to 48 hours to eliminate the radionuclide from the body. Also tell him to flush the toilet immediately after each voiding and to wash his hands with soap and water.
- Rubber gloves should be worn by caregivers every time urine is discarded after the procedure. Gloves should be considered nuclear waste and disposed of appropriately.
- The patient may resume a regular diet after the test, unless contraindicated.

Precautions

- This test is generally contraindicated during pregnancy or lactation because it exposes the fetus or infant to radiation.
- Personnel involved should also be aware of the risks and precautions of this radioactive test.

Normal findings

A normal HIDA scan shows the gallbladder to be normal in size, shape, and function; cystic and common bile ducts are patent.

Abnormal findings

Images may demonstrate acute or chronic cholecystitis, or common bile duct obstruction.

Interfering factors

- Patient's inability to remain still during the procedure
- Failure to observe pretest restrictions
- Presence of barium in GI tract (possible poor imaging)
- Increased bilirubin levels (decreased hepatic uptake)
- Fasting more than 24 hours, total parenteral nutrition, or alcoholism (decreased hepatic uptake)

15

Monitoring and catheterization

Fetal Monitoring

External Fetal Monitoring

In external fetal monitoring, a noninvasive test, an electronic transducer and a cardiotachometer amplify and record fetal heart rate (FHR) while a pressure-sensitive transducer (tocodynamometer) records uterine contractions. Fetal monitoring records the baseline FHR (average FHR over two contraction cycles or 10 minutes), periodic fluctuations in the baseline FHR, and beat-to-beat heart rate variability. (See *Understanding fetal monitoring terminology.*) External fetal monitoring is also used during other tests of fetal health, notably the nonstress test and the contraction stress test (CST).

Purpose

- To measure FHR and the frequency of uterine contractions
- To evaluate antepartum and intrapartum fetal health during stress and nonstress situations
- To detect fetal distress
- To determine the necessity for internal fetal monitoring

Patient preparation

- Explain to the patient that this test assesses fetal health.
- Explain the procedure to the patient and answer all questions. Assure the patient that external fetal monitoring is painless and won't hurt the fetus or interfere with normal labor.
- If monitoring is to be performed antepartum, instruct the patient to eat a meal just before the test to increase fetal activity, which decreases the test time.
- If the patient is still smoking, advise her to abstain for 2 hours before testing because smoking decreases fetal activity.
- Explain to the patient that she may have to restrict movement during baseline readings but that she may change position between the readings.
- Make sure the patient or a responsible family member has signed an informed consent form.

Equipment

Tocodynamometer (to measure uterine contractions); ultrasonic transducer (to amplify FHR); cardiotachymeter (to record FHR); mineral oil or ultrasound transmission jelly; elastic band, stockinette, or abdominal strap

Procedure and posttest care

- Place the patient in the semi-Fowler or left lateral position, with her abdomen exposed. Cover the ultrasound transducer receiver crystal with ultrasound transmission jelly.
- Palpate the patient's abdomen to identify the fetal chest area, locate the most distinct fetal heart sounds, and then secure the ultrasound transducer over this area with the elastic band, stockinette, or abdominal strap.
- Check the recording equipment to ensure an adequate printout and verify the fetal monitor's alarm boundaries.
- During monitoring, check the elastic band, stockinette, or abdominal strap to ensure that the fit is comfortable yet tight enough to produce a good tracing.
- As labor progresses, reposition the pressure transducer as necessary so that it remains on the fundal portion of the uterus. You may have to reposition the ultrasound transducer as fetal or maternal position changes.

Understanding fetal monitoring terminology

◆ **Baseline fetal heart rate:** Average fetal heart rate (FHR) over two contraction cycles or 10 minutes
◆ **Baseline changes:** Fluctuations in FHR unrelated to uterine contractions
◆ **Periodic changes:** Fluctuations in FHR related to uterine contractions
◆ **Amplitude:** Difference in beats per minute between baseline readings and fluctuation in FHR
◆ **Recovery time:** Difference between the end of the contraction and the return to the baseline FHR
◆ **Acceleration:** Transient rise in FHR lasting longer than 15 seconds and associated with a uterine contraction
◆ **Deceleration:** Transient fall in FHR related to a uterine contraction
◆ **Lag time:** Difference between the peak of the contraction and the lowest point of deceleration

Antepartum monitoring with nonstress tests

■ Tell the patient to hold the pressure transducer in her hand and to push it each time she feels the fetus move.

■ Within a 20-minute period, monitor baseline FHR until you record two fetal movements that last longer than 15 seconds each and cause heart rate accelerations of more than 15 beats/minute from the baseline. If you can't obtain two FHR accelerations within 30 minutes, shake the patient's abdomen to stimulate the fetus, and repeat the test.

Antepartum monitoring with CST

■ Induce contractions by oxytocin infusion or nipple stimulation (endogenous oxytocin).

■ When administering oxytocin, infuse a dilute solution at a rate of 1.0 mU/minute, increasing the oxytocin rate until the patient experiences three contractions within 10 minutes, each lasting longer than 45 seconds.

■ When using nipple stimulation, tell the patient to stimulate one nipple by hand until contractions begin. If a second contraction doesn't occur in 2 minutes, have her stimulate the nipple again. Stimulate both nipples if contractions don't occur in 15 minutes. Continue the test until contractions occur in 10 minutes.

■ If no decelerations occur during three contractions, the patient may be discharged. Late decelerations during any of the contractions require notification of the physician and further tests.

Intrapartum monitoring

■ Secure the pressure transducer with an elastic band, a stockinette, or an abdominal strap over the area of greatest uterine electrical activity during contractions (usually the fundus).

■ Adjust the machine to record 0 to 10 mm Hg pressure between palpable contractions.

■ Reposition the ultrasound and pressure transducers as necessary to ensure continuous accurate readings. Review the tracings frequently for baseline abnormalities, periodic changes, variability of changes, and uterine contraction abnormalities.

■ Record maternal movement, administration of drugs, and procedures performed directly on the tracing to assist evaluation of changes in the tracing.

■ Report abnormalities immediately.

■ Repeat antepartum monitoring weekly as long as indications, such as pregnancy over 42 weeks' gestation or fetal growth retardation, persist.

Precautions

- During CST, watch for fetal distress with oxytocin infusion or nipple stimulation.

Normal findings

Normal baseline FHR ranges from 120 to 160 beats/minute, with a variability of 5 to 25 beats/minute. For the antepartum nonstress test, the fetus is considered healthy and should remain so for another week if two fetal movements causing a heart rate acceleration of more than 15 beats/minute from baseline FHR occur in a 20-minute period. Nonstress testing is also done for postdate fetal well-being. A normal, healthy fetus usually has three rises in FHR within 10 to 15 minutes, but fetuses may sleep up to 45 minutes at a time. If there is no change in FHR in a 10-minute period, consider shaking the mother's abdomen gently, clapping loudly, or having the mother drink ice water or apple juice. If the FHR remains unchanged, a contraction stress test or biophysical profile test should be ordered. The fetus is assessed by watching fetal movements, muscle tone, fetal breathing, and the amniotic fluid index.

For the CST, the fetus is assumed to be healthy and should remain so for another week if three contractions occur during a 10-minute period, with no late decelerations.

Abnormal findings

Bradycardia (FHR ≤ 120 beats/minute) may indicate fetal heart block, malposition, or hypoxia. Fetal bradycardia may also be drug-induced. Tachycardia (FHR > 160 beats/minute) may result from maternal fever, tachycardia, hyperthyroidism, or use of vagolytic drugs or narcotics; early fetal hypoxia; or fetal infection or arrhythmia.

Decreased variability (a fluctuation of < 5 beats/minute in the FHR) may be caused by fetal arrhythmia or heart block; fetal hypoxia, central nervous system malformation, or infections; or vagolytic drugs. FHR accelerations may result from early hypoxia. They may precede or follow variable decelerations and may indicate that the fetus is in a breech position.

For the antepartum nonstress test, a positive result (fewer than two accelerations of FHR that last longer than 15 seconds each, with a heart rate acceleration of over 15 beats/minute) indicates an increased risk of perinatal morbidity and mortality and usually requires CST.

For the CST, persistent late decelerations during two or more contractions may indicate increased risk of fetal morbidity or mortality. Hyperstimulation (long or frequent uterine contractions) or suspicious results require biophysical profile assessment. If findings are unsatisfactory, cesarean birth may be indicated.

Interfering factors

- Maternal position, particularly if supine (may cause artifactual fetal distress)
- Drugs that affect the sympathetic and parasympathetic nervous systems (possible low FHR)
- Excessive maternal or fetal activity (possible difficulty in recording uterine contractions or FHR)
- Maternal obesity (possible difficulty due to density of abdominal wall)
- Loose or dirty leads or transducer connections (possible production of artifacts)

INTERNAL FETAL MONITORING

Internal fetal monitoring is an invasive procedure that involves attaching an electrode to the fetal scalp to directly monitor fetal heart rate (FHR). A catheter introduced into the uterine cavity measures the frequency and pressure of uterine contractions. Internal monitoring is performed only during labor, after the membranes have ruptured and the cervix has dilated 3 cm, with the fetal head lower than the –2 station and only if external monitoring provides inadequate data.

Internal monitoring provides more accurate information about fetal health than external monitoring and is especially useful in determining whether cesarean delivery is necessary. The procedure carries minimal risks to the mother (perforated uterus and intrauterine infection) and fetus (scalp abscess and hematoma).

Purpose

- To monitor FHR, especially beat-to-beat variability (short-term variability)
- To measure the frequency and pressure of uterine contractions to assess the progress of labor
- To evaluate intrapartum fetal health
- To supplement or replace external fetal monitoring

Patient preparation

- Explain to the patient that this test accurately assesses fetal health and uterine activity and that it doesn't necessarily mean that there's a problem. Describe the procedure and answer all questions.
- Warn the patient that she may feel mild discomfort when the uterine catheter and scalp electrode are inserted.
- Make sure the patient or a responsible family member has signed an informed consent form.

Equipment

Sterile fetal scalp electrode and guide tube, intrauterine pressure catheter, catheter guide, pressure transducer, fetal heart monitor

Procedure and posttest care

Measuring FHR

- Place the patient in the dorsal lithotomy position, and prepare her perineal area for a vaginal examination, explaining each step of the procedure as it's performed by a physician or certified nurse-midwife. As the procedure begins, ask the patient to breathe through her mouth and relax her abdominal muscles.
- After the vaginal examination, the fetal scalp is palpated and an appropriate site is identified. A plastic tube carrying the small electrode is introduced into the cervix, pressed firmly against the fetal scalp, and rotated clockwise to attach the electrode to the scalp. The electrode wire is tugged gently to ensure proper attachment and the tube is withdrawn, leaving the electrode in place.
- A conduction medium is applied to a leg plate, which is then strapped to the mother's thigh. Electrode wires are attached to the leg plate, and a cable from the leg plate is plugged into the fetal monitor. To check proper placement of the scalp electrode, the monitor is turned on and the ECG button is pressed; an FHR signal indicates proper electrode attachment.

Measuring uterine contractions

- Before inserting the uterine catheter, fill it with sterile normal saline solution

Normal intrauterine pressure readings during labor

STAGE OF LABOR	FREQUENCY (number of contractions per 10 minutes)	BASELINE PRESSURE (mm Hg)	PRESSURE DURING CONTRACTION (mm Hg)
Prelabor	1 to 2	None	25 to 40
First stage	3 to 5	8 to 12	30 to 40 (or more)
Second stage	5	10 to 20	50 to 80

to prevent air emboli. Explain each step of the procedure to the patient.

- Ask the patient to breathe deeply through her mouth and to relax her abdominal muscles.
- After the vagina has been examined and the presenting part of the fetus palpated, the catheter and catheter guide are inserted ⅜″ to ¾″ (1 to 2 cm) into the cervix, usually between the fetal head and the posterior cervix.
- The catheter is then gently advanced into the uterus until the black mark on the catheter is flush with the vulva. (The catheter guide should *never* be passed deeply into the uterus.)
- The guide is removed and the catheter is connected to a transducer that converts the intrauterine pressure, as measured by the fluid in the catheter, to an electrical signal.

Both procedures

- After removal of the fetal scalp electrode, apply antiseptic or antibiotic solution to the site of attachment.
- Watch for signs of fetal scalp abscess or maternal intrauterine infection.

Precautions

- Internal fetal monitoring is contraindicated if there's uncertainty about the fetus's presenting part or a technical impediment to attaching the lead.
- Prevent artifactual pressure readings by flushing the pressure transducer with normal saline solution; to relieve catheter obstruction (by vernix caseosa, for example), inject a small amount of sterile normal saline solution into the catheter while the transducer is isolated from the system.
- Make sure a low heart rate is actually the FHR, not the maternal heart rate.
- If FHR patterns indicate fetal distress, fetal oxygenation often can be improved by loading maternal fluids to increase placental perfusion, turning the mother on her side (preferably left) to alleviate supine hypotension, and administering oxygen to the mother. If these measures return heart rate patterns to normal, labor may continue. If abnormal patterns persist, cesarean birth may be necessary.
- Make sure the fetal scalp electrode and the uterine catheter are removed before cesarean delivery.

Reference values

Normal FHR ranges from 120 to 160 beats/minute, with a variability of 5 to 25 beats/minute. (See *Normal intrauterine pressure readings during labor.*)

Abnormal findings

Bradycardia (FHR < 120 beats/minute) may indicate fetal heart block, malposition, or hypoxia. Fetal bradycardia may also result from maternal ingestion of certain drugs, such as propranolol and narcotic analgesics.

Tachycardia (FHR > 160 beats/minute) may result from early fetal hypoxia, fetal infection or arrhythmia, prematurity, or maternal fever, tachycardia, hyperthyroidism, or use of vagolytic drugs.

Decreased variability (fluctuation of < 5 beats/minute from baseline) may result from fetal arrhythmia or heart block, hypoxia, central nervous system malformation, or infections, or from maternal use of narcotics or vagolytic drugs.

Early decelerations (slowing of FHR at the onset of a contraction with recovery to baseline within no more than 15 seconds after the contraction ends) are related to fetal head compression and usually ensure fetal health.

Late decelerations (slowing of FHR after a contraction begins, a lag time of more than 20 seconds, and a recovery time of more than 15 seconds) may be related to uteroplacental insufficiency, fetal hypoxia, or acidosis. Recurrent and persistently late decelerations with decreased variability usually indicate serious fetal distress, possibly resulting from conduction (spinal, caudal, or epidural) anesthesia or fetal hypoxia.

Variable decelerations (sudden precipitous drops in FHR unrelated to uterine contractions) are commonly related to cord compression. A severe drop in FHR (to < 70 beats/minute for more than 60 seconds) with a decrease in variability indicates fetal distress and may result in a compromised neonate. Poor beat-to-beat variability without periodic patterns may indicate fetal distress, requiring further evaluation such as analysis of fetal blood gas levels.

Decreased intrauterine pressure during labor that isn't progressing normally may require oxytocin stimulation. Elevated intrauterine pressure readings may indicate abruptio placentae or overstimulation from oxytocin, possibly resulting in fetal distress due to decreased placental perfusion.

Interfering factors

- Drugs that affect parasympathetic and sympathetic nervous systems

NEUROLOGIC MONITORING

ELECTROENCEPHALOGRAPHY

In EEG, electrodes attached to areas of the patient's scalp record the brain's electrical activity and transmit this information to an electroencephalograph, which records the resulting brain waves on recording paper. The procedure may be performed in a special laboratory or by a portable unit at the bedside. Ambulatory recording EEGs are available for the patient to wear at home or the workplace to record the patient as he performs his normal daily activities. Continuous-video EEG recording is available on an inpatient basis for the identification of epileptic discharges during clinical events or for localization of a seizure focus during a surgical evaluation of epilepsy. Intracranial electrodes are surgically implanted to record EEG changes for localization of the seizure focus.

Purpose

- To determine the presence and type of seizure disorder
- To aid diagnosis of intracranial lesions, such as abscesses and tumors
- To evaluate the brain's electrical activity in metabolic disease, cerebral ischemia, head injury, meningitis, encephalitis, mental retardation, psychological disorders, and drugs
- To evaluate altered states of consciousness or brain death

Patient preparation

- Explain to the patient that this test records the brain's electrical activity.
- Describe the procedure to the patient and family members, and answer all questions.
- Tell the patient that he must forgo caffeine before the test; other than this, there are no food or fluid restrictions. Tell him that skipping the meal before the test can cause relative hypoglycemia and alter the brain wave pattern.
- Thoroughly wash and dry the patient's hair to remove hair sprays, creams, and oils.
- Explain to the patient that during the test, he'll relax in a reclining chair or lie on a bed and that electrodes will be attached to his scalp with a special paste. Assure him that the electrodes won't shock him.
- If needle electrodes are used, explain to the patient that he'll feel a pricking sensation as they're inserted; however, flat electrodes are more commonly used.
- Do your best to allay the patient's fears because nervousness can affect brain wave patterns.
- Check the patient's medication history for drugs that may interfere with test results. Anticonvulsants, tranquilizers, barbiturates, and other sedatives should be withheld for 24 to 48 hours before the test as ordered by the physician. Infants and very young children occasionally require sedation to prevent crying and restlessness during the test, but sedation itself may alter test results.
- A patient with a seizure disorder may require a "sleep EEG." In this case, keep the patient awake the night before the test, and administer a sedative (such as chloral hydrate) to help him sleep during the test.
- If the test is performed to confirm brain death, provide family members with emotional support.

Procedure and posttest care

- Position the patient on the bed or in a reclining chair. Reassure him as the electrodes are attached to his scalp.
- Before the recording procedure begins, instruct the patient to close his eyes, relax, and remain still.
- During the recording, observe the patient carefully; note blinking, swallowing, talking, or other movements, and record these findings on the tracing. These activities may cause artifacts on the tracing and be misinterpreted as abnormal tracing.
- The recording may be stopped at intervals to let the patient rest or reposition himself. This is important because restlessness and fatigue can alter brain wave patterns.
- After an initial baseline recording, the patient may be tested under various stress-producing conditions to elicit patterns not observable while he's at rest. For example, he may be asked to breathe deeply and rapidly for 3 minutes (hyperventilation), which may elicit brain wave patterns typical of seizure disorders or other abnormalities. This technique is commonly used to detect absence seizures. Also, photic stimulation tests central cerebral activity in re-

sponse to bright light, accentuating abnormal activity in absence or myoclonic seizures. In this procedure, a strobe light placed in front of the patient is flashed 1 to 20 times/second; recordings are made with the patient's eyes opened and closed.

- Review carefully the reinstatement of anticonvulsant medication or other drugs withheld before the test.
- Carefully observe the patient for seizure activity, and provide a safe environment.
- Help the patient remove electrode paste from his hair.
- If the patient received a sedative before the test, take safety precautions such as raising the bed's side rails.
- If brain death is confirmed, provide emotional support for the family.
- If clinical events are found to be nonepileptic, a psychological evaluation may be needed.

Precautions

- Observe the patient carefully for seizure activity.
- If seizure activity occurs, record seizure patterns and be prepared to provide assistance. Have suction equipment readily available.

Normal findings

EEG records a portion of the brain's electrical activity as waves; some are irregular, whereas others demonstrate frequent patterns. Among the basic waveforms are the alpha, beta, theta, and delta rhythms.

Alpha waves occur at a frequency of 8 to 11 cycles/second in a regular rhythm. They're present only in the waking state when the patient's eyes are closed but he's mentally alert; usually, they disappear with visual activity or mental concentration. *Beta waves* (13 to 30 cycles/second)—generally associated with anxiety, depression, and use of sedatives—are seen most readily in the frontal and central regions of the brain. *Theta waves* (4 to 7 cycles/second) are most common in children and young adults and appear in the frontal and temporal regions. *Delta waves* (0.5 to 3.5 cycles/second) normally occur only in young children and during sleep.

Abnormal findings

Usually, about a 100′ to 200′ (30 to 60 m) strip of recordings is evaluated, with particular attention paid to basic waveforms, symmetry of cerebral activity, transient discharges, and responses to stimulation. A specific diagnosis depends on the patient's clinical status.

In patients with epilepsy, EEG patterns may identify the specific disorder. In *absence seizures,* the EEG shows spikes and waves at a frequency of 3 cycles/second. In *generalized tonic-clonic seizures,* it generally shows multiple, high-voltage, spiked waves in both hemispheres. In *temporal lobe epilepsy,* the EEG usually shows spiked waves in the affected temporal region. In patients with *focal seizures,* it usually shows localized, spiked discharges.

In patients with intracranial lesions, such as tumors or abscesses, the EEG may show slow waves (usually delta waves but possibly unilateral beta waves). Vascular lesions, such as cerebral infarcts and intracranial hemorrhages, generally produce focal abnormalities in the injured area.

Generally, any condition that causes a diminishing level of consciousness alters the EEG pattern in proportion to the degree of consciousness lost. For example, in a patient with a metabolic disorder, an inflammatory process (such as meningitis or encephalitis), or increased intracranial pressure, the EEG shows generalized, diffuse, and slow brain waves.

The most pathologic finding of all is an absent EEG pattern — a "flat" tracing (except for artifacts), which may indicate brain death.

Interfering factors

- Interference from extraneous electrical activity; head, body, eye, or tongue movement; or muscle contractions (possible production of excessive artifact)
- Anticonvulsants, barbiturates, tranquilizers, and other sedatives (possible masking of seizure activity)
- Acute drug intoxication or severe hypothermia resulting in loss of consciousness (flat EEG)

EVOKED POTENTIAL STUDIES

Evoked potential studies evaluate the integrity of visual, somatosensory, and auditory nerve pathways by measuring evoked potentials — the brain's electrical response to stimulation of the sensory organs or peripheral nerves. Evoked potentials are recorded as electronic impulses by surface electrodes attached to the scalp and skin over various peripheral sensory nerves. A computer extracts these low-amplitude impulses from background brain wave activity and averages the signals from repeated stimuli. (See *Visual and somatosensory evoked potentials.*)

Three types of responses are measured:

- *Visual evoked potentials,* produced by exposing the eye to a rapidly reversing checkerboard pattern, help evaluate demyelinating diseases, traumatic injury, and puzzling visual complaints.
- *Somatosensory evoked potentials,* produced by electrically stimulating a peripheral sensory nerve, help diagnose peripheral nerve disease and locate brain and spinal cord lesions.
- *Auditory brain stem evoked potentials,* produced by delivering clicks to the ear, help locate auditory lesions and evaluate brain stem integrity.

Purpose

- To aid diagnosis of nervous system lesions and abnormalities
- To assess neurologic function

Patient preparation

- Tell the patient that this group of tests measures the electrical activity of his nervous system. Explain who will perform the test and where it will take place.
- Tell the patient that he'll sit in a reclining chair or lie on a bed. If visual evoked potentials will be measured, electrodes will be attached to his scalp; if somatosensory evoked potentials will be measured, electrodes will be placed on his scalp, neck, lower back, wrist, knee, and ankle.
- Assure the patient that the electrodes won't hurt him. Encourage him to relax; tension can affect neurologic function and interfere with test results.
- Have the patient remove all jewelry and other metal objects.

Procedure and posttest care

- Position the patient in the reclining chair or on the bed, and tell him to relax and remain still.

Visual evoked potentials

- Electrodes are attached to the patient's scalp at occipital, parietal, and vertex sites; a reference electrode is placed on the midfrontal area or ear.
- The patient is positioned 3′ (1 m) from the pattern-shift stimulator.
- One eye is occluded, and the patient is instructed to fix his gaze on a dot in the center of the screen.

Visual and somatosensory evoked potentials

Visual (pattern-shift) evoked potentials: In this test, visual neural impulses are recorded as they travel along the pathway from the eye to the occipital cortex. Wave P100 is the most significant component of the resultant waveform. Normal P100 latency is about 100 milliseconds after the application of a visual stimulus, as shown in the top diagram. Increased P100 latency, shown in the bottom diagram, is an abnormal finding, indicating a lesion along the visual pathway.

NORMAL TRACING

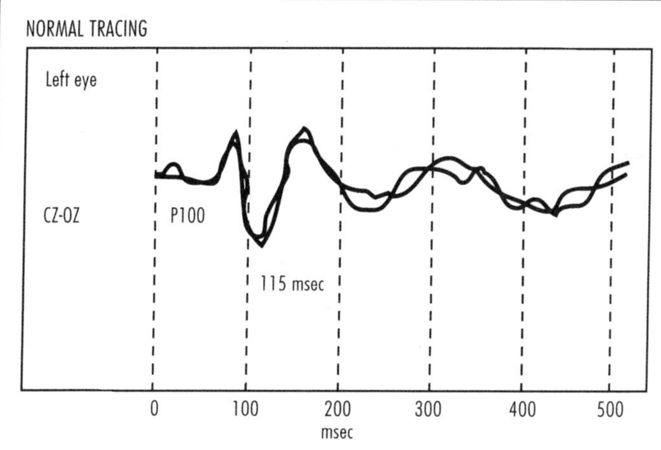

TRACING IN MULTIPLE SCLEROSIS

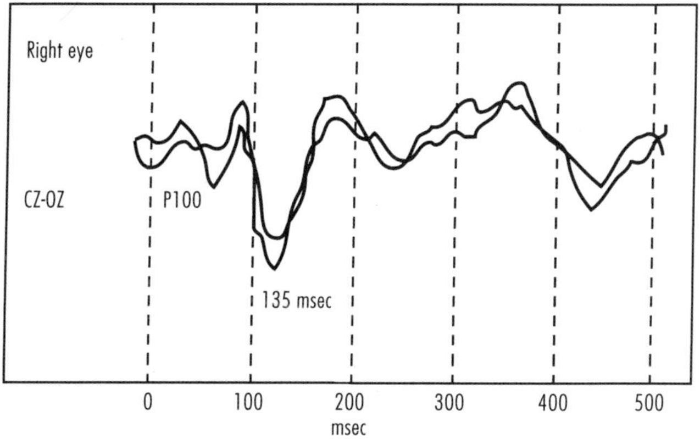

KEY: CZ = vertex; OZ = midocciput

(continued)

Visual and somatosensory evoked potentials *(continued)*

Somatosensory evoked potentials: These tests measure the conduction time of an electrical impulse traveling along a somatosensory pathway to the cortex. Interwave latency is the most significant component of the resultant waveform. On the set of upper- and lower-limb tracings shown below, the top tracings represent normal interwave latencies; the bottom tracings, typical abnormal latencies found in a patient with multiple sclerosis. Because of the close correlation between waveforms and the anatomy of somatosensory pathways, such tracings allow precise location of lesions that produce conduction defects.

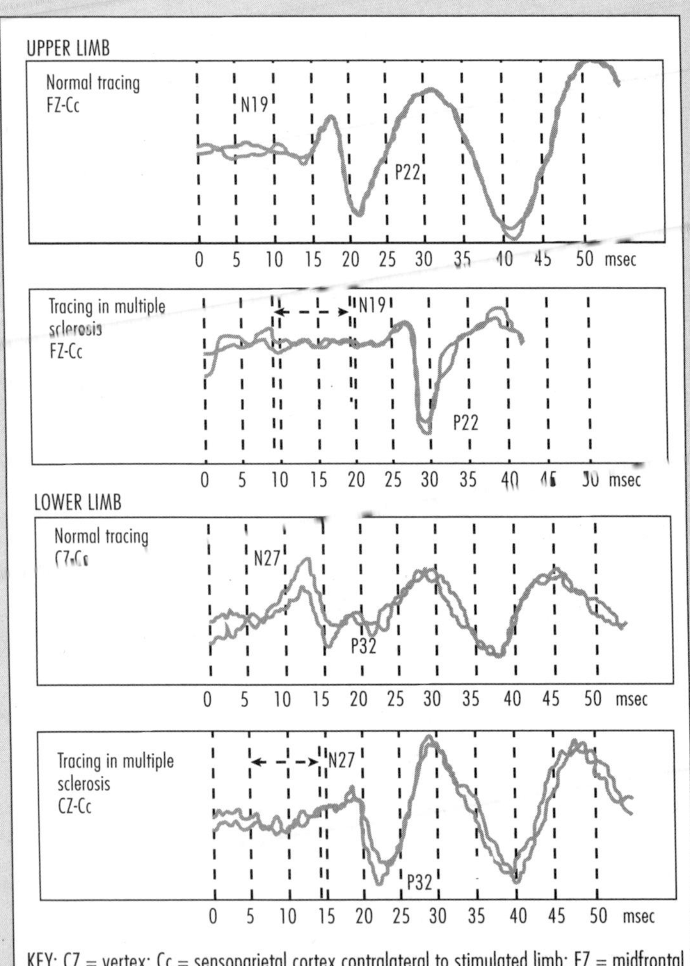

KEY: CZ = vertex; Cc = sensoparietal cortex contralateral to stimulated limb; FZ = midfrontal

- A checkerboard pattern is projected and then rapidly reversed or shifted 100 times, once or twice per second.
- A computer amplifies and averages the brain's response to each stimulus, and the results are plotted as a waveform.
- The procedure is repeated for the other eye.

Somatosensory evoked potentials

- Electrodes are attached to the patient's skin over somatosensory pathways — typically the wrist, knee, and ankle — to stimulate peripheral nerves. Recording electrodes are placed on the scalp over the sensory cortex of the hemisphere opposite the limb to be stimulated. Additional electrodes may be placed at Erb's point (above the clavicle overlying the brachial plexus), at the second cervical vertebra, and over the lower lumbar vertebrae. Midfrontal or noncephalic electrodes are placed for reference.
- Painless electrical stimulation is delivered to the peripheral nerve through the electrode. The intensity is adjusted to produce a minor muscle response such as a thumb twitch on median nerve stimulation at the wrist.
- Electrical stimuli are delivered 500 or more times at a rate of 5 per second.
- A computer measures and averages the time it takes for the electric current to reach the cortex; the results, expressed in milliseconds (msec), are recorded as waveforms.
- The test is repeated once to verify results; then the electrodes are repositioned, and the entire procedure is repeated for the other side.

Normal findings

Visual evoked potentials

On the waveform, the most significant wave is P100, a positive wave appearing about 100 msec after the pattern-shift stimulus is applied. The most clinically significant measurements are absolute P100 latency (the time between stimulus application and peaking of the P100 wave) and the difference between the P100 latencies of each eye. Because many physical and technical factors affect P100 latency, normal results vary greatly among laboratories and patients.

Somatosensory evoked potentials

Waveforms obtained vary, depending on locations of the stimulating and recording electrodes. The positive and negative peaks are labeled in sequence, based on normal time of appearance. For example, N19 is a negative peak normally recorded 19 msec after application of the stimulus. Each wave peak arises from a discrete location: N19 is generated mainly from the thalamus, P22 from the parietal sensory cortex, and so on. Interwave latencies (time between waves), rather than absolute latencies, are used as a basis for clinical interpretation. Latency differences between sides are significant.

Abnormal findings

Information from evoked potential studies is useful but insufficient to confirm a specific diagnosis. Test data must be interpreted in light of clinical information.

Visual evoked potentials

Generally, abnormal (extended) P100 latencies confined to one eye indicate a visual pathway lesion anterior to the optic chiasm. A lesion posterior to the optic chiasm usually doesn't produce abnormal P100 latencies. Because each eye projects to both occipital lobes, the unaffected pathway transmits sufficient impulses to produce a normal latency response. Bilateral abnormal P100 latencies have been found in patients with multiple sclerosis, optic neuritis, retinopathies, amblyopia (although abnormal latencies don't correlate well with impaired visual acuity), spinocerebellar degeneration, adrenoleukodystrophy, sarcoidosis, Parkinson's disease, and Huntington's disease.

Somatosensory evoked potentials
Because somatosensory evoked potential components are assumed to be linked in series, an abnormal interwave latency indicates a conduction defect between the generators of the two peaks involved. This often allows precise location of a neurologic lesion. Abnormal upper-limb interwave latencies may indicate cervical spondylosis, intracerebral lesions, or sensorimotor neuropathies. Abnormalities in the lower limb demonstrate peripheral nerve and root lesions, such as those in Guillain-Barré syndrome, compressive myelopathies, multiple sclerosis, transverse myelitis, and traumatic spinal cord injury.

Interfering factors

- Incorrect electrode placement or equipment failure
- Patient tension, inability to relax, or failure to cooperate
- Poor patient vision

ELECTROMYOGRAPHY

Electromyography (EMG) records the electrical activity of selected skeletal muscle groups at rest and during voluntary contraction. It involves percutaneous insertion of a needle electrode into a muscle. The electrical discharge of the muscle is then measured by an oscilloscope. Nerve conduction time is often measured simultaneously.

Purpose

- To aid differentiation between primary muscle disorders, such as the muscular dystrophies, and secondary disorders
- To help assess diseases characterized by central neuronal degeneration such as amyotrophic lateral sclerosis
- To aid diagnosis of neuromuscular disorders such as myasthenia gravis
- To aid in diagnosis of radiculomyopathies

Patient preparation

- Explain to the patient that this test measures the electrical activity of his muscles.
- Tell the patient that there are usually no restrictions on food or fluids (in some cases, cigarettes, coffee, tea, and cola may be restricted for 2 to 3 hours before the test).
- Describe the test, including who will perform it and where it will take place.
- Tell the patient that he may wear a hospital gown or any comfortable clothing that permits access to the muscles to be tested.
- Advise the patient that a needle will be inserted into selected muscles and that he may experience discomfort. Reassure him that adverse effects and complications are rare.
- Make sure the patient or a responsible family member has signed an informed consent form, if required.
- Check the patient's history for medications that may interfere with the results of the test, for example, cholinergics, anticholinergics, and skeletal muscle relaxants. If the patient is receiving such medications, note this on the chart and withhold medications as ordered.

Procedure and posttest care

- Position the patient on a stretcher or bed or in a chair, depending on the muscles to be tested. Position his arm or leg so that the muscle to be tested is at rest.
- The skin is cleaned with alcohol, the needle electrodes are quickly inserted,

and a metal plate is placed under the patient to serve as a reference electrode. Then the muscle's electrical signal (motor unit potential), recorded during rest and contraction, is amplified 1 million times and displayed on an oscilloscope screen or computer screen.

- The leadwires of the recorder are attached to an audio amplifier so that the fluctuation of voltage within the muscle can be heard.
- If the patient experiences residual pain, apply warm compresses and administer prescribed analgesics.
- Resume administration of any medications withheld for the test.

Precautions

- EMG is contraindicated in patients with bleeding disorders.

Normal findings

At rest, a normal muscle exhibits minimal electrical activity. During voluntary contraction, electrical activity increases markedly. A sustained contraction or one of increasing strength causes a rapid "train" of motor unit potentials that can be heard as a crescendo of sounds over the audio amplifier.

At the same time, the monitor displays a sequence of waveforms that vary in amplitude (height) and frequency. Waveforms that are close together indicate a high frequency, whereas waveforms that are far apart signify a low frequency.

Abnormal findings

In primary muscle diseases, such as muscular dystrophy, motor unit potentials are short (low amplitude), with frequent, irregular discharges. In disorders such as amyotrophic lateral sclerosis (as well as in peripheral nerve disorders), motor unit potentials are isolated and irregular but show increased amplitude and duration. In myasthenia gravis, motor unit potentials initially may be normal but progressively diminish in amplitude with continuing contractions. The interpreter distinguishes between waveforms that indicate a muscle disorder and those that indicate denervation. Findings must be correlated with the patient's history, clinical features, and the results of other neurodiagnostic tests.

Interfering factors

- Patient's inability to comply with instructions
- Drugs affecting myoneural junctions, such as cholinergics, anticholinergics, and skeletal muscle relaxants

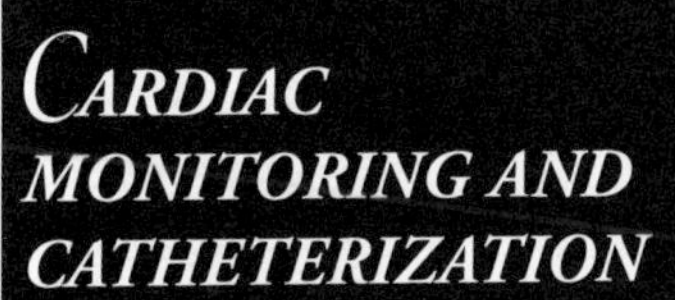

CARDIAC MONITORING AND CATHETERIZATION

ELECTROCARDIOGRAPHY

A common test for evaluating cardiac status, electrocardiography (ECG) graphically records the electric current (electrical potential) generated by the heart. This current radiates from the heart in all directions and, on reaching the skin, is measured by electrodes connected to an amplifier and strip chart recorder. The standard resting (scalar) ECG uses 5 electrodes to measure the electrical potential from 12 leads: the standard limb leads (I, II, III), the augmented limb leads (aV_R, aV_L, and aV_F), and the precordial, or chest, leads (V_1 through V_6).

New computerized ECG machines don't routinely use gel and suction bulbs. The electrodes are small tabs that peel off a sheet and adhere to the patient's skin. The leads coming from the ECG machine are clearly marked and applied to the electrodes with alligator clamps. The entire tracing is displayed on a screen so that abnormalities (loose leads or artifacts) can be corrected before the tracing is printed or transmitted to a central computer. The electrode tabs can remain on the patient's chest, arms, and legs to provide continuous lead placement for serial ECG studies.

Purpose

- To help identify primary conduction abnormalities, cardiac arrhythmias, cardiac hypertrophy, pericarditis, electrolyte imbalances, myocardial ischemia, and the site and extent of myocardial infarction (MI)
- To monitor recovery from MI
- To evaluate the effectiveness of cardiac medication (cardiac glycosides, antiarrhythmics, antihypertensives, and vasodilators)
- To assess pacemaker performance
- To determine the effectiveness of thrombolytic therapy and the resolution of ST-segment depression or elevation and T-wave changes

Patient preparation

- Explain to the patient that this test evaluates the heart's electrical activity.
- Tell the patient that he need not restrict food or fluids.
- Describe the test, including who will perform it, where it will take place, and how long it will last.
- Tell the patient that electrodes will be attached to his arms, legs, and chest and that the procedure is painless. Explain that during the test, he'll be asked to relax, lie still, and breathe normally.
- Advise the patient not to talk during the test because the sound of his voice may distort the ECG tracing.
- Check the patient's medication history for use of cardiac drugs, and note the use of such drugs on the test request form.

Equipment

ECG machine, recording paper, pregelled disposable electrodes, shaving supplies (if necessary), marking pen, moist cloth towel, sterile drape

Procedure and posttest care

- Place the patient in the supine position. If he can't tolerate lying flat, help him to assume the semi-Fowler position.
- Have the patient expose his chest, both ankles, and both wrists for electrode placement. If the patient is a woman, provide a chest drape until the chest leads are applied.
- Turn on the machine and check the paper supply.

Multichannel ECG

- Place electrodes on the inner aspect of the wrists, the medial aspect of the lower legs, and the chest. If using disposable electrodes, remove the paper backing before positioning.
- Connect the leadwires after all electrodes are in place.
- If frequent ECGs will be necessary, use a marking pen to indicate lead positions on the patient's chest to ensure consistent placement.
- Press the START button, and record any required information (for example, the patient's name and room number).
- The machine produces a printout showing all 12 leads simultaneously. Check to make sure all leads are represented in the tracing. If not, determine which one has come loose, reattach it, and restart the tracing.
- Make sure the wave doesn't peak beyond the top edge of the recording grid. If it does, adjust the machine to bring the wave inside the boundaries.

■ When the machine finishes the tracing, remove the electrodes and reposition the patient's gown and bed covers.

Single-channel ECG

■ Apply either disposable or standard electrodes to the inner aspect of the wrists and the medial aspect of the lower legs. Connect each leadwire to the corresponding electrode by inserting the wire prong into the terminal post and tightening the screw, if required.

■ Set the paper speed if required (usually 25 mm/second), and calibrate the machine by adjusting the sensitivity to normal. Recalibrate the machine after running each lead to provide a consistent test standard.

■ Turn the lead selector to I. Then mark the lead by writing "I" on the paper strip or by depressing the marking button on the machine (some machines do this automatically). Record for 3 to 6 seconds, and then return the machine to the standby mode. Repeat this procedure for leads II, III, aV_R, aV_L, and aV_F.

■ Determine proper placement for the chest electrodes. (If frequent ECGs are necessary, mark these spots on the patient's chest to ensure consistent placement.)

■ Connect the chest leadwire to the suction bulb, apply gel to each of the six chest positions, and then firmly press the suction bulb to attach the chest lead to the V_1 position. Mark the strips as before.

■ Turn the lead selector to V, and record V_1 for 3 to 6 seconds. Return the lead selector to standby. Reposition the electrode, and repeat the procedure for V_2 through V_6.

■ After completing V_6, run a rhythm strip on lead II for at least 6 seconds. Assess the quality of the tracings, and repeat any that are unclear.

■ Disconnect the equipment, remove the electrodes, and wipe the gel from the patient with a moist cloth towel. Wash the gel from the electrodes, and dry them thoroughly.

Both types

■ Label each ECG strip with the patient's name and room number (if applicable), date and time of the procedure, and physician's name. Note whether the ECG was performed during or on resolution of a chest pain episode.

■ Disconnect the equipment. The electrode patches are usually left in place if the patient is having recurrent chest pain or if serial ECGs are ordered, as with the use of thrombolytics.

■ Report any abnormal ECG findings to the physician.

Precautions

■ The recording equipment and other nearby electrical equipment should be properly grounded to prevent electrical interference.

■ Double-check color codes and lead markings to be sure connectors match.

■ Make sure the electrodes are firmly attached, and reattach them if loose skin contact is suspected. Don't use cables that are broken, frayed, or bare.

■ Make sure the patient is quiet and motionless during the test because talking and movement distort the recordings.

■ If the patient has a pacemaker in place, an ECG may be performed with or without a magnet. Indicate the presence of a pacemaker and whether a magnet is used. (Many pacemakers function only when the heartbeat falls below a preset rate; a magnet makes the pacemaker fire regularly, which permits evaluation of pacemaker performance.)

Normal findings

The lead II waveform, known as the rhythm strip, depicts the heart's rhythm more clearly than any other waveform.

Normal ECG waveforms

Because each lead takes a different view of heart activity, it generates its own characteristic tracing. The traces shown here are representative of each of the 12 leads. Leads aV_R, V_1, V_2, V_3, and V_4 normally show strong negative deflections below the baseline. Negative deflections indicate that the current is flowing away from the positive electrode; positive deflections, that the current is flowing toward the positive electrode.

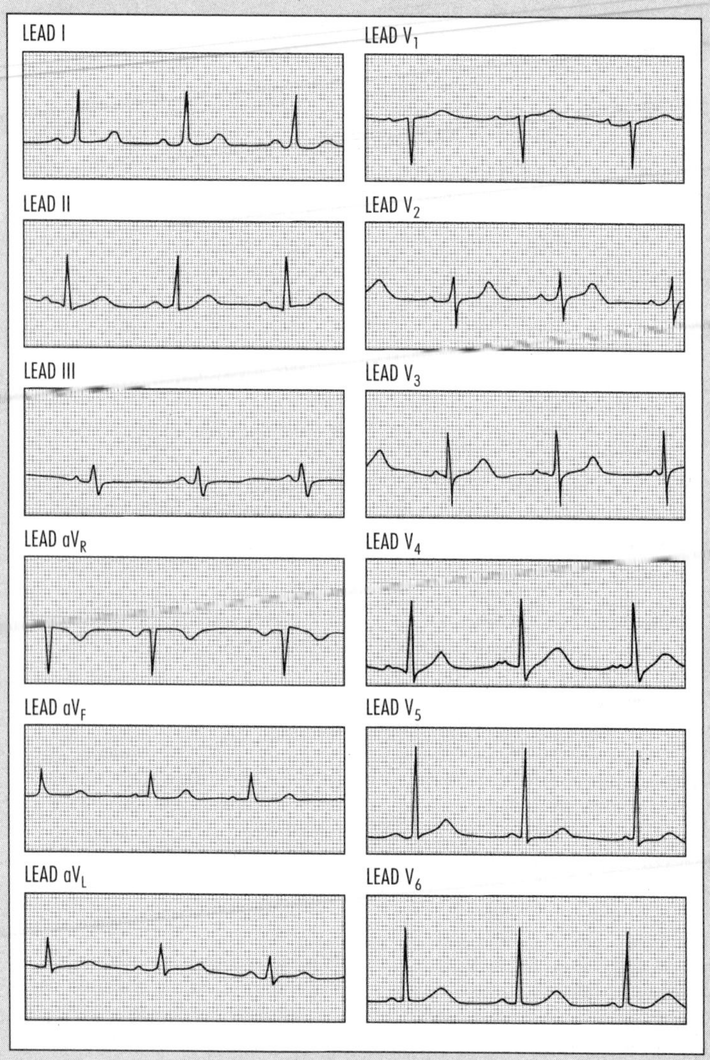

In lead II, the normal P wave doesn't exceed 2.5 mm (0.25 mV) in height or last longer than 0.12 second. The PR interval, which includes the P wave plus the PR segment, persists for 0.12 to 0.2 second for heart rates above 60 beats/minute. The QT interval varies with the heart rate and lasts 0.4 to 0.52 second for heart rates above 60 beats/minute; the voltage of the R wave in the V_1 through V_6 leads doesn't exceed 27 mm. The total QRS complex lasts 0.06 to 0.1 second. The ST segment is also useful for assessing myocardial ischemia. (See *Normal ECG waveforms.*)

Abnormal findings

An abnormal ECG may show MI, right or left ventricular hypertrophy, arrhythmias, right or left bundle-branch block, ischemia, conduction defects or pericarditis, electrolyte abnormalities (such as hypokalemia), and the effects of cardioactive drugs. Sometimes an ECG may reveal abnormal waveforms only during angina episodes or during exercise. (See *Abnormal ECG waveforms.*)

Interfering factors

- Inaccurate test results because of improper placement of electrodes, patient movement or muscle tremors, strenu-

(Text continues on page 706.)

Abnormal ECG waveforms

Premature ventricular contractions (PVCs) originate in an ectopic focus of the ventricular wall. They can be unifocal (having the same single focus), as shown in this tracing from lead V_1, or multifocal (arising from more than one ectopic focus). In PVCs, the P wave is absent and the QRS complex shows considerable distortion, usually deflecting in the opposite direction from the patient's normal QRS. The T wave also deflects in the opposite direction from the QRS complex, and the PVC usually precedes a compensatory pause. Some examples of abnormalities causing PVCs include electrolyte imbalances (especially hypokalemia), myocardial infarction (MI), reperfusion of a new MI or injury, hypoxia, and drug toxicity (cardiac glycosides, beta-adrenergics).

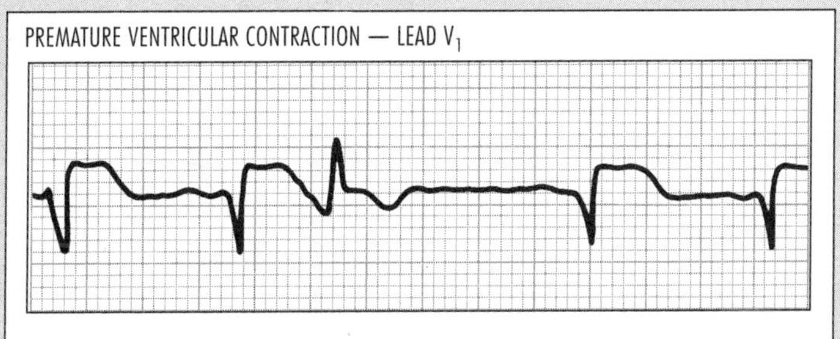

First-degree heart block, the most common conduction disturbance, occurs in healthy hearts as well as diseased hearts and usually is clinically insignificant. It's typically characteristic in elderly patients with chronic degeneration of the cardiac conduction system, and it occasionally

(continued)

Abnormal ECG waveforms *(continued)*

occurs in patients receiving cardiac glycosides or antiarrhythmic drugs, such as procainamide and quinidine. In children, first-degree heart block may be the earliest sign of acute rheumatic fever. In this lead V_1 tracing, the interval between the P wave and the QRS complex (the PR interval) exceeds 0.20 second.

FIRST-DEGREE HEART BLOCK — LEAD V_1

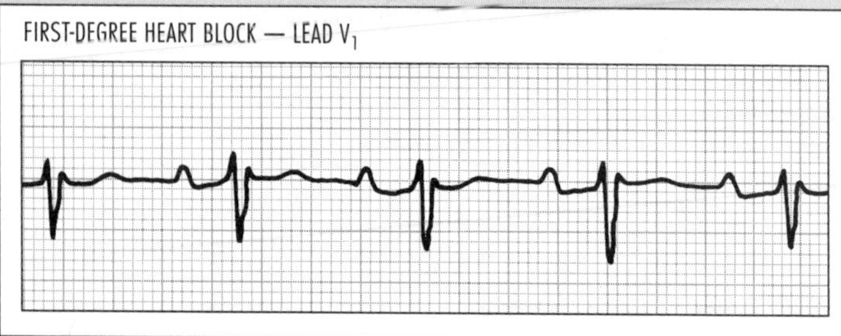

Hypokalemia is a common electrolyte imbalance that's caused by low serum potassium levels and affects the electrical activity of the myocardium. Mild hypokalemia may cause only muscle weakness, fatigue and, possibly, atrial or ventricular irritability; a severe imbalance causes pronounced muscle weakness, paralysis, atrial tachycardia with varying degrees of block, and PVCs that may progress to ventricular tachycardia and fibrillation.

Early signs of hypokalemia, as shown on this lead V_1 tracing, include prominent U waves, a prolonged QU interval, and flat or inverted T waves. Usually, T waves don't flatten or invert until potassium depletion becomes severe.

HYPOKALEMIA — LEAD V_1

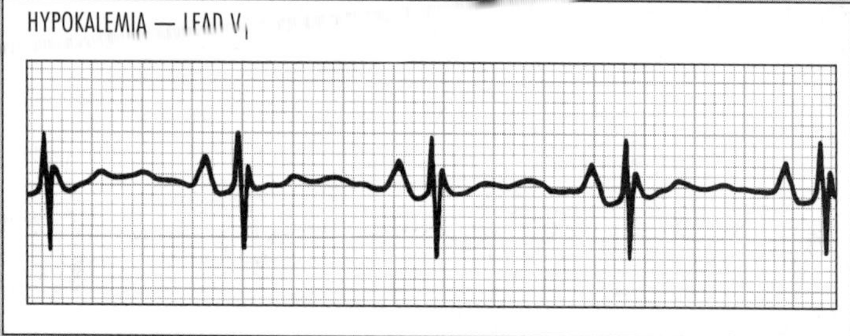

MI produces typical ECG changes in several leads at once, enabling the physician to accurately determine the location and extent of tissue damage. MI causes three changes: an inner zone of tissue necrosis (infarction), a surrounding zone of inflamed tissue, and an outer zone of ischemia (see diagram). As the infarction progresses, the first ECG change is an elevated ST segment, which indicates formation of an ischemic zone. Then the T wave begins to flatten and finally inverts, and enlarged Q waves appear, indicating developing necrosis — a true

Abnormal ECG waveforms *(continued)*

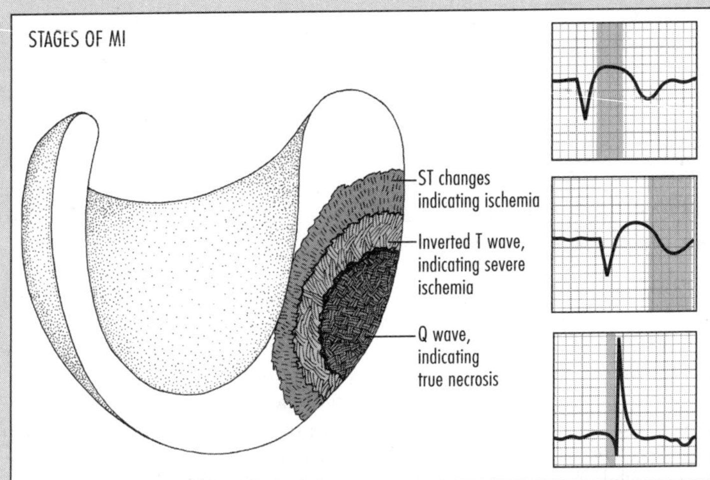

infarction. (Abnormal Q waves should be larger than one small square on the chart — 0.04 second by 0.1 mV.) The T wave may stay inverted for the rest of the patient's life or it can revert to normal, whereas the deep Q wave remains as a permanent indicator of necrosis. The infarction can be located by studying the characteristic ST-segment, T-wave, and Q-wave changes in various lead combinations. In the three tracings shown below, the ST-segment elevations in leads II, III, and aV_F indicate an infarction in the inferior (diaphragmatic) area of the heart.

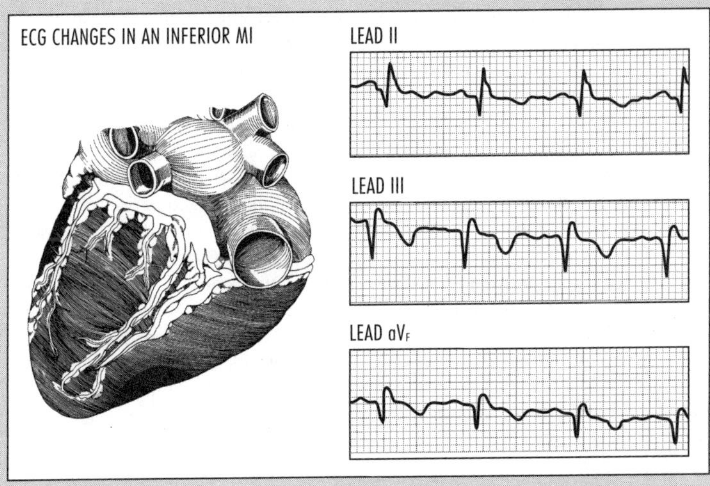

ous exercise before the test, or medication reactions

- Mechanical difficulties, such as ECG machine malfunction, faulty adherence of electrode patches (for example, due to diaphoresis), and electromagnetic interference (production of artifact)

EXERCISE ELECTROCARDIOGRAPHY

Also referred to as a stress test, an exercise electrocardiogram (ECG) evaluates the heart's response to physical stress, providing important diagnostic information that can't be obtained from a resting ECG alone.

An ECG and blood pressure readings are taken while the patient walks on a treadmill or pedals a stationary bicycle and his response to a constant or an increasing workload is observed. Unless complications develop, the test continues until the patient reaches the target heart rate (determined by an established protocol) or experiences chest pain or fatigue. The patient who has recently had a myocardial infarction (MI) or coronary artery surgery may walk the treadmill at a slow pace to determine his activity tolerance before discharge.

Purpose

- To help diagnose the cause of chest pain or other possible cardiac pain
- To determine the functional capacity of the heart after surgery or MI
- To screen for asymptomatic coronary artery disease (CAD), particularly in men over age 35
- To help set limitations for an exercise program
- To identify arrhythmias that develop during physical exercise
- To evaluate the effectiveness of antiarrhythmic or antianginal therapy
- To evaluate myocardial perfusion

Patient preparation

- Explain to the patient that this test records the heart's electrical activity and performance under stress.
- Instruct the patient not to eat, smoke, or drink alcoholic or caffeinated beverages for 3 hours before the test but to continue his prescribed drug regimen unless directed otherwise.
- Describe to the patient who will perform the test, where it will take place, and how long it will last.
- Tell the patient that the test will cause fatigue and that he'll be slightly breathless and sweaty, but assure him that the test poses few risks. He may, in fact, stop the test if he experiences fatigue or chest pain.
- Advise the patient to wear comfortable socks and shoes and loose, lightweight shorts or slacks. Men usually don't wear a shirt during the test, and women generally wear a bra and a lightweight short-sleeved blouse or a patient gown with a front closure.
- Explain to the patient that electrodes will be attached to several areas on his chest and, possibly, his back after the skin areas are cleaned and abraded. Reassure him that he won't feel any current from the electrodes; however, they may itch slightly.
- Tell the patient that his blood pressure will be checked periodically throughout the procedure, and assure him that his heart rate will be monitored continuously.
- If the patient is scheduled for a multistage *treadmill test,* explain that the speed and incline of the treadmill will increase at predetermined intervals and that he'll be informed of each adjustment.

- If the patient is scheduled for a *bicycle ergometer test,* explain that the resistance he experiences in pedaling increases gradually as he tries to maintain a specific speed.
- Encourage the patient to report his feelings during the test. Tell him that his blood pressure and ECG will be monitored for 10 to 15 minutes after the test.
- Check the patient's history for a recent physical examination (within 1 week) and for baseline 12-lead ECG results.
- Make sure the patient or a responsible family member has signed an informed consent form.

Procedure and posttest care

- The electrode sites are cleaned with an alcohol swab, and superficial epidermal cell layers and excess skin oils are removed with a gauze pad, fine sandpaper, or a dental burr. After thorough cleaning and abrading, adequately prepared sites will appear slightly red.
- Chest electrodes are placed according to the lead system selected and are secured with adhesive tape, if necessary. The leadwire cable is placed over the patient's shoulder, and the leadwire box is placed on his chest. The cable is secured by pinning it to the patient's clothing or taping it to his shoulder or back. Then the leadwires are connected to the chest electrodes.
- The monitor is started, and a stable baseline tracing is obtained. A baseline rhythm strip is checked for arrhythmias. A blood pressure reading is taken, and the patient is auscultated for the presence of S_3 or S_4 gallops or crackles.
- In a treadmill test, the treadmill is turned on to a slow speed, and the patient is shown how to step onto it and how to use the support railings to maintain balance but not support weight. Then the treadmill is turned off. The patient is instructed to step onto the treadmill, and it is turned on to slow speed until he gets used to walking on it. Intensity of exercise is then increased every 3 minutes by slightly increasing the speed of the machine and at the same time increasing the incline by 3%.
- For a bicycle ergometer test, the patient is instructed to sit on the bicycle while the seat and handlebars are adjusted to comfortable positions. The patient is instructed not to grip the handlebars tightly but to use them only for maintaining balance and to pedal until he reaches the desired speed, as shown on the speedometer.
- In both tests, a monitor is observed continuously for changes in the heart's electrical activity. The rhythm strip is checked at preset intervals for arrhythmias, premature ventricular contractions (PVCs), ST-segment changes, and T-wave changes. The test level and the time elapsed in the test level are marked on each strip. Blood pressure is monitored at predetermined intervals, usually at the end of each test level, and changes in systolic readings are noted. Some common responses to maximal exercise are dizziness, light-headedness, leg fatigue, dyspnea, diaphoresis, and a slightly ataxic gait. If symptoms become severe, the test is stopped.
- Usually, testing stops when the patient reaches the target heart rate. As the treadmill speed slows, he may be instructed to continue walking for several minutes to cool down. Then the treadmill is turned off, the patient is helped to a chair, and his blood pressure and ECG are monitored for 10 to 15 minutes or until the ECG returns to baseline.
- Auscultate for the presence of an S_3 or S_4 gallop. An S_4 gallop commonly develops after exercise because of increased blood flow volume and turbu-

lence. An S_3 gallop is more significant than an S_4 gallop, indicating transient left ventricular dysfunction.

- Tell the patient that he may resume any activities discontinued before the test.
- If any drugs were discontinued before the test, tell the patient that he may resume taking them.
- Remove electrodes and clean the electrode sites before the patient leaves.

Precautions

- Because an exercise ECG places considerable stress on the heart, it may be contraindicated in patients with ventricular aneurysm, dissecting aortic aneurysm, uncontrolled arrhythmias, pericarditis, myocarditis, severe anemia, uncontrolled hypertension, unstable angina, or heart failure.
- Stop the test immediately if the ECG shows three consecutive PVCs or any significant increase in ectopy, if the systolic blood pressure falls below resting level, if the heart rate falls to 10 beats/minute below resting level, or if the patient becomes exhausted. Depending on the patient's condition, the test may be stopped if the ECG shows bundle-branch block, ST-segment depression that exceeds 1.5 mm, persistent ST-segment elevation, or frequent or complicated PVCs; if blood pressure fails to rise above resting level; if systolic pressure exceeds 220 mm Hg; or if the patient experiences angina.

Normal findings

In a normal exercise ECG, the P and T waves, the QRS complex, and the ST segment change minimally; a slight ST-segment depression occurs in some patients, especially women. The heart rate rises in direct proportion to the workload and metabolic oxygen demand; blood pressure also rises as workload increases. The patient attains the endurance levels predicted by his age and the appropriate exercise protocol. (See *Exercise ECG tracings.*)

Abnormal findings

Although criteria for judging test results vary, two findings strongly suggest an abnormality: a flat or downsloping ST-segment depression of 1 mm or more for at least 0.08 second after the junction of the QRS and ST segments (J point) and a markedly depressed J point, with an upsloping but depressed ST segment of 1.5 mm below the baseline 0.08 second after the J point. T-wave inversion also signifies ischemia. Initial ST-segment depression on the resting ECG must be further depressed by 1 mm during exercise to be considered abnormal.

Hypotension resulting from exercise, ST-segment depression of 3 mm or more, downsloping ST segments, and ischemic ST segments appearing within the first 3 minutes of exercise and lasting 8 minutes into the posttest recovery period may indicate multivessel or left CAD. ST-segment elevation may indicate dyskinetic left ventricular wall motion or severe transmural ischemia.

The predictive value of this test for CAD varies with the patient's history and sex; false-negative and false-positive test results are common. This is often related to the effects of drugs, such as digoxin, or caffeine ingestion before testing. To detect CAD accurately, thallium imaging and stress testing, exercise multiple-gated acquisition scanning, or coronary angiography may be necessary.

Interfering factors

- Failure to observe pretest restrictions
- Inability to exercise to the target heart rate due to fatigue or failure to cooperate
- Wolff-Parkinson-White syndrome (anomalous atrioventricular excitation),

Exercise ECG tracings

These tracings are from an abnormal exercise electrocardiogram (ECG) obtained during a treadmill test performed on a patient who had just undergone a triple coronary artery bypass graft. The first tracing shows the heart at rest, with a blood pressure of 124/80 mm Hg. In the second tracing, the patient worked up to a 10% grade at 1.7 miles per hour before experiencing angina at 2 minutes, 25 seconds. The tracing shows a depressed ST segment; heart rate was 85 beats/minute, and blood pressure was 140/70 mm Hg. The third tracing shows the heart at rest 6 minutes after the test; blood pressure was 140/90 mm Hg.

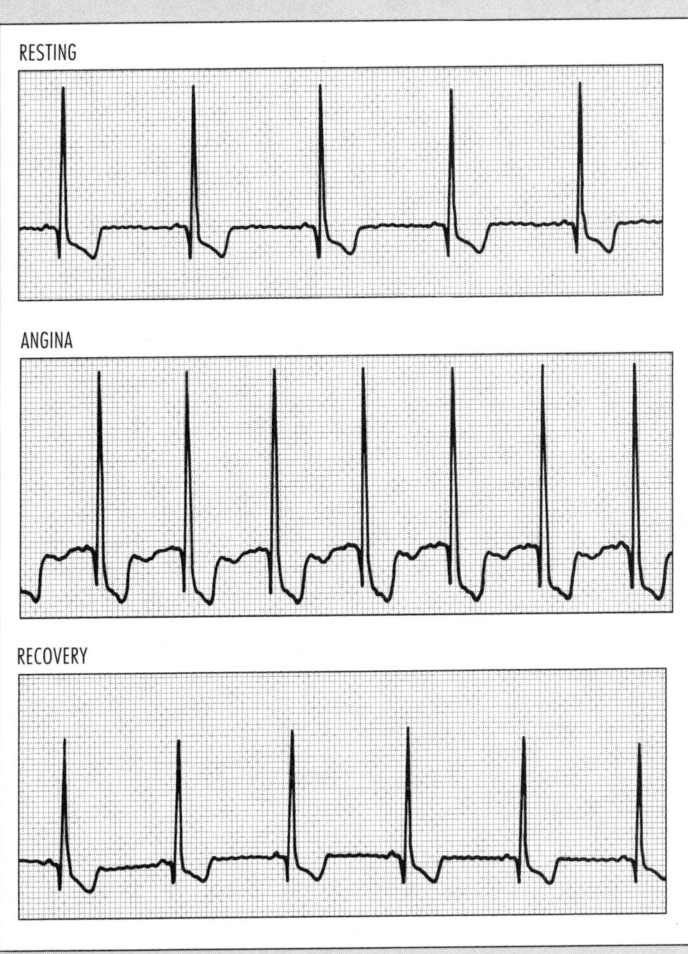

electrolyte imbalance, or use of a cardiac glycoside (possible false-positive)
- Conditions that affect left ventricular hypertrophy, such as congenital abnormalities and hypertension (possible interference with testing for ischemia)
- Beta-adrenergic blockers (may make test results difficult to interpret)

RADIOPHARMACEUTICAL MYOCARDIAL PERFUSION IMAGING

An imaging test also known as chemical stress imaging, radiopharmaceutical myocardial perfusion imaging is an alternative method of assessing coronary vessel function in patients who can't tolerate exercise electrocardiography (ECG).

In this test, I.V. infusion of a selected drug — for example, adenosine, dobutamine, or dipyridamole — is used to simulate the effects of exercise by increasing blood flow in the coronary arteries. Next, a radiopharmaceutical is injected I.V. to allow imaging that assists in evaluating the cardiac vessel's response to the drug-induced stress. Both resting and stress images are obtained to evaluate coronary perfusion.

Purpose

- To assess the presence and degree of coronary artery disease (CAD)
- To evaluate therapeutic procedures, such as bypass surgery or coronary angioplasty
- To evaluate myocardial perfusion

Patient preparation

- Describe the test, including who will perform it and where it will take place.
- Tell the patient that he'll need to arrive 1 hour before the test and that an I.V. line will be initiated before the test.
- If the patient will receive adenosine or dipyridamole, instruct him to avoid taking all theophylline medications for 24 to 36 hours and all caffeinated drinks for 12 hours before the test.
- If the patient will receive dobutamine, instruct him to withhold beta-adrenergic blockers for 48 hours before the test. Also tell him not to eat for 3 to 4 hours before the test, although he may have water. Instruct him to take his other medications as prescribed with sips of water.
- Tell the patient to continue taking antihypertensive medications. If his systolic blood pressure is higher than 200 mm Hg, the dobutamine stress test can't be done until his blood pressure is under control. Confirm that female patients aren't pregnant before performing the test.
- Tell the patient that a cardiologist, a nurse, an ECG technician, and a nuclear medicine technologist will be present for the medication infusion. Advise him that he'll be weighed first to determine the proper drug dose.
- Inform the patient that he may experience flushing, shortness of breath, dizziness, headache, chest pain, and increased heart rate during the infusion but that these will end as soon as the infusion ends and that emergency equipment will be available, if needed.
- Screen the patient for bronchospastic lung disease or asthma. Adenosine and dipyridamole are contraindicated in these patients; use dobutamine instead. Weigh the patient to determine the appropriate dosage.
- Make sure the patient or a responsible family member has signed an informed consent form.

Procedure and posttest care

- Place the patient on a bed or an examination table in the ECG or medical imaging department, and start an I.V. line.

- Apply 12 ECG leadwires to appropriate sites, and obtain baseline ECG and blood pressure readings.
- The selected chemical stress medication is infused, and blood pressure, pulse, and cardiac rhythm are monitored continuously.
- Tell the patient to report the symptoms he's feeling.
- At the appropriate time, the selected radiopharmaceutical is injected.
- Depending on which radiopharmaceutical is used, the patient either undergoes imaging immediately or is instructed to return for imaging 45 minutes to 2 hours later. Resting imaging may be done before stress imaging or 3 to 4 hours afterward, depending on the radiopharmaceutical used.
- Tell the patient when he needs to return and whether he should continue to fast.
- Remove the I.V. line after the images are completed.
- When all scans are completed, allow the patient to resume his regular diet.
- If the patient must return for further scanning, tell him to rest; he may also need to restrict foods and fluids in the interim.

Precautions

- This test is usually contraindicated in pregnant women.
- The use of adenosine or dipyridamole is contraindicated in bronchospastic lung disease or asthma.
- Keep resuscitation equipment available in case the patient experiences arrhythmias, angina, ST-segment depression, or bronchospasm.
- Aminophylline, the reversal agent for adenosine and dipyrimadole, can be administered to reverse severe adverse reactions.
- Contraindications include MI within 10 days of testing, acute myocarditis and pericarditis, unstable angina, arrhythmias, hypertension or hypotension, aortic or mitral stenosis, hyperthyroidism, and severe infection.
- Beta-adrenergic blockers, calcium channel blockers, and angiotensin-converting enzyme inhibitors should be withheld up to 36 hours before testing, as ordered. Nitrates should be withheld 6 hours before testing.

Normal findings

Imaging should reveal characteristic distribution of the radiopharmaceutical throughout the left ventrical and show no visible defects.

Abnormal findings

Cold spots are usually due to CAD but may result from myocardial fibrosis, attenuation due to soft tissue (for example, breasts and diaphragm), or coronary spasm. The absence of cold spots in the presence of CAD may result from insignificant artifact obstruction, single-vessel disease, or collateral circulation.

Interfering factors

- Certain drugs such as digoxin (may produce a false-positive reading)
- Cold spots due to artifacts, such as implants and electrodes
- Delayed imaging (may cause absence of cold spots in the presence of CAD)

AMBULATORY ELECTROCARDIOGRAPHY

Also called Holter monitoring or dynamic monitoring, ambulatory electrocardiography (ECG) involves the continuous recording of heart activity over a 24-hour period as the patient follows his normal routine. During this period, the patient wears a small reel-to-reel or cassette tape recorder connected to electrodes placed on his chest and keeps a diary of his activities and any associated symptoms. After the recording period, the tape is analyzed by a computer and a physician to correlate cardiac irregularities, such as arrhythmias and ST-segment changes, with the activities noted in the patient's diary.

Purpose

- To detect cardiac arrhythmias
- To evaluate chest pain
- To evaluate cardiac status after acute myocardial infarction (MI) or pacemaker implantation
- To evaluate the effectiveness of antiarrhythmic drug therapy
- To assess and correlate dyspnea, central nervous system symptoms (such as syncope and light-headedness), and palpitations with actual cardiac events and the patient's activities

Patient preparation

- Explain to the patient that this test helps determine how the heart responds to normal activity or, if appropriate, to cardioactive medication. Tell him that electrodes will be attached to his chest, that his chest may be shaved, and that he may experience some discomfort during preparation of the electrode sites.
- Explain that he'll wear a small tape recorder for 24 hours (for 5 to 7 days, if a patient-activated monitor is being used).
- Mention that a shoulder strap or a special belt will be provided to carry the recorder, which weights about 2 lb (1 kg). Show him how to position the recorder when he lies down.
- Encourage the patient to continue his routine activities during the monitoring period. Stress the importance of logging his usual activities (such as walking, climbing stairs, urinating, sleeping, and having sex), emotional upsets, physical symptoms (dizziness, palpitations, fatigue, chest pain, and syncope), and ingestion of medication; show the patient a sample diary.
- Tell the patient to wear loose-fitting clothing with front-buttoning tops during monitoring.
- Demonstrate the proper use of specific equipment, including how to mark the tape (if applicable) at the onset of symptoms.
- If a patient-activated monitor is being used, show the patient how to press the event button to activate the monitor if he experiences an unusual sensation. Instruct him not to tamper with the monitor or disconnect the leadwires or electrodes.
- Bathing instructions depend on the type of recorder being worn (certain equipment mustn't get wet).
- Advise the patient to avoid magnets, metal detectors, high-voltage areas, and electric blankets. Show him how to check the recorder to make sure it's working properly. Instruct him how to trouble-shoot problems if the monitor alarm sounds. Explain that if the monitor light flashes, one of the electrodes may be loose and he should depress the center of each one. Tell him to notify you if one comes off.
- If the patient won't be returning to the office or hospital immediately after the monitoring period, show him how to remove and store the equipment. Remind him to bring the diary when he returns.

Procedure and posttest care

- Clean and gently abrade the electrode sites. Peel the backings from the electrodes and apply them to the correct sites, making sure to press the sides and center of each electrode firmly to ensure proper adhesion.

- Attach the electrode cable securely to the monitor.
- Position the monitor and case as the patient will wear it, and then attach the leadwires to the electrodes. There shouldn't be too much slack or pull on the wires.
- Make sure the recorder has a new or fully charged battery, insert the tape, and turn on the recorder.
- Test the electrode attachment circuit by connecting the recorder to a standard ECG machine. Watch for artifacts while the patient moves normally (stands, sits).
- Remove all chest electrodes and clean the electrode sites after the test.

Precautions

- To eliminate muscle artifact, make sure the lead cable is plugged in firmly. Check to ensure that electrodes aren't placed over large muscle masses such as the pectorals.

Normal findings

When correlated with the patient's diary, the ECG pattern shows normal sinus rhythm with no significant arrhythmias or ST-segment changes. Changes in heart rate normally occur during various activities.

Abnormal findings

Abnormalities of the heart detected by ambulatory ECG include premature ventricular contractions (PVCs), conduction defects, tachyarrhythmias, bradyarrhythmias, and brady-tachy syndrome. Arrhythmias may be associated with dyspnea and central nervous system symptoms, such as dizziness and syncope.

During recovery from an MI, this test can monitor for PVCs to determine the prognosis and effectiveness of drug therapy.

ST-T wave changes associated with ischemia may coincide with chest pain or increased patient activity. ST-segment changes associated with an acute MI require careful study because smoking, eating, postural changes, certain drugs, Wolff-Parkinson-White syndrome, bundle-branch block, myocarditis, myocardial hypertrophy, anemia, hypoxemia, and abnormal hemoglobin binding can produce a similar tracing on the ECG. Monitoring the MI patient for 1 to 3 days before discharge and again 4 to 6 weeks after discharge may detect ST-T wave changes associated with ischemia or arrhythmias; such information aids patient therapy and rehabilitation and refines the prognosis. Monitoring a patient with an artificial pacemaker may detect an arrhythmia, such as bradycardia, that the pacemaker fails to override.

Although ambulatory ECG correlates patient symptoms and ECG changes, it doesn't always identify the symptoms' causes. If initial monitoring proves inconclusive, the test may be repeated.

Interfering factors

- Electrode placement over muscle mass, poor electrode contact with skin, or other failure to correctly apply the electrodes (possible muscle or movement artifact)
- Patient's failure to carefully record daily activities and symptoms, to maintain his normal routine, or to turn on the monitor during symptoms (if using a patient-activated monitor)
- Physiologic variation in arrhythmia frequency and severity (possible failure to detect arrhythmia during 24-hour Holter monitoring)

SIGNAL-AVERAGED ELECTRO-CARDIOGRAPHY

Signal averaging is the amplification, averaging, and filtering of an electrocardiogram (ECG) signal that's recorded on the body surface by orthogonal leads. The recording detects high-frequency, low-amplitude cardiac electrical signals in the last part of the QRS complex and in the ST segment. In patients who have survived an acute myocardial infarction (MI), these distinctive signals, called late potentials, may represent delayed disorganized activity in abnormal areas of the myocardium at the interface of fibrous scar tissue and normal tissue. This activity can lead to life-threatening ventricular arrhythmias.

In this computerized procedure, each electrode lead input is amplified, its voltage measured or sampled at intervals of 1 msec or less, and each sample converted into a digital number. The ECG is thereby converted from an analogue voltage waveform into a series of digital numbers that are, in essence, a computer-readable ECG of 100 or more QRS complexes.

Purpose

- To detect late potentials and evaluate the risk of life-threatening arrhythmias

Patient preparation

- Explain to the patient that this test is used to evaluate the electrical activity of his heart and his potential for developing a life-threatening arrhythmia.
- Inform the patient that the test will be performed by a technician who has been specially trained to monitor recording and computerized equipment used to analyze the signal-averaged ECG.
- Describe the test, including who will perform it, where it will take place, and how long it will last.
- Tell the patient that electrodes will be attached to his arms, legs, and chest and that the procedure is painless.
- Explain to the patient that during the test, he'll be asked to lie still and breathe normally. This is important because limb movement or the sound of his voice will distort the recording.
- Inform the patient that he need not restrict food or fluids before the test.
- Record on the patient's chart any use of antiarrhythmics.

Equipment

Recording paper, disposable electrodes or reusable electrodes with suction bulbs, conductive gel, rubber straps, 4″ × 4″ gauze pads, moist cloth towel, sterile drape, computer equipment for analyzing the recorded ECG

Procedure and posttest care

- Place the patient in the supine position. If he can't tolerate lying flat, help him into the semi-Fowler position.
- Have the patient expose his chest, both ankles, and both wrists for electrode placement. If the patient is a woman, provide a chest drape until the chest leads are applied.
- The test is performed by a technician who is specially trained to operate the recording and computer equipment used in analyzing the signal-averaged ECG.
- The technician gathers the multiple inputs necessary for signal averaging from standard orthogonal bipolar X, Y, and Z leads over a series of ECG cycles. The average is taken over a large number of beats, typically 100 or more.
- After the test is completed, disconnect the equipment. If suction cups were used, be sure to wash the conductive gel from the patient's skin.

Precautions

- The recording equipment and other nearby electrical equipment should be properly grounded to prevent electrical interference.
- Tissue-electrode artifacts can be minimized by lightly sanding the skin with fine sandpaper (no. 220), wiping with alcohol, and using silver-silver chloride electrodes.
- Urge the patient to lie as quiet and motionless as possible to avoid signal distortion.

Normal findings

A QRS complex without low potentials is considered normal.

The areas of interest in the signal-averaged ECG are:

- the duration of the filtered QRS complex (QRST), which indicates how long the completion of the QRS complex is delayed by late potentials
- the amount of energy in the late potentials, as indicated by the root mean square (RMS) voltage in the terminal 40 msec of the QRS complex (RMS40)
- the duration of the late potentials, as indicated by the duration of the low-amplitude signals of less than 40 μV in the terminal QRS region (LAS40).

The preceding values can be read either from the signal-averaged ECG itself or from the computer system.

Defining a late potential and scoring a signal-averaged ECG as normal or abnormal are highly dependent on technique. Representative criteria include when late potentials exist when the filtered QRS complex is longer than 114 msec; when there is less than 20 μV RMS of signal in the terminal 40 msec of the filtered QRS; or when the terminal portion of the filtered QRS remains below 40 μV for longer than 38 msec.

Abnormal findings

Identifying late potentials after the QRS complex indicates a risk of ventricular arrhythmias. Late potentials are most common and of greater prognostic value in patients who have sustained an MI. Those patients who don't have late potentials are at low risk for serious ventricular arrhythmias and sudden death. Although the predictive accuracy of a positive signal-averaged ECG is relatively low, it has been advocated as a screening test for patients who should undergo electrophysiologic testing.

Interfering factors

- Artifact from skeletal muscle movement (possible need to administer a muscle relaxant)
- Electromagnetic interference (possible need to shield and twist input cables to reduce noise)
- Poor tissue-electrode contact (production of artifact)
- Antiarrhythmic drugs

IMPEDANCE PLETHYSMOGRAPHY

Also called occlusive impedance phlebography, impedance plethysmography is a reliable, widely used, noninvasive test that measures venous flow in the limbs. Electrodes from a plethysmograph are applied to the patient's leg to record changes in electrical resistance (impedance) caused by blood volume variations that may result from respiration or venous occlusion.

Purpose

- To detect deep vein thrombosis (DVT) in the proximal deep veins of the leg

- To screen patients at high risk for thrombophlebitis
- To evaluate patients with suspected pulmonary embolism (because most pulmonary emboli are complications of DVT in the leg)

Patient preparation

- Explain to the patient that this test helps detect DVT.
- Inform the patient that he need not restrict food, fluid, or medications before the test.
- Explain that the test requires that both legs be tested and that three to five tracings may be made for each leg.
- Tell the patient who will perform the test and where it will take place.
- Assure the patient that the test is painless and safe.
- Emphasize that accurate testing requires that leg muscles be relaxed and breathing be normal. Reassure the patient that if he experiences pain that interferes with leg relaxation, a mild analgesic will be administered, if ordered.
- Just before the test, instruct the patient to void and to put on a hospital gown.

Procedure and posttest care

- Place the patient in the supine position, elevating the leg to be tested 30 to 35 degrees. To promote venous drainage, place the calf above heart level.
- Ask the patient to flex his knee slightly and to rotate his hips by shifting weight to the same side as the leg being tested.
- After the electrodes (connected to the plethysmograph) have been loosely attached to the calf about 3″ to 4″ (7.5 to 10 cm) apart, the pressure cuff (connected to the air pressure system) is wrapped snugly around the thigh about 2″ (5 cm) above the knee.
- The pressure cuff is inflated to 45 to 60 cm H_2O, allowing full venous distention without interfering with arterial blood flow. Pressure is maintained for 45 seconds or until the tracing stabilizes. (In a patient with reduced arterial blood flow, pressure is maintained for 2 minutes or longer, after which the pressure cuff is rapidly deflated.)
- The strip chart tracing, which records the increase in venous volume after cuff inflation and the decrease in venous volume 3 seconds after deflation, is checked. Then the test is repeated for the other leg. If necessary, three to five tracings for each leg are obtained to confirm full venous filling and outflow; the tracing showing the greatest rise and fall in venous volume is used as the test result.
- If the result is ambiguous, the position of the patient's leg as well as cuff and electrode placement are checked.
- Make sure the conductive gel is removed from the patient's skin after the test.

Normal findings

Temporary venous occlusion normally produces a sharp rise in venous volume; release of the occlusion produces rapid venous outflow.

Abnormal findings

When clots in a major deep vein obstruct venous outflow, the pressure in the distal leg (calf) veins rises and these veins become distended. Such veins are unable to expand further when additional pressure is applied with an occlusive thigh cuff. Blockage of major deep veins also decreases the rate at which blood flows from the leg. If significant thrombi are present in a major deep vein of the lower leg (popliteal, femoral, or iliac), both calf vein filling and venous outflow rate are reduced. In such cases, the physician will evaluate the need for further treatment, such as anticoagulant therapy, taking the patient's overall condition into consideration.

Interfering factors

- Decreased peripheral arterial blood flow due to shock, increased vasoconstriction, low cardiac output, or arterial occlusive disease
- Extrinsic venous compression, as from pelvic tumors, large hematomas, constricting clothing, or bandages
- Failure to breathe normally or to completely relax leg muscles due to pain
- Cold extremities due to cold room temperature

CARDIAC CATHETERIZATION

Cardiac catheterization involves passing a catheter into the right or left side of the heart. Catheterization can determine blood pressure and blood flow in the chambers of the heart, permit collection of blood samples, and record films of the heart's ventricles (contrast ventriculography) or arteries (coronary arteriography or angiography).

In catheterization of the left side of the heart, a catheter is inserted into an artery in the antecubital fossa or into the femoral artery through a puncture or cutdown procedure. Guided by fluoroscopy, the catheter is advanced retrograde through the aorta into the coronary artery orifices and left ventricle. Then a contrast medium is injected into the ventricle, permitting radiographic visualization of the ventricle and coronary arteries and filming (cineangiography) of heart activity.

Catheterization of the left side of the heart assesses the patency of the coronary arteries, mitral and aortic valve function, and left ventricular function. It aids diagnosis of left ventricular enlargement, aortic stenosis and insufficiency, aortic root enlargement, mitral insufficiency, aneurysm, and intracardiac shunt.

In catheterization of the right side of the heart, the catheter is inserted into an antecubital vein or the femoral vein and is advanced through the inferior vena cava or right atrium into the right side of the heart and the pulmonary artery. Catheterization of the right side of the heart assesses tricuspid and pulmonic valve function and pulmonary artery pressures.

Purpose

- To evaluate valvular insufficiency or stenosis, septal defects, congenital anomalies, myocardial function and blood supply, and cardiac wall motion

Patient preparation

- Explain to the patient that this test evaluates the function of the heart and its vessels.
- Instruct the patient to restrict food and fluids for at least 6 hours before the test but to continue his prescribed drug regimen unless directed otherwise.
- Describe the test, including who will perform it and where it will take place.
- Make sure the patient or a responsible family member has signed an informed consent form.
- Inform the patient that he may receive a mild sedative but will remain conscious during the procedure. He'll lie on a padded table as the camera rotates so that his heart can be examined from different angles.
- Tell the patient that the catheterization team will wear gloves, masks, and gowns to protect him from infection.
- Inform the patient that he'll have an I.V. needle inserted in his arm to administer medication. Assure him that

the electrocardiography (ECG) electrodes attached to his chest during the procedure will cause no discomfort.

■ Tell the patient that the catheter will be inserted into an artery or a vein in his arm or leg; if the skin above the vessel is hairy, it will be shaved and cleaned with an antiseptic.

■ Explain to the patient that he'll experience a transient stinging sensation when a local anesthetic is injected to numb the incision site for catheter insertion and that he may experience pressure as the catheter moves along the blood vessel. Assure him that these sensations are normal.

■ Inform the patient that injection of a contrast medium through the catheter may produce a hot, flushing sensation or nausea that quickly passes; instruct him to follow directions to cough or breathe deeply.

■ Explain to the patient that he'll be given medication if he experiences chest pain during the procedure and that he may also receive nitroglycerin periodically to dilate coronary vessels and aid visualization. Reassure him that complications, such as MI or thromboembolism, are rare.

■ Check the patient's history for hypersensitivity to shellfish, iodine, or the contrast media used in other diagnostic tests; notify the physician of any hypersensitivities.

■ Discontinue any anticoagulant therapy, as ordered, to reduce the risk of complications from venous bleeding.

■ Just before the procedure, tell the patient to void and put on a hospital gown.

Procedure and posttest care

■ The patient is placed in the supine position on a tilt-top table and secured by restraints. ECG leads are applied for continuous monitoring, and an I.V. line, if not already in place, is started with dextrose 5% in water or normal saline solution at a keep-vein-open rate.

■ After a local anesthetic is injected at the catheterization site, a small incision or percutaneous puncture is made into the artery or vein, and the catheter is passed through the needle into the vessel; the catheter is guided to the cardiac chambers or coronary arteries using fluoroscopy.

■ When the catheter is in place, the contrast medium is injected through it to visualize the cardiac vessels and structures.

■ The patient may be asked to cough or breathe deeply. Coughing helps counteract nausea or light-headedness caused by the contrast medium and can correct arrhythmias produced by its depressant effect on the myocardium; deep breathing can ease catheter placement into the pulmonary artery or the wedge position and moves the diaphragm downward, making the heart easier to visualize.

■ During the procedure, the patient may be given nitroglycerin to eliminate catheter-induced spasm or to measure its effect on the coronary arteries.

■ Monitor heart rate and rhythm, respiratory and pulse rates, and blood pressure frequently during the procedure.

■ After completion of the procedure, the catheter is removed and pressure should be applied to the incision site for about 30 minutes either manually or with a mechanical compression device. An adhesive bandage or clear occlusive dressing should be applied to protect the site and permit visualization for detection of bleeding or hematoma formation.

■ Monitor vital signs every 15 minutes for 2 hours after the procedure, every 30 minutes for the next 2 hours, and then every hour for 2 hours. If no hematoma or other problems arise, begin checking every 4 hours. If vital signs are unstable, check every 5 minutes and notify the physician.

- Observe the insertion site for a hematoma or blood loss. Additional compression may be necessary to control bleeding.
- Check the patient's color, skin temperature, and peripheral pulse below the puncture site. The brachial approach is associated with a higher incidence of vasospasm (characterized by cool fingers and hands and weak pulses on the affected side); this usually resolves within 24 hours.
- Enforce bed rest for 8 hours. If the femoral route was used for catheter insertion, keep the patient's leg extended for 6 to 8 hours; if the antecubital fossa was used, keep the patient's arm extended for at least 3 hours.
- If medications were withheld before the test, check with the physician about resuming administration.
- Administer prescribed analgesics.
- Unless the patient is scheduled for surgery, encourage intake of fluids high in potassium, such as orange juice, to counteract the diuretic effect of the contrast medium.
- Make sure a posttest ECG is scheduled to check for possible myocardial damage.

Precautions

- Coagulopathy, impaired renal function, and debilitation usually contraindicate catheterization of both sides of the heart. Unless a temporary pacemaker is inserted to counteract induced ventricular asystole, left bundle-branch block contraindicates catheterization of the right side of the heart.
- If the patient has valvular heart disease, prophylactic antimicrobial therapy may be indicated to guard against subacute bacterial endocarditis.

Normal findings

Cardiac catheterization should reveal no abnormalities of heart chamber size or configuration, wall motion or thickness, direction of blood flow, or valve motion; the coronary arteries should have a smooth and regular outline and vessels should be patent.

Cardiac catheterization provides information on pressures in the heart's chambers and vessels. Higher pressures than normal are clinically significant; lower pressures, except in shock, usually aren't significant. (See *Normal pressure curves,* page 720, and *Upper limits of normal pressures in cardiac chambers and great vessels in recumbent adults,* page 721.)

Abnormal findings

Common abnormalities confirmable by cardiac catheterization include coronary artery disease (CAD), myocardial incompetence, valvular heart disease, and septal defects.

In *CAD,* catheterization shows constriction of the lumen of the coronary arteries. Constriction greater than 70% is especially significant, particularly in proximal lesions. Narrowing of the left main coronary artery and occlusion or narrowing high in the left anterior descending artery are often indications for revascularization surgery. (This lesion responds best to coronary artery bypass grafting.)

Impaired wall motion can indicate *myocardial incompetence* from CAD, aneurysm, cardiomyopathy, or congenital anomalies. Comparing the size of the left ventricle in systole and diastole helps assess the efficiency of cardiac muscle contraction, segmental wall motion, chamber size, and ejection fraction. An ejection fraction under 35% generally increases the risk of complications and decreases the probability of successful surgery.

Normal pressure curves

Chambers of the right side of the heart
Two pressure complexes are represented for each chamber. Complexes at the far right in this diagram represent simultaneous recordings of pressures from the right atrium, right ventricle, and pulmonary artery.

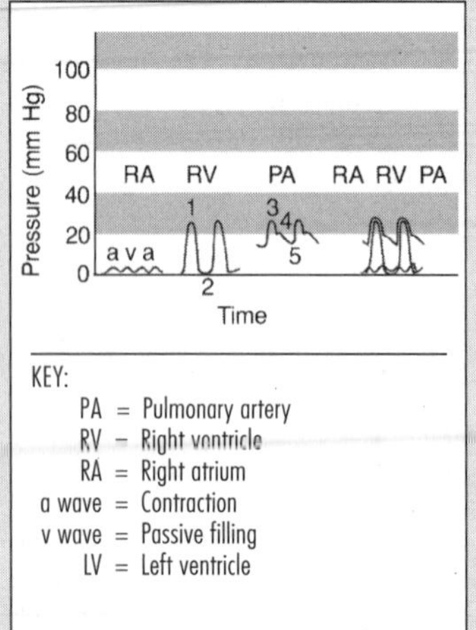

KEY:
PA = Pulmonary artery
RV = Right ventricle
RA = Right atrium
a wave = Contraction
v wave = Passive filling
LV = Left ventricle

Chambers of the left side of the heart
Overall pressure configurations are similar to those of the right side of the heart, but pressures in the left side of the heart are significantly higher because systemic flow resistance is much greater than pulmonary resistance.

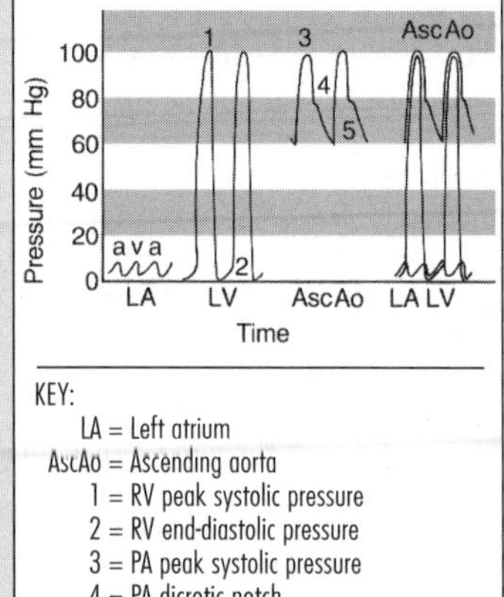

KEY:
LA = Left atrium
AscAo = Ascending aorta
1 = RV peak systolic pressure
2 = RV end-diastolic pressure
3 = PA peak systolic pressure
4 = PA dicrotic notch
5 = PA diastolic pressure

Valvular heart disease is indicated by a gradient, or difference in pressures, above and below a heart valve. For example, systolic pressure measurements on both sides of a stenotic aortic valve show a gradient across the valve. The higher the gradient, the greater the degree of stenosis. If left ventricular systolic pressure measures 200 mm Hg and aortic systolic pressure measures 120 mm Hg, the gradient across the valve is 80 mm Hg. Because these pressures should normally be equal during systole, when the aortic valve is open, a gradient of this magnitude indicates the need for corrective surgery. Incompetent valves can be visualized during ventriculography by watching retrograde flow of the contrast medium across the valve during systole.

Septal defects (both atrial and ventricular) can be confirmed by measuring blood oxygen content in both sides of the heart. Elevated blood oxygen levels on the right side indicate a left-to-right atrial or ventricular shunt; decreased oxygen levels on the left side indicate a right-to-left shunt.

Cardiac output can be measured by analyzing blood oxygen levels in the cardiac chambers. This may be accomplished by drawing blood from cardiac chambers or by injecting contrast medium into the venous circulation and

Upper limits of normal pressures in cardiac chambers and great vessels in recumbent adults

CHAMBER OR VESSEL	PRESSURE (mm Hg)
Right atrium	6 (mean)
Right ventricle	30/6*
Pulmonary artery	30/12* (mean, 18)
Left atrium	12 (mean)
Left ventricle	140/12*
Ascending aorta	140/90* (mean, 105)
Pulmonary artery wedge	Almost identical (±1 to 2 mm Hg) to left atrial mean pressure

* Peak systolic and end-diastolic

measuring its concentration as it moves past a thermodilution catheter.

Interfering factors

- Improperly functioning equipment and poor technique
- Patient anxiety (increase in heart rate and cardiac chamber pressures)

PULMONARY ARTERY CATHETERIZATION

In pulmonary artery (PA) catheterization, also known as Swan-Ganz catheterization, a balloon-tipped, flow-directed catheter is threaded through the right atrium to provide intermittent occlusion of the pulmonary artery. PA catheterization permits measurement of both pulmonary artery pressure (PAP) and pulmonary artery wedge pressure (PAWP).

The PAWP reading accurately reflects left atrial pressure and left ventricular end-diastolic pressure, although the catheter itself never enters the left side of the heart. Obtaining this information is possible because the heart momentarily relaxes during diastole as it fills with blood from the pulmonary veins; at this instant, the pulmonary vasculature, left atrium, and left ventricle act as a single chamber, and all have identical pressures. Thus, changes in PAP and PAWP reflect changes in left ventricular filling pressure, permitting detection of left ventricular impairment.

The procedure is usually performed at bedside in an intensive care unit. The catheter is inserted through the cephalic vein in the antecubital fossa or the subclavian (sometimes femoral) vein. In addition to measuring atrial and PA pressures, this procedure evaluates pulmonary vascular resistance and tissue oxygenation, as indicated by mixed venous oxygen content. It should be performed cautiously in patients with left bundle-branch block or implanted pacemakers.

Purpose

- To help assess right and left ventricular function
- To monitor therapy for myocardial infarction, cardiogenic shock, septic shock, pulmonary edema, fluid-related hypovolemia and hypotension, systolic murmur, unexplained sinus tachycardia, and various cardiac arrhythmias
- To monitor fluid status in patients with serious burns, renal disease, noncardiogenic pulmonary edema, or adult respiratory distress syndrome
- To monitor the effects of cardiovascular drugs, such as nitroglycerin and nitroprusside
- To establish baseline pressures preoperatively in patients with existing cardiac disease and then adjust I.V. medications for optimal surgical success
- To differentiate between pulmonary and cardiac pulmonary edema

Patient preparation

- Explain to the patient that this test evaluates heart function and provides data necessary to determine appropriate therapy or manage fluid status.
- Tell the patient that he need not restrict food or fluids before the test.
- Describe the test, including who will perform it and where it will take place.
- Tell the patient that he'll be conscious during catheterization and that he may experience discomfort from administration of the local anesthetic.
- Explain that catheter insertion takes about 30 minutes but that the catheter will remain in place, causing little or no discomfort.
- Instruct the patient to report any discomfort immediately.
- Explain that after insertion he'll need to have a portable chest X-ray to confirm proper placement of the PA catheter.
- Make sure the patient or a responsible family member has signed an informed consent form.

Equipment

Pressure cuff; balloon-tipped, flow-directed PA catheter; bag of heparinized normal saline solution (usually 500 ml of normal saline solution with 500 to 1,000 units of heparin, if ordered); alcohol sponges; medication-added label; pressure bag; pressure tubing with flush device and disposable transducer; monitor and monitor cable; I.V. pole with transducer mount; ECG monitor and electrodes; emergency resuscitation equipment; armboard (for antecubital insertion); lead aprons (if fluoroscope is used during insertion); sutures; 4″ × 4″ gauze pads or other dry occlusive dressing material; prepackaged introducer kit; optional: dextrose 5% in water, shaving materials

If a prepackaged introducer kit is unavailable, obtain the following: introducer (one size larger than the catheter), sterile tray containing instruments for procedure, masks, sterile gowns and gloves, povidone-iodine ointment, sutures, two 10-ml syringes, local anesthetic (1% to 2% lidocaine), one 5-ml syringe, 25G needle, ½″ needle, 1″ and 3″ tape.

Procedure and posttest care

- Choose an appropriate flexible PA catheter. Catheters used in this test come in two- to five-lumen modes and in various lengths. In the two-lumen catheter, one lumen contains the balloon, 1 mm behind the catheter tip; the other lumen, which opens at the tip, measures pressure in front of the balloon. The two-lumen catheter measures PAP and PAWP and can be used to sample mixed venous blood and to infuse I.V. solutions. The three-lumen catheter has an additional proximal lumen that opens 12″ (30.5 cm) behind the tip; when the tip is in the main pulmonary artery, the proximal lumen lies in the right atrium, permitting administration of fluids or monitoring of right atrial pressure (central venous pressure). The four-lumen type includes a transistorized thermistor for monitoring blood temperature and allows measurement of cardiac output. A four-lumen catheter with thermodilution and pacer port mode is used in critical care settings to allow for pacing, if necessary. The introducer part of the system may also be used to infuse large amounts of fluids.

- Before catheterization, set up the equipment according to the manufacturer's directions and the facility's protocol.
- If the insertion site is being prepared for a cutdown procedure, prepare the patient's skin and cover it with a sterile drape.
- Assist the patient to the supine position. For antecubital insertion, his arm is abducted with the palm upward on an overbed table for support; for subclavian insertion, the patient is placed in the supine position with his head and shoulders slightly lower than his trunk to make the vein more accessible. If the patient can't tolerate the supine position, assist him to the semi-Fowler position. During the test, monitor all pressures with the patient in the same position.
- Check the catheter balloon for defects, using sterile technique, and flush all ports to ensure patency.
- The catheter introducer is inserted into the vein percutaneously or by cutdown.
- Then the catheter is inserted through the introducer and directed to the right atrium, and the catheter balloon is partially inflated so that venous flow carries the catheter tip through the right atrium and tricuspid valve into the right ventricle and the PA.
- Observe the monitor for characteristic waveform changes. Obtain a printout of each stage of catheter insertion. (See *PA catheterization: Insertion sites and associated waveforms,* page 724.)
- Instruct the patient to extend the appropriate arm (or leg, if the catheter is inserted into the femoral vein).
- As the catheter is passed into the chambers of the right side of the heart, observe the monitor screen for frequent premature ventricular contractions or tachycardia (including ventricular tachycardia), which may result from right ventricular catheter irritation. If irritation occurs, the catheter may be partially withdrawn or medication administered to suppress the arrhythmia or right bundle-branch block.
- To record the PAWP, carefully inflate the catheter balloon with the specified amount of air; the catheter tip will float into the wedge position, as indicated by an altered waveform on the monitor screen. If a PAWP waveform occurs with less than the recommended inflation volume, don't inflate the balloon further.
- After the balloon is inflated, record the PAWP. Then allow the balloon to deflate passively. This allows the catheter to float back into the PA. Observe the monitor screen for a PA waveform.
- The 1.5-ml syringe that comes in the introducer kit has an indentation along

PA catheterization: Insertion sites and associated waveforms

As the pulmonary artery (PA) catheter is directed through the chambers on the right side of the heart to its wedge position, it produces distinctive waveforms on the oscilloscope screen that are important indicators of the catheter's position in the heart.

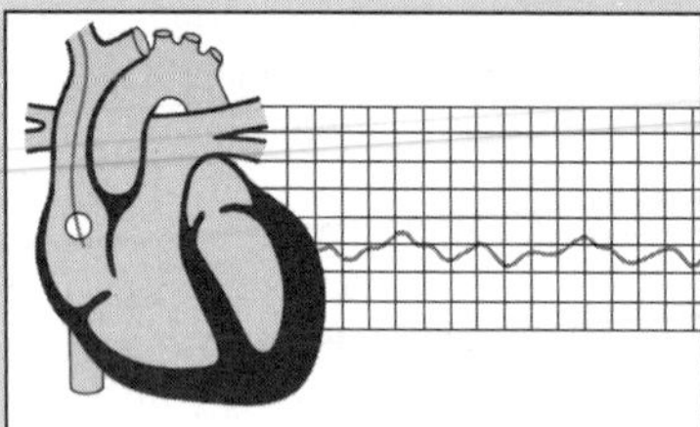

RIGHT ATRIAL PRESSURE
When the catheter tip reaches the right atrium from the superior vena cava, the waveform on the oscilloscope screen or readout strip resembles the one shown. When this waveform appears, the physician inflates the catheter balloon, which floats the tip through the tricuspid valve into the right ventricle.

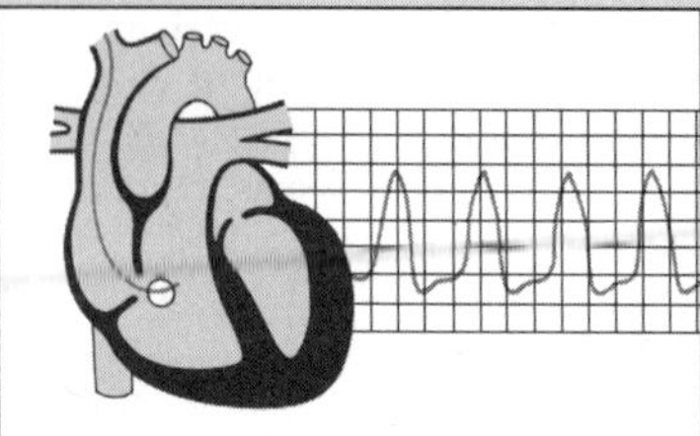

RIGHT VENTRICULAR PRESSURE
When the catheter tip reaches the right ventricle, the waveform looks like the one shown at left.

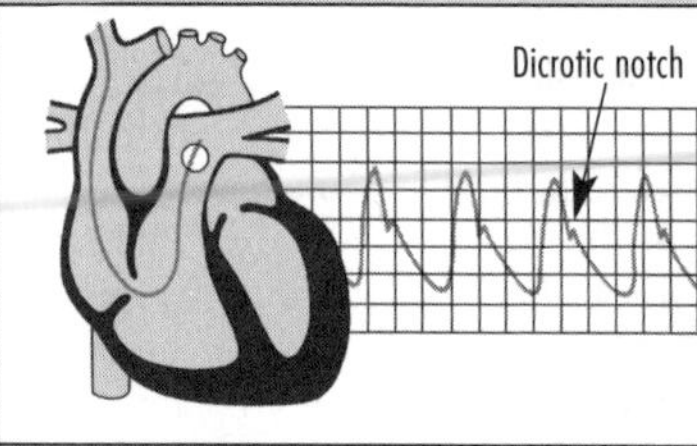

PULMONARY ARTERY PRESSURE
A waveform that resembles the one shown at left indicates that the balloon has floated the catheter tip through the pulmonic valve into the pulmonary artery. A dicrotic notch should be visible in the waveform, indicating the closing of the pulmonic valve.

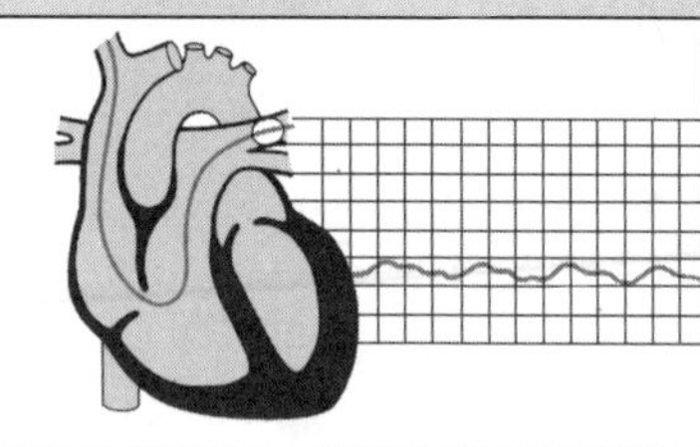

PULMONARY ARTERY WEDGE PRESSURE
Blood flow in the pulmonary artery then carries the catheter balloon into one of the pulmonary artery's many smaller branches. When the vessel becomes too narrow for the balloon to pass through, the balloon wedges in the vessel, occluding it. The monitor then displays a pulmonary artery wedge pressure waveform such as the one shown at left.

the barrel that won't allow you to inject more than 1.5 cc of air, to prevent overinflation. The stopcock should be turned so that it's perpendicular to the insertion port to prevent air from the syringe from accidentally inflating the balloon.

- Don't overinflate the balloon catheter. Overinflation could distend the PA, causing vessel rupture.
- If the balloon can't be fully deflated after recording the PAWP, don't reinflate it unless the physician is present; balloon rupture may cause a life-threatening air embolism. Check all connections for air leaks that may have prevented balloon inflation, particularly if the patient is confused or uncooperative.
- When the catheter's correct positioning and function are established, it's sutured to the skin. Antimicrobial ointment and an airtight dressing are applied to the insertion site according to facility policy.
- A chest X-ray is obtained, as ordered, to verify catheter placement.
- Set alarms on the electrocardiogram (ECG) and pressure monitors.
- Monitor vital signs as ordered or per facility protocol.
- Document PAP waveforms at the beginning of each shift, and monitor them frequently throughout each shift and with changes in treatment. Check PAWP and cardiac output as ordered (usually every 6 to 8 hours).
- Take routine aseptic precautions to prevent infection.
- When the catheter is no longer needed, the dressing is removed and the catheter is slowly withdrawn after ensuring that the balloon is deflated. The ECG is monitored for arrhythmias. In some facilities, the physician is required to remove the catheter.
- After the catheter is withdrawn, the catheter tip is often sent for analysis.
- Apply a sterile dressing over the catheter introducer.
- Observe the site for signs of infection, such as redness, swelling, and discharge.
- Watch for complications, such as pulmonary emboli, PA perforation, heart murmurs, thrombi, and arrhythmias.

Precautions

- Before obtaining a PAWP reading, flush the monitoring system and recalibrate the system per facility protocol.
- After obtaining a PAWP, make sure the balloon is completely deflated.
- Maintain 300 mm Hg of pressure in the pressure bag to permit a fluid flow of 3 to 6 ml/hour. Instruct the patient to extend the appropriate arm (or leg, if the catheter is inserted in the femoral vein).
- If a damped waveform occurs, the catheter may need to be adjusted. Pulmonary infarct may occur if the catheter is allowed to remain in a wedged position.
- Make sure the stopcocks are properly positioned and the connections are secure. Loose connections may introduce air into the system or cause blood backup, leakage of deoxygenated blood, or inaccurate pressure readings.
- Make sure the lumen hubs are properly identified to serve the appropriate catheter ports.
- Don't add or remove fluids from the distal PA port; this could cause pulmonary extravasation or damage the artery.
- If the catheter hasn't been sutured to the skin, tape it securely to prevent dislodgment.
- Observe the catheter insertion site for signs of infection, such as redness, swelling, and discharge.
- If the patient shows signs of sepsis, treat the catheter as the source of infec-

tion and send it for culture when removed.

■ Watch for complications, such as pulmonary emboli, pulmonary artery perforation, heart murmurs, thrombi, and arrhythmias.

Reference values

Normal pressures are as follows:

■ *right atrial pressure:* 1 to 6 mm Hg
■ *systolic right ventricular pressure:* 20 to 30 mm Hg
■ *end-diastolic right ventricular pressure:* < 5 mm Hg
■ *systolic PAP:* 20 to 30 mm Hg
■ *diastolic PAP:* 10 to 15 mm Hg
■ *mean PAP:* < 20 mm Hg
■ *PAWP:* 6 to 12 mm Hg
■ *left atrial pressure:* about 10 mm Hg.

Abnormal findings

An abnormally high right atrial pressure can indicate pulmonary disease, right-sided heart failure, fluid overload, cardiac tamponade, tricuspid stenosis and insufficiency, or pulmonary hypertension.

Elevated right ventricular pressure can result from pulmonary hypertension, pulmonary valvular stenosis, right-sided heart failure, pericardial effusion, constrictive pericarditis, chronic heart failure, or ventricular septal defects.

An abnormally high PAP is characteristic in increased pulmonary blood flow, as occurs in a left-to-right shunt secondary to atrial or ventricular septal defect; increased PA resistance, as occurs in pulmonary hypertension or mitral stenosis; chronic obstructive pulmonary disease; pulmonary edema or embolus; and left ventricular failure from any cause. PA systolic pressure is the same as right ventricular systolic pressure. PA diastolic pressure is the same as left atrial pressure, except in patients with severe pulmonary disease causing pulmonary hypertension; in such patients, catheterization is still important diagnostically.

Elevated PAWP can result from left ventricular failure, mitral stenosis and insufficiency, cardiac tamponade, or cardiac insufficiency; depressed PAWP can result from hypovolemia.

Interfering factors

■ Malfunctioning monitoring and recording devices, loose connections, clot formation at the catheter tip, air in the fluid column, or a ruptured balloon
■ Mechanical ventilation with positive pressure, causing increased intrathoracic pressure (increase in catheter pressure)
■ Incorrect catheter placement, causing excessive movement called catheter fling (damped pressure tracing)
■ Migration of the catheter against a vessel wall (possible constant occlusion, or wedging, of the PA)
■ Extreme patient agitation

ELECTROPHYSIOLOGY STUDIES

Electrophysiological studies (also known as His' bundle electrography) permit measurement of discrete conduction intervals by recording electrical conduction during the slow withdrawal of a bipolar or tripolar electrode catheter from the right ventricle through the bundle of His to the sinoatrial node. The catheter is introduced into the femoral vein, passing through the right atrium and across the septal leaflet of the tricuspid valve.

Purpose

■ To diagnose arrhythmias and conduction anomalies

- To determine the need for an implanted pacemaker, an internal cardioverter-defibrillator, and cardioactive drugs and to evaluate their effects on the conduction system and ectopic rhythms
- To locate the site of a bundle-branch block, especially in asymptomatic patients with conduction disturbances
- To determine the presence and location of accessory conducting structures

Patient preparation

- Explain to the patient that this test will help evaluate his heart's conduction system.
- Tell the patient not to eat or drink anything for at least 6 hours before the test.
- Describe the test, including who will perform it and where it will take place.
- Inform the patient that after the groin area is shaved, a catheter will be inserted into the femoral vein and an I.V. line may be started. Assure him that the ECG electrodes attached to his chest during the test will cause no discomfort.
- Explain to the patient that he'll experience a stinging sensation when a local anesthetic is injected to numb the incision site for catheter insertion and that he may experience pressure on catheter insertion.
- Inform the patient that he'll be conscious during the test, and urge him to report any discomfort or pain.
- Make sure the patient or a responsible family member has signed an informed consent form.
- Check the patient's history, and inform the physician of any ongoing drug therapy.
- Just before the procedure, ask the patient to void and to put on a hospital gown.

Procedure and posttest care

- Help the patient into the supine position on a padded table.
- Limb electrodes and precordial leads are applied for continuous monitoring. If not already in place, an I.V. line is started and dextrose 5% in water or normal saline solution is administered at a keep-vein-open rate.
- After a local anesthetic is injected at the catheterization site, a small incision or percutaneous puncture is made and a J-tip electrode is introduced I.V. into the femoral vein (or into the antecubital fossa). The catheter is guided to the cardiac chambers using fluoroscopy. The catheter is advanced until it crosses the tricuspid valve and enters the right ventricle. Then the catheter is slowly withdrawn from the tricuspid area, and recordings of conduction intervals are made from each pole of the catheter, either simultaneously or sequentially.
- Monitor the patient's vital signs frequently during the test, noting especially a drop in blood pressure during an arrhythmia.
- The catheter is removed and a pressure dressing is applied after completion of the procedure.
- Monitor vital signs every 15 minutes for 1 hour after the procedure and then every hour for 4 hours until stable. If unstable, check every 15 minutes and notify the physician.
- Observe for shortness of breath, chest pain, pallor, or changes in pulse or blood pressure.
- Enforce bed rest for 4 to 6 hours.
- Check the catheter insertion site for bleeding, as ordered, usually every 30 minutes for 8 hours. If bleeding occurs, notify the physician and apply a pressure bandage until the bleeding stops.
- Advise the patient that he may resume his usual diet.
- Make sure a 12-lead resting ECG is scheduled to assess for changes.

Precautions

■ Electrophysiology studies are contraindicated in patients with severe coagulopathy, recent thrombophlebitis, or acute pulmonary embolism.

■ Have emergency medication and resuscitation equipment available in case the patient develops arrhythmias during the test.

Normal findings

Normal conduction intervals in adults are as follows: HV interval, 35 to 55 msec; AH interval, 45 to 150 msec; and PA interval, 20 to 40 msec.

Abnormal findings

■ A prolonged HV interval (the conduction time from the bundle of His to the Purkinje fibers) can result from acute or chronic disease.

■ Atrioventricular nodal (AH interval) delays can stem from atrial pacing, chronic conduction system disease, carotid sinus pressure, recent myocardial infarction, and use of certain drugs.

■ Intra-atrial (PA interval) delays can result from acquired, surgically induced, or congenital atrial disease and atrial pacing.

Interfering factors

■ Malfunctioning recording equipment and improper catheter positioning

PULSE OXIMETRY

Pulse oximetry is a continuous noninvasive study of arterial blood oxygen saturation (SaO_2) using a clip or probe attached to a sensor site (usually the earlobe or fingertip). The percentage expressed is the ratio of oxygen to hemoglobin.

Purpose

■ To monitor the oxygenation of the tissues and organs perioperatively and during an acute illness

■ To monitor oxygenation in patients with higher oxygen needs (such those on a ventilator or those receiving a high percentage of oxygen) or when weaning from an oxygen source

■ To monitor oxygen saturation during activities to determine patient tolerance

■ To determine the effectiveness of bronchodilators

■ To monitor oxygenation during testing for sleep apnea

Patient preparation

■ Explain to the patient that this test assesses oxygen content in the hemoglobin. Describe the procedure and answer all questions.

■ Explain who will perform the test, where it will take place, and how long it will last.

■ Make sure the patient has no false fingernails or nail polish.

■ Explain to the patient that the area where the clip or probe is attached must be massaged to increase blood flow.

Procedure and posttest care

■ Place the probe or clip over the finger or other intended sensor site so that the light beams and sensors are opposite each other.

■ Turn on the monitor, and ensure that it accurately detects the patient's pulse and reads the percentage of oxygen.

■ If the monitor is to remain on continuously, ensure that the skin remains intact under the probe or clip and that the circulation is adequate. Select alternate sensor sites if the skin doesn't remain intact.

■ Remove the probe and clean it with alcohol after the test.

Precautions

- Closely observe the monitor, and report decreasing or abnormal SaO_2 levels.

Normal findings

SaO_2 levels are normally greater than 95%.

Abnormal findings

Hypoxemia with levels less than 95% indicate impaired cardiopulmonary function or abnormal gas exchange.

Interfering factors

- Movement of the finger, ear, or alternate sensor site
- Improper placement of the probe or clip
- Anemic conditions, vasoconstriction, certain medications (such as vasopressors), hypotension, vessel obstruction, nail polish or false fingernails, administrations of lipid emulsions, elevated carboxyhemoglobin (carbon monoxide) levels in the blood

16

Special function tests

Eyes and Vision

Visual Acuity Tests

A visual acuity test evaluates the patient's ability to distinguish the form and detail of an object. In this test, the patient is asked to read letters on a standardized visual chart, commonly called the Snellen chart, from a distance of 20′ (6.1 m). Charts showing the letter "E" in various positions and sizes are used for young children and other people who can't read. The smaller the symbol the patient can identify, the sharper his visual acuity. A patient's near (reading) vision may be tested as well, using a standardized chart such as the Jaeger card (a card with print in graded sizes).

The Snellen test should be performed on all patients with eye complaints. Near-vision test is routine for those complaining of eyestrain or reading difficulty and for everyone over age 40. Results serve as a baseline for treatments, follow-up examinations, and referrals.

Purpose

- To test distance and near visual acuity
- To identify refractive errors in vision

Patient preparation

- Tell the patient that these tests evaluate distant and near vision.
- Tell the patient that the tests take only a few minutes. If he wears glasses, tell him to bring them to the examination.

Equipment

Standardized eye charts, including the Snellen or E chart to test distance visual acuity, and the Jaeger card to test near visual acuity; occlusion supplies, including a handheld occluder and disposable tissues for insertion between the patient's eyes and glasses; disposable eye patches; standard 20′ (6.1-m) room or equipment to simulate correct distance (mirrors or chart with proportionately reduced letters); illumination (10′ to 30′ candles)

Procedure and posttest care

Distance visual acuity

- Have the patient sit 20′ (6.1 m) away from the eye chart. If he's wearing glasses, tell him to remove them so his uncorrected vision can be tested first.
- Begin with the right eye unless vision in the left eye is known to be more acute. Have the patient occlude the left eye; then ask him to read the smallest line of letters he can see on the chart. Encourage him to try to read lines he can't see clearly because intelligent guesses usually indicate that the patient can recognize some of the symbols' details.
- Record the number of the smallest line the patient can read. This number is expressed as a fraction. The numerator is the distance between the patient and the chart; the denominator is the distance from which a patient with normal vision can read the line. The greater the denominator, the poorer the vision.
- If the patient makes an error on a line, record the results with a minus number. For example, if the patient reads the 20/40 line but makes one error, record his vision as 20/40–1. If the patient reads the 20/40 line and one symbol on the next line, record his vision as 20/40+1.
- Have the patient occlude the right eye; then repeat the test for the left eye. To minimize recall, use a different set of symbols or have the patient read the lines backward.
- If the patient wears glasses, test his corrected vision using the same proce-

Special procedures for testing vision

The following tests may be performed if the patient can't identify the largest letter on the Snellen chart.

Pinhole test. If the patient's visual acuity is less than 20/20, this test can determine whether the cause is refractive error or organic disease. In this test, the patient is asked to look through a pinhole in the center of a disk at the visual acuity chart. Looking through the tiny opening eliminates peripheral light rays and improves the patient's vision if impairment is related to refractive error. If impairment results from organic disease, vision fails to improve.

Changing the distance. If the patient can't identify the largest letter or symbol on the chart (line 20/200), tell him to walk toward the chart until he can correctly identify it. Record the distance at which the patient can identify the symbol as the numerator. For example, 2/200 means the patient can identify at 2′ (61 cm) a symbol that a person with normal vision can identify at 200′ (61 m).

Counting fingers. If the patient can't identify the largest symbol at any distance, hold up your fingers at various distances in front of his eyes. When the patient correctly identifies the number of fingers in front of him, note the distance, for example 4′/CF.

Hand motion. If the patient can't identify the number of fingers at any distance, wave your hand in front of his eyes at various distances. If he can detect hand movement, note the distance, for example 2′/HM.

Light projection. If the patient can't identify hand motion at any distance, darken the room and tell him to look straight ahead. Shine a penlight in each quadrant — nasal, temporal, superior, and inferior — of each eye. Note in which quadrants the patient can perceive light, for example, light projection/superior and nasal quadrants.

Light perception. If the patient can't perceive light projection at all, ask if he can tell whether the light is on or off. If the patient has no light perception, note NLP; otherwise, note that light perception exists.

dure. If he normally wears glasses but doesn't have them with him, note this on the test results.

■ In recording the patient's responses, indicate which eye was tested and whether it was tested with or without corrective lenses.

■ If the patient can't read the largest letter on the chart, further testing is necessary. (See *Special procedures for testing vision.*)

Near visual acuity

■ Have the patient remove his glasses and occlude the left eye. Ask him to read the Jaeger card at his customary reading distance. Both eyes are tested with and without corrective lenses.

■ In reporting near visual acuity, specify both the size of the smallest print legible to the patient and the nearest distance at which reading is possible.

Normal findings

Most charts for distance visual acuity are read at 20′ (6.1 m). If the patient's vision is normal, results are expressed as 20/20, which means that the smallest symbol he can identify at 20′ is the same symbol a patient with normal vision can identify from the same distance.

Abnormal findings

If the patient can read the 20/20 line on the Snellen chart, he has normal distance visual acuity. If the denominator is more than 20 (for example, 40), his visual acuity is less than normal. In this case, it means he reads at 20′ what a person with normal vision can read at 40′ (12.2 m). A person with visual acuity of 20/200 in the better corrected eye is considered legally blind. Similarly, if the denominator is less than 20, the patient's distance visual acuity is better than normal. For example, 20/15 vision means that the patient can read at 20′ what a person with normal visual acuity can see at 15′ (4.6 m).

Normal near visual acuity is usually recorded as 14/14 because standard testing charts, such as the Jaeger card, are generally held 14″ (36 cm) from the patient's eyes.

Decreased near visual acuity is indicated by a larger denominator. For example, 14/20 near vision means that the patient can read at 14″ what a person with normal vision can read at 20″ (51 cm).

Normal or better-than-normal visual acuity doesn't necessarily indicate normal vision. For example, a visual field defect may be present if the patient consistently misses the letters on one side of all the lines. A field defect is present if the patient states that one or more of the letters disappear or become illegible when he is looking at a nearby letter. Such findings indicate the need for further visual field testing, such as the Amsler's chart test and the tangent screen examination.

Patients with less-than-normal visual acuity require further testing, including refraction and a complete ophthalmologic examination, to determine whether visual loss is due to injury, disease, or a need for corrective lenses.

Interfering factors

- Patient's failure to bring glasses to the examination
- Glasses improperly prescribed or outdated in their degree of correction (possible to have better visual acuity without them)
- Patient's inability to cooperate

SLIT-LAMP EXAMINATION

The slit lamp is an instrument equipped with a special lighting system and a binocular microscope that allows an ophthalmologist to visualize in detail the anterior segment of the eye, including the eyelids, eyelashes, conjunctiva, sclera, cornea, tear film, anterior chamber, iris, crystalline lens, and vitreous face. To evaluate normally transparent or near-transparent ocular fluids and tissues, the size, shape, intensity, and depth of the light source as well as the magnification of the microscope may be altered. If abnormalities are noted, special devices are attached to the slit lamp to allow more detailed investigation.

Purpose

- To detect and evaluate abnormalities of anterior segment tissues and structures

Patient preparation

- Tell the patient that this examination evaluates the front portion of the eyes. Tell him that the test requires that he remain still. Reassure him that the examination is painless.
- If the patient wears contact lenses, tell him to remove them for the test, unless the test is being performed to evaluate the fit of the lens.
- If the test calls for dilating eyedrops, check the patient's history for adverse reactions to mydriatics or for the presence of narrow-angle glaucoma before administering the drops. Dilating eyedrops aren't used in routine eye examinations; however, some diseases require pupillary dilation before slit-lamp examination.

Procedure and posttest care

- Seat the patient in the examining chair. Have him place both feet on the floor and position his chin on the rest and his forehead against the bar. Dim the lights in the room.
- The ophthalmologist examines the patient's eyes starting with the lids and lashes and progressing to the vitreous face, altering light and magnification as necessary. In some cases, a special camera can be attached to the slit lamp to photograph portions of the eye.
- If dilating drops were instilled, tell the patient that his near vision will be blurred for up to 2 hours.

Precautions

- Don't instill mydriatic drops into the eyes of a patient who has had a hypersensitivity reaction to them or who has angle-closure glaucoma.

Normal findings

Slit-lamp examination should reveal no abnormalities of anterior segment tissues and structures.

Abnormal findings

Slit-lamp examination may detect pathologic conditions, such as corneal abrasions and ulcers, lens opacities, iritis, and conjunctivitis, as well as irregularly shaped corneas. A parchmentlike consistency of the lid skin, with redness, minor swelling, and moderate itching, may indicate a hypersensitivity reaction. If a corneal abrasion or ulcer is detected, a fluorescein stain may be applied to allow better viewing of the area. If a tearing deficiency is suspected, the ophthalmologist may examine the eye after applying a fluorescein or rose bengal stain; he may also perform Schirmer's test. Some abnormal findings may indicate impending disorders. For example, early-stage lens opacities may signal the development of cataracts.

Interfering factors

- Patient's inability to cooperate

OPHTHALMOSCOPY

Ophthalmoscopy allows magnified examination of the vascular and nerve tissue of the fundus, including the optic disk, retinal vessels, macula, and retina. This test is conducted with either a direct or an indirect ophthalmoscope — one of the most important diagnostic tools in ophthalmology. Generally, examiners use the direct ophthalmoscope, a small, handheld instrument consisting of a light source, a viewing device, a reflecting device to channel light into the patient's eyes, and spherical lenses to correct refractive error of the patient or examiner. If a slit lamp isn't available, the examiner may also use the ophthalmoscope to examine the patient's cornea, iris, and lens.

If an abnormality of the retina is suspected, further testing, such as fluores-

Fluorescein angiography

Fluorescein angiography is a special diagnostic test that's used to visualize and photograph the vascular structures of the eye. A fluorescein angiogram may be used to rule out retinal disease or to follow the progression of retinal disorders.

A fundus camera system rapidly photographs the retina after an I.V. injection of sodium fluorescein dye. The dye enters the arteries of the eye and gives a clear view of the vasculature. Then the angiogram is carefully examined to detect the precise location of abnormalities, such as leakage from diabetic retinopathy and age-related macular degeneration.

cein angiography, may be necessary. (See *Fluorescein angiography.*)

Purpose

- To detect and evaluate eye disorders as well as ocular manifestations of systemic disease

Patient preparation

- Explain to the patient that this test permits examination of the back of the eye.
- Describe the test, including who will perform it, where it will take place, and how long it will last.
- Advise the patient that eyedrops may be used to dilate the pupils for a clearer examination, but reassure him that he'll experience no discomfort during the test.
- When using eyedrops, check the patient's history for previous use of dilating eyedrops, indications of possible hypersensitivity, and angle-closure glaucoma.

Procedure and posttest care

- Routine examination of the ocular media and fundus is usually conducted without dilating the pupil if there's sufficient light in the ophthalmoscope and room lighting is subdued. If indicated, two instillations of mydriatic eyedrops are usually necessary to achieve maximum dilation.
- The patient sits upright in the examination chair and the room lights are dimmed to keep irregular reflections from interfering with the examination.
- The examiner sits about 2′ (60 cm) away from the patient and slightly to his right. The examination begins with the patient's right eye. The ophthalmoscope is held in the right hand in front of the examiner's right eye. A small adjustment near the forefinger allows him to select different lenses quickly.
- While sitting slightly to the patient's right, the examiner's right index finger is positioned on the lens selection dial to facilitate rapid lens changes.
- The illuminated dial should be set to zero, and the patient told to look straight ahead at a specific object 20′ (6.1 m) away—for example, a large symbol on a standardized vision chart—for the duration of the examination.
- Remaining on the patient's right side, the examiner moves forward until he's within 6″ (15 cm) of the patient. At this point, he directs the light beam into the pupil and looks for the red reflex (red reflection from the fundus), which is visible without magnification. Then he focuses on the optic disk, noting its size, shape, and color.
- Next, the examiner looks for a white central depression in the optic disk—the physiologic cup—and observes the retinal vessels that emerge from the disk.

■ Finally, the examiner focuses on the macula — a yellowish depression slightly below the center of the optic disk — and its center, the fovea. The examiner tells the patient to look up, down, and to each side to examine the extreme periphery. The superior, inferior, temporal, and nasal portions of the retina are examined respectively.

■ This procedure is then repeated for the left eye, with the examiner moving slightly to the patient's left side and holding the ophthalmoscope in the left hand and in front the examiner's left eye.

Precautions

■ Don't administer dilating eyedrops to a patient who has a history of hypersensitivity reactions to them or who has angle-closure glaucoma.

■ Make sure the patient maintains fixation throughout the procedure.

Normal findings

With the beam of light from the ophthalmoscope is directed into the patient's pupil, the red reflex should be visible through the aperture. The slightly oval optic disk lies to the nasal side of the fundus center. Although its color varies widely, it's usually pink, with darker edges at its nasal border. The physiologic cup, a pale depression in the center of the optic disk, varies widely in size; it tends to be larger in patients with myopia and smaller in those with hyperopia.

The semitransparent retina surrounds the optic disk. Branching out from the disk are the retinal vessels, including the venules and the slightly smaller arterioles. Vessel diameter progressively decreases with distance from the optic disk. Retinal arterioles generally have a medium red color; venules appear dark red or blue.

The macula is the most darkly pigmented area of the retina. In its center lies a small, even darker spot — the fovea. A tiny light reflex can be seen at the center of the fovea, caused by reflection of the ophthalmoscopic light from the concave inner surface of the area.

Abnormal findings

An absent or a diminished red reflex may be due to gross corneal lesions, dense opacities of the aqueous or vitreous (such as from blood after hemorrhage), cataracts, or detached retina. A cloudy vitreous that obscures the fundus may be caused by inflammatory disease of the optic disk, retina, or uvea. Fundal lesions should be sketched or photographed for further study.

Optic neuritis causes the optic disk to become elevated and more vascular; small hemorrhages may also occur. Optic nerve atrophy causes the disk to appear white. Papilledema, which may result from increased intracranial pressure, causes abnormal elevation of the disk, blurring of disk margins, engorged vessels, and hemorrhages.

In glaucoma, the physiologic cup may appear enlarged and gray, with white edges. A milky white retina characterizes the acute phase of a central retinal artery occlusion; the fovea, in contrast to the ischemic macula, appears as a bright red spot. Central retinal vein occlusion is marked by widespread retinal hemorrhaging, patches of white exudate, and disk elevation.

Retinal detachments appear as gray elevated areas, possibly with areas of red vascular choroid exposed by retinal tears. A choroidal tumor appears as a dark lesion.

The integrity of retinal vessels is commonly evaluated to aid diagnosis of systemic disease. Hypertension, for example, causes vasospasm, sclerosis, and eventual occlusion of retinal arterioles, leading to retinal edema and hemorrhage and papilledema. Diabetes mellitus may be complicated by retinal fibroses, patches of white exudate, and microaneurysms. Other systemic disorders present similar findings.

Interpretation of ophthalmoscopic findings depends largely on the examiner's knowledge and experience because an abnormality can arise from several sources. After an ophthalmoscopic evaluation, referral for complete medical evaluation may be necessary.

Interfering factors

- Room not sufficiently dark, inadequate light source, or other condition improper for examination
- Patient's inability to cooperate
- Conditions prohibiting a good view of the fundus, such as insufficient dilation, dense cataracts, cloudy media, and gross nystagmus

CORNEAL STAINING

Corneal staining with fluorescein dye allows a detailed view of the anterior part of the eye that can't ordinarily be seen during slit-lamp examination. A special attachment is used during the slit-lamp examination to enhance visualization.

Purpose

- To detect the depth and pattern of injuries to the corneal surface of the eye
- To diagnose corneal injuries

Patient preparation

- Describe the procedure to the patient. Explain that this test evaluates the eye surface and is painless.
- Tell the patient who will perform the test and where it will take place.
- Ask the patient for a detailed history of the eye injury and the symptoms associated with the injury.
- Ask the patient to remove glasses or contact lenses before the test.

Procedure and posttest care

- Seat the patient in the examination chair.
- Stain the patient's eye surface with the fluorescein dye by touching the tip of the fluorescein strip to the lower conjunctival sac.
- Ask the patient to close his eye to help spread the dye over the corneal surface.
- Have the patient sit properly in the examination chair with his forehead placed against the bar apparatus.
- Instruct the patient to look straight ahead while his eyes are examined with the slit lamp.
- Defects are recorded while the eye is being examined with a bright light.
- Inform the patient that any blurring of vision will gradually disappear within 2 hours.

Precautions

- Monitor the patient for allergic reaction to the fluorescein dye.
- Because the dye used in this test causes blurred vision, ensure that the patient has a responsible person to take him home.

Normal findings

The normal cornea is convex in shape and has a smooth, shiny appearance. No scratches or indentations are noted.

Abnormal findings

Abnormal findings include corneal scratches, abrasions, ulcerations, and keratitis.

Interfering factors

- Patient's inability to remain still during the examination
- Allergy to the fluorescein dye

TONOMETRY

Tonometry allows indirect measurement of intraocular pressure and serves as an effective screen for early detection of glaucoma, which strikes 2% of people over age 40 and is a common cause of blindness. Indentation tonometry tests this resistance by measuring how deeply a known weight depresses the cornea; applanation tonometry provides the same information by measuring the amount of force required to flatten a known area of the cornea. Both procedures necessitate corneal anesthetization and careful examination technique. Patients with intraocular pressure problems can now monitor their pressure at home with a portable tonometer. If the intraocular pressure is elevated, other tests, such as applanation tonometry, visual field testing, and ophthalmoscopy, must confirm diagnosis.

Purpose

- To measure intraocular pressure
- To aid diagnosis and follow-up evaluation of glaucoma

Patient preparation

- Explain to the patient that this test measures the pressure within his eyes.
- Tell the patient that the test takes only a few minutes and requires that his eyes be anesthetized, but reassure him that the procedure is painless.
- If the patient wears contact lenses, instruct him to remove them before the test or until the anesthetic wears off completely.
- Ask the patient to assume a supine position. Make sure he's relaxed and have him loosen restrictive clothing around his neck. Instruct him not to cough or squeeze his eyelids together.

Equipment

Indentation tonometer (Schiøtz's tonometer is the most popular), sterilized or used with disposable sterile tonofilms; topical anesthetic

Procedure and posttest care

- Ask the patient to look down. Raise his superior eyelid with your thumb, place one drop of the topical anesthetic at the top of the sclera, and have the patient blink.
- Check the tonometer for a zero reading on the steel test block that comes with the instrument. Make sure the plunger moves freely. The first measurement on each eye is obtained with the 5.5-g weight.
- Have the patient look up and stare at a spot on the ceiling. Then ask him to open his mouth, take a deep breath, and exhale slowly for distraction.
- With the thumb and forefinger of one hand, hold the lids of his right eye open against the orbital rim.
- Hold the tonometer vertically with the thumb and forefinger of the other hand, and rest the footplate on the apex of the cornea.
- With the footplate in place, check the indicator needle for a rhythmic transmission caused by the ocular pulse; then record the calibrated scale reading that converts to a measurement of intraocular pressure. If the reading doesn't exceed 4, add an additional weight (7.5, 10, or 15 g) to obtain a reliable result.
- Repeat the procedure on the left eye, and record the time the test is performed.

- Tell the patient not to rub his eyes for at least 20 minutes after the test to prevent corneal abrasion.
- If the patient wears contact lenses, tell him not to reinsert them for at least 2 hours.
- If the tonometer moved across the cornea during the test, tell the patient he may feel a slight scratching sensation in the eye when the anesthetic wears off. This sensation should disappear within 24 hours because most abrasions resulting from tonometry affect only the epithelium, which regenerates in 24 hours.

Precautions

- Tonometry should never be performed on a patient with a corneal ulcer or infection, except by a skilled examiner and only in an emergency such as suspected acute angle-closure glaucoma.
- Avoid resting your fingers on the cornea or pressing on the cornea because this increases intraocular pressure.
- Don't touch the lashes; this could trigger a blink response or Bell's phenomenon (upward movement of the eyes with forced closure of the lids), which can cause the footplate to move and scratch the cornea.

Normal findings

Intraocular pressure normally ranges from 12 to 20 mm Hg, with diurnal variations. The highest point is reached at the time of waking; the lowest point, in the evening.

Abnormal findings

Elevated intraocular pressure requires further testing for glaucoma. Because intraocular pressure varies diurnally, findings must be supplemented with serial measurements obtained at different times on different days.

Interfering factors

- Poor patient cooperation
- Deformed corneal curvature that prevents proper placement of the footplate
- Corneoscleral rigidity or flaccidity, as determined by an ophthalmologist (falsely elevated or depressed readings)

EARS AND HEARING

OTOSCOPY

Otoscopy is the direct visualization of the external auditory canal and the tympanic membrane through an otoscope. It's a basic part of physical examination of the ear and should be performed before other auditory or vestibular tests. Otoscopy indirectly provides information about the eustachian tube and the middle ear cavity.

Purpose

- To visualize inner ear structures
- To detect foreign bodies, cerumen, or stenosis in the external canal
- To detect external or middle ear pathology, such as infection or tympanic membrane perforation

Patient preparation

- Describe the procedure to the patient, and explain that this test permits visualization of the ear canal and eardrum.
- Reassure the patient that the examination is usually painless.
- Tell the patient that his ear will be pulled upward and backward to straighten the canal, to facilitate insertion of the otoscope.
- If the patient will undergo pneumatic otoscopy, tell him that he may expe-

Common abnormalities of the tympanic membrane

Visual examination of the tympanic membrane may reveal abnormal findings. This chart lists some of the more common findings as well as their typical causes.

ABNORMAL FINDINGS	USUAL CAUSE
Bright red color	Inflammation (otitis media)
Yellowish color	Pus or serum behind the tympanic membrane (acute or chronic otitis media)
Bubble behind the tympanic membrane	Serous fluid in middle ear (serous otitis media)
Absent light reflection	Bulging tympanic membrane (acute otitis media)
Absent or diminishing landmarks	Thickened tympanic membrane (chronic otitis media, otitis externa, or tympanosclerosis)
Oval dark areas	Perforated or scarred tympanic membrane (otitis media or trauma)
Prominent malleus	Retracted tympanic membrane (nonfunctional eustachian tube)
Reduced mobility	Stiffened middle ear system (serous otitis media or, less frequently, middle ear adhesions)

ience dizziness with nystagmus, a positive fistula sign.

Procedure and posttest care

- When assembling the otoscope, test the lamp and be sure to attach the largest speculum that fits comfortably into the patient's ear.
- With the patient seated, tilt his head slightly away from you so that the ear to be examined is pointed upward.
- Pull the auricle up and back (pull downward if the patient is under age 3); insert the otoscope gently into the ear canal with a downward and forward motion. If insertion is difficult, replace the speculum with a smaller one.
- If you still feel resistance, withdraw the otoscope and tell the physician.
- Look through the lens and gently advance the speculum until you see the tympanic membrane. Obtain as full a view as possible, and note redness, swelling, lesions, discharge, foreign bodies, and scaling in the canal. Check the tympanic membrane for color, scarring, contours, perforation, and a cone of light that appears at the 5 o'clock position in the right ear and at the 7 o-clock position in the left; this is a reflection of the otoscope lamp.

■ Locate the malleus, partially visible through the translucent tympanic membrane. Examine the membrane itself and the surrounding fibrous rim (annulus).

Precautions

■ The otoscope should be advanced slowly and gently through the medial portion of the ear canal to avoid irritation of the canal lining, especially if an infection is suspected.
■ Continuing to insert an otoscope against resistance may cause perforation of the tympanic membrane.

Normal findings

The normal tympanic membrane is thin, translucent, shiny, and slightly concave. It appears as a pearl gray or pale pink disk that reflects light in its inferior portion. The short process, manubrium mallei, and umbo should be visible but not prominent.

Abnormal findings

Scarring, discoloration, or retraction or bulging of the tympanic membrane indicates a pathologic condition. (See *Common abnormalities of the tympanic membrane.*) Movement of the tympanic membrane in tandem with respiration suggests abnormal patency of the eustachian tube.

Normal light reflex extends inferiorly and anteriorly from the umbo. However, an altered or absent light reflex isn't a reliable indicator of disease because there can be many normal variations of the tympanic membrane and posterior bony ear canal.

Interfering factors

■ Obstruction of the ear canal by cerumen or foreign matter
■ Recumbent position during otoscopy (possible masking of serous otitis media)

TUNING FORK TESTS

The Weber, Rinne, and Schwabach tuning fork tests are quick, valuable screening tools for detecting hearing loss and obtaining preliminary information as to its type. The Weber test determines whether a patient lateralizes the tone of the tuning fork to one ear. The Rinne test compares air and bone conduction in both ears. The Schwabach test compares the patient's bone conduction response with that of the examiner, who is assumed to have normal hearing.

Test results are most reliable when a low-frequency tuning fork is used; results aren't definitive because they depend on subjective factors, such as the examiner's ability to strike the fork with equal force each time and the patient's ability to report audible tones correctly.

Results of the Weber test may be misleading, and the Rinne test frequently doesn't detect a mild conductive hearing loss (10 to 35 dB). Thus, abnormal test results require confirmation by pure tone audiometry.

Purpose

■ To screen for or confirm hearing loss
■ To help distinguish conductive from sensorineural hearing loss

Patient preparation

■ Describe the procedure to the patient, and explain that these tests help detect and assess hearing loss. Tell him who will conduct the tests, and reassure him that they're painless.
■ Explain to the patient that concentration and prompt responses are essential for accurate testing. Have the patient use hand signals to indicate whether a tone is louder in his right ear

or left ear and when he stops hearing the tone.

■ Inform the patient that tuning fork tests aren't definitive and that further testing may be necessary to confirm abnormal results.

Procedure and posttest care

■ Using a low-frequency tuning fork (256 or 512 Hz), practice achieving a consistent tone by gently striking a prong against your elbow or the heel of your hand, by stroking the prongs upward, or by pinching them together.

■ When performing each test, be careful to strike the tuning fork with equal force. Hold the fork at its base to allow the prongs to vibrate freely. Record the name of the test, the result, and the vibrating frequency of the tuning fork.

Weber test

■ Vibrate the fork, and place its base on the midline of the patient's skull at the forehead.

■ Ask the patient whether the tone is louder in his left ear or his right ear or is equally loud in both. Describe the results as Weber left, Weber right, or Weber midline, according to his response.

Rinne test

■ Test bone conduction by holding the tuning fork between your thumb and index finger and placing the base of the vibrating fork against the patient's mastoid process.

■ Test air conduction by moving the vibrating prongs next to (but not touching) the external ear. Ask the patient which location has the louder or longer sound. Repeat the procedure for the other ear.

■ Record results as Rinne-positive, if the air-conducted sound is heard louder or longer, or Rinne-negative, if the bone-conducted sound is heard louder or longer.

Schwabach test

■ Holding the tuning fork between thumb and index finger, place the base of the vibrating tuning fork against the patient's left mastoid process and ask whether he hears the tone. If he does, immediately place the tuning fork on your left mastoid process and listen for the tone.

■ Alternate the tuning fork between the patient's left mastoid process and your own until one of you stops hearing the sound. Record the length of time the patient continues to hear it.

■ Repeat the procedure on the right mastoid process.

All tests

■ Refer the patient for further audiologic testing if the tuning fork tests suggest a hearing loss.

Precautions

■ Tonometry should never be performed on a patient with a corneal ulcer or infection, except by a skilled examiner, and only in an emergency, such as suspected acute angle-closure glaucoma.

■ Avoid resting your fingers on the cornea or pressing the cornea because this increases intraocular pressure.

■ Don't touch the lashes; this could trigger a blink response or Bell's phenomenon (upward movement of the eyes with forced closure of the lids), which can cause the footplate to move and scratch the cornea.

Normal findings

A patient with normal hearing will respond to the Weber test by hearing the same tone equally loudly in both ears (Weber midline result); to the Rinne test by hearing the air-conducted tone louder or longer than the bone-conducted tone (Rinne-positive result); and to the Schwabach test by hearing the tone for the same duration as the examiner.

Abnormal findings

In the Weber test, lateralization of the tone to one ear suggests a conductive loss on that side or a sensorineural loss on the other side. Lateralization results if the tone is louder in one ear (Stenger effect) or reaches one ear sooner (phase effect). If one ear has a sensorineural loss, the Stenger effect causes lateralization to the unaffected ear; if one ear has a conductive loss, either the Stenger or the phase effect produces lateralization to that ear. If a patient's hearing loss is unilateral, the Weber test may suggest the type of loss. If a patient's hearing loss is bilateral, this test may help to identify the ear with the better bone conduction.

In the Rinne test, hearing the bone-conducted tone louder or longer than the air-conducted tone indicates a conductive loss. In unilateral hearing loss, the tone may be heard louder when conducted by bone, but in the opposite ear; this is a false-negative Rinne test result. A sensorineural loss is indicated when the sound is heard louder by air conduction.

In the Schwabach test, hearing the tone longer than the examiner hears it suggests a conductive loss; conversely, a shorter duration indicates a sensorineural loss. A conductive loss attenuates (decreases the energy of) air-conducted sound in a room with ambient noise, enabling patients with this type of loss to hear bone-conducted sound longer than the examiner can hear such sound.

If the patient has abnormal results on retesting, pure tone audiometry is indicated to confirm hearing loss and determine its type and severity.

Interfering factors

- Failure to strike the tuning fork with equal force or to hold it correctly during the procedure
- Striking the tuning fork on a hard surface rather than on the elbow or knee
- Failure to use either the 512-Hz frequency tuning fork or the more sensitive 256-Hz tuning fork
- Inaccurate patient response due to poor understanding of his task
- Undetected hearing loss in the examiner

PURE TONE AUDIOMETRY

Pure tone audiometry, performed with an audiometer, provides a record of the thresholds (the lowest intensity levels) at which a patient can hear a set of test tones introduced through earphones or a bone conduction (sound) vibrator. The energy of these pure tones is concentrated at discrete frequencies. The octave frequencies between 125 and 8,000 Hz are used to obtain air conduction thresholds; frequencies between 250 and 4,000 Hz are used to obtain bone conduction thresholds.

Comparison of air and bone conduction thresholds can suggest a conductive, sensorineural, or mixed hearing loss but doesn't indicate the cause of the loss; further audiologic and vestibular tests and X-rays may be needed. Pure tone audiometry results may also suggest a need to consult an audiologist for evaluation of communication difficulties. (See *Interpreting pure tone audiograms,* page 744.)

Pure tone audiometry is indicated for any patient who requires quantitative hearing assessment. There are no contraindications; however, results depend on the patient's cooperation. Acoustic emission test results may provide additional information.

Interpreting pure tone audiograms

Sensorineural hearing loss depresses both air (circles) and bone (arrows) conduction thresholds to about the same degree. No matter how sound vibrations reach the inner ear, they must be transmitted to higher neural centers through the sensorineural system.

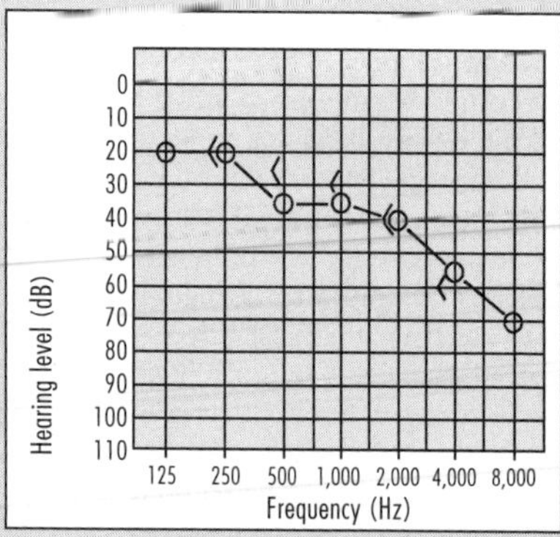

Conductive hearing loss, produced by interference with the conductive mechanism, depresses air conduction thresholds but generally doesn't affect bone thresholds.

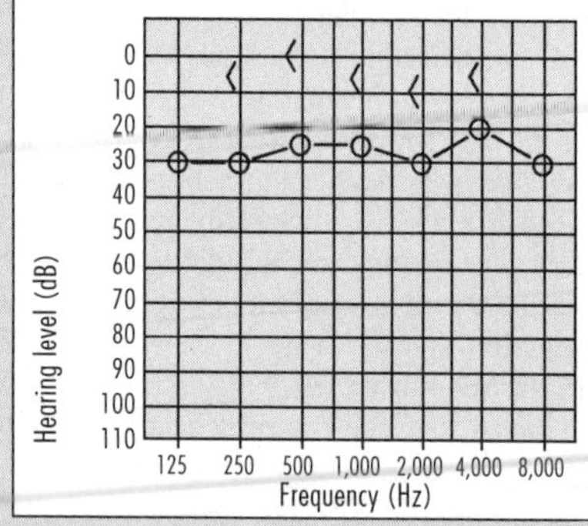

Mixed hearing loss involves abnormal air and bone conduction thresholds. Air conduction thresholds demonstrate a greater loss due to a conductive lesion.

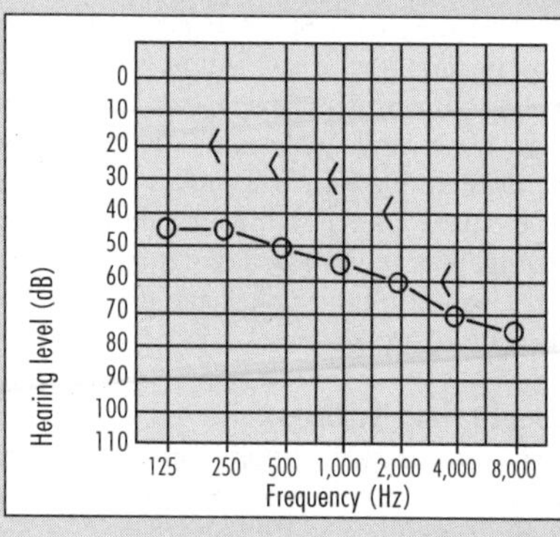

Purpose

- To determine the presence, type, and degree of hearing loss
- To assess communication abilities and rehabilitation needs
- To accurately determine pure tone and speech reception threshold

Patient preparation

- Describe the procedure to the patient, and explain that this test determines the presence and degree of hearing loss. Explain who will perform the test and where it will take place.
- Tell the patient that each ear will be tested, beginning with the ear with the better hearing acuity. Explain that he'll hear tones at various intensities and that he should signal (or press the response button) each time he hears the tone. Emphasize that he should respond even if the tone is faint.
- Just before the test, ask the patient to remove any jewelry or apparel that obstructs proper earphone placement.
- Postpone the test if the patient has been exposed to loud noises (loud enough to cause tinnitus or to make face-to-face communication difficult) within the past 16 hours.

Equipment

Otoscope, calibrated audiometer with earphones, and bone conduction vibrator. Note that the test environment must be quiet; a sound-treated room is recommended.

Procedure and posttest care

- The patient's ear canal is checked with the otoscope for impacted cerumen.
- The examiner presses a finger on the auricle and then the tragus to rule out possible closure of the ear canal under pressure from the earphones. If the canal tends to close, a stiff-walled plastic tube is carefully inserted into the canal. This modification is recorded on the audiogram.
- The earphones are positioned properly and the headband is tightened.
- A test tone is presented to the patient's better ear.

Air conduction testing

- A 1,000-Hz tone is presented to the patient's better ear. The intensity of the tone is decreased in 10-dB steps until the patient fails to respond. Then intensity is increased in 5-dB steps until he hears the tone again. Sequences of 10-dB decrements and 5-dB increments are repeated until the patient responds to at least two of three presentations at a single level. The threshold level is the lowest decibel level at which the response rate is at least 50%.
- Using this procedure, tones are presented to the better ear in this order: 1,000 Hz, 2,000 Hz, 4,000 Hz, 8,000 Hz, 1,000 Hz, 500 Hz, and 250 Hz.
- After testing the better ear, the other ear is tested. In each ear, test or retest differences may be + or –5 dB. If the difference between the first and second threshold at 1,000 Hz is greater than 10 dB, test results are unreliable; equipment should be checked for malfunction, and the patient should be reinstructed and retested.
- Many audiologists sample hearing only at octave points. Others may prefer the detail resulting from testing the mid-octave frequencies. The American Speech-Language-Hearing Association recommends testing the better ear first and that mid-octave points be tested when a difference of 20 dB or greater is seen in the thresholds at adjacent octaves.

Bone conduction testing

- The earphones are removed, and the vibrator is placed on the mastoid process of the better ear (the auricle shouldn't touch the vibrator).

Relating pure tone average to hearing loss and speech audibility

The patient's pure tone average helps determine his degree of hearing loss as well as the audibility of speech in a quiet environment.

PURE TONE AVERAGE (dB)	DEGREE OF HEARING LOSS	SPEECH AUDIBILITY
0 to 25	Normal limits	No significant difficulty
26 to 40	Mild	Difficulty with faint or distant speech
41 to 55	Moderate	Difficulty with conversational speech
56 to 70	Moderately severe	Speech must be loud; difficulty with group conversation
71 to 90	Severe	Difficulty with loud speech; understands only shouted or amplified speech
91+	Profound	May not understand amplified speech

- Ascending and descending tones are presented, as in air conduction testing, using 250, 500, 1,000, 2,000, and 4,000 Hz.

Both tests

- Refer the patient to an audiologist if test results are inconsistent or are confounded by possible crossover.

Precautions

- Any modifications of standard testing procedure—such as inserting a plastic tube to prevent ear canal collapse—must be recorded on the audiogram.
- Be on the alert for false responses; they can be misleading and influence interpretation of test results. False responses include failure to indicate when a tone has been heard or responding when no tone has been heard.

Normal findings

The normal range of hearing sensitivity is 0 to 25 dB for adults and 0 to 15 dB for children. Normal test results don't rule out a hearing disorder; a mild middle ear infection or other disorder may exist without interfering with auditory function.

Abnormal findings

The pure tone average—the average of pure tone air conduction thresholds obtained at 500, 1,000, and 2,000 Hz—quantifies the degree of hearing loss. When these three thresholds vary widely, the mean of the best two, known as the Fletcher average, indicates the degree of hearing loss.

The relation between threshold responses for air and bone conduction tones determines the type of hearing loss. In *sensorineural hearing loss,* both thresholds are depressed; in *conductive hearing loss,* air thresholds are depressed, but bone thresholds are unchanged; and in *mixed hearing loss,* both thresholds are abnormal, with air conduction more depressed than bone conduction. (See *Relating pure tone average to hearing loss and speech audibility.*)

Interfering factors

- Impacted cerumen or a closed ear canal (possible 35- to 40-dB artifactual conductive hearing loss)
- Patient's confusion of vibrotactile with auditory sensation or tinnitus with the signal (invalid results)
- Cracked or poorly fitting earphones (low-frequency leakage and false-high thresholds)
- Uncalibrated audiometer or background noise (possible invalidation)
- Presenting extraneous cues to the patient, such as a rhythmic pattern of test tones or hand movement near the attenuator dial (possible invalidation)
- Patient uncooperative or inattentive (possible invalidation)
- Ear infection

VESTIBULAR AND CEREBELLAR DYSFUNCTION

A patient who reports disequilibrium, dizziness, or nystagmus may undergo screening tests for vestibular or cerebellar dysfunction. These tests evaluate balance and coordination as the patient performs various maneuvers with eyes open and closed. Abnormal results suggest the need for further evaluation.

Purpose

- To help identify vestibular or cerebellar disorders that affect the entire body (balance tests)
- To help identify vestibular or cerebellar disorders that affect the arms (coordination tests)

Patient preparation

- Explain to the patient that these tests help identify neurologic dysfunction and that some evaluate his sense of balance.
- Describe the tests, including who will perform them, where they will take place, and how long they will last.
- Reassure the patient that he's in no danger of falling during the test.
- Assess the patient's general physical condition, which will influence his ability to perform the maneuvers.
- Check the patient's history for use of drugs that affect the central nervous system (CNS) and for recent alcohol consumption.

Procedure and posttest care

To assess balance

- Ask the patient to perform as many of the following test maneuvers as possible, and observe for a tendency to sway or fall.
- Have the patient stand with his feet together, arms at his sides, and eyes open for 20 seconds. Tell him to maintain this position for another 20 seconds with his eyes closed.
- Have the patient stand on one foot for 5 seconds and then on the other foot for 5 seconds; instruct him to repeat the procedure with his eyes closed.
- Tell the patient to stand heel to toe for 20 seconds with his eyes open and then to maintain the same position with his eyes closed for another 20 seconds.
- Instruct the patient to walk forward and backward in a straight line, heel to

toe, first with his eyes open and then with them closed.

To assess coordination

- With the patient seated and facing you, hold out your index finger at his shoulder level.
- Tell the patient to touch your finger with his right index finger.
- Then tell the patient to lower his arm and close his eyes. Have him touch your finger again.
- The patient then repeats the entire maneuver using his left index finger.
- Failure to perform this maneuver rapidly and accurately is called past-pointing. Observe the degree and direction of past-pointing.
- Another test of coordination requires the patient to touch his thumb to each of his fingers, both forward and backward as quickly as possible; repeat using the left hand.

Precautions

- Any of these tests may be contraindicated if the patient is physically incapable of performing some or all of the required maneuvers.
- When assessing balance, the examiner should stand close to the patient to catch him if he falls. If the patient is tall or heavy, someone should assist the examiner.

Normal findings

During tests for balance, a healthy person maintains his balance with his eyes open and closed. When testing coordination, a healthy person touches the examiner's finger with his eyes open and closed; past-pointing doesn't occur.

Abnormal findings

A peripheral vestibular lesion can cause swaying or falling in the direction opposite to the nystagmus when the patient's eyes are closed; a cerebellar lesion causes swaying or falling when the eyes are open or closed.

A labyrinthine disorder can lead to past-pointing in the direction opposite to the nystagmus when the patient's eyes are closed; a cerebellar lesion can lead to past-pointing when the eyes are open or closed; and a lateralized lesion can lead to past-pointing with the arm on the affected side only.

Interfering factors

- Alcohol or drugs that affect the CNS, such as stimulants, antianxiety agents, sedatives, and medications to relieve vertigo

GASTROINTESTINAL FUNCTION

ESOPHAGEAL ACIDITY

The esophageal acidity test evaluates the competence of the lower esophageal sphincter — the major barrier to reflux — by measuring intraesophageal pH with an electrode attached to a manometric catheter.

Purpose

- To evaluate the competence of the lower esophageal sphincter

Patient preparation

- Explain to the patient that this test evaluates the function of the sphincter between the esophagus and the stomach. Tell him to fast and avoid smoking after midnight before the test.
- Describe the test, including who will perform it and where it will take place.
- Tell the patient that a tube will be passed through his mouth into his

stomach and that he may experience slight discomfort, a desire to cough, or a gagging sensation.

■ Just before the test, check the patient's pulse rate and blood pressure, and instruct him to void.

■ Withhold antacids, anticholinergics, cholinergics, beta-adrenergic blockers, alcohol, corticosteroids, cimetidine, and reserpine for 24 hours before the test. If they must be continued, note this on the laboratory request.

■ Make sure the patient or a responsible family member has signed an informed consent form.

Procedure and posttest care

■ After the patient is placed in the high Fowler position, the catheter with the electrode is introduced into his mouth.

■ The patient is instructed to swallow when the electrode reaches the back of his throat.

■ Using a manometer, the examiner locates the lower esophageal sphincter. The catheter is raised ¾″ (1.9 cm). The patient is told to perform Valsalva's maneuver or lift his legs to stimulate reflux. After he does so, intraesophageal pH is measured.

■ If the pH is normal, the catheter is passed into the patient's stomach. A prescribed acid solution (300 ml of 0.1 N HCl) is instilled over 3 minutes (100 ml/minute). Then the catheter is raised ¾″ above the sphincter. Again, the patient is asked to perform Valsalva's maneuver or lift his legs and intraesophageal pH is measured.

■ After the test, tell the patient that he may resume his usual diet and restart any medications withheld for the test, as ordered.

■ Provide lozenges if the patient complains of a sore throat.

Precautions

■ During insertion, the electrode may enter the trachea instead of the esophagus. If the patient develops cyanosis or paroxysms of coughing, move the electrode immediately.

■ Observe the patient closely during insertion because arrhythmias may develop.

■ Clamp the catheter before removing it, to prevent aspiration of fluid into the lungs.

Reference values

The pH of the esophagus normally exceeds 5.0.

Abnormal findings

An intraesophageal pH of 1.5 to 2 indicates gastric acid reflux resulting from incompetence of the lower esophageal sphincter. Persistent reflux leads to chronic reflux esophagitis. Additional studies, such as barium swallow and esophagogastroduodenoscopy, are necessary to diagnose and determine the extent of esophagitis.

Interfering factors

■ Failure to adhere to pretest restrictions

■ Antacids, anticholinergics, histamine-2 blockers, and proton pump inhibitors (possible lowering of intraesophageal pH because of decrease in gastric secretions or acidity)

■ Alcohol, cholinergics, reserpine, adrenergic blockers, and corticosteroids (possible elevation of intraesophageal pH because of reflux from a relaxed lower esophageal sphincter or an increase in gastric secretions)

ACID PERFUSION TEST

Also called the Bernstein test, the acid perfusion test helps to distinguish pain caused by esophagitis (burning epigastric or retrosternal pain that radiates to the back or arms) from pain caused by angina pectoris or other disorders. It requires perfusion of saline and acidic solutions into the esophagus through a nasogastric (NG) tube.

Purpose

- To distinguish chest pains caused by esophagitis from those caused by cardiac disorders

Patient preparation

- Tell the patient that this test helps determine the cause of heartburn.
- Explain to the patient the following restrictions: no antacids for 24 hours before the test, no food for 12 hours before the test, and no fluids or smoking for 8 hours before the test.
- Describe the test, including who will perform it, where it will take place, and how long it will last.
- Explain that the test involves passing a tube through his nose into the esophagus and that he may experience some discomfort, a desire to cough, or a gagging sensation during tube passage.
- Tell the patient that liquid is slowly perfused through the tube into the esophagus and that he should immediately report any pain or burning during perfusion.
- Just before the test, check the patient's pulse rate and blood pressure. Ask him whether he's experiencing any heartburn and, if so, to describe it.
- Make sure the patient or a responsible family member has signed an informed consent form.

Procedure and posttest care

- After the patient is seated, insert an NG tube that has been marked 12″ (30.5 cm) from the tip into his stomach. Attach a 20-ml syringe to the tube and aspirate stomach contents. Withdraw the tube into the esophagus (to the 12″ mark).
- Hang labeled containers of normal saline solution and a prescribed acidic solution (0.1 N HCl) on an I.V. pole behind the patient; then connect the NG tube to I.V. tubing.
- Open the line from the normal saline solution, and infuse it at a rate of 60 to 120 drops/minute. Continue perfusion for 5 to 10 minutes.
- Ask the patient whether he's experiencing any discomfort, and record his response.
- Without the patient's knowledge, close the line from the normal saline solution and open the line from the acidic solution. Infuse the acidic solution into the esophagus at the same rate used for the saline solution. Continue perfusion for 30 minutes.
- Ask the patient again whether he's experiencing any discomfort, and record his response.
- If the patient experiences discomfort, close the line from the acidic solution immediately and open the line from the normal saline solution. Continue to perfuse this solution until the discomfort subsides.
- If ordered, repeat perfusion of the acidic solution to verify the patient's response. If this isn't required, or if the patient experiences no discomfort after perfusion of the acidic solution for 30 minutes, stop the solution and withdraw the NG tube.
- If the patient complains of pain or burning, administer an antacid as ordered. If he complains of a sore throat, provide soothing lozenges or obtain an order for an ice collar.

■ Instruct the patient to resume his usual diet and medication schedule as ordered.

Precautions

■ The acid perfusion test is contraindicated in patients with esophageal varices, heart failure, acute myocardial infarction, or other cardiac disorders.
■ During intubation, make sure the tube enters the esophagus and not the trachea. Withdraw the tube immediately if the patient develops cyanosis or paroxysmal coughing.
■ Assess the patient's pulse rate and rhythm to detect any arrhythmias that may develop.
■ Clamp the tube before removing it, to prevent aspiration of fluid into the lungs.

Normal findings

Absence of pain or burning during perfusion of either solution indicates a healthy esophageal mucosa.

Abnormal findings

In patients with esophagitis, the acidic solution causes pain or burning, and the normal saline solution should produce no adverse effects. Occasionally, both solutions cause pain in patients with esophagitis, but they may cause no pain in patients with asymptomatic esophagitis.

Interfering factors

■ Failure to adhere to pretest restrictions
■ Beta-adrenergic blockers, anticholinergics, reserpine, corticosteroids, histamine-2 blockers, and acid pump inhibitors may affect test results.

RENAL FUNCTION

UROFLOMETRY

Uroflometry, a simple, noninvasive test, uses a uroflometer to detect and evaluate dysfunctional voiding patterns. The uroflometer, contained in a funnel into which the patient voids, measures flow rate (volume of urine voided per second), continuous flow (time of measurable flow), and intermittent flow (total voiding time, including any interruptions).

Types of uroflometers include rotary disc, electromagnetic, spectrophotometric, and gravimetric systems. The gravimetric system, which weighs urine as it's voided and plots the weight against time, is the simplest to use.

Purpose

■ To evaluate lower urinary tract function
■ To demonstrate bladder outlet obstruction

Patient preparation

■ Explain to the patient that this test evaluates his pattern of urination. Advise him not to urinate for several hours before the test and to increase fluid intake so that he'll have a full bladder and a strong urge to void.
■ Describe the test, including who will perform it and where it will take place.
■ Instruct the patient to remain still while voiding during the test to help ensure accurate results. Assure him that he'll have complete privacy during the test.
■ As ordered, discontinue drugs that may affect bladder and sphincter tone, such as urinary spasmolytics and anticholinergics.

Equipment

Commode chair with funnel containing a uroflometer, beaker to hold urine, transducer, start and flow cables, data recording module

Procedure and posttest care

- Check cable connections before the test.
- Remind the patient not to strain while voiding.
- Ask a male patient to void while standing and a female patient to void while sitting.
- The patient pushes the START button on the commode chair, counts for 5 seconds (1 one-thousand, 2 one-thousand, and so on), and voids. When finished, he counts for 5 seconds and pushes the button again. The volume of urine voided is then recorded and plotted as a curve over the time of voiding. The patient's position and the route of fluid intake (oral or I.V.) are noted.
- Instruct the patient to resume any medications discontinued for the test.
- Monitor the patient for urine retention or bladder distension. Also monitor intake and output. If neurogenic bladder is diagnosed, teach self-catheterization, if indicated; provide bladder training as needed.

Precautions

- The transducer must be level, and the beaker must be centered beneath the funnel.
- The beaker must be large enough to hold all urine; overflow can invalidate results and damage the transducer.

Reference values

Flow rate varies according to the patient's age and sex and the volume of urine voided. The chart at the top of the next column lists the minimum volumes needed to obtain adequate recordings.

AGE	MIN. VOL. (ml/sec)	MALE (ml/sec)	FEMALE (ml/sec)
4 to 7	100	10	10
8 to 13	100	12	15
14 to 45	200	21	18
46 to 65	200	12	15
66 to 80	200	9	10

Abnormal findings

Increased flow rate indicates reduced urethral resistance, possibly associated with external sphincter dysfunction. (See *Characteristic uroflow curves.*) A high peak on the curve plotted over the voiding time indicates decreased outflow resistance, possibly due to stress incontinence. Decreased flow rate indicates outflow obstruction or hypotonia of the detrusor muscle. More than one distinct peak in a normal curve indicates abdominal straining, possibly due to pushing against an obstruction to empty the bladder.

Interfering factors

- Drugs that affect bladder and sphincter tone, such as urinary spasmolytics and anticholinergics
- Strong drafts (possible effect on transducer function)
- Patient movement while seated on the commode chair (possible inaccuracy of flow recording)
- Presence of toilet tissue in the beaker (invalidation)
- Straining to void

Characteristic uroflow curves

Normal curve

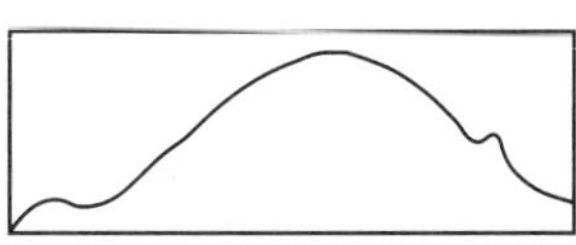

Normal peak with hesitancy may result from the patient's embarrassment or advanced age.

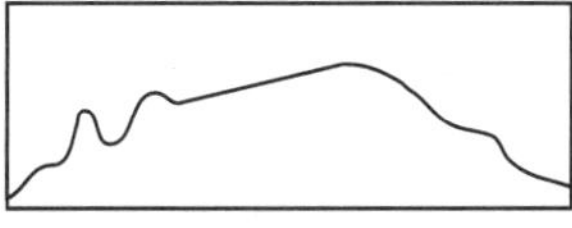

High peak flow over short voiding time may indicate incontinence.

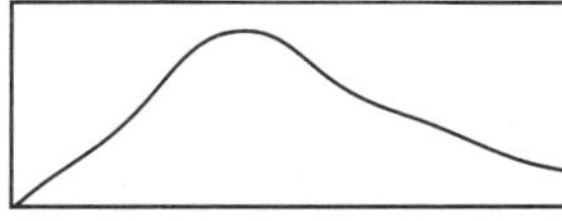

Many peaks over normal voiding time indicate abdominal straining and detrusor muscle weakness.

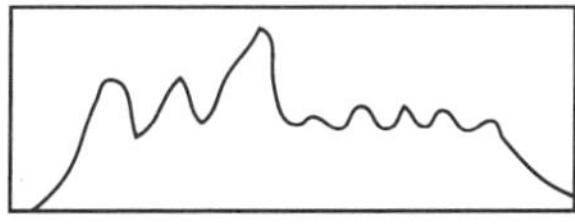

Low peak with long voiding time and urethral dribbling indicates obstruction.

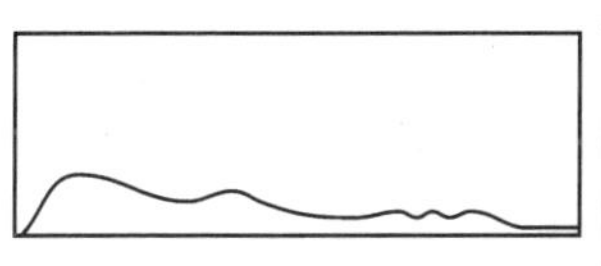

CYSTOMETRY

Cystometry assesses the bladder's neuromuscular function by measuring efficiency of the detrusor muscle reflex, intravesical pressure and capacity, and the bladder's reaction to thermal stimulation. Because results from cystometry can be ambiguous, they're typically supported by results of other tests, such as cystourethrography, excretory urography, and voiding cystourethrography.

Purpose

- To evaluate detrusor muscle function and tonicity
- To help determine the cause of bladder dysfunction

Patient preparation

- Explain to the patient that this test evaluates bladder function.
- Tell the patient that he need not restrict food or fluid before the test.
- Describe the procedure, including who will perform it, where it will take place, and how long it will last.
- Tell the patient that he'll feel a strong urge to void during the test and that he may feel embarrassed or uncomfortable. Provide reassurance.
- Make sure the patient or a responsible family member has signed an informed consent form.
- Check the patient's medication history for drugs that may affect test results, such as antihistamines.
- Tell the patient to urinate just before the procedure.

Equipment

Four-channel gas cystometer, set of catheters

Procedure and posttest care

- Place the patient in the supine position on the examination table.
- A catheter is passed into the bladder to measure residual urine level. Any difficulty with insertion of the catheter may reflect meatal or urethral obstruction.
- To test the patient's response to thermal sensation, 30 ml of room-temperature physiologic saline solution or sterile water is instilled into the bladder. Then an equal volume of warm (110° to 115° F [43.3° to 46.1° C]) fluid is instilled into the bladder. The patient is asked to report his sensations, such as the need to void, nausea, flushing, discomfort, and a feeling of warmth.
- After the fluid is drained from the patient's bladder, the catheter is connected to the cystometer, and normal saline solution, sterile water, or gas (usually carbon dioxide) is slowly introduced into the bladder. The flow of gas is adjusted automatically to the desired reading (100 ml/minute) by a four-channel cystometer.
- The patient is asked to indicate when he *first* feels an urge to void and then when he feels he *must* urinate. The related pressure and volume are automatically plotted on the graph.
- When the bladder reaches its full capacity, the patient is asked to urinate so that the maximal intravesical voiding pressure can be recorded. The patient's bladder is then drained and, if no additional tests are required, the catheter is removed; otherwise, the catheter is left in place to measure urethral pressure profile or to provide supplemental findings.
- If abnormal bladder function is caused by muscle incompetence or disrupted innervation, an anticholinergic (atropine) or cholinergic medication (bethanechol) may be injected and the study repeated in 20 to 30 minutes.
- Encourage the patient to drink lots of fluids, unless contraindicated, to relieve burning on urination, a common adverse effect of the procedure.
- Short-term antibiotics are commonly given to prevent infection.
- Administer a sitz bath or warm tub bath if the patient experiences discomfort after the test.
- Measure fluid intake and urine output for 24 hours. Watch for hematuria that persists after the third voiding and for signs of sepsis (such as fever or chills).

Precautions

- Cystometry is contraindicated in patients with acute urinary tract infections because uninhibited contractions may cause erroneous readings and the test may lead to pyelonephritis and septic shock.
- Tell the patient not to strain at voiding; it can cause ambiguous cystometric readings.
- If the patient has a spinal cord injury that has caused motor impairment, transport him on a stretcher so that the test can be performed without transferring him to the examination table.

Findings

(For characteristic findings, see *Normal and abnormal cystometry findings.*)

Interfering factors

- Failure to follow instructions because of misunderstanding or embarrassment
- Inability to urinate in the supine position
- Concurrent use of drugs such as antihistamines (possible interference with bladder function)
- Cystometry performed within 6 to 8 weeks after surgery for spinal cord injury (inconclusive results)

Normal and abnormal cystometry findings

Because cystometry assesses micturition and vesical function, it can aid diagnosis of neurogenic bladder dysfunction. The five main types of neurogenic bladder, as presented in the following chart, result from lesions of the central or peripheral nervous system. Uninhibited neurogenic bladder results from a lesion to the upper motor neuron and causes frequent, often uncontrollable micturition in the presence of even a small amount of urine. A complete upper motor neuron lesion characterizes reflex neurogenic bladder and causes total loss of conscious sensation and vesical control

FEATURE OR RESPONSE	NORMAL BLADDER FUNCTION	UNINHIBITED NEUROGENIC BLADDER (mildly spastic, incomplete upper motor neuron lesion)	REFLEX NEUROGENIC BLADDER (completely spastic, complete upper motor neuron lesion)
Micturition			
Start	+	+/0	0
Stop	+	0	0
Residual urine	0	0	+
Vesical sensation	+	+	0
First urge to void	150 to 200 ml	E (<150 ml)	0
Bladder capacity	400 to 500 ml	↓	↓
Bladder contractions	0	+	+
Intravesical pressure	L	↑	↑
Bulbocavernosus reflex	+	+	↑
Saddle sensation	+	+	0
Bethanechol test (exaggerated response)	0	+	0
Ice water test	+	+	+
Anal reflex	+	+	+
Heat sensation and pain	+	+	0

KEY:
+ = Present/Positive
0 = Absent/Negative
↑ = Increased
↓ = Decreased
V = Variable
E = Early
D = Delayed
L = Low

(continued)

Normal and abnormal cystometry findings *(continued)*

In autonomous neurogenic bladder, a lower motor neuron lesion produces a flaccid bladder that fills without contracting. The patient can't perceive bladder fullness or initiate and maintain urination without applying external pressure. Lower motor neuron lesions can cause sensory or motor paralysis of the bladder. In sensory paralysis, the patient experiences chronic urine retention because he can't perceive bladder fullness. In motor paralysis, the patient has full sensation but can't initiate or control urination.

FEATURE OR RESPONSE	AUTONOMOUS NEUROGENIC BLADDER (flaccid, incomplete lower motor neuron lesion)	SENSORY PARALYTIC BLADDER (lower motor neuron lesion)	MOTOR PARALYTIC BLADDER (lower motor neuron lesion)
Micturition			
Start	0	+	0
Stop	0	+	0
Residual urine	+	+	++
Vesical sensation	0	0	+
First urge to void	0	D	+
Bladder capacity	↑	↑ (<1,000 ml)	V
Bladder contractions	0	0	0
Intravesical pressure	↓	↓	L
Bulbocavernosus reflex	0	+/↓/0	+
Saddle sensation	0	V	+
Bethanechol test (exaggerated response)	+	+	0
Ice water test	0	0	0
Anal reflex	0	V	V
Heat sensation and pain	0	0	+

KEY:
+ = Present/Positive
0 = Absent/Negative
↑ = Increased
↓ = Decreased
V = Variable
E = Early
D = Delayed
L = Low

EXTERNAL SPHINCTER ELECTROMYOGRAPHY

External sphincter electromyography measures electrical activity of the external urinary sphincter using needle electrodes inserted in perineal or periurethral tissues, electrodes in an anal plug, or skin electrodes. Skin electrodes are the most common method used.

Incontinence is the primary indication for external sphincter electromyography. Often, the test is done with cystometry and voiding urethrography as part of a full urodynamic study.

Purpose

- To assess neuromuscular function of the external urinary sphincter
- To assess the functional balance between bladder and sphincter muscle activity

Patient preparation

- Explain to the patient that this test will determine how well his bladder and sphincter muscles work together.
- Describe the test, including who will perform it, where it will take place, and how long it will last.
- If skin electrodes are used, describe their placement and explain the preparatory procedure, which may include shaving a small area.
- If needle electrodes are used, describe their placement to the patient and explain that the discomfort is equivalent to an I.M. injection. Assure him that he'll feel discomfort only during insertion. Explain that wires connect the needles to the recorder but pose no danger of electric shock. If the patient is a woman, tell her that she may notice slight bleeding at the first voiding.
- If an anal plug is used, tell the patient that only the tip of the plug will be inserted into the rectum and that he may feel fullness but no discomfort.
- Check the patient's history for use of cholinergic or anticholinergic drugs, and note such use.
- Make sure the patient or a responsible family member has signed an informed consent form.

Equipment

Electromyograph and recorder; skin, needle, or anal plug electrodes; ground plate; electrode paste; tape; antiseptic solution such as povidone-iodine; preparatory tray if shaving is necessary.

Procedure and posttest care

- Place the patient in the lithotomy position for electrode placement. After placement, he may lie in the supine position. Record the patient's position, the type of electrode and measuring equipment used, and any other tests done at the same time.
- Electrode paste is applied to the ground plate, which is taped to the thigh and grounded. The electrodes are positioned and connected to electrode adapters.
- When using skin electrodes, clean the skin with antiseptic solution and then dry the area. If necessary, shave a small area to optimize electrode contact. Apply electrode paste and tape the electrodes in place. For women, electrodes are placed in the periurethral area; for men, in the perineal area beneath the scrotum.
- To position needle electrodes on a male patient, a gloved finger is inserted in the rectum. The needles and wires are inserted through the perineal skin toward the apex of the prostate. Needle positions are 3 o'clock and 9 o'clock. The needles are withdrawn, and the

wires are held in place and then taped to the thigh.

- To position needle electrodes on a female patient, the labia are spread and the needles and wires are inserted periurethrally at the 2 o'clock and 10 o'clock positions. The needles are withdrawn, and the wires are taped to the thigh.
- When using anal plug electrodes, the plug is lubricated and the patient is asked to breathe slowly and deeply and to relax the anal sphincter to accommodate the plug by bearing down.
- After electrode placement, the adapters are inserted in the preamplifier and recording starts. The patient is asked to alternately relax and tighten the sphincter.
- When sufficient data have been recorded, the patient is asked to bear down and exhale while the anal plug and needle electrodes are removed. Remove skin electrodes gently to avoid pulling hair and tender skin.
- Clean and dry the area before the patient dresses.
- In some urodynamic laboratories, cystometrography is done with electromyography (EMG) for a thorough evaluation of detrusor and sphincter coordination.
- For women, watch for and report hematuria after the first voiding, if needle electrodes were used.
- Watch for and report symptoms of mild urethral irritation, such as dysuria, hematuria, and urinary frequency.
- Advise the patient to take a warm sitz bath, and encourage him to drink 2 to 3 L (2 to 3 qt) of fluids daily, unless contraindicated.

Precautions

- Insert the needles quickly to minimize discomfort.
- The ground plate should be properly applied and anchored; wires should be taped securely to prevent artifacts.

Normal findings

The EMG shows increased muscle activity when the patient tightens the external urinary sphincter and decreased muscle activity when he relaxes it. If EMG and cystometrography are performed simultaneously, a comparison of results shows that muscle activity of the normal sphincter increases as the bladder fills. During voiding and bladder contraction, muscle activity decreases as the sphincter relaxes. This comparison is important in assessing external sphincter efficiency and functional balance between bladder and sphincter muscle activity.

Abnormal findings

Failure of the sphincter to relax or increased muscle activity during voiding demonstrates detrusor–external sphincter dyssynergia. Confirmation of such muscle activity by EMG may indicate neurogenic bladder, spinal cord injury, multiple sclerosis, Parkinson's disease, or stress incontinence.

Interfering factors

- Patient movement (possible distortion)
- Effect of anticholinergic or cholinergic drugs on detrusor and sphincter activity
- Improperly placed and anchored electrodes

Miscellaneous Tests

Tensilon Test

The Tensilon test involves careful observation of the patient after I.V. administration of Tensilon (edrophonium chloride), a rapid, short-acting anticholinesterase that improves muscle strength by increasing muscle response to nerve impulses.

Purpose

- To aid diagnosis of myasthenia gravis
- To aid in differentiation between myasthenic and cholinergic crises
- To monitor oral anticholinesterase therapy

Patient preparation

- Explain to the patient that this test helps determine the cause of muscle weakness.
- Describe the test, including who will perform it, where it will take place, and how long it will last.
- Don't describe the exact response that will be evaluated; foreknowledge can affect the test's objectivity.
- Explain to the patient that a small tube will be inserted into a vein in his arm and that a drug will be administered periodically. He'll be asked to make repetitive muscle movements, and his reactions will be observed. To ensure accuracy, the test may be repeated several times.
- Advise the patient that Tensilon may produce some unpleasant adverse effects, but reassure him that someone will be with him at all times and that any reactions will quickly disappear.
- Check the patient's history for medications that affect muscle function, anticholinesterase therapy, drug hypersensitivities, and respiratory disease. Withhold medications as ordered. If the patient is receiving anticholinesterase therapy, note this on the requisition request; include the time of the most recent dose.
- Make sure the patient or a responsible family member has signed an informed consent form.

Equipment

Standard: 10 mg Tensilon, 0.4 mg atropine (may be prescribed for patients with respiratory distress), one tuberculin and one 3-ml syringe, I.V. infusion set, 50-ml bag of I.V. solution (dextrose 5% in water [D_5W] or normal saline solution), tape, tourniquet, alcohol swabs

Emergency: 0.5 to 1 mg atropine I.V. for cholinergic crisis, 0.5 to 2 mg neostigmine methylsulfate I.V. for myasthenic crisis (may be repeated up to a total of 5 mg), extra tuberculin and 3-ml syringes (for atropine or neostigmine injections), resuscitation equipment, including a tracheotomy tray

Procedure and posttest care

- Begin an I.V. infusion of D_5W or normal saline solution.
- When performing the test on an adult patient suspected of having myasthenia gravis, 2 mg of Tensilon are administered initially. Before the rest of the dose is administered, the physician may want to fatigue the muscles by asking the patient to perform various exercises, such as looking up until ptosis develops, counting to 100 until his voice diminishes, or holding his arms above his shoulders until they drop. When the muscles are fatigued, the remaining 8 mg of Tensilon are administered over 30 seconds.

■ Some physicians may prefer to begin the test with a placebo injection to evaluate the patient's muscle response more accurately. The placebo isn't necessary if cranial muscles are being tested, because cranial strength can't be simulated voluntarily.

■ After Tensilon is administered, the patient is asked to perform repetitive muscle movements, such as opening and closing his eyes and crossing and uncrossing his legs. Closely observe the patient for improved muscle strength. If muscle strength doesn't improve within 3 to 5 minutes, the test may be repeated.

■ To differentiate between myasthenic crisis and cholinergic crisis, 1 to 2 mg of Tensilon is infused. After infusion, continually monitor the patient's vital signs. Watch closely for respiratory distress, and be prepared to provide respiratory assistance.

■ If muscle strength doesn't improve, more Tensilon is infused cautiously, 1 mg at a time up to a maximum of 5 mg, and the patient is observed for distress.

■ Neostigmine is administered immediately if the test demonstrates myasthenic crisis; atropine is administered for cholinergic crisis.

■ To evaluate oral anticholinesterase therapy, 2 mg of Tensilon is infused 1 hour after the patient's last dose of the anticholinesterase. The patient is observed carefully for adverse effects and muscle response.

■ After Tensilon administration, the I.V. line is kept open at a rate of 20 ml/hour until all of the patient's responses have been evaluated.

■ When the test is complete, discontinue the I.V. and check the patient's vital signs.

■ Check the puncture site for hematoma, excessive bleeding, and swelling.

■ As ordered, tell the patient to resume any medications withheld for the test.

Precautions

■ Because of the systemic adverse reactions Tensilon may produce, this test may be contraindicated in patients with hypotension, bradycardia, apnea, and mechanical obstruction of the intestine or urinary tract.

■ Patients with respiratory ailments, such as asthma, should receive atropine during the test to minimize adverse reactions to Tensilon.

■ Stay with the patient during the test, and observe him closely for adverse reactions.

■ Keep resuscitation equipment handy in case of respiratory failure.

Normal findings

People who don't have myasthenia gravis usually develop fasciculation in response to Tensilon. The physician must interpret the responses carefully to distinguish a normal person from one with myasthenia gravis.

Abnormal findings

If the patient has myasthenia gravis, muscle strength should improve promptly after administration of Tensilon. The degree of improvement depends on the muscle group being tested; improvement is usually obvious within 30 seconds. Although the maximum benefit lasts only several minutes, lingering effects may persist — for example, up to 2 hours in a patient receiving prednisone. All patients with myasthenia gravis show improved muscle strength in this test; some patients respond slightly, and the test may need to be repeated to confirm the diagnosis.

The test may yield inconsistent results if myasthenia gravis affects only ocular muscles, as in mild or early forms of the disorder. It may produce a positive response in motor neuron disease and in some neuropathies and myopathies. The response is usually less dramatic and less consistent than in myasthenia gravis.

Patients in myasthenic crisis show brief improvement in muscle strength after Tensilon administration. Patients in cholinergic crisis (anticholinesterase overdose) may experience exaggerated muscle weakness. If Tensilon increases the patient's muscle strength without increasing adverse effects, oral anticholinesterase therapy can be increased. If Tensilon decreases muscle strength in a person with severe adverse reactions, therapy should be reduced. If the test shows no change in muscle strength and only mild adverse effects occur, therapy should remain the same.

Interfering factors

- Prednisone (possible delay of Tensilon's effect on muscle strength)
- Quinidine and anticholinergics (inhibit the action of Tensilon)
- Procainamide and muscle relaxants (inhibit normal muscle response)

COLD STIMULATION TEST FOR RAYNAUD'S SYNDROME

The cold stimulation test for Raynaud's syndrome demonstrates Raynaud's syndrome by recording temperature changes in the patient's fingers before and after submersion in ice water. Note that digital blood pressure recording or examination of the arteries in the arm and palmar arch should precede this test to rule out arterial occlusive disease.

Purpose

- To detect Raynaud's syndrome, an arteriospastic disorder characterized by intense vasospasm of the small cutaneous arteries and arterioles of the hands after exposure to cold or stress

Patient preparation

- Explain to the patient that this test detects vascular disorders.
- Tell the patient that he need not restrict food or fluids for the test.
- Describe the test, including who will perform it, where it will take place, and how long it will last.
- Explain to the patient that he may experience discomfort when his hands are briefly immersed in ice water.
- Have the patient remove his watch and other jewelry, and encourage him to relax.

Procedure and posttest care

- To minimize extraneous environmental stimuli, make sure the test room is neither too warm nor too cold.
- Tape a thermistor to each of the patient's fingers, and record the temperature.
- Have the patient submerge his hands in an ice-water bath for 20 seconds.
- When the patient removes his hands from the water, record the temperature of his fingers immediately and every 5 minutes thereafter until it returns to the baseline temperature.

Precautions

- The cold stimulation test is contraindicated in patients with gangrenous fingers or open, infected wounds.

Normal findings

Normally, digital temperature returns to baseline levels within 15 minutes.

Abnormal findings

If digital temperature takes longer than 20 minutes to return to the baseline level, Raynaud's syndrome is indicated.

Its benign form, Raynaud's disease, requires no specific treatment and has no serious sequelae. Its more serious form, Raynaud's phenomenon, is associated with connective tissue disorders that may not be clinically apparent for several years, such as scleroderma, systemic lupus erythematosus, and rheumatoid arthritis. Distinguishing between Raynaud's phenomenon and Raynaud's disease is difficult.

Interfering factors

- Excessively warm or cold test environment

PULMONARY FUNCTION TESTS

Pulmonary function tests (volume, capacity, and flow rate tests) are a series of measurements that evaluate ventilatory function through spirometric measurements; they're performed on patients with suspected pulmonary dysfunction.

Of the seven tests used to determine volume, tidal volume (V_T) and expiratory reserve volume (ERV) are direct spirographic measurements; minute volume (MV), carbon dioxide (CO_2) response, inspiratory reserve volume (IRV), and residual volume (RV) are calculated from the results of other pulmonary function tests; and thoracic gas volume (TGV) is calculated from body plethysmography.

Of the pulmonary capacity tests, vital capacity (VC), inspiratory capacity (IC), functional residual capacity (FRC), total lung capacity (TLC), and forced expiratory flow (FEF) may be measured directly or calculated from the results of other tests. Forced vital capacity (FVC), flow-volume curve, forced expiratory volume (FEV), peak expiratory flow rate (PEFR), and maximal voluntary ventilation (MVV) are direct spirographic measurements. Diffusing capacity for carbon monoxide (DL_{CO}) is calculated from the amount of carbon monoxide exhaled. (See *Interpreting pulmonary function tests.*)

Purpose

- To determine the cause of dyspnea
- To assess the effectiveness of specific therapeutic regimens
- To determine whether a functional abnormality is obstructive or restrictive
- To measure pulmonary dysfunction
- To evaluate a patient before surgery
- To evaluate as part of a job screening (firefighting, for example)

Patient preparation

- Explain to the patient that these tests evaluate pulmonary function. Instruct him to eat only a light meal before the tests and not to smoke for 12 hours before the tests.
- Describe the tests and equipment. Explain who will perform the tests, where they will take place, and how long they will last.
- Describe the operation of a spirometer.
- Advise the patient that the accuracy of the tests depends on his cooperation.
- Assure the patient that the procedures are painless and that he'll be able to rest between tests.
- Inform the laboratory if the patient is taking an analgesic that depresses respiration.
- As ordered, withhold bronchodilators for 8 hours.
- Just before the test, tell the patient to void and to loosen tight clothing. If he wears dentures, tell him to wear them during the test to help form a seal around the mouthpiece. Advise him to

(Text continues on page 766.)

Interpreting pulmonary function tests

Pulmonary function tests are interpreted after data are collected and calculated. The implications are reviewed in the chart below.

PULMONARY FUNCTION TEST	METHOD OF CALCULATION	IMPLICATIONS
Tidal volume (VT): amount of air inhaled or exhaled during normal breathing	Determining the spirographic measurement for 10 breaths and then dividing by 10	Decreased V_T may indicate restrictive disease and requires further testing, such as full pulmonary function studies or chest X-rays.
Minute volume (MV): total amount of air expired per minute	Multiplying V_T by the respiratory rate	Normal MV can occur in emphysema; decreased MV may indicate other diseases such as pulmonary edema. Increased MV can occur with acidosis, increased CO_2, decreased partial pressure of arterial oxygen, exercise, and low compliance states.
Carbon dioxide (CO_2) response: increase or decrease in MV after breathing various CO_2 concentrations	Plotting changes in MV against increasing inspired CO_2 concentrations	Reduced CO_2 response may occur in emphysema, myxedema, obesity, hypoventilation syndrome, and sleep apnea.
Inspiratory reserve volume (IRV): amount of air inspired over above-normal inspiration	Subtracting V_T from inspiratory capacity	Abnormal IRV alone doesn't indicate respiratory dysfunction; IRV decreases during normal exercise.
Expiratory reserve volume (ERV): amount of air exhaled after normal expiration	Direct spirographic measurement	ERV varies, even in healthy people, but usually decreases in obese people.
Residual volume (RV): amount of air remaining in the lungs after forced expiration	Subtracting ERV from functional residual capacity (FRC)	RV > 35% of TLC after maximal expiratory effort may indicate obstructive disease.

(continued)

Interpreting pulmonary function tests *(continued)*

PULMONARY FUNCTION TEST	METHOD OF CALCULATION	IMPLICATIONS
Vital capacity (VC): total volume of air that can be exhaled after maximum inspiration	Direct spirographic measurement or adding V_T, IRV, and ERV	Normal or increased VC with decreased flow rates may indicate any condition that causes a reduction in functional pulmonary tissue, such as pulmonary edema. Decreased VC with normal or increased flow rates may indicate decreased respiratory effort resulting from neuromuscular disease, drug overdose, or head injury; decreased thoracic expansion; or limited movement of the diaphragm.
Inspiratory capacity (IC): amount of air that can be inhaled after normal expiration	Direct spirographic measurement or adding IRV and V_T	Decreased IC indicates restrictive disease.
Thoracic gas volume (TGV): total volume of gas in the lungs from both ventilated and nonventilated airways	Body plethysmography	Increased TGV indicates air trapping, which may result from obstructive disease.
Functional residual capacity (FRC): amount of air remaining in the lungs after normal expiration	Nitrogen washout, helium dilution technique, or adding ERV and RV	Increased FRC indicates overdistention of lungs, which may result from obstructive pulmonary disease.
Total lung capacity (TLC): total volume of the lungs when maximally inflated	Adding V_T, IRV, ERV, and RV; or FRC and IC; or VC and RV	Low TLC indicates restrictive disease; high TLC indicates overdistended lungs caused by obstructive disease.
Forced vital capacity (FVC): amount of air exhaled forcefully and quickly after maximum inspiration	Direct spirographic measurement; expressed as a percentage of the total volume of gas exhaled	Decreased FVC indicates flow resistance in the respiratory system from obstructive disease, such as chronic bronchitis, or from restrictive disease such as pulmonary fibrosis.

Interpreting pulmonary function tests *(continued)*

PULMONARY FUNCTION TEST	METHOD OF CALCULATION	IMPLICATIONS
Flow-volume curve (also called flow-volume loop): greatest rate of flow (V_{max}) during FVC maneuvers versus lung volume change	Direct spirographic measurement at 1-second intervals; calculated from flow rates (expressed in L/second) and lung volume changes (expressed in liters) during maximal inspiratory and expiratory maneuvers	Decreased flow rates at all volumes during expiration indicate obstructive disease of the small airways, such as emphysema. A plateau of expiratory flow near TLC, a plateau of inspiratory flow at mid-VC, and a square wave pattern through most of VC indicate obstructive disease of large airways. Normal or increased PEFR, decreased flow with decreasing lung volumes, and markedly decreased VC indicate restrictive disease.
Forced expiratory volume (FEV): volume of air expired in the 1st, 2nd, or 3rd second of an FVC maneuver	Direct spirographic measurement; expressed as a percentage of FVC	Decreased FEV_1 and increased FEV_2 and FEV_3 may indicate obstructive disease; decreased or normal FEV_1 may indicate restrictive disease.
Forced expiratory flow (FEF): average rate of flow during the middle half of FVC	Calculated from the flow rate and the time needed for expiration of the middle 50% of FVC	Low FEF (25% to 75%) indicates obstructive disease of the small and medium-sized airways.
Peak expiratory flow rate (PEFR): V_{max} during forced expiration	Calculated from the flow-volume curve or by direct spirographic measurement, using a pneumotachometer or electronic tachometer with a transducer to convert flow to electrical output display	Decreased PEFR may indicate a mechanical problem, such as upper airway obstruction, or obstructive disease. PEFR is usually normal in restrictive disease but decreases in severe cases. Because PEFR is effort dependent, it's also low in a person who has poor expiratory effort or doesn't understand the procedure.

(continued)

Interpreting pulmonary function tests *(continued)*

PULMONARY FUNCTION TEST	METHOD OF CALCULATION	IMPLICATIONS
Maximal voluntary ventilation (MVV) (also called maximum breathing capacity): the greatest volume of air breathed per unit of time	Direct spirographic measurement	Decreased MVV may indicate obstructive disease; normal or decreased MVV may indicate restrictive disease, such as myasthenia gravis.
Diffusing capacity for carbon monoxide (DL_{CO}): milliliters of carbon monoxide diffused per minute across the alveolocapillary membrane	Calculated from analysis of the amount of carbon monoxide exhaled compared with the amount inhaled	Decreased DL_{CO} due to a thickened alveolocapillary membrane occurs in interstitial pulmonary diseases, such as pulmonary fibrosis, asbestosis, and sarcoidosis; DL_{CO} is reduced in emphysema because of the loss of alveolocapillary membrane.

put on the noseclip so that he can adjust to it before the test.

Equipment

For direct spirography: spirometer, noseclip, mouthpiece

For body plethysmography: body plethysmograph, mouthpiece, transducer

Procedure and posttest care

- When measuring *tidal volume,* tell the patient to breathe normally into the mouthpiece 10 times.
- When measuring *expiratory reserve volume,* tell the patient to breathe normally for several breaths and then to exhale as completely as possible.
- When measuring *vital capacity,* tell the patient to inhale as deeply as possible and to exhale into the mouthpiece as completely as possible. This procedure is repeated three times, and the test result showing the largest volume is used.
- When measuring *inspiratory capacity,* tell the patient to breathe normally for several breaths and then to inhale as deeply as possible.
- When measuring *functional residual capacity,* tell the patient to breathe normally into a spirometer that contains a known concentration of an insoluble gas (usually helium or nitrogen) in a known volume of air. After a few breaths, the concentrations of gas in the spirometer and in the lungs reach equilibrium. Then the point of equilibrium and the concentration of gas in the spirometer are recorded.
- When measuring *thoracic gas volume,* the patient is put in an airtight box (or

body plethysmograph) and told to breathe through a tube connected to a transducer. At end-expiration, the tube is occluded, the patient is told to pant, and changes in intrathoracic and plethysmographic pressures are measured. The results are used to calculate total TGV and FRC.

- When measuring *forced vital capacity* and *forced expiratory volume,* tell the patient to inhale as slowly and deeply as possible and then exhale into the mouthpiece as quickly and completely as possible. This procedure is repeated three times, and the largest volume is recorded. The volume of air expired at 1 second (FEV_1), at 2 seconds (FEV_1), and at 3 seconds (FEV_3) during all three repetitions is also recorded.
- When measuring *maximal voluntary ventilation,* tell the patient to breathe into the mouthpiece as quickly and deeply as possible for 15 seconds.
- When measuring *diffusing capacity for carbon monoxide,* the patient inhales a gas mixture with a low concentration of carbon monoxide and then holds his breath for 10 seconds before exhaling.
- After the tests, instruct the patient to resume his usual activities, diet, and medication schedule as ordered.

Precautions

- Pulmonary function tests are contraindicated in patients with acute coronary insufficiency, angina, or recent myocardial infarction.
- Watch for respiratory distress, changes in pulse rate and blood pressure, and coughing or bronchospasm.

Reference values

Normal values are predicted for each patient based on age, height, weight, and sex and are expressed as a percentage. Usually, results are considered abnormal if they're less than 80% of these values.

The following reference values can be calculated at bedside with a portable spirometer: V_T, 5 to 7 ml/kg of body weight; ERV, 25% of VC; IC, 75% of VC; FEV_1, 83% of VC (after 1 second); FEV_2, 94% of VC (after 2 seconds); and FEV_3, 97% of VC (after 3 seconds).

Abnormal findings

See the accompanying chart.

Interfering factors

- Hypoxia, metabolic disturbances, or lack of patient cooperation
- Pregnancy or gastric distention (possible displacement of lung volume)
- Narcotic analgesic or sedative (possible decrease in inspiratory and expiratory forces)
- Bronchodilators (possible temporary improvement in pulmonary function)

D-XYLOSE ABSORPTION

The D-xylose absorption test evaluates patients with symptoms of malabsorption, such as weight loss and generalized malnutrition, weakness, and diarrhea. D-xylose is a pentose sugar that's absorbed in the small intestine without the aid of pancreatic enzymes, passes through the liver without being metabolized, and is excreted in the urine. Because of its absorption in the small intestine without digestion, measurement of D-xylose in the urine and blood indicates the absorptive capacity of the small intestine.

Purpose

- To aid differential diagnosis of malabsorption
- To determine the cause of malabsorption syndrome

Patient preparation

- Tell the patient that this test helps evaluate digestive function by analyzing blood samples and urine specimens after ingestion of a sugar solution.
- Explain to the patient that he must fast overnight before the test and that he'll have to fast and remain in bed during the test.
- Tell the patient that the test requires several blood samples. Explain who will perform the venipunctures and when.
- Explain to the patient that he may experience discomfort from the needle punctures and the tourniquet.
- Inform the patient that all his urine will be collected for 5 or 24 hours as ordered.
- Withhold medications that alter test results, such as aspirin and indomethacin, as ordered. Record any medications the patient is taking on the laboratory request.

Equipment

Tourniquet, venipuncture equipment, 10-ml tube without additives, sterile urine specimen container, specimen labels, gloves, biohazard transport bags (per facility protocol)

Procedure and posttest care

- Perform a venipuncture to obtain a fasting blood sample, and collect the sample in a 10-ml tube without additives. Collect a first-voided morning urine specimen. Label these specimens, and send them to the laboratory immediately to serve as a baseline.
- Give the patient 25 g of D-xylose dissolved in 8 oz (240 ml) of water, followed by an additional 8 oz of water. If the patient is a child, administer 0.5 g of D-xylose per pound of body weight, up to 25 g. Record the time of D-xylose ingestion.
- For an adult, draw a blood sample 2 hours after D-xylose ingestion; for a child, 1 hour after ingestion. Collect the sample in a 10-ml tube without additives. Occasionally, a 5-hour sample may be drawn to support the findings of the 1- or 2-hour sample.
- Collect and pool all urine during the 5 or 24 hours after D-xylose ingestion.
- If a hematoma develops at the venipuncture site, apply warm soaks.
- Observe the patient for abdominal discomfort or mild diarrhea caused by D-xylose ingestion.
- Instruct the patient to resume his usual diet and medication schedule as ordered.

Precautions

- Handle the sample gently to prevent hemolysis.
- Tell the patient not to contaminate the urine specimens with toilet tissue or stool.
- Be sure to collect all urine and refrigerate the specimen during the collection period.
- Because patients age 65 and older and those with borderline or elevated creatinine levels tend to have low 5-hour urine levels but normal 24-hour levels, the physician will have to establish the length of the collection period. At the end of the collection period, send the urine specimen to the laboratory immediately.
- Maintain bed rest and withhold food and fluids (other than D-xylose) throughout the test period.

Reference values

Normal values are as follows:

- *children:* blood concentration > 30 mg/dl in 1 hour; urine, 16% to 33% of ingested D-xylose excreted in 5 hours

■ *adults:* blood concentration 25 to 40 mg/dl in 2 hours; urine, > 3.5 g excreted in 5 hours (age 65 or older, > 5 g in 24 hours).

Abnormal findings

Depressed blood and urine D-xylose levels most commonly result from malabsorption disorders that affect the proximal small intestine, such as sprue and celiac disease. Depressed levels may also result from regional enteritis involving the jejunum, Whipple's disease, multiple jejunal diverticula, myxedema, diabetic neuropathic diarrhea, rheumatoid arthritis, alcoholism, severe heart failure, and ascites.

Interfering factors

■ Failure to adhere to pretest restrictions
■ Aspirin (decreased D-xylose excretion by the kidneys)
■ Indomethacin (decreased intestinal D-xylose absorption)
■ Failure to obtain a complete urine specimen or to collect blood samples at designated times
■ Intestinal overgrowth of bacteria, renal insufficiency, or renal retention of urine (possible drop in urine levels)

DEXAMETHASONE SUPPRESSION

The dexamethasone suppression test requires administration of dexamethasone, an oral steroid. Dexamethasone suppresses levels of circulating adrenal steroid hormones in normal people but fails to suppress them in patients with Cushing's syndrome and some forms of clinical depression.

Purpose

■ To diagnose Cushing's syndrome
■ To aid diagnosis of clinical depression

Patient preparation

■ Explain to the patient the purpose of the test.
■ Inform the patient that the test requires two blood samples drawn after administration of dexamethasone. Explain who will perform the venipunctures and when.
■ Explain to the patient that he may experience discomfort from the needle punctures and the tourniquet.
■ Restrict food and fluids for 10 to 12 hours before the test.

Procedure and posttest care

■ On the first day, give the patient 1 mg of dexamethasone at 11 p.m. On the next day, collect blood samples at 4 p.m. and 11 p.m. More frequent sampling may increase the likelihood of measuring a nonsuppressed cortisol peak.
■ If a hematoma develops at the venipuncture site, apply warm soaks.

Precautions

Many medications, including corticosteroids, oral contraceptives, lithium, methadone, aspirin, diuretics, morphine, and monoamine oxidase (MAO) inhibitors, can affect the accuracy of test results. If possible, don't administer any of these medications for 24 to 48 hours before the test, as ordered.

Reference values

A cortisol level of 5 g/dl (140 nmol/L) or greater indicates failure of dexamethasone suppression.

Abnormal findings

A normal test result doesn't rule out major depression, but an abnormal result strengthens a clinically based diagnosis. Failure of suppression occurs in patients with Cushing's syndrome, severe stress, and depression that's likely to respond to treatment with antidepressants.

Interfering factors

- Diabetes mellitus, pregnancy, and severe stress, such as trauma, severe weight loss, dehydration, and acute alcohol withdrawal (possible false-positive)
- Certain drugs, particularly barbiturates or phenytoin, within 3 weeks of the test (possible false-positive)
- Caffeine consumed after midnight the night before the test (possible false-positive)
- Failure to withhold corticosteroids, oral contraceptives, lithium, methadone, aspirin, diuretics, morphine, or MAO inhibitors for 24 to 48 hours before the test

SLEEP STUDIES

Also known as polysomnography, sleep studies are tests used to help in the differential diagnosis of sleep-disordered breathing. Several parameters are evaluated for the patient being tested for sleep disorder; these include cardiac rate and rhythm, chest and abdominal wall movement, nasal and oral airflow, oxygen saturation, muscle activity, retinal function, and brain activity during the sleep phase.

Purpose

- To diagnose breathing disorders in persons with a history of excessive snoring, narcolepsy, excessive daytime sleepiness, insomnia, cardiac rhythm disorders, and restless leg spasms

Patient preparation

- Explain to the patient the purpose of the test and have him maintain normal sleep schedules so that he's neither deprived of sleep nor overrested.
- Inform the patient that sleep studies are usually scheduled for the evening and night hours, usually 10 p.m. to 6 a.m. and take place in a designated sleep laboratory.
- Explain to the patient that he should abstain from caffeinated products and naps for 2 to 3 days before the test.
- Tell the patient that he may bathe or shower before the test.

Procedure and posttest care

- Electrodes are secured to the patient's skin, depending on the type of monitoring being used.
- Ensure the patient's comfort, and tell him that normal body movements won't interfere with the electrodes.
- The lights are turned off and the EEG monitored for a baseline reading before the patient falls asleep.
- Ensure that the recording and video equipment record the sleep events as they occur.
- Monitoring of the patient during sleep continues until the test is completed.

Precautions

- For the patient with known sleep apnea, split-night studies may be ordered. These include monitoring the patient for the first half of the night, then using continuous positive airway pressure or nasal ventilation to open the obstructed airway during the second half of the night.
- Monitor the patient for respiratory distress.

Normal findings

A normal sleep study shows a respiratory disturbance index (or apnea-hypopnea index) of fewer than 5 to 10 episodes per study period and normal electrocardiogram (cardiac rate and rhythm), impedance (chest and abdominal wall motion), airway (nasal and oral airflow), arterial oxygen saturation (oximetry), leg electromyogram (for muscle activity), electro-oculogram (for retinal function), and EEG (for brain activity).

Abnormal findings

Abnormal recordings reveal obstructive sleep apnea syndrome. Abnormal movement during sleep indicates a seizure or movement disorder.

Interfering factors

- Electrophysiologic artifacts, defective electrodes, diaphoresis, environmental noises
- Patient's inability to fall asleep

TILT-TABLE TEST

The tilt-table test is used for patients with recurrent syncope or pre-syncope (near syncope) to determine the cause of orthostatic hypotension, which is a drop in blood pressure associated with an overreaction of the nerves resulting in neural mediated syncope. The patient is placed on a table with a foot support and slowly raised to a more vertical position while his blood pressure, pulse, and other symptoms are noted. Tilt-table testing may be performed when other causes of syncopal attacks, such as heart disease, have been ruled out.

Purpose

- To detect the cause of orthostatic hypotension (postural hypotension)

Patient preparation

- Explain to the patient that this test helps determine the cause of fainting.
- Instruct the patient to restrict food or fluids for a specified time (usually 4 hours) prior to the test to prevent nausea. For early morning testing, instruct the patient to fast beginning at midnight the night before the test.
- Tell the patient who will perform the test, where it will take place, and how long it will last.
- Tell the patient that an I.V. line will be inserted prior to the test to provide fluids or medications prescribed during the test.
- Tell the patient that he'll be asked to lie on a special tilt-table and that, after he's secured to the table with safety straps, the table will be tilted slightly while his blood pressure, pulse, heart rate, and oxygenation are monitored closely.
- Tell the patient that the lights may be dimmed or soft music played to help him relax.
- Tell the patient that he may experience transient feelings of light-headedness, nausea, sweating, or weakness and to tell the staff if he experiences these feelings.
- Tell the patient that he may receive an adrenalin-like medication that will increase his heart rate (as if he were exercising) and may cause his heart to pound. Assure him that this is expected and that he will feel normal once the medication is stopped.
- Tell the patient that there are no activity restrictions after the test is completed but that he'll need someone to take him home after the test.
- Make sure the patient or a responsible family member has signed an informed consent form.
- Review the patient's medication history, and alert the physician to medications the patient may be taking.

Procedure and posttest care

- The patient is placed in a supine position on the tilt table and secured to the table with safety straps.
- The patient is connected to an ECG, pulse oximeter, and blood pressure monitoring device. An I.V. line is inserted.
- Lights are dimmed or soft music played to help the patient relax.
- Baseline vital signs are obtained for approximately 10 minutes while the patient rests supine on the table.
- Inform the patient that the table is going to be tilted and that he'll be monitored closely; reiterate the need for him to express any discomfort he experiences. Reassure appropriately.
- With the patient's head up, the table is tilted to 30 degrees. Vital signs are monitored for 5 minutes in this position.
- With the patient's head up, the table is tilted to 60 degrees. Vital signs are monitored for 45 minutes in this position. (Usually a drop in blood pressure occurs within 30 minutes of this position.)
- If the patient becomes extremely uncomfortable, the test is stopped. If the test can be completed, the table is lowered until the patient is flat and the second part of the test begins.
- Tell the patient that the adrenaline-like medication will be administered. Remind him that he may feel his heart pounding, much like he's exercising.
- An isoproterenol infusion is begun slowly, as ordered, while vital signs are monitored. It's increased as necessary according to facility protocol. Once the appropriate dose is determined, the table is tilted (patient's head up) to 60 degrees and the patient is observed for 15 minutes.
- If the test is completed, the table may be returned to flat, the dose of isoproterenol increased, and the test repeated with the table tilted (patient's head up) to 60 degrees for a third time, then returned to the supine position.
- Monitoring continues until vital signs return to baseline, per facility protocol.

Precautions

- Stop the test when the patient develops symptoms of syncope with a significant drop in blood pressure.
- The patient may require close monitoring and treatment for syncopal symptoms.
- Ensure that safety straps are secured in case the patient faints during the test.

Normal findings

Blood pressure remains normal despite symptoms such as light-headedness and dizziness.

Abnormal findings

The test is positive if the patient develops a drop in blood pressure associated with symptoms. A borderline test is determined if the protocol is completed and the patient experiences a drop in blood pressure without developing symptoms.

Interfering factors

- Failure to follow pretest restrictions
- Medications that produce syncopal symptoms, such as anti-hypertensives and beta-adrenergic blockers

APPENDICES

INDEX

APPENDIX A NORMAL LABORATORY TEST VALUES

HEMATOLOGY

Bleeding time
Template: 3 to 6 minutes (SI, 3 to 6 m)
Ivy: 3 to 6 minutes (SI, 3 to 6 m)
Duke: 1 to 3 minutes (SI, 1 to 3 m)

Clot retraction
50%

Erythrocyte sedimentation rate
Males: 0 to 15 mm/hour (SI, 0 to 10 mm/hour)
Females: 0 to 20 mm/hour (SI, 0 to 20 mm/hour)

Fibrin split products
Screening assay: < 10 µg/ml (SI, < 10 mg/L)
Quantitative assay: < 3 µg/ml (SI, < 3 mg/L)

Fibrinogen, plasma
200 to 400 mg/dl (SI, 2 to 4 g/L)

Hematocrit
Males: 42% to 52% (SI, 0.42 to 0.52)
Females: 36% to 48% (SI, 0.36 to 0.48)

Hemoglobin, total
Males: 14 to 17.4 g/dl (SI, 140 to 174 g/L)
Females: 12 to 16 g/dl (SI, 120 to 160 g/L)

Partial thromboplastin time
21 to 35 seconds (SI, 21 to 35 s)

Platelet aggregation
3 to 5 minutes (SI, 3 to 5 m)

Platelet count
140,000 to 400,000/µl (SI, 140 to 400 × 10^9/L)

Prothrombin time
10 to 14 seconds (SI, 10 to 14 s); INR for patients on warfarin therapy, 2 to 3 (SI, 2.0 to 3.0) (those with prosthetic heart valve, 2.5 to 3.5 [SI, 2.5 to 3.5])

Red blood cell count
Males: 4.5 to 5.5 million/ml (SI, 4.5 to 5.5 × 10^{12}/L) venous blood
Females: 4 to 5 million/ml (SI, 4 to 5 × 10^{12}/L) venous blood

Red cell indices
Mean corpuscular volume: 82 to 98 µm^3
Mean corpuscular hemoglobin: 26 to 34 pg/cell
Mean corpuscular hemoglobin concentration: 31 to 37 g/dl

Reticulocyte count
0.5% to 2.5% (SI, 0.005 to 0.025) of total red blood cell count

Thrombin time, plasma
10 to 15 seconds

White blood cell differential, blood
Neutrophils: 54% to 75% (SI, 0.54 to 0.75)
Lymphocytes: 25% to 40% (SI, 0.25 to 0.40)
Monocytes: 2% to 8% (SI, 0.02 to 0.08)
Eosinophils: up to 4% (SI, up to 0.04)
Basophils: up to 1% (SI, up to 0.01)

BLOOD CHEMISTRY

Acid phosphatase, serum
0 to 3.7 ng/ml (SI, 0 to 3.7 U/L)

Alanine aminotransferase
Adults: 8 to 50 U/L (SI, 0.14 to 0.85 µkat/L)
Children: 10 to 35 U/L (SI, 0.10 to 0.35 µkat/L)

Amylase, serum
≥ 18 years: 25 to 85 U/L (SI, 0.39 to 1.45 μkat/L)

Arterial blood gases
pH: 7.35 to 7.45 (SI, 7.35 to 7.45)
$PaCO_2$: 35 to 45 mm Hg (SI, 4.7 to 5.3 kPa)
PaO_2: 80 to 100 mm Hg (SI, 10.6 to 13.3 kPa)
HCO_3^-: 22 to 26 mEq/L (SI, 22 to 25 mmol/L)
SaO_2: 94% to 100% (SI, 0.94 to 1.00)

Aspartate aminotransferase
Males: 8 to 46 U/L (SI, 0.14 to 0.78 μkat/L)
Females: 7 to 34 U/L (SI, 0.12 to 0.58 μkat/L)

Bilirubin, serum
Adults, total: 0.2 to 1 mg/dl (SI, 3.5 to 17 μmol/L)
Neonates, total: 2 to 12 mg/dl (SI, 34 to 205 μmol/L)
Neonates, unconjugated indirect: 0.2 to 0.8 mg/dl (SI, 3.5 to 14 μmol/L)

Blood urea nitrogen
8 to 20 mg/dl (SI, 2.9 to 7.5 mmol/L)

Calcium, serum
Adults: 8.2 to 10.2 mg/dl (SI, 2.05 to 2.54 mmol/L)
Children: 8.6 to 11.2 mg/dl (SI, 2.15 to 2.79 mmol/L)

Carbon dioxide, total, blood
22 to 26 mEq/L (SI, 22 to 26 mmol/L)

Cholesterol, total, serum
Men: < 205 mg/dl (SI, < 5.30 mmol/L) (desirable)
Women: < 190 mg/dl (SI,< 4.90 mmol/L) (desirable)

C-reactive protein, serum
Negative or < 0.8 mg/dl (SI, < 8 mg/L)

Creatine kinase, isoenzymes
CK-BB: none
CK-MB: 0 to 7 U/L (SI, 0 to 7 ug/L)
CK-MM: 5 to 7 U/L (SI, 5 to 7 ug/L)

Creatinine, serum
Adults: 0.6 to 1.3 mg/dl (SI, 53 to 115 μmol/L)

Glucose, plasma, fasting
70 to 110 mg/dl (SI, 3.9 to 6.1 mmol/L)

Glucose, plasma, 2-hour postprandial
< 145 mg/dl (SI, < 8mmol/L)

Iron, serum
Males: 50 to 150 μg/dl (SI, 11.6 to 31.3 μmol/L)
Females: 35 to 145 μg/dl (SI, 9.0 to 30.4 μmol/L)

Lactate dehydrogenase
Total: 71 to 207 U/L in adults (SI, 1.2 to 3.52 μkat/L)
LD_1: 14% to 26% (SI, 0.14 to 0.26)
LD_2: 29% to 39% (SI, 0.29 to 0.39)
LD_3: 20% to 26% (SI, 0.20 to 0.26)
LD_4: 8% to 16% (SI, 0.08 to 0.16)
LD_5: 6% to 16% (SI, 0.06 to 0.16)

Lipase
< 160 U/L (SI, < 2.72 μkat/L)

Lipoproteins, serum
HDL cholesterol:
– *Males:* 37 to 70 mg/dl (SI, 0.96 to 1.8 mmol/L)
– *Females:* 40 to 84 mg/dl (SI, 1.03 to 2.2 mmol/L)
LDL cholesterol: < 130 mg/dl (SI, < 3.36 mmol/L)

Magnesium, serum
1.3 to 2.1 mg/dl (SI, 0.65 to 1.05 mmol/L)

Phosphates, serum
2.7 to 4.5 mg/dl (SI, 0.87 to 1.45 mmol/L)

Potassium, serum
3.8 to 5 mEq/L (SI, 3.5 to 5 mmol/L)

Protein, serum
Total: 6.3 to 8.3 g/dl (SI, 64 to 83 g/L)
Albumin fraction: 3.5 to 5 g/dl (SI, 35 to 50 g/L)
Alpha$_1$-globulin: 0.1 to 0.3 g/dl (SI, 1 to 3 g/L)
Alpha$_2$-globulin: 0.6 to 1 g/dl (SI, 6 to 10 g/L)
Beta globulin: 0.7 to 1.1 g/dl (SI, 7 to 11 g/L)
Gamma globulin: 0.8 to 1.6 g/dl (SI, 8 to 16 g/L)

Sodium, serum
135 to 145 mEq/L (SI, 135 to 145 mmol/L)

Thyroxine, total, serum
5 to 13.5 μg/dl (SI, 60 to 165 mmol/L)

Triglycerides, serum
Males > 20 years: 40 to 180 mg/dl (SI, 0.11 to 2.01 mmol/L)
Females > 20 years: 10 to 190 mg/dl (SI, 0.11 to 2.21 mmol/L)

Triiodothyronine
80 to 200 ng/dl (SI, 1.2 to 3.0 nmol/L)

Uric acid, serum
Males: 3.4 to 7 mg/dl (SI, 202 to 416 μmol/L)
Females: 2.3 to 6 mg/dl (SI, 143 to 357 μmol/L)

URINE CHEMISTRY

Amylase, urine
1 to 17 U/hour (SI, 0.017 to 0.29 μkat/hour)

Bence Jones protein, urine
Negative

Bilirubin, urine
Negative

Calcium, urine
100 to 300 mg/24 hours (SI, 2.50 to 7.50 mmol/day)

Chloride, urine
110 to 250 mEq/24 hours (SI, 110 to 250 mmol/day)

Creatinine, urine
Males: 14 to 26 mg/kg/body weight/24 hours (SI, 124 to 230 μmol/kg/body weight/day)
Females: 11 to 20 mg/kg/body weight/24 hours (SI, 97 to 177 μmol/kg/body weight/day)

Glucose, urine
Negative

17-hydroxycorticosteroids, urine
Males: 4.5 to 12 mg/24 hours (SI, 12.4 to 33.1 μmol/day)
Females: 2.5 to 10 mg/24 hours (SI, 6.9 to 27.6 μmol/day)

17-ketogenic steroids, urine
Males: 4 to 14 mg/24 hours (SI, 13 to 49 μmol/day)
Females: 2 to 12 mg/24 hours (SI, 7 to 42 μmol/day)

Ketones, urine
Negative

17-Ketosteroids, urine
Males: 10 to 25 mg/24 hours (SI, 35 to 87 μmol/day)
Females: 4 to 6 mg/24 hours (SI, 4 to 21 μmol/day)

Protein, urine
50 to 80 mg/24 hours (SI, 50 to 80 mg/day)

Red blood cells, urine
0 to 3 per high-power field

Sodium, urine
40 to 220 mEq/L/24 hours (SI, 40 to 220 mmol/day)

Sodium chloride, urine
110 to 250 mEq/L (SI, 110 to 250 mmol/day)

Urinalysis, routine
Color: straw
Appearance: clear
Specific gravity: 1.005 to 1.035
pH: 4.5 to 8
Epithelial cells: few
Casts: occasional hyaline casts
Crystals: present

Urine osmolality
24-hour urine: 300 to 900 mOsm/kg
Random urine: 50 to 1,400 mOsm/kg

Urobilinogen, urine
$<$ 4 mg/24 hours (SI, $<$ 4.0 EU/day)

Vanillylmandelic acid, urine
$<$ 8 mg/24 hours

White blood cell count, urine
0 to 4 per high-power field

MISCELLANEOUS

Cerebrospinal fluid
Pressure: 50 to 180 mm H_2O
Appearance: clear, colorless
Gram stain: no organisms

Lupus erythematosus cell preparation
Negative

Occult blood, fecal
$\leq$ 2 mg total Hb/g feces

Rheumatoid factor, serum
Negative

Venereal Disease Research Laboratory, serum
Negative

APPENDIX B
NORMAL AND ABNORMAL SERUM DRUG LEVELS

DRUG NAME AND THERAPEUTIC VALUE*	PURPOSE OF TEST	SIGNIFICANCE OF ABNORMAL VALUE
Acetaminophen < 50 mcg/ml (SI, < 330 μmol/L)	Monitoring for overdose	◆ Increased value (≥ 120 mcg/ml [SI, ≥ 794 μmol/L]) signifies overdose. ◆ Decreased value shows that drug has little therapeutic effect.
Amikacin Peak: 20 to 25 mcg/ml (SI, 43 to 60 μmol/L) Trough: 5 to 10 mcg/ml (SI, 6.8 to 13.7 μmol/L)	Monitoring drug therapy	◆ Adjust time or amount of dose or both.
Amitriptyline 75 to 200 ng/ml (SI, 289 to 903 nmol/L)	Monitoring drug therapy	◆ Decreased value shows that drug has little therapeutic effect. ◆ Higher levels may signify toxicity.
Digoxin 0.5 to 2 ng/ml (SI, 0.64 to 2.8 nmol/L)	Monitoring drug therapy	◆ Increased value (≥ 3 ng/ml [SI, ≥ 3.8 nmol/L]) may signify toxicity. ◆ Decreased value shows that drug may have decreased therapeutic effect.
Ethanol 0 (legal limit for blood alcohol level for drivers varies from state to state)	Detecting ethanol in bloodstream (degree of alcohol in blood correlates to level of intoxication)	◆ Value > 300 mcg/ml (SI, > 86.8 mmol/L) suggests alcohol ingestion. ◆ Value > 3,000 mcg/ml (SI, > 866 mmol/L) depresses respirations and can be considered lethal.
Ethosuximide 40 to 100 mcg/ml (SI, 280 to 710 μmol/L)	Monitoring drug therapy	◆ Increased value (≥ 100 mcg/ml [SI, ≥ 710 μmol/L)] may signify toxicity. ◆ Decreased value shows that drug may have decreased therapeutic effect.

* *These values are for adults.*

DRUG NAME AND THERAPEUTICVALUE*	PURPOSE OF TEST	SIGNIFICANCE OF ABNORMAL VALUE
Ethylene glycol 0	Monitoring for overdose	◆ Increased value (≥ 2 mEq/L) may signify toxicity. ◆ Value > 20 mEq/L is considered lethal.
Gentamicin Peak: 4 to 8 mcg/ml (SI, 12 to 17 μmol/L) Trough: 1 to 2 mcg/ml (SI, 2 to 4 μmol/L)	Monitoring drug therapy	◆ Adjust time or amount of dose or both.
Lidocaine 2 to 5 mcg/ml (SI, 6.4 to 25.6 μmol/L)	Monitoring drug therapy and evaluating toxicity	◆ Increased value (≥ 6 mcg/ml [SI, ≥ 26 μmol/L]) may signify toxicity. ◆ Decreased value shows that drug may have decreased therapeutic effect.
Lithium Trough: 0.8 to 1.2 mEq/L (SI, 0.6 to 1.2 nmol/L)	Monitoring drug therapy and evaluating toxicity	◆ Increased value (trough >1.5 mEq/L [SI, > 1.5 mmol/L]) may signify toxicity. ◆ Decreased value shows that drug may have decreased therapeutic effect.
Methotrexate < 10 micromol 24 hour postdose < 1 micromol 48 hour postdose < 0.2 micromol 72 hour postdose	Monitoring drug therapy	◆ Adjust time or amount of dose or both.
Nitroprusside (thiocyanate level) 4 to 20 mcg/dl	Evaluating toxicity	◆ Increased value (≥ 60 mcg/ml) may signify toxicity. ◆ Decreased value shows that drug may have decreased therapeutic effect.
Nortriptyline 50 to 150 ng/ml (SI, 190 to 570 nmol/L)	Monitoring drug therapy	◆ Decreased value shows that drug has little therapeutic effect. ◆ Increased levels can cause depression.

** These values are for adults.*

DRUG NAME AND THERAPEUTIC VALUE*	PURPOSE OF TEST	SIGNIFICANCE OF ABNORMAL VALUE
Phenobarbital 1 to 5 mcg/ml (SI, 4 to 22 μmol/L)	Monitoring drug therapy, evaluating toxicity, and evaluating for possible abuse	◆ Increased value (≥ 10 mcg/ml [SI, ≥ 44 μmol/L]) may signify toxicity; 30 to 40 mcg/ml (SI, 132 to 176 μmol/L) is used to reduce intracranial pressure but requires artificial respiratory support. ◆ Decreased value shows that drug may have decreased therapeutic effect.
Phenytoin Plasma: 10 to 20 mcg/ml (40 to 79 μmol/L)	Monitoring drug therapy and evaluating toxicity	◆ Increased value (> 20 mcg/ml [SI, > 79 μmol/L]) may signify toxicity. ◆ Decreased value shows that drug may have decreased therapeutic effect.
Procainamide 4 to 8 mcg/ml (SI, 17 to 42 μmol/L)	Monitoring drug therapy and evaluating toxicity	◆ Increased value (> 16 mcg/ml [SI, > 84 μmol/L]) may signify toxicity. ◆ Decreased value shows that drug may have decreased therapeutic effect.
Propafenone 0.5 to 2 mcg/ml	Monitoring drug therapy	◆ Adjust time or amount of dose or both.
Quinidine 2 to 5 mcg/ml (SI, 6 to 15 μmol/L)	Monitoring drug therapy and evaluating toxicity	◆ Increased value (≥ 7 mcg/ml [SI, ≥ 18 μmol/L]) may signify toxicity. ◆ Decreased value shows that drug may have decreased therapeutic effect.
Salicylate 2 to 20 mg/dl (SI, 1.09 to 2.17 mmol/L)	Monitoring drug therapy and evaluating toxicity	◆ Increased value (≥ 50 mg/dl [SI, ≥ 3.62 mmol/L]) may signify toxicity. ◆ Decreased value shows that drug may have decreased therapeutic effect.
Theophylline 10 to 20 mcg/ml (SI, 44 to110 μmol/L)	Monitoring drug therapy and evaluating toxicity	◆ Increased value (≥ 20 mcg/ml [SI, > 110 μmol/L]) may signify toxicity. ◆ Decreased value shows that drug may have decreased therapeutic effect.

** These values are for adults.*

DRUG NAME AND THERAPEUTIC VALUE*	PURPOSE OF TEST	SIGNIFICANCE OF ABNORMAL VALUE
Tobramycin Peak: 4 to 8 mcg/ml (SI, 12 to 17 mg/L) Trough: 1 to 2 mcg/ml (SI, 2 to 4 µmol/L)	Monitoring drug therapy	◆ Adjust time or amount of dose or both.
Valproic acid Trough: > 40 mcg/ml (SI, > 278 µmol/L)	Monitoring drug therapy	◆ Increased value (≥ 120 mcg/ml [SI, ≥ 832 µmol/L]) may signify toxicity. Adverse effects may occur at levels > 125 mcg/ml (SI, > 866 µmol/L). ◆ Decreased value shows that drug may have decreased therapeutic effect.
Vancomycin Peak: 20 to 40 mcg/ml (SI, 14 to 28 µmol/L) Trough: 5 to 10 mcg/ml (SI, 3 to 7 µmol/L)	Monitoring drug therapy	◆ Increased value (≥ 100 mcg/ml [SI, ≥ 69 µmol/L]) may signify toxicity. ◆ Decreased value shows that drug may have decreased therapeutic effect.
Verapamil 50 to 200 ng/ml (SI, 100 to 410 nmol/L)	Monitoring drug therapy	◆ Increased value (peak ≥ 400 ng/ml [SI, ≥ 810 nmol/L]) may signify toxicity. ◆ Decreased value shows that drug may have decreased therapeutic effect.

* *These values are for adults.*

APPENDIX C
ILLUSTRATED GUIDE TO HOME TESTING

In recent years, the number of diagnostic tests that people can perform themselves at home has greatly increased. The teaching aids on the following pages describe how to accurately perform several of the most common home tests, including tests for blood cholesterol levels, pacemaker function, and the presence of human immunodeficiency virus.

When you review these tests with your patient, be sure to:

- stress the importance of following the manufacturer's instructions exactly
- explain unfamiliar terms
- review any special forms that the patient must complete such as the diary needed when using a Holter monitor
- discuss how to follow up on test results.

Testing your blood glucose level

Dear Patient:
Testing your blood glucose levels daily will tell you whether your diabetes is under control. Follow these steps to learn how to obtain blood for testing and how to perform the test.

Getting ready

1. Begin by assembling the necessary equipment: your glucose meter, a lancet, an alcohol pad, gauze pads, and a vial with reagent strips.
2. Remove a reagent strip from the vial. Then replace the cap, making sure that it's tight.
3. Turn on the glucose meter and, if necessary, calibrate the machine according to the manufacturer's instructions. Then wait for the display window to show that the meter is ready for the blood sample.

Obtaining blood

1. Wash your hands thoroughly and dry them. Choose a site on the end or side of any fingertip. To enhance blood flow, hold your finger under warm water for a minute or two.
2. Hold your hand below your heart, and press the blood toward the fingertip you plan to pierce by squeezing that fingertip with the thumb of the same hand. Wipe the designated fingertip with an alcohol pad, and dry it with a gauze pad. Then place your fingertip (with your thumb still pressed against it) on a firm surface such as a table.

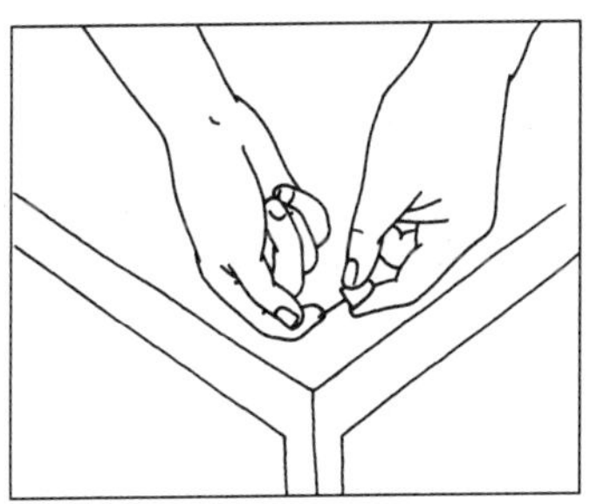

3. Twist off the lancet's protective cap. Then grasp the lancet and quickly pierce your fingertip just to the side of the finger pad, where you have more blood vessels and fewer nerve endings.
4. Next, push the sharp end of the lancet into the protective cap to avoid accidental sticks. Place the device in a sharps container (a coffee can or a 2-L plastic soda bottle).
5. Remove your thumb from your fingertip to permit blood flow. Then gently press your finger until you get a large, hanging drop of blood.

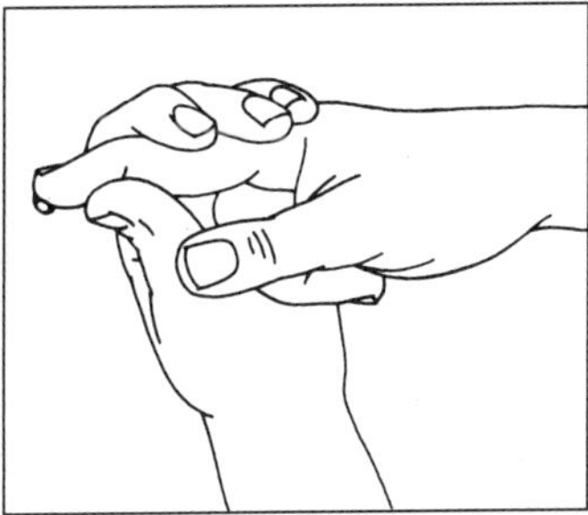

Testing blood

1. When the display window indicates that the meter is ready, touch the drop of blood to the reagent strip at the indicated spot, and insert the strip into the glucose meter. In most cases, the drop of blood will automatically start the meter's timer. Apply pressure to the puncture site with a dry gauze pad to stop the bleeding.
2. After the meter has finished the test, you can read the results from the display window. The meter will automatically store the date, time, and results of the test.

Collecting a urine specimen: For males

Dear Patient:
Your doctor wants you to have your urine tested. A urine test can tell whether you have an infection or too much or too little of certain substances in your body. To make sure that test results are accurate, your urine shouldn't contain "outside germs" from your hands or penis.

Follow these directions carefully. Read them through to the end before collecting the specimen.

1. Wash your hands thoroughly. Open the package of disposable wipes that the nurse gave you, and place it on a clean, dry surface nearby.

2. Remove the lid from the specimen cup and place it flat side down. Don't touch the inside of the cup or lid.

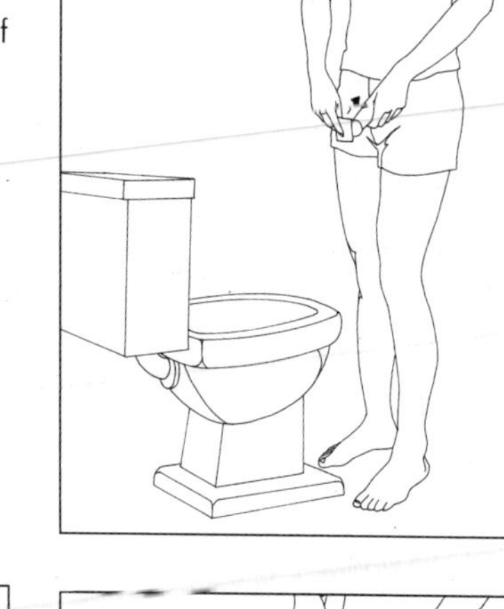

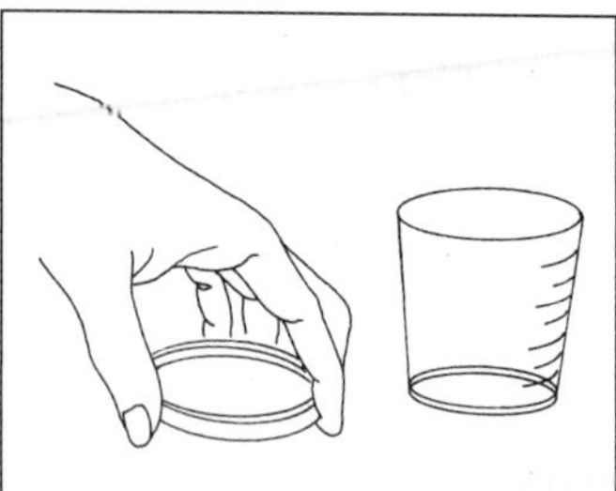

3. Prepare to urinate. (If you're uncircumcised, first pull back your foreskin.) Using a disposable wipe, clean the head of your penis from the urethral opening toward you (as shown at the top of the next column). Then discard the used wipe.

4. Urinate a small amount into the toilet. After 1 or 2 seconds, catch about 1 oz (30 ml) of urine in the specimen cup. The nurse will tell you how far to fill the cup. As a rule, you'll fill it about one-fourth or more full. Don't allow the cup to touch your penis at any time. When you're done, place the lid on the cup and return it to the nurse.

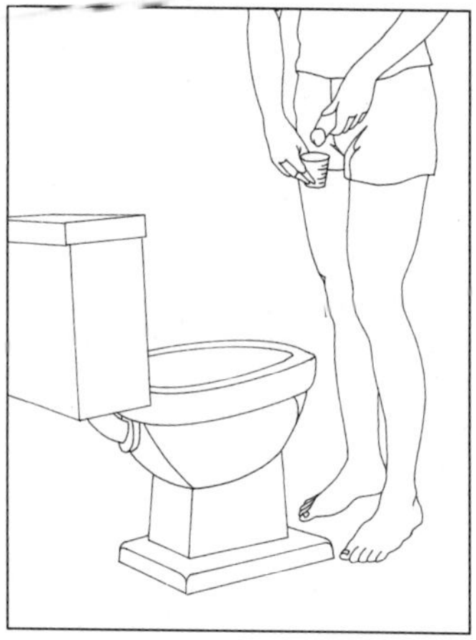

Note: Don't drink a lot of water before the test. This could affect the accuracy of the test results.

Collecting a urine specimen: For females

Dear Patient:
Your physician has asked you to provide a urine specimen for testing. The specimen can tell whether you have an infection or too much or too little of certain substances in your body. To make sure that the test results are accurate, your urine shouldn't contain "outside germs" from your hands, labia, or urethral opening.

Follow these directions carefully. Read them through to the end before collecting the specimen.

1. Wash your hands thoroughly. Open the package of disposable wipes that the nurse gave you, and place it on a clean, dry, surface nearby.
2. Remove the lid from the specimen cup and place it flat side down. Don't touch the inside of the cup or lid.
3. Sit as far back on the toilet as possible. Spread your labia apart with one hand (as shown below), keeping the folds separated for the rest of the procedure.

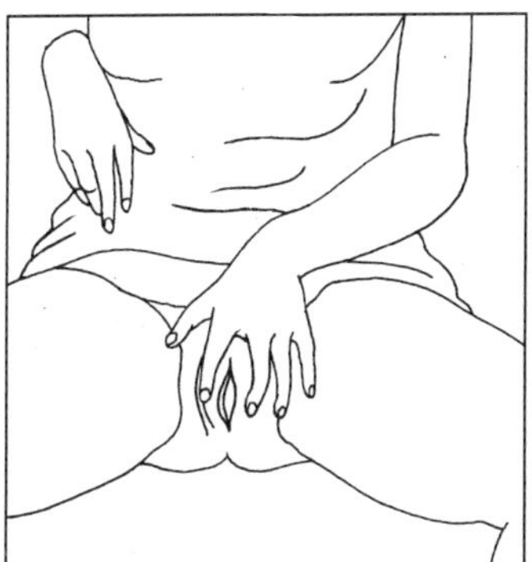

4. Using the disposable wipes, clean the area between the labia and around the urethra thoroughly from front to back (as shown at the top of the next column). Use a new wipe for each stroke. Discard the used wipes.

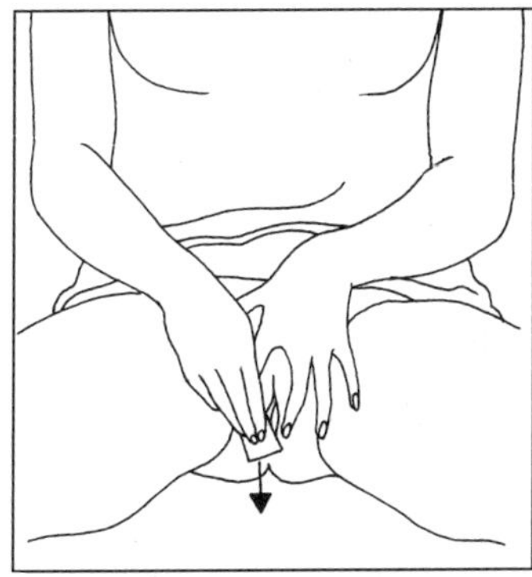

5. Urinate a small amount into the toilet. After 1 or 2 seconds, hold the specimen cup below your urine stream (as shown below) and catch about 1 oz (30 ml) of urine in the cup. Don't allow the cup to touch your skin at any time.

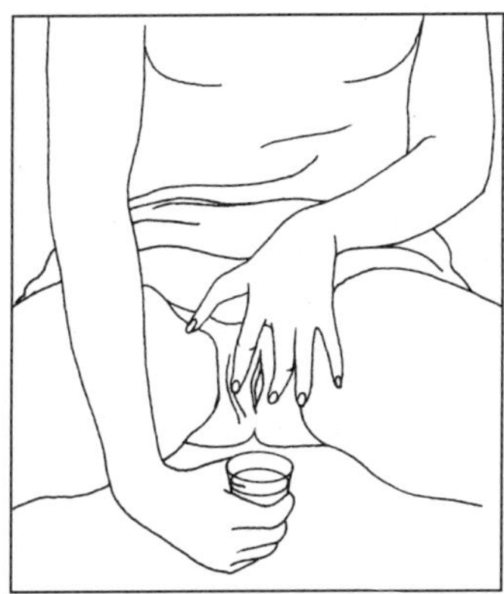

6. When you're done, place the lid on the cup and return it to the nurse.
Note: Don't drink a lot of water before the test. This could affect the accuracy of the test results.

Testing for blood in your stool

Dear Patient:
A home fecal occult blood test is an easy, inexpensive way to detect blood in your stool. For accurate results, follow the directions given by the nurse or physician, read the instructions included with the test kit, and review these guidelines.

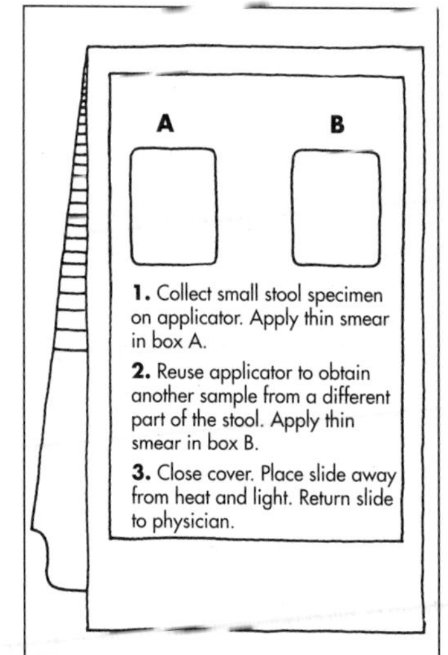

Getting ready
Don't eat red meat or raw fruits or vegetables for 3 days before you take the test and during the test period. Also avoid diet supplements containing iron or vitamin C and painkillers containing aspirin or ibuprofen (such as Advil and Nuprin) for the same time period. All of these substances can affect test results.

Increase your intake of high-fiber foods, such as whole grain breads and cereals. Your physician may also ask you to eat popcorn or nuts.

Performing the test
1. Make sure all your supplies are in one place. They may include your test cards (or slides), a chemical developer, a wooden applicator, and a watch with a second hand.
2. Obtain a stool sample. You can do this by laying a long sheet of clear plastic wrap across the toilet bowl to catch the stool, or by removing stool from the bowl. Flush the remaining stool down the toilet.

Use the applicator to smear a thin film of the sample onto the slot marked "A" on the front of the test card. Smear a thin film of a second sample from a *different area of the same stool* onto the slot marked "B" on the same side of the card.
3. *If the physician or a laboratory will be analyzing the test samples,* close slots A and B, put your name and the date on the test kit, and return the card (or slide) to the physician or laboratory as soon as possible.

If you're doing the test yourself, turn the card over and open the back window. Apply two drops of the chemical developer to the paper covering each sample. Wait 1 minute; then read the results.

If either slot has a bluish tint, the test results are positive for blood in the stool. *If neither slot looks blue,* the test results are normal. Write down the results. Discard the used applicator and wash your hands thoroughly.
4. Repeat the test on your next two bowel movements. Report the results of all of the tests to the physician. Even if only one of the six test results is positive, the physician may recommend other tests.

Using a Holter monitor

Dear Patient:
Your physician has ordered you to wear a Holter monitor for 24 hours. It works like a continuous electrocardiogram (ECG) by recording any irregular heartbeats you may have. The information from this recording will help your physician determine if abnormal heartbeats are causing your symptoms, such as chest pain or discomfort, dizziness, or weakness. If you're taking a heart medication, the Holter monitor can also help your physician evaluate how well the medication is working.

The monitor has adhesive patches (called *leads*) that the nurse will attach to your skin. She'll also show you how to wear the monitor on a belt or over your shoulder. If one of the leads becomes loose, secure it with a piece of tape.

While wearing the monitor, you can perform most of your usual activities. You'll even wear it to bed.

Practice these safety measures while wearing the Holter monitor:

◆ Don't get the monitor wet — don't shower, bathe, or swim with it on.

◆ Avoid high-voltage areas, strong magnetic fields, and microwave ovens.

While you're wearing the monitor, you'll write down your activities and feelings. This diary will help your physician establish a connection between your monitor tracing and your activities and feelings. Jot down the time of day when you perform any activity, such as taking medication, eating, drinking, moving your bowels, urinating, engaging in sexual activity, exercising, and sleeping, or experience any strong emotions, such as anger or fear. (See the sample entries below.)

If your monitor has an event button, the nurse will show you how to press it in case you experience anything unusual such as a sudden, rapid heartbeat.

Tuesday	10:30 am	Rode from hospital in car	Legs tired, some shortness
			of breath
	11:30 am	Watched TV in living room	Comfortable
	12:15 pm	Ate lunch, took Inderal	Indigestion
	1:30 pm	Walked next door to see neighbor	Shortness of breath
	2:45 pm	Walked home	Very tired, legs hurt
	3:00-4:00pm	Urinated, took nap	Comfortable
	5:30 pm	Ate dinner, slowly	Comfortable
	7:20 pm	Had bowel movement	Shortness of breath
	9:00 pm	Watched TV-drank 1 beer	Heart beating fast for
			about one minute, no pain
	11:00 pm	Took Inderal, urinated, went to bed	Tired
Wednesday	8:15 am	Awoke, urinated, washed face and arms	Very tired, rapid heartbeat
			for about 30 seconds
	10:30 am	Returned to hospital	Felt better

Checking your pacemaker by telephone

Dear Patient:
Your physician wants to check your pacemaker regularly by telephone. Doing this helps him monitor how well the pacemaker is working and the strength of the battery while you stay at home. Here's how to use your pacemaker's transmitter.

Inserting the battery

Before using your transmitter for the first time, remove the battery cover and insert the battery supplied by the manufacturer. You'll need to replace the battery every 2 to 3 months, according to the manufacturer's instructions.

Setting up the transmitter

When you're ready, take the transmitter out of its case. Also remove the electrode cable from the case, and plug the cable into the jack on the transmitter.

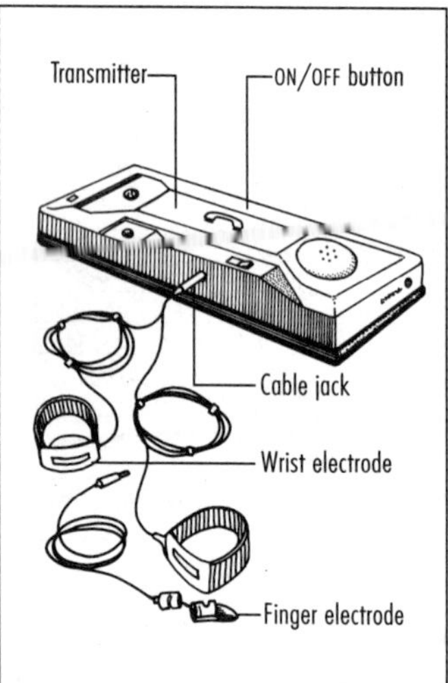

Place the electrodes on your fingers or on your wrists. Then turn on the transmitter and listen for the tones indicating that the power is on.

Phoning in your electrocardiogram

Dial the telephone number of your physician's office or the pacemaker clinic, and listen for instructions.

When directed, place the telephone handset in the pacemaker transmitter. Stay still (for up to 60 seconds) to minimize interference with the signals from your heart.

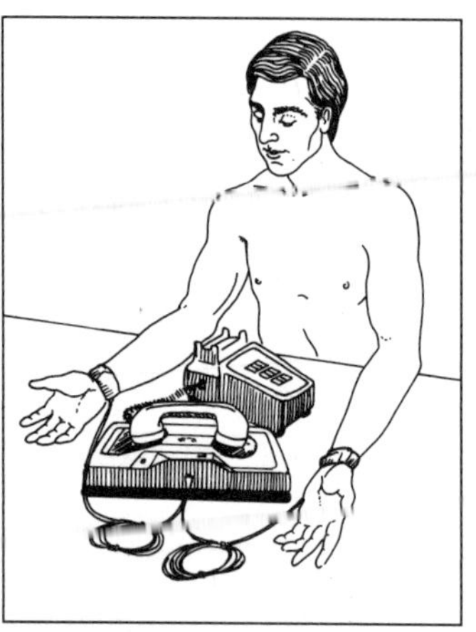

Wait for further instructions. For example, the physician may ask you to use a special magnet that's in the transmitter's case. To do so, simply hold the magnet over the pacemaker and transmit your electrocardiogram as before.

When you finish transmitting, take off the electrodes and turn off the transmitter. Place the equipment in the storage case until the next time you use it.

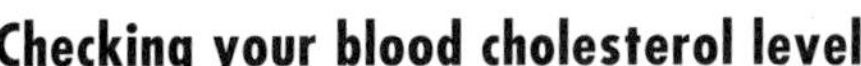

Checking your blood cholesterol level

Dear Patient:
Testing your blood cholesterol level can tell you whether you're at risk for heart disease. If you take cholesterol-lowering medication or are on a low-cholesterol diet, testing your blood cholesterol level will help you determine if your cholesterol is under control. If you have any questions about test results or the risk factors associated with heart disease, always consult your physician.

Follow these steps to learn how to obtain a blood sample and how to perform the test. Remember, because cholesterol levels can change from day to day and can be affected by stress, weight loss, illness, or pregnancy, one cholesterol reading may not be final.

Getting ready

1. Begin by assembling the necessary equipment included in the packet: the test device, the test result chart, and a lancet, plus an alcohol pad and gauze pads.
2. Read the instructions thoroughly.

Obtaining blood

1. Wash your hands thoroughly and dry them. Choose a site on the end or side of any fingertip. To enhance blood flow, hold your finger under warm water for a minute or two.
2. Hold your hand below your heart, and press the blood toward the fingertip you plan to pierce by squeezing that fingertip with the thumb of the same hand. Wipe the designated fingertip with an alcohol pad, and dry it with a gauze pad. Place your fingertip (with your thumb still pressed against it) on a firm surface such as a table.
3. Twist off the lancet's protective cap. Then grasp the lancet and quickly pierce your fingertip just to the side of the finger pad, where you have more blood vessels and fewer nerve endings.
4. Push the sharp end of the lancet into the protective cap to avoid accidental sticks. Place the device in a sharps container (such as a coffee can or a 2-L plastic soda bottle).
5. Remove your thumb from your fingertip to permit blood flow. Apply gentle pressure to your finger until you get a large, hanging drop of blood.
6. Point your finger down directly over the blood well, and place the hanging drop of blood into the blood well, making sure that you fill the black circle completely. Then wait at least 2 but no more than 4 minutes. Press the puncture site with a dry gauze pad to stop the bleeding.

Reading the results

When the display windows indicate that the test is complete, read the results. Compare the reading on the testing device with the chart included in the packet for your cholesterol level. Remember to inform your physician about the results.

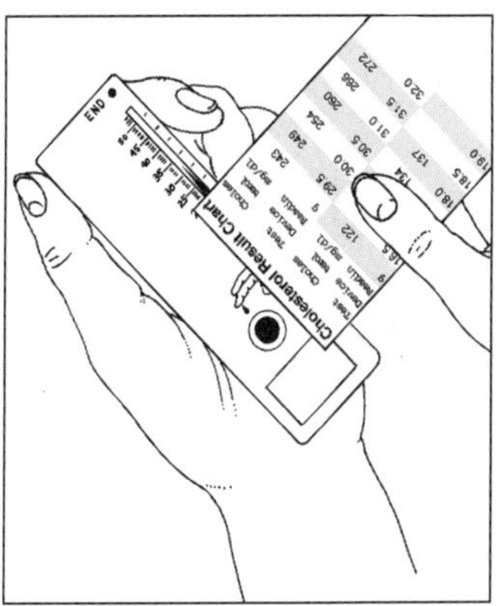

Performing a home ovulation test

Dear Patient:
A home ovulation test helps you determine the best time to try to become pregnant. It works by monitoring the amount of luteinizing hormone (LH) that's found in your urine.

Normally, during each menstrual cycle, levels of this hormone rise suddenly (LH surge), causing an egg to be released from the ovary 24 to 36 hours later. The release of the egg is known as *ovulation.* Ovulation normally occurs once a month, about 2 weeks before your period, and lasts about 24 hours. This is your most fertile period — the only time each month that you can become pregnant.

Follow these directions to test your urine for the presence of LH and to determine when you're most likely to become pregnant. To know when to begin testing, you'll need to know the length of your menstrual cycle. Count from the beginning of one period to the beginning of the next period. (Count the first day of bleeding as day 1). Use the chart below to determine when to begin testing.

Length of cycle	Start test this many days after your last period begins	Length of cycle	Start test this many days after your last period begins
21	5	31	14
22	5	32	15
23	6	33	16
24	7	34	17
25	8	34	18
26	9	36	19
27	10	37	20
28	11	38	21
29	12	39	22
30	13	40	23

Getting ready

1. Read the instructions thoroughly before you perform the test. This test can be performed any time of the day or night but should be performed at the same time each day.

Note: Don't urinate for at least 4 hours before taking this test, and don't drink a lot of liquids for several hours before testing.

2. Remove the test stick from the package and remove the cap.

Performing the test

1. Sit on the toilet. Direct the absorbent tip of the test stick downward and directly into your urine stream for at least 5 seconds or until it's thoroughly wet. *Don't urinate on the windows of the stick.* You can also urinate into a clean, dry cup or container and dip the test stick (absorbent tip only) into the urine for at least 5 seconds.

2. Lay the test stick on a clean, dry, flat surface.

Reading the results

1. Wait at least 5 minutes to read the results. When the test is finished, a line will appear in the small window (control window).

2. *If there's no line in the large rectangular window (test window) or if the line is lighter than the line in the small rectangular window,* you haven't begun your LH surge. You should continue with daily testing.

3. *If you see one line in the large window that's similar to or darker than the line in the small window* (as shown at right), you've detected an LH surge. This means that you should ovulate within the next 24 to 36 hours.

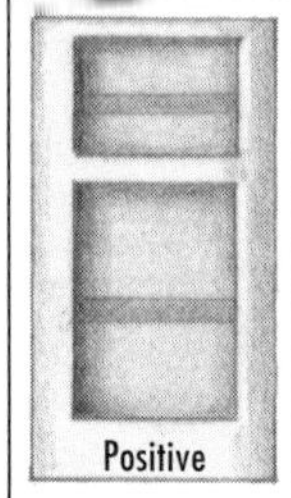

Positive

Once you've determined that you're about to ovulate, you know you're at the start of the most fertile time of your cycle.

Performing a home HIV test

Dear Patient:
Human immunodeficiency virus (HIV) is a virus that attacks your immune system and causes acquired immunodeficiency syndrome (AIDS). By testing your blood, you can determine if you've been infected with HIV. Remember that even if you've been exposed to the HIV virus, it may not become evident in your blood for 6 months. If you have any questions about your test results or the risk factors associated with HIV, *always* consult a physician.

Follow these steps to learn how to obtain a blood sample and how to perform the test.

Getting ready

1. Begin by assembling the necessary equipment included in the packet: a lancet, a test card with your personal identification number (to receive the confidential and anonymous test results), and the envelope in which to send the test card to the laboratory. Also gather an alcohol pad and gauze pads.

2. Read the instructions thoroughly before you stick your finger. Remove the personal identification card from the bottom of the test card, and place it in a safe place.

Obtaining blood

1. Wash your hands thoroughly and dry them. Choose a site on the end or side of any fingertip. To enhance blood flow, hold your finger under warm water for a minute or two.

2. Hold your hand below your heart, and press the blood toward the finger-tip you plan to pierce by squeezing that fingertip with the thumb of the same hand. Wipe the designated fingertip with an alcohol pad, and dry it with a gauze pad. Place your fingertip (with your thumb still pressed against it) on a firm surface such as a table.

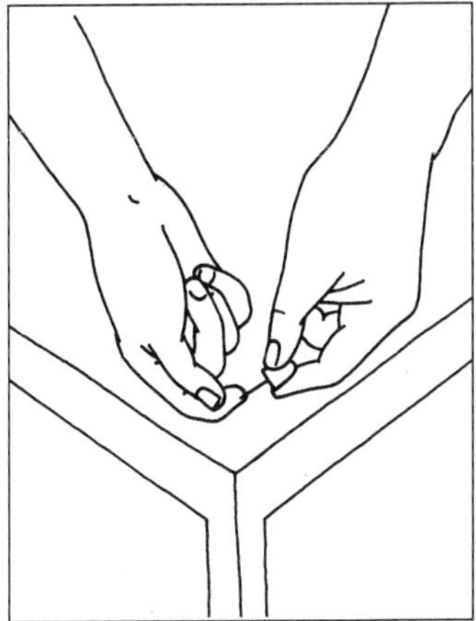

3. Twist off the lancet's protective cap. Then grasp the lancet and quickly pierce your fingertip just to the side of the finger pad, where you have more blood vessels and fewer nerve endings.

4. Push the sharp end of the lancet into the protective cap to avoid accidental sticks.

5. Remove your thumb from your fingertip to permit blood flow. Then apply gentle pressure to your finger until you get a large, hanging drop of blood.

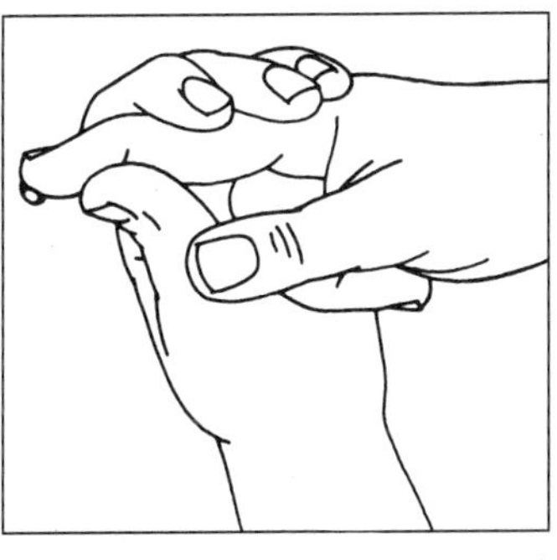

(continued)

Performing a home HIV test *(continued)*

6. Point your finger down directly over the three circles on the test card (as shown at right). Completely fill each circle with blood from your finger.
7. Place any used lancets in the containers attached to the mailing card. Slip the test card in the postage-paid mailer, seal the mailer, and send it to the address printed on the front. Save the part of the card that lists the toll-free number to call for results.

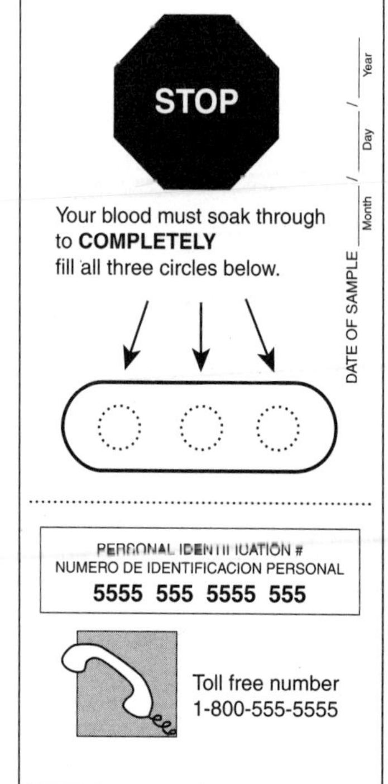

Obtaining the results

In about 1 week, call the toll-free number on the identification card. Give your identification number to the person who answers, and wait for the results. *If your test is positive for HIV,* a specially trained counselor will advise you what to do next and will tell you about HIV and AIDS organizations nationwide. *If your test results are negative for HIV,* the trained counselor will advise you how to maintain your negative HIV status.

Remember, a negative test result doesn't necessarily mean you're free from HIV infection. It may simply mean that the antibodies aren't yet present in your blood. To be certain, repeat the test with a new package in 6 months.

INDEX

i refers to an illustration; t refers to a table; **bold text** refers to main entries.

i refers to an illustration; t refers to a table; **bold text** refers to main entries.

C

i refers to an illustration; t refers to a table; **bold text** refers to main entries.

i refers to an illustration; t refers to a table; **bold text** refers to main entries.

i refers to an illustration; t refers to a table; **bold text** refers to main entries.

E

i refers to an illustration; t refers to a table; **bold text** refers to main entries.

i refers to an illustration; t refers to a table; **bold text** refers to main entries.

i refers to an illustration; t refers to a table; **bold text** refers to main entries.

I

i refers to an illustration; t refers to a table; **bold text** refers to main entries.

i refers to an illustration; t refers to a table; **bold text** refers to main entries.

i refers to an illustration; t refers to a table; **bold text** refers to main entries.

i refers to an illustration; t refers to a table; **bold text** refers to main entries.

i refers to an illustration; t refers to a table; **bold text** refers to main entries.

i refers to an illustration; t refers to a table; **bold text** refers to main entries.

i refers to an illustration; t refers to a table; **bold text** refers to main entries.

i refers to an illustration; t refers to a table; **bold text** refers to main entries.

W

X

Y

Z